VOLUME EIGHTY-NINE

VITAMINS AND HORMONES

Sleep Hormones

VOLUME EIGHTY-NINE

VITAMINS AND HORMONES

Sleep Hormones

Editor-in-Chief

GERALD LITWACK

Toluca Lake, North Hollywood, California

ELSEVIER

AMSTERDAM • BOSTON • HEIDELBERG • LONDON
NEW YORK • OXFORD • PARIS • SAN DIEGO
SAN FRANCISCO • SINGAPORE • SYDNEY • TOKYO
Academic Press is an imprint of Elsevier

Cover photo credit:
Tsunematsu,T., and Yamanaka, A.
The Role of Orexin/Hypocretin in the Central Nervous System and Peripheral Tissues
Vitamins and Hormones (2012) **89**, pp. 19–34

Academic Press is an imprint of Elsevier
32 Jamestown Road, London, NW1 7BY, UK
Radarweg 29, PO Box 211, 1000 AE Amsterdam, The Netherlands
Linacre House, Jordan Hill, Oxford OX2 8DP, UK
225 Wyman Street, Waltham, MA 02451, USA
525 B Street, Suite 1900, San Diego, CA 92101-4495, USA

First edition 2012

ISBN: 978-0-12-394623-2
ISSN: 0083-6729

For information on all Academic Press publications
visit our website at elsevierdirect.com

Printed and bound by CPI Group (UK) Ltd, Croydon, CR0 4YY

Transferred to digital print 2012

Contents

Contributors

Ernest Adeghate
Department of Anatomy, Faculty of Medicine & Health Sciences, United Arab Emirates University, Al Ain, United Arab Emirates

Morio Azuma
Laboratory of Regulatory Biology, Graduate School of Science and Engineering, University of Toyama, Toyama, Japan

Corey Baimel
Department of Anesthesiology, Pharmacology & Therapeutics, University of British Columbia, Vancouver, British Columbia, Canada

Stephanie L. Borgland
Department of Anesthesiology, Pharmacology & Therapeutics, University of British Columbia, Vancouver, British Columbia, Canada

Michelle Cao
Division of Sleep Medicine, Stanford University School of Medicine, Stanford, California, USA

William Corrigall
Department of Psychiatry, University of Minnesota, Minneapolis, Minnesota, USA

Rodrigo A. España
Department of Neurobiology and Anatomy, Drexel University College of Medicine, Philadelphia, Pennsylvania, USA

Ozhan Eyigor
Department of Histology and Embryology, Faculty of Medicine, Uludag University, Bursa, Turkey

Eric Frenette
Department of Neurology, University of Sherbrooke, Sherbrooke, Quebec, Canada

Xiao-Bing Gao
Section of Comparative Medicine, Program in Integrative Cell Signaling and Neurobiology of Metabolism, Yale University School of Medicine, New Haven, Connecticut, USA

Tomoko Ishizuka[1]
Department of Medical Science and Technology, Graduate School of Allied Health Sciences, Faculty of Medicine, Osaka University, Osaka, Japan

Kathryn A. Jewett
WWAMI Medical Education Program, Sleep and Performance Research Center, Spokane, and Department of Veterinary and Comparative Anatomy, Pharmacology and Physiology, Washington State University, Pullman, Washington, USA

Ilker M. Kafa
Department of Anatomy, Faculty of Medicine, Uludag University, Bursa, Turkey

Tadeusz Kaminski
Department of Animal Physiology, University of Warmia and Mazury in Olsztyn, Oczapowskiego 1A, Olsztyn-Kortowo, Poland

Ki Sung Kang[2]
Department of Anatomy, Showa University School of Medicine, Tokyo, Japan

Hiroshi Katsuki
Department of Chemico-Pharmacological Sciences, Graduate School of Pharmaceutical Sciences, Kumamoto University, Kumamoto, Japan

James M. Krueger
WWAMI Medical Education Program, Sleep and Performance Research Center, Washington State University, Spokane, Washington, USA

Tomoyuki Kuwaki
Department of Physiology, Kagoshima University Graduate School of Medical and Dental Sciences, Sakuragaoka 8-35-1, Kagoshima, Japan

Alben Lui
Stanford University Medical Center, Stanford, California, USA

Kouhei Matsuda
Laboratory of Regulatory Biology, Graduate School of Science and Engineering, and Laboratory of Regulatory Biology, Graduate School of Innovative Life Science, University of Toyama, Toyama, Japan

Vijayakumar Mavanji
Minnesota Obesity Prevention Training Program, School of Public Health, University of Minnesota and Minneapolis VA Health Care System, Minneapolis, Minnesota, USA

[1] Present address: Department of Pharmacology, Osaka Dental University, 8-1 Kuzuhahanazono-cho, Hirakata, Osaka 573-1121, Japan.
[2] Present address: Natural Products Research Center, Korea Institute of Science and Technology, Gangneung, Gangwon-do, South Korea.

Shotaro Michinaga
Laboratory of Pharmacology, Faculty of Pharmacy, Osaka Ohtani University, Osaka, Japan

Zehra Minbay
Department of Histology and Embryology, Faculty of Medicine, Uludag University, Bursa, Turkey

Tomotaka Murotani[3]
Department of Medical Science and Technology, Graduate School of Allied Health Sciences, Faculty of Medicine, Osaka University, Osaka, Japan

Katsunori Nonogaki
Department of Lifestyle Medicine, Translational Research Center, Tohoku University Hospital, Sendai, Miyagi, Japan

Paul M. Pilowsky
Australian School of Advanced Medicine, Macquarie University, Sydney, Australia

Ahmed A. Rahman
Australian School of Advanced Medicine, Macquarie University, Sydney, Australia, and Pharmacy Discipline, Life Science School, Khulna University, Khulna, Bangladesh

Israt Z. Shahid
Australian School of Advanced Medicine, Macquarie University, Sydney, Australia, and Pharmacy Discipline, Life Science School, Khulna University, Khulna, Bangladesh

Nina Smolinska
Department of Animal Physiology, University of Warmia and Mazury in Olsztyn, Oczapowskiego 1A, Olsztyn-Kortowo, Poland

Susumu Tanaka
Department of Psychiatry and Behavioral Science, Tokyo Metropolitan Institute of Medical Science, Kamikitazawa 2-1-6, Setagaya-ku, Tokyo, Japan

Jennifer A. Teske
Department of Nutritional Sciences, University of Arizona and Southern Arizona VA Health Care System, Tucson, Arizona, and Department of Food Science and Nutrition, University of Minnesota, Saint Paul, Minnesota, USA

Tomomi Tsunematsu
Division of Cell Signaling, National Institute for Physiological Sciences, Okazaki, Japan

[3] Present address: Kobe University School of Medicine, 7-5-1 Kusunoki-cho, Chuo-ku, Kobe, Hyogo 650-0017, Japan.

Hélène Volkoff
Department of Biology, and Department of Biochemistry, Memorial University of Newfoundland, St John's, Newfoundland, Canada

Akihiro Yamanaka
Division of Cell Signaling, National Institute for Physiological Sciences; Department of Physiological Sciences, The Graduate University for Advanced Studies, Okazaki, and PRESTO, JST, Kawaguchi, Japan

Atsushi Yamatodani
Department of Medical Science and Technology, Graduate School of Allied Health Sciences, Faculty of Medicine, Osaka University, Osaka, Japan

Wei Zhang[4]
Department of Physiology, Kagoshima University Graduate School of Medical and Dental Sciences, Sakuragaoka 8-35-1, Kagoshima, Japan

[4] Present address: Department of Surgery, University of Alabama at Birmingham, Birmingham, Alabama, USA.

Preface

Orexins A and B (also known as hypocretins 1 and 2) are the sleep hormones. These two neurohormones with 50% sequence identity are derived from a single precursor polypeptide chain (preproorexin). Orexin A has 33 amino acids in its chain and orexin B has 28 amino acids in its chain. These hormones are manufactured in the hypothalamus and through projections are distributed throughout the brain. Orexin A binds to two G protein-coupled receptors (OX1R and OX2R), while orexin B binds less avidly to the second receptor. Not only do these hormones promote wakefulness and sleep, but also they have many other activities and these together with basic information about the hormones are described in this volume.

Chapter 1 concerns "Neurohormones and sleep" by E. Frenette, A. Lui, and M. Cao. "The role of orexin/hypocretin in the central nervous system and peripheral tissues" is a contribution by T. Tsunematsu and A. Yamanaka. X.-B. Gao reviews "Plasticity in neurons synthesizing wake/arousal promoting hormone hypocretin/orexin." T. Kaminski and N. Smolinska report on "Expression of orexin receptors in the pituitary." This is followed by "Transcriptional regulation of the hypocretin/orexin gene" by S. Tanaka. Energy relationships are considered by J. A. Teske and V. Mavanji in "Energy expenditure: role of orexin." E. Adeghate reports on "Orexins: tissue localization, functions, and its relation to insulin secretion and diabetes mellitus." "Orexin neurons and emotional stress" is discussed by T. Kuwaki and W. Zhang. I. Z. Shahid, A. A. Rahman, and P. M. Pilowsky are the authors of "Orexin and central regulation of cardiorespiratory system." R. A. España contributes "Hypocretin/orexin involvement in reward and reinforcement." This is followed by a treatise on "Glutamate and orexin neurons" by O. Eyigor, Z. Minbay, and I. M. Kafa. Next, K. Nonogaki covers "Serotonin conflict in sleep-feeding." "Humoral sleep regulation; interleukin-1 and tumor necrosis factor" is reported by K. A. Jewett and J. M. Krueger.

In three chapters, various drug effects on orexin neurons and actions are discussed. "Action of modafinil through histaminergic and orexinergic neurons" is the topic of T. Ishizuka, T. Murotani, and A. Yamatodani. The second paper in this category is "Anti-Parkinson drugs and orexin neurons" by H. Katsuki and S. Michinaga. Last, C. Baimel, S. L. Borgland, and W. Corrigall offer "Cocaine and nicotine research illustrates a range of hypocretin mechanisms in addiction."

The final two chapters deal with nonmammalian organisms. H. Volkoff discusses "Sleep and orexins in nonmammalian vertebrates." Finally, "Orexin system in teleost fish" is the subject of K. Matsuda, M. Azuma, and K. S. Kang.

I thank Mary Ann Zimmerman and Sarah Latham of Elsevier for continual help in completing books in this serial.

The figure on the cover is a reproduction of Figure 2.1 from Chapter 2 entitled: "The role of orexin/hypocretin in the central nervous system and peripheral tissues" by T. Tsunematsu and A. Yamanaka.

Gerald Litwack
Toluca Lake, CA
February 7, 2012

CHAPTER ONE

Neurohormones and Sleep

Eric Frenette,* Alben Lui,† *and* Michelle Cao‡

Contents

Abstract

Mutual interactions between neurohormones, sleep, and the circadian system have been extensively studied. Hormonal secretion is either influenced by sleep and is independent of circadian timing or is closely coupled with the light–dark cycle, although both processes ultimately interact with each other.

Sleep has a strong effect on the levels of some hormones (e.g., growth hormone) but little effect on others that are primarily regulated by the circadian system (e.g., melatonin). The exact mechanisms through which sleep affects circulating hormonal levels are not well understood. Much more is known about

* Department of Neurology, University of Sherbrooke, Sherbrooke, Quebec, Canada
† Stanford University Medical Center, Stanford, California, USA
‡ Division of Sleep Medicine, Stanford University School of Medicine, Stanford, California, USA

Vitamins and Hormones, Volume 89
ISSN 0083-6729, http://dx.doi.org/10.1016/B978-0-12-394623-2.00001-9

how the circadian system influences the secretion of hormones. Under normal circumstances, behaviors and the circadian system are synchronized with an optimal phase relationship, and consequently, hormonal systems are exquisitely regulated. Every bit of information constitutes but one small component of a broader, more global neurohormonal picture. In this review, we attempt to divide this analysis into sections including the pineal gland, adenohypophysis, neurohypophysis, describing the reciprocal influence regarding sleep and various neurohormones.

I. Introduction

According to a simple definition, sleep is a reversible behavioral state of perceptual disengagement from and unresponsiveness to the environment, a reduction of motor output and the absence of consciousness. (Carskadon and Dement, 2005). Humans spend approximately one-third of their lives sleeping, but the function of this behavior is not well understood. Nevertheless, sleep deprivation studies indicate that sleep is required for proper cognitive, motor, and physiological function (Buxton *et al.*, 2010; Pilcher and Huffcutt, 1996; Rechtschaffen *et al.*, 1989).

Sleep is regulated by circadian rhythm and homeostatic drive, the so-called processes C and S, respectively. Process C is found in the alternating pattern of night and day over an approximately 24-h period. Process S is mainly influenced by prior sleep or lack thereof (Achermann and Borbély, 2003).

Sleep is divided into non-rapid eye movement (NREM) sleep and rapid eye movement (REM) sleep (Carskadon and Dement, 1996). Sleep also cycles roughly every 90 min after falling asleep until waking up in a classic ultradian pattern. Usually four or five cycles are encountered on a normal sleep night. NREM and REM sleep alternate on a regular basis, and the occurrence of both makes up a cycle. NREM is furthermore divided into four stages labeled 1, 2, 3, and 4 according to the so-called R&K criteria (Rechtschaffen and Kales, 1968). In 2007, the American Academy of Sleep Medicine (AASM) has proposed a new classification of NREM sleep, dividing it into three stages, N1, N2, and N3, the last one lumping together R&K stages 3 and 4. REM sleep is characterized by REMs, decreased or absent muscle tone, EEG desynchronization, and autonomic instability. The new classification proposes stage R as terminology (American Academy of Sleep Medicine, 2007). It is important to understand the differences of the two scoring systems, as older studies use the R&K criteria for staging sleep and the newer ones will most likely use the new terminology.

II. Pineal Gland

A. Melatonin

Melatonin (structurally 5-methoxy-*N*-acetyltryptamine) is a hormone secreted by the pineal gland of the brain and is released into the blood and cerebrospinal fluid. It plays an important role in regulation of sleep and circadian rhythm. Melatonin is synthesized within the pineal gland from the essential amino acid tryptophan (Axelrod *et al.*, 1969; Fig. 1.1). Tryptophan is first converted to 5-hydroxytryptophan by tryptophan hydroxylase and to

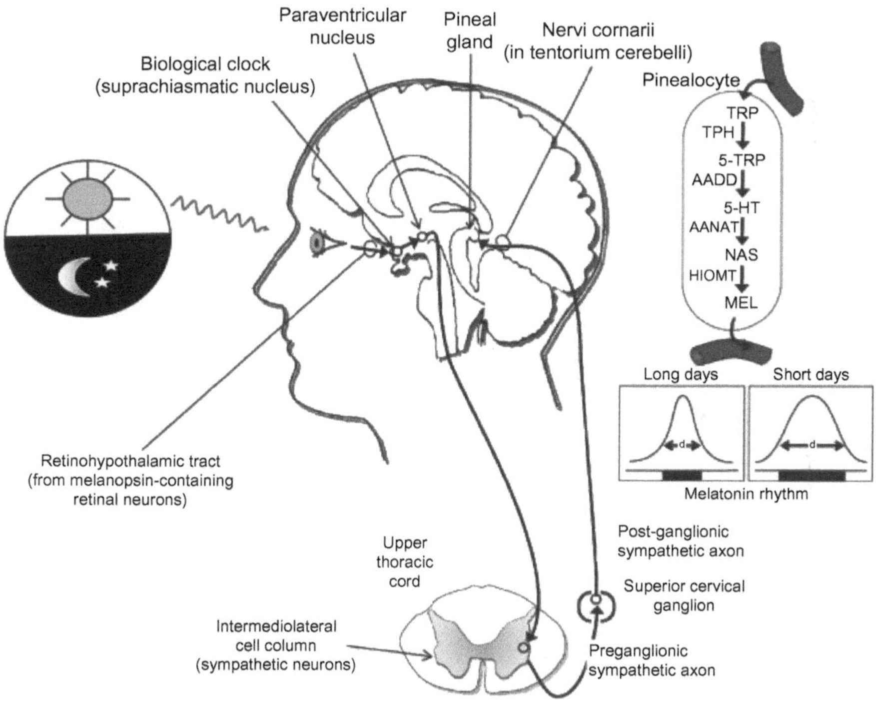

Figure 1.1 Neural pathway connecting the eyes (the melanopsin-containing ganglion cells of the retina) with the pineal gland and the synthesis of melatonin (MEL) from tryptophan (TRP) in a pinealocyte. Just prior to their entrance into the pineal gland the postganglionic fibers form discrete nerve bundles in the tentorium cerebelli, the meninges that lie between the cerebrum and cerebellum. TPH, tryptophan hydroxylase; 5-TRP, 5-hydroxytryptophan; AADD, L-amino acid decarboxylase; 5-HT, serotonin; AANAT, arylalkylamine *N*-acetyltransferase; NAS, *N*-acetylserotonin; HIOMT, hydroxyindole-*O*-methyltransferase. The duration of the nocturnal elevation of melatonin varies with the season of the year. Adapted from Reiter *et al.* (2010).

serotonin by L-amino acid decarboxylase. Serotonin is then converted by arylalkylamine *N*-acetyltransferase (AANAT) to *N*-acetylserotonin before the final step of being converted to melatonin by hydroxyindole-*O*-methyltransferase (HIOMT).

B. Regulation and function of melatonin

It has been well demonstrated that melatonin synthesis is regulated by light exposure in both animal (Deguchi, 1982; Klein and Moore, 1979; Klein and Weller, 1970; Moore and Klein, 1974) and human (Lewy *et al.*, 1980) subjects. In humans, light inhibits melatonin during the day. Therefore, melatonin increases at the onset of dim light, peaking during the nocturnal sleep period and diminishing with exposure to bright light (Stickgold, 2009). The nighttime rise in melatonin is related to maximal fatigue, minimal degree of alertness, and physical and mental performance. Melatonin is inversely related to the body temperature. That is, the endogenous nocturnal melatonin peak in humans is accompanied by a drop in core body temperature (Reiter *et al.*, 2010). As the length of daylight varies between seasons, the cycle of melatonin also varies (see Fig. 1.1). It is thought that the cycle length of melatonin may serve as an internal "calendar" for the body. This is important for certain animals such as seasonal breeders.

The mechanism of melatonin regulation is complex and begins with a specialized group of retinal ganglion that relates light-related signal to the suprachiasmatic nuclei (SCN) of the anterior hypothalamus via the retinohypothalamic tract (Moore, 1996). The SCN sends axonal projection first to the periventricular nucleus (PVN); axons from the PVN descend to the intermediolateral cell column of the thoracic spinal cord to the preganglionic sympathetic nuclei. Subsequent projections ascend via the sympathetic trunk to the superior cervical ganglia, from where the postganglionic sympathetic axons synapse on the pineal gland (Fig. 1.1). SCN induces production of melatonin through synaptic norepinephrine release at the sympathetic nerve endings at the pinealocytes, activating the enzymes responsible for the final steps of melatonin synthesis, AANAT and HIOMT.

C. Melatonin in clinical use

Despite the fact that minimal, if any, melatonin is found in the human diet (Van Tassel *et al.*, 2001), melatonin is marketed in the United States as a "dietary supplement." Melatonin preparations have been widely used for the treatment of insomnia and sleep phase disorders such as delayed sleep phase syndrome and jet lag, especially given its rather mild side effect profile and relatively lack of potential for dependence. Melatonin taken in the evening typically advances sleep phase, while administration in the morning delays sleep phase (Reiter *et al.*, 2010). Whether exogenous melatonin increases sleep duration varies between studies. A recent meta-analysis (Brzezinski *et al.*, 2005) concluded that with melatonin administration, there is a significant reduction in sleep latency by 4 min, increase in sleep efficiency by 2.2%, and increase in total sleep duration by 12.8 min in a total of 284 subjects. However, the doses of melatonin used between studies vary greatly, between 0.1 and 80 mg.

One of the issues with exogenous melatonin is the widely variable dosing. A commonly marketed dose is between 1 and 10 mg of melatonin. Because only very low dose (0.1–0.3 mg) of exogenous melatonin is enough to reach the physiologic nocturnal peak concentration of melatonin in young adults (Dollins *et al.*, 1994), the commonly marketed doses would elevate plasma melatonin concentration to many folds its normal physiologic value.

There have been several studies documenting potential adverse reaction and nonphysiological phenomena with high-dose melatonin administration including increased prolactin (Waldhauser *et al.*, 1987), hypothermia (Deacon and Arendt, 1995), and daytime sleepiness. However, currently, there are no data concerning the potential effects of long-term melatonin use. Some animal studies have demonstrated melatonin receptor desensitization (Gerdin *et al.*, 2004a,b), which raises the possibility of tolerance. Ramelteon is a synthetic melatonin agonist recently approved by the FDA in the United States as a prescription medication for insomnia.

III. Adenohypophysis

A. Growth hormone axis

Four hormones are involved in growth hormone axis regulation and sleep (growth hormone-releasing hormone, GHRH; growth hormone, GH; somatostatin release-inhibiting factor, SRIF; and ghrelin).

GHRH is synthesized by cells of the arcuate nucleus of the hypothalamus. It is secreted into the hypophyseal portal system at the median eminence to bind to its receptor on the anterior pituitary gland. GH is then released into the bloodstream. Somatostatin is released by the paraventricular nucleus of the hypothalamus, and although it does not seem to directly prevent GH synthesis, it modulates the pituitary response to GHRH by decreasing the amplitude of GH bursts. Ghrelin has only recently been isolated. It is mainly, but not exclusively, produced by the stomach. It is the only naturally occurring substance known to bind to the secretagogue receptor. Stimulation of the secretagogue receptor enhances GH release but needs GHRH-primed pituitary gland to do so (Sam and Frohman, 2008).

GH is released in a pulsatile manner, with the largest surge occurring in the first sleep cycle, when slow-wave sleep (SWS) is at its peak. Although GH and slow wave are closely intertwined, GHRH seems ultimately responsible for this association, as GHRH receptor blockade suppresses GH secretion while not altering SWS production (Jessup *et al.*, 2004). Studies have identified sleep as the major influence in GH production, regardless of the circadian timing of the sleep episode, characterizing it as a truly homeostatic response (Van Cauter *et al.*, 1992). However, a minor circadian influence also seems to be present (Van Cauter, 2005).

Both men and women have their highest surge of GH during the first episode of SWS. The key difference is related to the distribution of GH secretion on a 24-h period. However, in female, this does not account for the majority of its daily secretion, as opposed to men (Jaffe *et al.*, 1998).

With sleep deprivation, studies have shown blunting of the GH pulse associated with sleep. However, the GH pulses become more evenly distributed throughout the 24 h with individual pulses being larger. The total amount of GH secreted in normal sleep and in sleep deprivation is found to be similar (Brandenberger *et al.*, 2000). This finding argues against GH deficiency being a cause of growth inhibition in children with sleep disorders.

The different peptides involved in the GH cascade are known to exert specific effects on sleep. However, results of studies can be difficult to generalize, as methodological differences are seen between them. It is usually accepted that GHRH increases SWS and GH secretion in young males (Steiger *et al.*, 1992). Effects on REM sleep are less robust. In women, the effects of GHRH infusion on sleep architecture are different compared to men, with data showing a decrease in both NREM stage 4 and REM sleep, even though GH secretion is identical to that seen in men (Mathias *et al.*, 2007).

SRIF infusion in older individuals has yielded identical results in both sexes, decreasing total sleep time and REM sleep, especially the length of the last REM sleep episode (Frieboes *et al.*, 1997).

Intravenous ghrelin administration seems to have gender specificities, as it increases GH levels and SWS but decreases REM sleep in young adult men; however, it does not change sleep architecture in age-matched women (Weikel *et al.*, 2003). This noticeable difference is present even though overall effects of ghrelin on GH and cortisol secretion, when given in a pulsatile fashion at the commencement of nighttime sleep, are identical in both males and females (Kluge *et al.*, 2007; Weikel *et al.*, 2003). It is postulated that the effect of ghrelin on SWS is mediated through stimulation of GHRH secretion, which promotes SWS in humans (Steiger *et al.*, 1992).

B. Hypothalamic–pituitary–adrenal axis

Parvonuclear cells of the paraventricular nucleus of the hypothalamus release corticotropin-releasing hormone (CRH) into the hypophyseal portal system at the median eminence. CRH reaches the anterior pituitary gland, which allows for corticotropin levels to increase and stimulate the adrenal glands to release cortisol. Both corticotropin and cortisol act as a negative feedback on CRH production (Buckley and Schatzberg, 2005).

In normal individuals, the nadir or quiescent period of cortisol production is seen around sleep onset. The peak or acrophase is reached at midmorning. In between these two extremes, cortisol levels start to rise a couple of hours before the scheduled awakening. Overall, cortisol levels are mainly reflected by circadian rhythmicity. Sleep deprivation does not change the pattern of cortisol secretion. The only differences amount in lower peak and higher trough levels, presumably by a lack of the enhancing effects seen at sleep onset for the nadir and at arousal for the peak. Consequently, homeostatic regulation does exist, but its exerted influence is less prevalent than that of the circadian cycle (Van Cauter, 2005).

CRH inhibits SWS in the first part of the sleep episode. Its effects on REM sleep are more debatable, as it does seem to increase REM sleep in animal but not in humans, where REM sleep is actually reduced (Holsboer *et al.*, 1998). This effect on REM sleep in humans is also shared by corticotropin and cortisol (Fehm *et al.*, 1993; Friess *et al.*, 1994). However, the main result might be more the consequence of cortisol suppression of REM sleep, as infusion of corticotropin when cortisol production is blocked does not yield any change in REM sleep architecture (Jahn *et al.*, 2003). Cortisol also increases SWS through CRH inhibition, a condition not seen with corticotropin (Steiger, 2007).

CRH and GHRH effects seem to be balanced with one another and vary in a reciprocal fashion. When GHRH level is at its peak, CRH level is low. This favors SWS in the first part of the night as maximal GH concentration is documented. In the latter part of the night, as GH levels decline, the equilibrium shifts toward cortisol production, leading ultimately to arousal from sleep (Steiger, 2007).

One study has shown gender differences, as women demonstrate greater cortisol production at the beginning of the night as opposed to men. This was also accompanied by a lesser amount of SWS in women than in men, contrary to what is usually seen (Antonijevic *et al.*, 1999).

C. Gonadal axis

Gonadotropin-releasing hormone (GnRH)-secreting neurons, located in the preoptic area of the hypothalamus, release GnRH into the hypophyseal portal system at the median eminence. Subsequently, the anterior pituitary gland is activated to generate follicle-stimulating hormone (FSH) and/or luteinizing hormone (LH). These hormones stimulate their end-organ to produce testosterone in men and estradiol and progesterone in women (Degroot and Jameson, 2005).

Prepubertal individuals of either sex exhibit low FSH and LH levels, a low LH to FSH ratio, and a low LH pulse amplitude and frequency. At sleep onset, small surge of LH is seen but is in itself insufficient to alter significantly sex hormone production (Apter *et al.*, 1993). Puberty is associated with an increase GnRH pulses, possibly through release of central inhibition (McCartney, 2010). This is closely associated with sleep and creates an increase in LH pulse amplitude and frequency (Wu *et al.*, 1996). It is followed by morning increases of testosterone in boys and estradiol and progesterone in girls. By late puberty, daytime occurrence of LH surges supplants nighttime secretion (McCartney, 2010).

Adult women exhibit the menstrual cycle, which is closely related to changes in hormonal response. Initially, a sleep-related decrease in LH pulse frequency, coupled with an increase in pulse amplitude, is seen in the early follicular phase in postpubertal women. Sleep deprivation clearly inhibits this pattern (Rossmanith, 1998). The reduction in pulse frequency favors FSH production. Secretion of estradiol and inhibin in mid/late-follicular phase prepares for increase in LH secretion and the luteal phase. Progesterone increases through the luteal phase, having a negative feedback on GnRH pulse frequency, thus preparing the body for the next follicular phase (McCartney, 2010).

During the menstrual cycle, there are no significant alterations of the major sleep parameters. An increase in spindle activity has been reported in the luteal phase, possibly through the action of progesterone and its metabolites. A shortened REM sleep activity has also been shown in the luteal phase. A change in basal temperature rather than a direct hormonal effect might be the cause (Driver *et al.*, 1996). Sleep architecture in women suffering from severe premenstrual syndrome does not seem to differ from healthy controls, although sleep complaints are higher in the former group (Baker *et al.*, 2007).

Menopause brings the menstrual cycle to an end. LH and FSH no longer vary according to the luteal cyclic pattern. However, studies have shown that residual LH pulsatility and secretion, mainly present during nighttime sleep, can persist. It may be involved in the pathogenesis of the disturbed sleep exhibited in menopausal women, such as reduced total sleep time, increased wake after sleep onset, early morning awakening, although no clear correlation with estradiol levels has been shown (Murphy and Campbell, 2007).

Sleep-disordered breathing is significantly more common in postmenopausal than in premenopausal women and may contribute to the daytime symptoms of tiredness and sleepiness encountered by many (Young *et al.*, 2003). Hormone replacement therapy, either with estrogen or with a combination of estrogen and progestin, has not yielded consistent results, although some studies have shown an improvement of the respiratory disturbance index (RDI) with usage of estrogen alone (Manber *et al.*, 2003). In presence of obstructive sleep apnea, this type of therapeutic intervention is not currently recommended by the AASM (Morgenthaler *et al.*, 2006).

In men, LH secretion is pulsatile with increased amplitude of the LH surge in NREM sleep and decreased amplitude in REM sleep, consistent with an ultradian cycle (Fehm *et al.*, 1991). In older men, LH levels rarely surpass the ones seen in younger men, and LH secretion becomes more erratic and less organized and synchronized (Veldhuis, 2000).

In young adult men, testosterone levels peak in the early morning, evolving from a sleep onset nadir (Axelsson *et al.*, 2005). Studies using REM deprivation protocols have shown a blunted nocturnal testosterone level (Luboshitzky *et al.*, 2001). This robust association may be interpreted as a homeostatic effect of sleep on testosterone secretion.

D. Thyroid axis

TRH, synthesized by the paraventricular nucleus of the hypothalamus, is released into the hypophyseal portal system at the median eminence and ensures production of thyrotropin by the anterior pituitary gland. Thyrotropin then reaches the bloodstream where it can exert its effects on the thyroid gland to stimulate synthesis of thyroid hormones (T3/T4) (Degroot and Jameson, 2005).

Thyrotropin level is low throughout the day and normally rises early in the evening to reach maximal concentration at usual sleep onset. Decline occurs afterwards, accelerating in the latter part of the night to attain its lowest point after morning arousal. Its rhythm matches the circadian clock. Homeostatic sleep drive also does exert an effect on thyrotropin blood levels but more so modulate its secretion than modify the pattern. For example, total sleep deprivation enhances the nocturnal peak of thyrotropin. Thus, sleep decreases thyrotropin secretion, whereas total sleep deprivation lifts this partial inhibition (Brabant *et al.*, 1990). Thyrotropin production has to be present in order for sleep to affect blood levels, as low thyrotropin levels are not further decreased by daily naps. However, partial sleep deprivation, as exemplified by short sleep nights, does not seem to alter thyrotropin or thyroid hormones secretion pattern (Kessler *et al.*, 2010). The nocturnal peak of thyrotropin is lessened when the homeostatic sleep drive is enhanced by prior sleep deprivation. SWS rebound may exert an inhibitory effect on the thyrotropin peak (Brabant *et al.*, 1990).

Data are lacking regarding the effects of the thyroid cascade on sleep itself. One investigator studied the consequence of TRH administration on normal men and did not find any significant effect, albeit a minute decrease in total sleep time (Hemmeter *et al.*, 1998).

E. Prolactin axis

Lactotrope cells located in the anterior pituitary gland synthesize and secrete prolactin. They are under the regulatory control of the dopaminergic neurons situated in the arcuate nucleus of the hypothalamus, which inhibit prolactin secretion. Thyrotropin-releasing hormone (TRH) enhances prolactin release (Degroot and Jameson, 2005).

Change in prolactin levels is essentially driven by sleep itself. The levels quickly rise after sleep onset to reach their peak concentration in the middle of the sleep episode, independently of the circadian timing, thus confirming the homeostatic effect of sleep itself, regardless of the time of day. The nadir is normally found at midday (Spiegel *et al.*, 1994). However, there seems to be a weak circadian effect, as shown in studies of phase advance and phase delay. Maximal levels of prolactin are achieved when both homeostatic drive and circadian rhythm are synchronized. Otherwise, the sleep-related peaks will be reduced in amplitude. This modest effect is less prominent in men than in women (Waldstreicher *et al.*, 1996).

The influence of prolactin on sleep itself is subject to debate. Clear data for REM sleep regulation in human subjects are still missing (Roky *et al.*, 1995). Prolactin has also been postulated to increase SWS, as seen in some patients with prolactinomas (Frieboes *et al.*, 1998). Contradictory results abound and the issue is yet to be elucidated.

IV. Neurohypophysis Axis

A. Vasopressin

Magnocellular neurons of the supraoptic and paraventricular nuclei of the hypothalamus terminate in the posterior pituitary gland. Vasopressin, or arginine vasopressin (AVP) (sometimes called antidiuretic hormone [ADH]), reaches systemic circulation via the inferior hypophyseal artery, a branch of the internal carotid artery. The release of AVP from the posterior pituitary is controlled by three main factors of physiologic importance: (1) plasma osmolality, (2) effective blood volume, and (3) blood pressure. Although pulsatile secretion of vasopressin is documented, no role of sleep has been identified (Brandenberger *et al.*, 1998). Studies in animal models have implicated, in late night sleep period, the decrease firing of suprachiasmatic nucleus, which relieves the inhibition on supraoptic neurons and allows for osmoregulated AVP secretion (Trudel and Bourque, 2010).

B. Oxytocin

Oxytocin is the other hormone produced by the neurohypophysis. Sleep is not known to exert any influence on circulating levels of this hormone (Forsling, 2000).

V. Other Hormones

A. Leptin

Leptin is primarily produced in fat cells and plays an important role in appetite regulation. Large fat cells produce more leptin than small fat cells. The serum leptin concentration is strongly correlated with body fat content (Considine *et al.*, 1996). Leptin functions to signal the brain, specifically in the arcuate nucleus of the hypothalamus, about the quantity of stored fat. In animal studies, systemic leptin administration reduces food intake (Van Heek *et al.*, 1997). There are human subjects with congenital leptin deficiency due to mutation in the leptin gene. These individuals develop early-onset massive obesity and hyperphagia. These symptoms respond to subcutaneous administration of leptin (Farooqi *et al.*, 2002). Leptin is also known to be important for reproductive functions.

Leptin release has been shown to be related to sleep and circadian rhythm (Saad *et al.*, 1998; Simon *et al.*, 1998). Plasma leptin concentration increases during the daytime and reaches a nocturnal peak between 22:00 and 03:00. The nadir of leptin concentration is between around 08:00 and 17:40. When human subjects underwent total sleep deprivation, a circadian-related leptin release is still observed at night. A study of sleep curtailment (Spiegel *et al.*, 2004) (two nights of 4 h in bed) demonstrates an overall reduction of leptin level by 18%. There is a corresponding increase in reported hunger by 23% and an increase in appetite for foods with high carbohydrate by 30%. The consequence of these observations is consistent with increased caloric intake in subjects who are sleep deprived (Brondel *et al.*, 2010). These findings may provide partial explanation for the association between short sleep time and higher BMI. However, leptin is not found to be significantly abnormal in patients with obstructive sleep apnea (Papaioannou *et al.*, 2011).

B. Insulin and glucose

Insulin is a peptide hormone secreted by pancreatic beta cells in the islets of Langerhans. Insulin secretion is primarily regulated by plasma glucose concentration. Insulin is secreted in response to a rise in blood glucose concentration.

Although insulin secretion is primarily regulated by blood glucose concentration, there is some evidence that insulin secretion is controlled by circadian rhythm as well. It has been well established that glucose tolerance and insulin responses to glucose and meals are higher in the morning than at night. Insulin secretion rises during the early morning hours, reaching a peak in the early afternoon, and declines throughout the evening and night (Boden *et al.*, 1996). More recently, there have been accumulating evidence that melatonin exerts an inhibitory effect on the pancreatic beta cells via direct binding of melatonin receptors on the beta-cell surface (Peschke and Muhlbauer, 2010). This finding provides an explanation for the decrease in insulin secretion at night, when plasma melatonin concentration is high.

Sleep deprivation in general has been associated with reduced pancreatic beta-cell responsiveness to glucose, leading to lower glucose tolerance (Morselli *et al.*, 2010). Although it has been proposed that obstructive sleep apnea may be a risk factor for impaired glucose tolerance, only one of three randomized controlled trials showed a small benefit on glucose metabolism when obstructive sleep apnea is treated (Clarenbach *et al.*, 2011).

VI. Summary

Sleep is regulated by two separate processes, circadian rhythm and homeostatic drive. Sleep, circadian, and homeostatic processes are involved in the regulation of many hormones. In turn, these hormones also regulate the circadian process. Levels of many hormones vary across day and night. Such fluctuations are attributable not only to changes in sleep and wakefulness and other behaviors but also to the circadian system. Under normal circumstances, sleep, behaviors, and the circadian system are synchronized with an optimal phase relationship, and consequently, hormonal systems are exquisitely regulated. Desynchronization of this intimately regulated process involving sleep, the circadian, and homeostatic systems, and various hormones may lead to consequences on the metabolic function and health-related problems.

REFERENCES

Achermann, P., and Borbély, A. A. (2003). Mathematical models of sleep regulation. *Front. Biosci.* **8,** s683–s693.

American Academy of Sleep Medicine (2007). AASM Manual for the Scoring of Sleep and Associated Events: Rules, Terminology and Technical Specifications. American Academy of Sleep Medicine, Westchester, IL.

Antonijevic, I. A., Murck, H., Frieboes, R., Holsboer, F., and Steiger, A. (1999). On the gender differences in sleep-endocrine regulation in young normal humans. *Neuroendocrinology* **70,** 280–287.

Apter, D., Bützow, T. L., Laughlin, G. A., and Yen, S. S. (1993). Gonadotropin-releasing hormone pulse generator activity during pubertal transition in girls: Pulsatile and diurnal patterns of circulating gonadotropins. *J. Clin. Endocrinol. Metab.* **76**(4), 940–949.

Axelrod, J., Shein, H. M., and Wurtman, R. J. (1969). Stimulation of C14-melatonin synthesis from C14-tryptophan by noradrenaline in rat pineal in organ culture. *Proc. Natl. Acad. Sci. U.S.A.* **62,** 544–549.

Axelsson, J., Ingre, M., Akerstedt, T., and Holmback, U. (2005). Effects of acutely displaced sleep on testosterone. *J. Clin. Endocrinol. Metab.* **90,** 4530–4535.

Baker, F. C., Kahan, T. L., Trinder, J., and Colrain, I. M. (2007). Sleep quality and the sleep electroencephalogram in women with severe premenstrual syndrome. *Sleep* **30,** 1283–1291.

Boden, G., Ruiz, J., Urbain, J. L., and Chen, X. (1996). Evidence for a circadian rhythm of insulin secretion. *Am. J. Physiol.* **271,** E246–E252.

Brabant, G., Prank, K., Ranft, U., Schuermeyer, T., Wagner, T. O., Hauser, H., Kummer, B., Feistner, H., Hesch, R. D., and von zur Mühlen, A. (1990). Physiological regulation of circadian and pulsatile thyrotropin secretion in normal man and woman. *J. Clin. Endocrinol. Metab.* **70,** 403–409.

Brandenberger, G., Charloux, A., Gronfier, C., and Otzenberger, H. (1998). Ultradian rhythms in hydromineral hormones. *Horm. Res.* **49,** 131–135.

Brandenberger, G., Gronfier, C., Chapotot, F., Simon, C., and Piquard, F. (2000). Effect of sleep deprivation on overall 24 h growth-hormone secretion. *Lancet* **356,** 1408.

Brondel, L., Romer, M. A., Nougues, P. M., Touyarou, P., and Davenne, D. (2010). Acute partial sleep deprivation increases food intake in healthy men. *Am. J. Clin. Nutr.* **91,** 1550–1559.

Brzezinski, A., Vangel, M. G., Wurtman, R. J., Norrie, G., Zhdanova, I., Ben-Shushan, A., and Ford, I. (2005). Effects of exogenous melatonin on sleep: A meta-analysis. *Sleep Med. Rev.* **9,** 41–50.

Buckley, T. M., and Schatzberg, A. F. (2005). On the interactions of the hypothalamic-pituitary-adrenal (HPA) axis and sleep: Normal HPA axis activity and circadian rhythm, exemplary sleep disorders. *J. Clin. Endocrinol. Metab.* **90,** 3106–3114.

Buxton, O. M., Pavlova, M., Reid, E. W., Wang, W., Simonson, D. C., and Adler, G. K. (2010). Sleep restriction for 1 week reduces insulin sensitivity in healthy men. *Diabetes* **59,** 2126–2133.

Carskadon, M. A., and Dement, W. C. (1996). Normal human sleep: An overview. *In* "Principles and Practice of Sleep Medicine," (M. H. Kryger, *et al.*, Eds.), pp. 16–25. Saunders, Philadelphia, PA.

Carskadon, M. A., and Dement, W. C. (2005). Normal human sleep: An overview. *In* "Principles and Practice of Sleep Medicine," (M. H. Kryger, T. Roth, and W. C. Dement, Eds.). 4th edn, Saunders, Philadelphiap. 13.

Clarenbach, C. F., West, S. D., and Kohler, M. (2011). Is obstructive sleep apnea a risk factor for diabetes? *Discov. Med.* **12,** 17–24.

Considine, R. V., Sinha, M. K., Heiman, M. L., Kriauciunas, A., Stephens, T. W., Nyce, M. R., Ohannesian, J. P., Marco, C. C., McKee, L. J., Bauer, T. L., *et al.* (1996). Serum immunoreactive-leptin concentrations in normal-weight and obese humans. *N. Engl. J. Med.* **334,** 292–295.

Deacon, S., and Arendt, J. (1995). Melatonin-induced temperature suppression and its acute phase-shifting effects correlate in a dose-dependent manner in humans. *Brain Res.* **688,** 77–85.

Degroot, L. and Jameson, L. J. (Eds.) (2005). *In* Endocrinology, 5th edn Saunders, Philadelphia.

Deguchi, T. (1982). Sympathetic regulation of circadian rhythm of serotonin N-acetyltransferase activity in pineal gland of infant rat. *J. Neurochem.* **38,** 797–802.

Dollins, A. B., Zhdanova, I. V., Wurtman, R. J., Lynch, H. J., and Deng, M. H. (1994). Effect of inducing nocturnal serum melatonin concentrations in daytime on sleep, mood, body temperature, and performance. *Proc. Natl. Acad. Sci. U.S.A.* **91,** 1824–1828.

Driver, H. S., Dijk, D. J., Werth, E., Biedermann, K., and Borbély, A. A. (1996). Sleep and the sleep electroencephalogram across the menstrual cycle in young healthy women. *J. Clin. Endocrinol. Metab.* **81,** 728–735.

Farooqi, I. S., Matarese, G., Lord, G. M., Keogh, J. M., Lawrence, E., Agwu, C., Sanna, V., Jebb, S. A., Perna, F., Fontana, S., Lechler, R. I., DePaoli, A. M., *et al.* (2002). Beneficial effects of leptin on obesity, T cell hyporesponsiveness, and neuroendocrine/metabolic dysfunction of human congenital leptin deficiency. *J. Clin. Invest.* **110,** 1093–1103.

Fehm, H. L., Clausing, J., Kern, W., Pietrowsky, R., and Born, J. (1991). Sleep-associated augmentation and synchronization of luteinizing hormone pulses in adult men. *Neuroendocrinology* **54,** 192–195.

Fehm, H. L., Späth-Schwalbe, E., Pietrowsky, R., Kern, W., and Born, J. (1993). Entrainment of nocturnal pituitary-adrenocortical activity to sleep processes in man—A hypothesis. *Exp. Clin. Endocrinol.* **101,** 267–276.

Forsling, M. L. (2000). Diurnal rhythms in neurohypophysial function. *Exp. Physiol.* **85,** 179–186.

Frieboes, R. M., Murck, H., Schier, T., Holsboer, F., and Steiger, A. (1997). Somatostatin impairs sleep in elderly human subjects. *Neuropsychopharmacology* **16,** 339–345.

Frieboes, R. M., Murck, H., Stalla, G. K., Antonijevic, I. A., and Steiger, A. (1998). Enhanced slow wave sleep in patients with prolactinoma. *J. Clin. Endocrinol. Metab.* **83,** 2706–2710.

Friess, E., V Bardeleben, U., Wiedemann, K., Lauer, C. J., and Holsboer, F. (1994). Effects of pulsatile cortisol infusion on sleep-EEG and nocturnal growth hormone release in healthy men. *J. Sleep Res.* **3,** 73–79.

Gerdin, M. J., Masana, M. I., and Dubocovich, M. L. (2004a). Melatonin-mediated regulation of human MT(1) melatonin receptors expressed in mammalian cells. *Biochem. Pharmacol.* **67,** 2023–2030.

Gerdin, M. J., Masana, M. I., Rivera-Bermudez, M. A., Hudson, R. L., Earnest, D. J., Gillette, M. U., and Dubocovich, M. L. (2004b). Melatonin desensitizes endogenous MT2 melatonin receptors in the rat suprachiasmatic nucleus: Relevance for defining the periods of sensitivity of the mammalian circadian clock to melatonin. *FASEB J.* **18,** 1646–1656.

Hemmeter, U., Rothe, B., Guldner, J., Holsboer, F., and Steiger, A. (1998). Effects of thyrotropin-releasing hormone on the sleep EEG and nocturnal hormone secretion in male volunteers. *Neuropsychobiology* **38,** 25–31.

Holsboer, F., von Bardeleben, U., and Steiger, A. (1998). Effects of intravenous corticotropin-releasing hormone upon sleep-related growth hormone surge and sleep EEG in man. *Neuroendocrinology* **48,** 32–38.

Jaffe, C. A., Ocampo-Lim, B., Guo, W., Krueger, K., Sugahara, I., DeMott-Friberg, R., Bermann, M., and Barkan, A. L. (1998). Regulatory mechanisms of growth hormone secretion are sexually dimorphic. *J Clin Invest* **102,** 153–164.

Jahn, H., Kiefer, F., Schick, M., Yassouridis, A., Steiger, A., Kellner, M., and Wiedemann, K. (2003). Sleep-endocrine effects of the 11-b-hydroxasteroiddehydrogenase inhibitor metyrapone. *Sleep* **26,** 823–829.

Jessup, S. K., Malow, B. A., Symons, K. V., and Barkan, A. L. (2004). Blockade of endogenous growth hormone-releasing hormone receptors dissociates nocturnal growth hormone secretion and slow-wave sleep. *Eur. J. Endocrinol.* **151,** 561–566.

Kessler, L., Nedeltcheva, A., Imperial, J., and Penev, P. D. (2010). Changes in serum TSH and free T4 during human sleep restriction. *Sleep* **33,** 1115–1118.

Klein, D. C., and Moore, R. Y. (1979). Pineal N-acetyltransferase and hydroxyindole-O-methyltransferase: Control by the retinohypothalamic tract and the suprachiasmatic nucleus. *Brain Res.* **174,** 245–262.

Klein, D. C., and Weller, J. L. (1970). Indole metabolism in the pineal gland: A circadian rhythm in N-acetyltransferase. *Science* **169,** 1093–1095.

Kluge, M., Schüssler, P., Zuber, V., Kleyer, S., Yassouridis, A., Dresler, M., Uhr, M., and Steiger, A. (2007). Ghrelin enhances the nocturnal secretion of cortisol and growth hormone in young females without influencing sleep. *Psychoneuroendocrinology* **32,** 1079–1085.

Lewy, A. J., Wehr, T. A., Goodwin, F. K., Newsome, D. A., and Markey, S. P. (1980). Light suppresses melatonin secretion in humans. *Science* **210,** 1267–1269.

Luboshitzky, R., Zabari, Z., Shen-Orr, Z., Herer, P., and Lavie, P. (2001). Disruption of the nocturnal testosterone rhythm by sleep fragmentation in normal men. *J. Clin. Endocrinol. Metab.* **86,** 1134–1139.

Manber, R., Kuo, T. F., Cataldo, N., and Colrain, I. M. (2003). The effects of hormone replacement therapy on sleep-disordered breathing in postmenopausal women: A pilot study. *Sleep* **26,** 163–168.

Mathias, S., Held, K., Ising, M., Weikel, J. C., Yassouridis, A., and Steiger, A. (2007). Systemic growth hormone-releasing hormone (GHRH) impairs sleep in healthy young women. *Psychoneuroendocrinology* **32,** 1021–1027.

McCartney, C. R. (2010). Maturation of sleep-wake gonadotrophin-releasing hormone secretion across puberty in girls: Potential mechanisms and relevance to the pathogenesis of polycystic ovary syndrome. *J. Neuroendocrinol.* **22,** 701–709.

Moore, R. Y. (1996). Neural control of the pineal gland. *Behav. Brain Res.* **73,** 125–130.

Moore, R. Y., and Klein, D. C. (1974). Visual pathways and the central neural control of a circadian rhythm in pineal serotonin N-acetyltransferase activity. *Brain Res.* **71,** 17–33.

Morgenthaler, T. I., Kapen, S., Lee-Chiong, T., Alessi, C., Boehlecke, B., Brown, T., Coleman, J., Friedman, L., Kapur, V., Owens, J., Pancer, J., Swick, T., *et al.* (2006). Practice parameters for the medical therapy of obstructive sleep apnea. *Sleep* **29,** 1031–1035.

Morselli, L., Leproult, R., Balbo, M., and Spiegel, K. (2010). Role of sleep duration in the regulation of glucose metabolism and appetite. *Best Pract. Res. Clin. Endocrinol. Metab.* **24,** 687–702.

Murphy, P. J., and Campbell, S. S. (2007). Sex hormones, sleep, and core body temperature in older postmenopausal women. *Sleep* **30,** 1788–1794.

Papaioannou, I., Patterson, M., Twigg, G. L., Vazir, A., Ghatei, M., Morrell, M. J., and Polkey, M. I. (2011). Lack of association between impaired glucose tolerance and appetite regulating hormones in patients with obstructive sleep apnea. *J. Clin. Sleep. Med.* **7**(5), 486–492.

Peschke, E., and Muhlbauer, E. (2010). New evidence for a role of melatonin in glucose regulation. *Best Pract. Res. Clin. Endocrinol. Metab.* **24,** 829–841.

Pilcher, J. J., and Huffcutt, A. I. (1996). Effects of sleep deprivation on performance: A meta-analysis. *Sleep* **19,** 318–326.

Rechtschaffen, A., and Kales, A. (1968). A Manual of Standardized Terminology: Techniques and Scoring Systems for Sleep Stages of Human Subjects. UCLA Brain Information Service/Brain Research Institute, Neurological Information Network, Los Angeles. National Institutes of Health Publications No. 204.

Rechtschaffen, A., Bergmann, B. M., *et al.* (1989). Sleep deprivation in the rat: X. Integration and discussion of the findings. *Sleep* **12**(1), 68–87.

Reiter, R. J., Tan, D. X., and Fuentes-Broto, L. (2010). Melatonin: A multitasking molecule. *Prog. Brain Res.* **181,** 127–151.

Roky, R., Obál, F., Jr., Valatx, J. L., Bredow, S., Fang, J., Pagano, L. P., and Krueger, J. M. (1995). Prolactin and rapid eye movement sleep regulation. *Sleep* **18,** 536–542.

Rossmanith, W. G. (1998). The impact of sleep on gonadotropin secretion. *Gynecol. Endocrinol.* **12,** 381–389.

Saad, M. F., Riad-Gabriel, M. G., Khan, A., Sharma, A., Michael, R., Jinagouda, S. D., Boyadjian, R., and Steil, G. M. (1998). Diurnal and ultradian rhythmicity of plasma leptin: Effects of gender and adiposity. *J. Clin. Endocrinol. Metab.* **83,** 453–459.

Sam, S., and Frohman, L. A. (2008). Normal physiology of hypothalamic pituitary regulation. *Endocrinol. Metab. Clin. North Am.* **37,** 1–22.

Simon, C., Gronfier, C., Schlienger, J. L., and Brandenberger, G. (1998). Circadian and ultradian variations of leptin in normal man under continuous enteral nutrition: Relationship to sleep and body temperature. *J. Clin. Endocrinol. Metab.* **83,** 1893–1899.

Spiegel, K., Follenius, M., Simon, C., Saini, J., Ehrhart, J., and Brandenberger, G. (1994). Prolactin secretion and sleep. *Sleep* **17,** 20–27.

Spiegel, K., Tasali, E., Penev, P., and Van Cauter, E. (2004). Brief communication: Sleep curtailment in healthy young men is associated with decreased leptin levels, elevated ghrelin levels, and increased hunger and appetite. *Ann. Intern. Med.* **141,** 846–850.

Steiger, A. (2007). Neurochemical regulation of sleep. *J. Psychiatr. Res.* **41,** 537–552.

Steiger, A., Guldner, J., Hemmeter, U., Rothe, B., Wiedemann, K., and Holsboer, F. (1992). Effects of growth hormone-releasing hormone and somatostatin on sleep EEG and nocturnal hormone secretion in male controls. *Neuroendocrinology* **56,** 566–573.

Stickgold, R. (2009). The Neuroscience of Sleep. Elsevier, Boston, MA.

Trudel, E., and Bourque, C. W. (2010). Central clock excites vasopressin neurons by waking osmosensory afferents during late sleep. *Nat. Neurosci.* **13,** 467–474.

Van Cauter, E. (2005). Endocrine physiology. *In* "Principles and Practice of Sleep Medicine," (M. H. Kryger, T. Roth, and W. C. Dement, Eds.), 4th edn, pp. 266–282. Saunders, Philadelphia.

Van Cauter, E., Kerkhofs, M., Caufriez, A., Van Onderbergen, A., Thorner, M. O., and Copinschi, G. (1992). A quantitative estimation of growth hormone secretion in normal man: Reproducibility and relation to sleep and time of day. *J. Clin. Endocrinol. Metab.* **74,** 1441–1450.

Van Heek, M., Compton, D. S., France, C. F., Tedesco, R. P., Fawzi, A. B., Graziano, M. P., Sybertz, E. J., Strader, C. D., and Davis, H. R., Jr. (1997). Diet-induced obese mice develop peripheral, but not central, resistance to leptin. *J. Clin. Invest.* **99,** 385–390.

Van Tassel, D. L., Roberts, N., Lewy, A., and O'Neill, S. D. (2001). Melatonin in plant organs. *J. Pineal Res.* **31,** 8–15.

Veldhuis, J. D. (2000). Recent neuroendocrine facets of male reproductive aging. *Exp. Gerontol.* **35,** 1281–1308.

Waldhauser, F., Lieberman, H. R., Lynch, H. J., Waldhauser, M., Herkner, K., Frisch, H., Vierhapper, H., Waldhausl, W., Schemper, M., Wurtman, R. J., *et al.* (1987). A pharmacological dose of melatonin increases PRL levels in males without altering those of GH, LH, FSH, TSH, testosterone or cortisol. *Neuroendocrinology* **46,** 125–130.

Waldstreicher, J., Duffy, J. F., Brown, E. N., Rogacz, S., Allan, J. S., and Czeisler, C. A. (1996). Gender differences in the temporal organization of proclactin (PRL) secretion: Evidence for a sleep-independent circadian rhythm of circulating PRL levels—A clinical research center study. *J. Clin. Endocrinol. Metab.* **81,** 1483–1487.

Weikel, J. C., Wichniak, A., Ising, M., Brunner, H., Friess, E., Held, K., Mathias, S., Schmid, D. A., Uhr, M., and Steiger, A. (2003). Ghrelin promotes slow-wave sleep in humans. *Am. J. Physiol. Endocrinol. Metab.* **284,** 407–415.

Wu, F. C., Butler, G. E., Kelnar, C. J., Huhtaniemi, I., and Veldhuis, J. D. (1996). Ontogeny of pulsatile gonadotropin releasing hormone secretion from midchildhood, through puberty, to adulthood in the human male: A study using deconvolution analysis and an ultrasensitive immunofluorometric assay. *J. Clin. Endocrinol. Metab.* **81,** 1798–1805.

Young, T., Finn, L., Austin, D., and Peterson, A. (2003). Menopausal status and sleep-disordered breathing in the Wisconsin Sleep Cohort Study. *Am. J. Respir. Crit. Care Med.* **167,** 1181–1185.

CHAPTER TWO

The Role of Orexin/Hypocretin in the Central Nervous System and Peripheral Tissues

Tomomi Tsunematsu* *and* Akihiro Yamanaka*,†,‡

Contents

Abstract

Orexin, also called hypocretin, is a neuropeptide produced in neurons sparsely distributed in the lateral hypothalamic area. Orexin exhibits its physiological effects after binding two G-protein-coupled receptors, orexin 1 receptor and orexin 2 receptor. Impairment of the orexin signal, either by deletion of the

* Division of Cell Signaling, National Institute for Physiological Sciences, Okazaki, Japan
† Department of Physiological Sciences, The Graduate University for Advanced Studies, Okazaki, Japan
‡ PRESTO, JST, Kawaguchi, Japan

Vitamins and Hormones, Volume 89
ISSN 0083-6729, http://dx.doi.org/10.1016/B978-0-12-394623-2.00002-0

prepro-orexin or orexin 2 receptor gene or by the ablation of orexin neurons, results in a sleep disorder similar to narcolepsy, suggesting that the orexin system plays an important role in the regulation of sleep/wakefulness. In addition, previous studies have suggested that orexin is involved in energy and fluid homeostasis, emotion regulation, stress responsiveness, and reward. However, growing evidence also suggests that orexin affects the function of peripheral tissues via direct activation of orexin receptors or through activation of autonomic nervous or endocrine systems. In this review, we discuss the physiological roles of orexin not only in the central nervous system but also in the peripheral tissues.

I. Introduction

The neuropeptides orexin A and orexin B (also known as hypocretin 1 and hypocretin 2, respectively) were initially identified as endogenous ligands for two orphan G-protein-coupled receptors (GPCRs; de Lecea *et al.*, 1998; Sakurai *et al.*, 1998). They were initially recognized as regulators of feeding behavior due to their exclusive production in the lateral hypothalamic area (LHA), which is a well-known feeding center. Moreover, intracerebroventricular (i.c.v.) injection of synthetic orexin peptide induces feeding behavior (Edwards *et al.*, 1999; Haynes *et al.*, 1999; Sakurai *et al.*, 1998).

Subsequent studies demonstrated that the orexin system also plays a crucial role in the regulation of sleep/wakefulness states since orexin deficiency in humans and animals produces characteristic symptoms of the sleep disorder narcolepsy (Chemelli *et al.*, 1999; Hara *et al.*, 2001; Lin *et al.*, 1999; Peyron *et al.*, 2000; Thannickal *et al.*, 2000). Further investigation suggested roles for orexin in the coordination of emotion, energy and fluid homeostasis, reward, and arousal (Boutrel *et al.*, 2005; Harris *et al.*, 2005; Mieda *et al.*, 2004; Narita *et al.*, 2006; Tsunematsu *et al.*, 2008; Yamanaka *et al.*, 2003). Additionally, the orexin system also regulates autonomic functions, including blood pressure and heart rate and neuroendocrine axes, including the hypothalamic–pituitary–adrenal (HPA) axis (Jaszberenyi *et al.*, 2000; Kuru *et al.*, 2000; Sakamoto *et al.*, 2004; Sakurai *et al.*, 1998; Samson *et al.*, 1999; Shirasaka *et al.*, 1999). These findings suggest that orexin neurons play a critical, adaptive role in the coordination of central and peripheral states according to the environment, which is beneficial for survival.

In this review, we briefly discuss the basic biology of orexin and orexin receptors and then focus on the role of orexin neural systems in the regulation of feeding behavior, energy homeostasis, and neuroendocrine function.

II. Orexin and Orexin Receptors

A. Identification of orexin

Orexin/hypocretin was independently identified by two different groups in 1998 utilizing completely different methodologies. Orexin A and B were identified as endogenous ligands for two orphan GPCRs by a method called "reverse pharmacology" (Sakurai *et al.*, 1998). Orexin-producing neurons (orexin neurons) were localized to the LHA, a region known as a feeding center. Further, i.c.v. injection of synthetic orexin peptide increased food consumption. Therefore, these neuropeptides were named orexin after the Greek word *orexis*, meaning "appetite" (Edwards *et al.*, 1999; Haynes *et al.*, 1999; Sakurai *et al.*, 1998). At the same time, de Lecea and colleagues identified a novel mRNA specifically expressed in the hypothalamus and the putative mature peptides were termed as hypocretin-1 and -2 (de Lecea *et al.*, 1998). Since these independent discoveries, it is now known that orexin and hypocretin are synonymous names for the same set of peptides.

Orexins constitute a novel peptide family with no significant homology with any previously described peptides. Orexin A and B are produced from a common precursor polypeptide, prepro-orexin, by enzymatic cleavage (Fig. 2.1). Orexin A is a 33-amino acid peptide of 3562 Da, with an

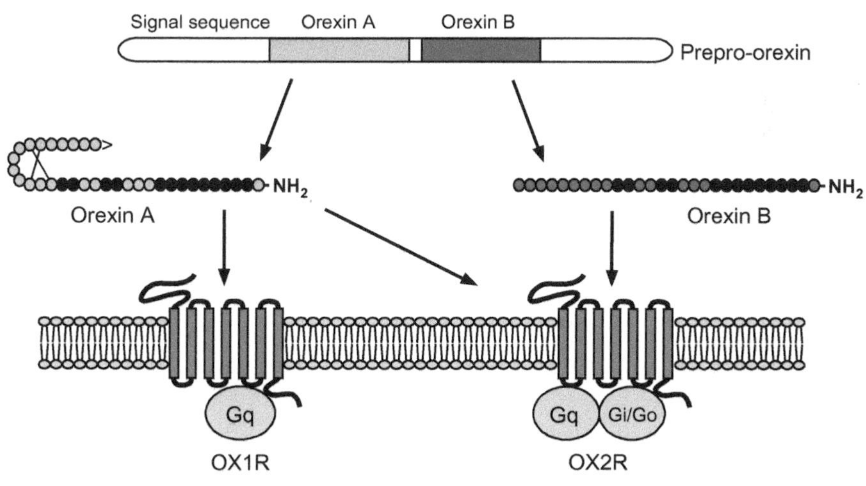

Figure 2.1 An overview of orexin peptide and orexin receptor systems. Orexin A and orexin B are derived from a common precursor peptide, prepro-orexin. The actions of orexins are mediated via two G-protein-coupled receptors, OX1R and OX2R. OX1R is selective for orexin A, whereas OX2R shows a similar sensitivity for both orexin A and orexin B. OX1R is coupled exclusively to the Gq subclass of G proteins, whereas OX2R is coupled to the G_i and/or G_q subclass.

N-terminal pyroglutamyl residue and C-terminal amidation. The four Cys residues of orexin A form two sets of intrachain disulfide bonds. This structure is completely conserved across several mammalian species (human, rat, mouse, cow, sheep, dog, and pig). On the other hand, rat orexin B is a 28-amino acid, C-terminally amidated linear peptide of 2937 Da, which is 46% identical to orexin A. The C-terminal half of orexin B is very similar to that of orexin A (73% identical), although the N-terminal half is more variable. Mouse orexin B is identical to rat orexin B. Compared to the rodent sequence, human orexin B has two amino acid substitutions within a 28-residue stretch (Sakurai *et al.*, 1998).

B. Orexin receptors

The actions of orexins are mediated via two types of GPCRs, orexin 1 receptor (OX1R) and orexin 2 receptor (OX2R) (also known as Hcrtr1 and Hcrtr2, respectively). The amino acid similarity between full-length OX1R and OX2R sequences is 64%. OX1R has an order of magnitude greater affinity for orexin A versus orexin B. On the other hand, OX2R has similar affinity for both orexin A and orexin B (Sakurai *et al.*, 1998) (Fig. 2.1). OX1R couples to the $G_{q/11}$ class of G-proteins, which results in activation of phosopholipase C and subsequent triggering of the phosphatidylinositol cascade. In contrast, OX2R couples to both $G_{q/11}$ and G_i classes of G-proteins in neuronal cell lines (Zhu *et al.*, 2003).

C. Distribution of orexin neurons

Orexin neurons are sparsely located in the LHA and perifornical area in the brain and widely project throughout the entire brain, excluding the cerebellum (Date *et al.*, 1999; Nambu *et al.*, 1999; Peyron *et al.*, 1998). This anatomical distribution suggests that the activity of orexin neurons influences multiple brain functions. Particularly, dense orexin-immunoreactive nerve endings are found in the paraventricular nucleus (PVN), arcuate nucleus of the hypothalamus (Arc), raphe nuclei, tuberomammillary nucleus (TMN), and locus coeruleus (LC) (Fig. 2.2). Orexin neurons also contain dynorphin (Chou *et al.*, 2001), galanin (Hakansson *et al.*, 1999), prolactin (Risold *et al.*, 1999), neuronal activity-regulated pentraxin (Reti *et al.*, 2002), and glutamate (Abrahamson *et al.*, 2001). In contrast, orexin neurons do not express glutamic acid decarboxylase (GAD)-67 mRNA, suggesting that orexin neurons are not GABAergic neurons (Rosin *et al.*, 2003).

D. Distribution of orexin receptors

Consistent with the broad projection of orexin neurons, OX1R and OX2R mRNAs are widely distributed throughout the central nervous system. The expression of OX1R and OX2R shows partially overlapping but largely

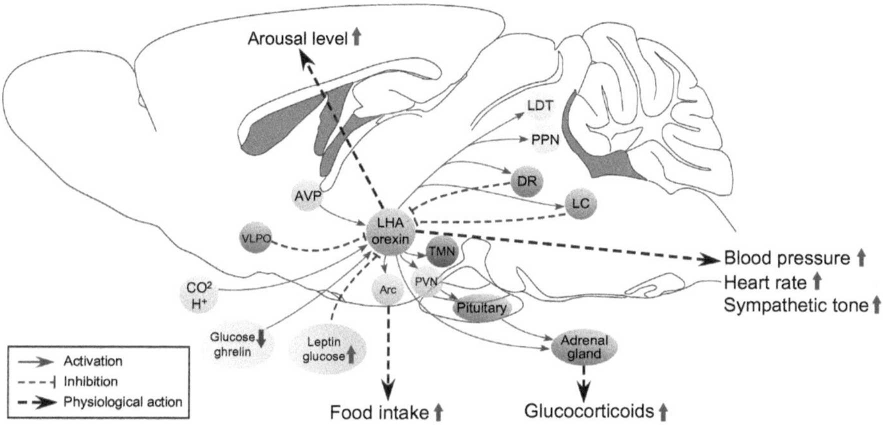

Figure 2.2 Interaction of orexin neurons with other brain regions and peripheral tissues. Orexin neurons are exclusively located in the lateral hypothalamic area and project throughout the brain. Dashed blue lines show inhibitory projections. Red arrows show excitatory projections. Dashed black arrows show physiological actions of the orexin system. Arc, arcuate nucleus; DR, dorsal raphe nuclei; LC, locus coeruleus; LDT, laterodorsal tegmental nucleus; LHA, lateral hypothalamic area; PPN, pedunculopontine nucleus; PVN, paraventricular nucleus; TMN, tuberomammillary nucleus; VLPO, ventrolateral preoptic nucleus. (See Color Insert.)

distinct and complementary distribution patterns, suggesting that they play different physiological roles. OX1Rs are expressed in the prefrontal and infralimbic cortex, hippocampus (cornu ammonis 2), amygdala, bed nucleus of the stria terminalis (BST), PVN, anterior hypothalamus, dorsal raphe nucleus (DR), ventral tegmental area, LC, and laterodorsal tegmental nucleus (LDT)/pedunculopontine nucleus (PPN) (Lu *et al.*, 2000; Marcus *et al.*, 2001; Trivedi *et al.*, 1998). OX2Rs are also expressed in the amygdala, BST, PVN, DR, and LDT/PPN. In addition to these regions, OX2Rs are abundantly expressed in the Arc, TMN, dorsomedial hypothalamic nucleus, PVN, LHA, hippocampus (cornu ammonis 3), and medial septal nucleus (Lu *et al.*, 2000; Marcus *et al.*, 2001; Trivedi *et al.*, 1998). These histological studies suggest that orexins and their receptors are likely to play a broad regulatory role in the central nervous system and could regulate feeding, sleep, emotion, and reward functions. Additionally, OX1Rs are also distributed in peripheral tissues, such as the kidney, adrenal gland, thyroid, testis, ovaries, and jejunum. OX2Rs are found in the adrenal gland, lung, and pituitary (Johren *et al.*, 2001).

E. Orexin and narcolepsy

It is well known that the LHA, where orexin neurons are localized, is involved in food intake and energy homeostasis. Initially, orexins were recognized as regulators of feeding behavior since i.c.v. injection of orexin during the light period induced increases in food intake in rats and mice (Edwards *et al.*, 1999; Haynes *et al.*, 1999, 2000; Sakurai *et al.*, 1998; Yamanaka *et al.*, 1999). In addition to the role in feeding behavior, previous studies using genetically modified animals revealed that compromised orexin systems produce a narcolepsy-like phenotype. Narcolepsy is a sleep disorder characterized by a primary disorganization of the sleep/wakefulness cycle. Onset of narcoleptic conditions is usually seen during adolescence. A main symptom of the disorder is excessive daytime sleepiness, which manifests itself primarily when the subject falls asleep at inappropriate times, called a sleep attack. Narcolepsy patients also often suffer from cataplexy, which is a sudden weakening of bilateral postural muscle tone. These attacks are often triggered by emotional stimuli, such as laughter, excitement, and pleasure.

Mice lacking the prepro-orexin gene or dogs with null mutations in the OX2R gene show phenotypes remarkably similar to humans with narcolepsy (Chemelli *et al.*, 1999; Lin *et al.*, 1999). Studies have also demonstrated that *prepro-orexin* knockout mice, orexin neuron-ablated mice (*orexin/ataxin-3* transgenic mice), *OX2R* knockout mice, and *OX1R/OX2R* double knockout mice exhibit similar narcolepsy-like phenotypes that strongly parallel human narcolepsy, characterized by behavioral arrests similar to cataplexy, occasional direct transitions to rapid eye movement sleep from wakefulness, and severe fragmentation of the sleep/wakefulness cycle (Chemelli *et al.*, 1999; Hara *et al.*, 2001; Willie *et al.*, 2001, 2003). A postmortem study of human narcolepsy subjects consistently shows an 80–100% reduction in the number of neurons in the LHA. Additionally, orexin peptide levels in the cerebrospinal fluid are decreased to undetectable levels in narcoleptic patients (Nishino *et al.*, 2000; Peyron *et al.*, 2000). These results strongly suggest that the orexin system plays an important role in the regulation of sleep/wakefulness states, particularly in the maintenance of wakefulness.

III. Function of Orexins in Feeding Behavior and Energy Homeostasis

A. Pharmacological effects of orexin on feeding behavior

Initially, orexin neurons were thought to be involved in the regulation of feeding behavior due to their exclusive localization to the LHA and their pharmacological effects on feeding behavior. I.c.v. injection of orexin peptides during the light period induces feeding behavior (Edwards *et al.*, 1999; Haynes *et al.*, 2000, 2002; Sakurai *et al.*, 1998). Supporting this result, i.c.v. injection of an anti-orexin antibody or OX1R selective antagonist (SB334867) reduces spontaneous food consumption (Haynes *et al.*, 2000; Yamada *et al.*, 2000). Additionally, orexin mRNA expression is significantly increased during fasting (Sakurai *et al.*, 1998).

Studies using genetically modified mice have shown that orexin plays a role in the regulation of energy homeostasis as well. Orexin neuron-ablated mice show hypophagia but also display late onset obesity (Hara *et al.*, 2001, 2005). Similarly, human narcoleptic patients have decreased caloric intake but an increased body mass index (Gallopin *et al.*, 2000). These results suggest that the orexin system likely positively regulates feeding activity and basal energy expenditure. These facts might explain the reason why narcoleptic mice and humans show increased body weight despite hypophagia.

B. Interaction with other feeding-related hypothalamic neurons

Excess caloric intake increases the amount of adipose tissue. This result in an increase in serum levels of leptin, a potent suppressant of feeding released from adipocytes. The Arc, which is implicated in the regulation of feeding behavior (Elias *et al.*, 1999), is thought to be a major target for leptin-induced hypophagia. The Arc contains neuropeptide Y (NPY)/agouti-related protein (AgRP)-coexpressing neurons as well as proopiomelanocortin (POMC)/ cocaine and amphetamine-related transcript (CART)-coexpressing neurons. NPY/AgRP neurons stimulate feeding, whereas POMC/CART neurons suppress feeding behavior. Consistent with the dense projection of orexin neurons to the Arc (Date *et al.*, 1999; Peyron *et al.*, 1998), several studies have suggested that an increase in food intake following i.c.v. injection of orexin is at least partly mediated via activation of NPY/AgRP neurons in the Arc (Fig. 2.2). For example, c-Fos expression is induced in NPY/AgRP neurons by i.c.v. injection of orexin, and the orexin A-induced increase in food intake is partly inhibited by prior administration of an NPY-Y1 receptor selective antagonist (Yamanaka *et al.*, 2000). Other pathways by which orexin induces feeding might include inhibition of POMC/CART neurons (Muroya *et al.*, 2004). The OX1R-selective antagonist SB334867 ameliorated the obesity observed in leptin-deficient *ob/ob* mice, suggesting that leptin deficiency activates the orexin pathway to increase food intake (Haynes *et al.*, 2002). In addition, the orexin system stimulates feeding-associated glucose utilization in skeletal muscle by activation of the sympathetic nervous system through actions on the ventromedial hypothalamic nucleus (Shiuchi *et al.*, 2009)

C. Regulation of orexin neurons by feeding-related humoral factors

The activity of orexin neurons is also affected by humoral and neuroendocrine factors that are known indicators of energy balance. Among them, the most important factor is glucose concentration. It was reported that the activity of orexin neurons is regulated by extracellular glucose levels

(Yamanaka *et al.*, 2003). Concentrations of glucose in the blood and in the cerebrospinal fluid change in parallel (Dunn-Meynell *et al.*, 2002). Increasing extracellular glucose concentrations or leptin administration induces a marked hyperpolarization and cessation of action potentials in orexin neurons. In contrast, declining extracellular glucose concentrations induce depolarization and increase the frequency of action potentials in orexin neurons (Burdakov *et al.*, 2005; Yamanaka *et al.*, 2003) (Fig. 2.2). These facts suggest that orexin neurons are glucose-sensitive neurons that play an important role in both feeding and energy expenditure within the LHA. Orexin neuron-ablated transgenic mice (*orexin/ataxin-3* mice) fail to respond to fasting in terms of increased locomotor activity and increased waking time. Although it was originally demonstrated that the mechanism for inhibition of orexin neurons by glucose is mediated by tandem-pore K^+ (K_{2p}) channels (Burdakov *et al.*, 2006), further studies found that deletion of these channel subunit genes did not abolish the glucose responsiveness of orexin neurons (Gonzalez *et al.*, 2009; Guyon *et al.*, 2009). Thus, the responsible molecular element involved in glucose-induced hyperpolarization of orexin neurons has not yet been identified. Interestingly, i.c.v. injection of orexin induces increases in water intake as well as food intake (Kunii *et al.*, 1999). This result suggests a role for orexin neurons in fluid homeostasis. Additionally, arginine-vasopressin (AVP), also known as antidiuretic hormone, activates orexin neurons via the V1a receptor (Tsunematsu *et al.*, 2008). What is the physiological role of activation of orexin neurons by these factors related to energy and fluid homeostasis? The evidence indicates that reduced food or water availability (in emergency situations) adaptively increases general arousal levels through the activation of orexin neurons. These findings are consistent with the idea that orexin neurons play an important role in coordinating the behavioral state of animals according to environmental changes, which is beneficial for survival. For example, in a condition where food and water is not available, orexin neurons are activated and orexin is released in the brain. This would cause an increase in general arousal levels and locomotor activity and might help animals expand a search of their territory. As a result, this might increase the chances of finding food or a new water source. The orexin system might thus contribute to an increased probability of survival in nature.

IV. Function of Orexins in Peripheral Tissues

A. The effect of orexin on the autonomic nervous system

Several studies have reported that central administration of orexin induces the expression of c-Fos, a marker of neuronal activation, in the LC, Arc, central gray, raphe nuclei, nucleus of the solitary tract, supraoptic nucleus, and PVN. These regions are known to be involved in the regulation of autonomic and neuroendocrine function in rats (Date *et al.*, 1999; Kuru *et al.*, 2000). It was also demonstrated that i.c.v. injection of orexin increases blood pressure, heart rate, and renal sympathetic nerve activity. These effects were abolished by administration of α- or β-adrenoceptor antagonists (Shirasaka *et al.*, 1999). Additionally, a high dose of orexin increased plasma noradrenaline (NA) concentration (Shirasaka *et al.*, 1999). Therefore, it is likely that orexin increases sympathetic nerve tone. Which orexin receptor subtype is involved in this response? The autonomic response induced by orexin A is larger than that induced by orexin B (Chen *et al.*, 2000; Shirasaka *et al.*, 1999). Additionally, OX1R selective antagonism markedly attenuates increases in blood pressure, heart rate, and plasma NA concentration induced by orexin A in rats (Hirota *et al.*, 2003). These results suggest that orexin A positively regulates sympathetic nerve tone mainly through the OX1R. In addition, orexin knockout mice display 10–15 mmHg lower blood pressure than wild-type littermates (Kayaba *et al.*, 2003). This result suggests that orexins stimulate sympathetic outflow under physiological conditions. Therefore, orexin deficiency might decrease sympathetic tone, resulting in decreases in energy expenditure.

B. Orexin in the regulation of the HPA axis

There is much evidence showing that orexins might play a role in the regulation of the HPA axis via a central mechanism (Al-Barazanji *et al.*, 2001; Brunton and Russell, 2003; Jaszberenyi *et al.*, 2000; Kuru *et al.*, 2000). I.c.v. injection of both orexin A and orexin B was shown to activate neurons in the PVN and to increase plasma adrenocorticotrophin (ACTH) and corticosteroid levels in rats (Al-Barazanji *et al.*, 2001; Kuru *et al.*, 2000; Nanmoku *et al.*, 2002; Russell *et al.*, 2001) (Fig. 2.2). In contrast, intraperitoneal injection of orexin was ineffective in causing these effects, suggesting that orexin activates the HPA system only through the central nervous system (Jaszberenyi *et al.*, 2000). This response might be mediated by corticotropin-releasing hormone (CRH) and AVP in the PVN. Orexin neurons innervate the PVN, in which OX2R is abundantly expressed (Lu *et al.*, 2002; Marcus *et al.*, 2001). Orexin also enhances c-Fos expression and CRH and AVP mRNA expression in the PVN (Al-Barazanji *et al.*, 2001; Brunton and Russell, 2003; Kuru *et al.*, 2000). The effect of centrally injected orexins on HPA axis function was completely inhibited by a CRH receptor antagonist, demonstrating the ability of orexins to activate hypothalamic CRH neurons in the PVN, most likely via the OX2R, with subsequent activation of the HPA axis.

However, other studies suggest that orexins might activate adrenocortical cells without an involvement of the HPA axis. Interestingly, chronic administration of orexin for 1 week did not affect plasma ACTH levels, but increased plasma cortisol and aldosterone levels (Malendowicz *et al.*, 2001). In addition, orexin increases cortisol secretion in a dose-dependent manner using freshly dispersed normal and adenomatous human adrenocortical cells (Spinazzi *et al.*, 2005). This evidence suggests that orexins might modulate HPA axis responsiveness to different types of stress not only via CRH and AVP neurons in the PVN but also by direct activation of orexin receptors expressed in adrenocortical cells. In fact, it was reported that narcoleptic patients display blunted ACTH and cortisol secretion (Kok *et al.*, 2002).

V. Conclusions and Future Directions

Over more than a decade of research, it has been demonstrated that the orexin peptide system plays a crucial role in the regulation of energy balance, emotion, reward function, and arousal through activation of OX1Rs and/or OX2Rs. Orexin receptors are expressed not only in the central nervous system but also in a variety of organs in peripheral tissues. However, the mechanism of action of orexins in peripheral tissues has not been completely clarified. Orexin peptide is present at detectable levels in the serum (Arihara *et al.*, 2001; Johren *et al.*, 2001). However, the source of orexin in peripheral tissue is still unclear. Is orexin directly released into the blood stream or leaked from the cerebrospinal fluid? One possibility is that orexin is released from the pituitary since orexin-immunoreactive fibers are present in the median eminence and pituitary (Date *et al.*, 1999; Nambu *et al.*, 1999). The other possibility is that orexin is produced directly in peripheral tissues. Orexin-immunoreactive cells are observed in the gastrointestinal tract and pancreas (Johren *et al.*, 2001; Kirchgessner and Liu, 1999; Nakabayashi *et al.*, 2003). However, the question of orexin synthesis in peripheral tissue is still under discussion. Further studies are needed to better understand orexin physiology in peripheral tissues.

Taken together, orexin neurons play an important role in coordinating central and peripheral states according to environmental changes, which is highly beneficial to survival in nature.

Acknowledgments

This study was supported by JST PRESTO program and a Grant-in-Aid for Scientific Research (B) (23300142), Grant-in-Aid for Scientific Research on Innovative Area "Mesoscopic Neurocircuitry" (23115103) from the Ministry of Education, Culture, Sports, Science, and Technology (MEXT) of Japan (A. Y.) and the Japan Society for Promotion of Science (JSPS) postdoctoral fellowship (T. T.).

REFERENCES

Abrahamson, E. E., Leak, R. K., and Moore, R. Y. (2001). The suprachiasmatic nucleus projects to posterior hypothalamic arousal systems. *Neuroreport* **12,** 435–440.

Al-Barazanji, K. A., Wilson, S., Baker, J., Jessop, D. S., and Harbuz, M. S. (2001). Central orexin-A activates hypothalamic-pituitary-adrenal axis and stimulates hypothalamic corticotropin releasing factor and arginine vasopressin neurones in conscious rats. *J. Neuroendocrinol.* **13,** 421–424.

Arihara, Z., Takahashi, K., Murakami, O., Totsune, K., Sone, M., Satoh, F., Ito, S., and Mouri, T. (2001). Immunoreactive orexin-A in human plasma. *Peptides* **22,** 139–142.

Boutrel, B., Kenny, P. J., Specio, S. E., Martin-Fardon, R., Markou, A., Koob, G. F., and de Lecea, L. (2005). Role for hypocretin in mediating stress-induced reinstatement of cocaine-seeking behavior. *Proc. Natl. Acad. Sci. U.S.A.* **102,** 19168–19173.

Brunton, P. J., and Russell, J. A. (2003). Hypothalamic-pituitary-adrenal responses to centrally administered orexin-A are suppressed in pregnant rats. *J. Neuroendocrinol.* **15,** 633–637.

Burdakov, D., Gerasimenko, O., and Verkhratsky, A. (2005). Physiological changes in glucose differentially modulate the excitability of hypothalamic melanin-concentrating hormone and orexin neurons in situ. *J. Neurosci.* **25,** 2429–2433.

Burdakov, D., Jensen, L. T., Alexopoulos, H., Williams, R. H., Fearon, I. M., O'Kelly, I., Gerasimenko, O., Fugger, L., and Verkhratsky, A. (2006). Tandem-pore K+ channels mediate inhibition of orexin neurons by glucose. *Neuron* **50,** 711–722.

Chemelli, R. M., Willie, J. T., Sinton, C. M., Elmquist, J. K., Scammell, T., Lee, C., Richardson, J. A., Williams, S. C., Xiong, Y., Kisanuki, Y., Fitch, T. E., Nakazato, M., *et al.* (1999). Narcolepsy in orexin knockout mice: Molecular genetics of sleep regulation. *Cell* **98,** 437–451.

Chen, C. T., Hwang, L. L., Chang, J. K., and Dun, N. J. (2000). Pressor effects of orexins injected intracisternally and to rostral ventrolateral medulla of anesthetized rats. *Am. J. Physiol. Regul. Integr. Comp. Physiol.* **278,** R692–R697.

Chou, T. C., Lee, C. E., Lu, J., Elmquist, J. K., Hara, J., Willie, J. T., Beuckmann, C. T., Chemelli, R. M., Sakurai, T., Yanagisawa, M., Saper, C. B., and Scammell, T. E. (2001). Orexin (hypocretin) neurons contain dynorphin. *J. Neurosci.* **21,** RC168.

Date, Y., Ueta, Y., Yamashita, H., Yamaguchi, H., Matsukura, S., Kangawa, K., Sakurai, T., Yanagisawa, M., and Nakazato, M. (1999). Orexins, orexigenic hypothalamic peptides, interact with autonomic, neuroendocrine and neuroregulatory systems. *Proc. Natl. Acad. Sci. U.S.A.* **96,** 748–753.

de Lecea, L., Kilduff, T. S., Peyron, C., Gao, X., Foye, P. E., Danielson, P. E., Fukuhara, C., Battenberg, E. L., Gautvik, V. T., Bartlett, F. S., 2nd, Frankel, W. N., van den Pol, A. N., *et al.* (1998). The hypocretins: Hypothalamus-specific peptides with neuroexcitatory activity. *Proc. Natl. Acad. Sci. U.S.A.* **95,** 322–327.

Dunn-Meynell, A. A., Routh, V. H., Kang, L., Gaspers, L., and Levin, B. E. (2002). Glucokinase is the likely mediator of glucosensing in both glucose-excited and glucose-inhibited central neurons. *Diabetes* **51,** 2056–2065.

Edwards, C. M., Abusnana, S., Sunter, D., Murphy, K. G., Ghatei, M. A., and Bloom, S. R. (1999). The effect of the orexins on food intake: Comparison with neuropeptide Y, melanin-concentrating hormone and galanin. *J. Endocrinol.* **160,** R7–R12.

Elias, C. F., Aschkenasi, C., Lee, C., Kelly, J., Ahima, R. S., Bjorbaek, C., Flier, J. S., Saper, C. B., and Elmquist, J. K. (1999). Leptin differentially regulates NPY and POMC neurons projecting to the lateral hypothalamic area. *Neuron* **23,** 775–786.

Gallopin, T., Fort, P., Eggermann, E., Cauli, B., Luppi, P. H., Rossier, J., Audinat, E., Muhlethaler, M., and Serafin, M. (2000). Identification of sleep-promoting neurons in vitro. *Nature* **404,** 992–995.

Gonzalez, J. A., Jensen, L. T., Doyle, S. E., Miranda-Anaya, M., Menaker, M., Fugger, L., Bayliss, D. A., and Burdakov, D. (2009). Deletion of TASK1 and TASK3 channels disrupts intrinsic excitability but does not abolish glucose or pH responses of orexin/hypocretin neurons. *Eur. J. Neurosci.* **30,** 57–64.

Guyon, A., Tardy, M. P., Rovere, C., Nahon, J. L., Barhanin, J., and Lesage, F. (2009). Glucose inhibition persists in hypothalamic neurons lacking tandem-pore K+ channels. *J. Neurosci.* **29,** 2528–2533.

Hakansson, M., de Lecea, L., Sutcliffe, J. G., Yanagisawa, M., and Meister, B. (1999). Leptin receptor- and STAT3-immunoreactivities in hypocretin/orexin neurones of the lateral hypothalamus. *J. Neuroendocrinol.* **11,** 653–663.

Hara, J., Beuckmann, C. T., Nambu, T., Willie, J. T., Chemelli, R. M., Sinton, C. M., Sugiyama, F., Yagami, K., Goto, K., Yanagisawa, M., and Sakurai, T. (2001). Genetic ablation of orexin neurons in mice results in narcolepsy, hypophagia, and obesity. *Neuron* **30,** 345–354.

Hara, J., Yanagisawa, M., and Sakurai, T. (2005). Difference in obesity phenotype between orexin-knockout mice and orexin neuron-deficient mice with same genetic background and environmental conditions. *Neurosci. Lett.* **380,** 239–242.

Harris, G. C., Wimmer, M., and Aston-Jones, G. (2005). A role for lateral hypothalamic orexin neurons in reward seeking. *Nature* **437,** 556–559.

Haynes, A. C., Jackson, B., Overend, P., Buckingham, R. E., Wilson, S., Tadayyon, M., and Arch, J. R. (1999). Effects of single and chronic intracerebroventricular administration of the orexins on feeding in the rat. *Peptides* **20,** 1099–1105.

Haynes, A. C., Jackson, B., Chapman, H., Tadayyon, M., Johns, A., Porter, R. A., and Arch, J. R. (2000). A selective orexin-1 receptor antagonist reduces food consumption in male and female rats. *Regul. Pept.* **96,** 45–51.

Haynes, A. C., Chapman, H., Taylor, C., Moore, G. B., Cawthorne, M. A., Tadayyon, M., Clapham, J. C., and Arch, J. R. (2002). Anorectic, thermogenic and anti-obesity activity of a selective orexin-1 receptor antagonist in ob/ob mice. *Regul. Pept.* **104,** 153–159.

Hirota, K., Kushikata, T., Kudo, M., Kudo, T., Smart, D., and Matsuki, A. (2003). Effects of central hypocretin-1 administration on hemodynamic responses in young-adult and middle-aged rats. *Brain Res.* **981,** 143–150.

Jaszberenyi, M., Bujdoso, E., Pataki, I., and Telegdy, G. (2000). Effects of orexins on the hypothalamic-pituitary-adrenal system. *J. Neuroendocrinol.* **12,** 1174–1178.

Johren, O., Neidert, S. J., Kummer, M., Dendorfer, A., and Dominiak, P. (2001). Prepro-orexin and orexin receptor mRNAs are differentially expressed in peripheral tissues of male and female rats. *Endocrinology* **142,** 3324–3331.

Kayaba, Y., Nakamura, A., Kasuya, Y., Ohuchi, T., Yanagisawa, M., Komuro, I., Fukuda, Y., and Kuwaki, T. (2003). Attenuated defense response and low basal blood pressure in orexin knockout mice. *Am. J. Physiol. Regul. Integr. Comp. Physiol.* **285,** R581–R593.

Kirchgessner, A. L., and Liu, M. (1999). Orexin synthesis and response in the gut. *Neuron* **24,** 941–951.

Kok, S. W., Roelfsema, F., Overeem, S., Lammers, G. J., Strijers, R. L., Frolich, M., Meinders, A. E., and Pijl, H. (2002). Dynamics of the pituitary-adrenal ensemble in hypocretin-deficient narcoleptic humans: Blunted basal adrenocorticotropin release and evidence for normal time-keeping by the master pacemaker. *J. Clin. Endocrinol. Metab.* **87,** 5085–5091.

Kunii, K., Yamanaka, A., Nambu, T., Matsuzaki, I., Goto, K., and Sakurai, T. (1999). Orexins/hypocretins regulate drinking behaviour. *Brain Res.* **842,** 256–261.

Kuru, M., Ueta, Y., Serino, R., Nakazato, M., Yamamoto, Y., Shibuya, I., and Yamashita, H. (2000). Centrally administered orexin/hypocretin activates HPA axis in rats. *Neuroreport* **11,** 1977–1980.

Lin, L., Faraco, J., Li, R., Kadotani, H., Rogers, W., Lin, X., Qiu, X., de Jong, P. J., Nishino, S., and Mignot, E. (1999). The sleep disorder canine narcolepsy is caused by a mutation in the hypocretin (orexin) receptor 2 gene. *Cell* **98,** 365–376.

Lu, X. Y., Bagnol, D., Burke, S., Akil, H., and Watson, S. J. (2000). Differential distribution and regulation of OX1 and OX2 orexin/hypocretin receptor messenger RNA in the brain upon fasting. *Horm. Behav.* **37,** 335–344.

Lu, J., Bjorkum, A. A., Xu, M., Gaus, S. E., Shiromani, P. J., and Saper, C. B. (2002). Selective activation of the extended ventrolateral preoptic nucleus during rapid eye movement sleep. *J. Neurosci.* **22,** 4568–4576.

Malendowicz, L. K., Hochol, A., Ziolkowska, A., Nowak, M., Gottardo, L., and Nussdorfer, G. G. (2001). Prolonged orexin administration stimulates steroid-hormone secretion, acting directly on the rat adrenal gland. *Int. J. Mol. Med.* **7,** 401–404.

Marcus, J. N., Aschkenasi, C. J., Lee, C. E., Chemelli, R. M., Saper, C. B., Yanagisawa, M., and Elmquist, J. K. (2001). Differential expression of orexin receptors 1 and 2 in the rat brain. *J. Comp. Neurol.* **435,** 6–25.

Mieda, M., Williams, S. C., Sinton, C. M., Richardson, J. A., Sakurai, T., and Yanagisawa, M. (2004). Orexin neurons function in an efferent pathway of a food-entrainable circadian oscillator in eliciting food-anticipatory activity and wakefulness. *J. Neurosci.* **24,** 10493–10501.

Muroya, S., Funahashi, H., Yamanaka, A., Kohno, D., Uramura, K., Nambu, T., Shibahara, M., Kuramochi, M., Takigawa, M., Yanagisawa, M., Sakurai, T., Shioda, S., *et al.* (2004). Orexins (hypocretins) directly interact with neuropeptide Y, POMC and glucose-responsive neurons to regulate Ca^{2+} signaling in a reciprocal manner to leptin: Orexigenic neuronal pathways in the mediobasal hypothalamus. *Eur. J. Neurosci.* **19,** 1524–1534.

Nakabayashi, M., Suzuki, T., Takahashi, K., Totsune, K., Muramatsu, Y., Kaneko, C., Date, F., Takeyama, J., Darnel, A. D., Moriya, T., and Sasano, H. (2003). Orexin-A expression in human peripheral tissues. *Mol. Cell. Endocrinol.* **205,** 43–50.

Nambu, T., Sakurai, T., Mizukami, K., Hosoya, Y., Yanagisawa, M., and Goto, K. (1999). Distribution of orexin neurons in the adult rat brain. *Brain Res.* **827,** 243–260.

Nanmoku, T., Isobe, K., Sakurai, T., Yamanaka, A., Takekoshi, K., Kawakami, Y., Goto, K., and Nakai, T. (2002). Effects of orexin on cultured porcine adrenal medullary and cortex cells. *Regul. Pept.* **104,** 125–130.

Narita, M., Nagumo, Y., Hashimoto, S., Khotib, J., Miyatake, M., Sakurai, T., Yanagisawa, M., Nakamachi, T., Shioda, S., and Suzuki, T. (2006). Direct involvement of orexinergic systems in the activation of the mesolimbic dopamine pathway and related behaviors induced by morphine. *J. Neurosci.* **26,** 398–405.

Nishino, S., Ripley, B., Overeem, S., Lammers, G. J., and Mignot, E. (2000). Hypocretin (orexin) deficiency in human narcolepsy. *Lancet* **355,** 39–40.

Peyron, C., Tighe, D. K., van den Pol, A. N., de Lecea, L., Heller, H. C., Sutcliffe, J. G., and Kilduff, T. S. (1998). Neurons containing hypocretin (orexin) project to multiple neuronal systems. *J. Neurosci.* **18,** 9996–10015.

Peyron, C., Faraco, J., Rogers, W., Ripley, B., Overeem, S., Charnay, Y., Nevsimalova, S., Aldrich, M., Reynolds, D., Albin, R., Li, R., Hungs, M., *et al.* (2000). A mutation in a case of early onset narcolepsy and a generalized absence of hypocretin peptides in human narcoleptic brains. *Nat. Med.* **6,** 991–997.

Reti, I. M., Reddy, R., Worley, P. F., and Baraban, J. M. (2002). Selective expression of Narp, a secreted neuronal pentraxin, in orexin neurons. *J. Neurochem.* **82,** 1561–1565.

Risold, P. Y., Griffond, B., Kilduff, T. S., Sutcliffe, J. G., and Fellmann, D. (1999). Preprohypocretin (orexin) and prolactin-like immunoreactivity are coexpressed by neurons of the rat lateral hypothalamic area. *Neurosci. Lett.* **259,** 153–156.

Rosin, D. L., Weston, M. C., Sevigny, C. P., Stornetta, R. L., and Guyenet, P. G. (2003). Hypothalamic orexin (hypocretin) neurons express vesicular glutamate transporters VGLUT1 or VGLUT2. *J. Comp. Neurol.* **465,** 593–603.
Russell, S. H., Small, C. J., Dakin, C. L., Abbott, C. R., Morgan, D. G., Ghatei, M. A., and Bloom, S. R. (2001). The central effects of orexin-A in the hypothalamic-pituitary-adrenal axis in vivo and in vitro in male rats. *J. Neuroendocrinol.* **13,** 561–566.
Sakamoto, F., Yamada, S., and Ueta, Y. (2004). Centrally administered orexin-A activates corticotropin-releasing factor-containing neurons in the hypothalamic paraventricular nucleus and central amygdaloid nucleus of rats: Possible involvement of central orexins on stress-activated central CRF neurons. *Regul. Pept.* **118,** 183–191.
Sakurai, T., Amemiya, A., Ishii, M., Matsuzaki, I., Chemelli, R. M., Tanaka, H., Williams, S. C., Richardson, J. A., Kozlowski, G. P., Wilson, S., Arch, J. R., Buckingham, R. E., *et al.* (1998). Orexins and orexin receptors: A family of hypothalamic neuropeptides and G protein-coupled receptors that regulate feeding behavior. *Cell* **92,** 573–585.
Samson, W. K., Gosnell, B., Chang, J. K., Resch, Z. T., and Murphy, T. C. (1999). Cardiovascular regulatory actions of the hypocretins in brain. *Brain Res.* **831,** 248–253.
Shirasaka, T., Nakazato, M., Matsukura, S., Takasaki, M., and Kannan, H. (1999). Sympathetic and cardiovascular actions of orexins in conscious rats. *Am. J. Physiol.* **277,** R1780–R1785.
Shiuchi, T., Haque, M. S., Okamoto, S., Inoue, T., Kageyama, H., Lee, S., Toda, C., Suzuki, A., Bachman, E. S., Kim, Y. B., Sakurai, T., Yanagisawa, M., *et al.* (2009). Hypothalamic orexin stimulates feeding-associated glucose utilization in skeletal muscle via sympathetic nervous system. *Cell Metab.* **10,** 466–480.
Spinazzi, R., Rucinski, M., Neri, G., Malendowicz, L. K., and Nussdorfer, G. G. (2005). Preproorexin and orexin receptors are expressed in cortisol-secreting adrenocortical adenomas, and orexins stimulate in vitro cortisol secretion and growth of tumor cells. *J. Clin. Endocrinol. Metab.* **90,** 3544–3549.
Thannickal, T. C., Moore, R. Y., Nienhuis, R., Ramanathan, L., Gulyani, S., Aldrich, M., Cornford, M., and Siegel, J. M. (2000). Reduced number of hypocretin neurons in human narcolepsy. *Neuron* **27,** 469–474.
Trivedi, P., Yu, H., MacNeil, D. J., Van der Ploeg, L. H., and Guan, X. M. (1998). Distribution of orexin receptor mRNA in the rat brain. *FEBS Lett.* **438,** 71–75.
Tsunematsu, T., Fu, L. Y., Yamanaka, A., Ichiki, K., Tanoue, A., Sakurai, T., and van den Pol, A. N. (2008). Vasopressin increases locomotion through a V1a receptor in orexin/hypocretin neurons: Implications for water homeostasis. *J. Neurosci.* **28,** 228–238.
Willie, J. T., Chemelli, R. M., Sinton, C. M., and Yanagisawa, M. (2001). To eat or to sleep? Orexin in the regulation of feeding and wakefulness. *Annu. Rev. Neurosci.* **24,** 429–458.
Willie, J. T., Chemelli, R. M., Sinton, C. M., Tokita, S., Williams, S. C., Kisanuki, Y. Y., Marcus, J. N., Lee, C., Elmquist, J. K., Kohlmeier, K. A., Leonard, C. S., Richardson, J. A., *et al.* (2003). Distinct narcolepsy syndromes in orexin receptor-2 and orexin null mice: Molecular genetic dissection of Non-REM and REM sleep regulatory processes. *Neuron* **38,** 715–730.
Yamada, H., Okumura, T., Motomura, W., Kobayashi, Y., and Kohgo, Y. (2000). Inhibition of food intake by central injection of anti-orexin antibody in fasted rats. *Biochem. Biophys. Res. Commun.* **267,** 527–531.
Yamanaka, A., Sakurai, T., Katsumoto, T., Yanagisawa, M., and Goto, K. (1999). Chronic intracerebroventricular administration of orexin-A to rats increases food intake in daytime, but has no effect on body weight. *Brain Res.* **849,** 248–252.

Yamanaka, A., Kunii, K., Nambu, T., Tsujino, N., Sakai, A., Matsuzaki, I., Miwa, Y., Goto, K., and Sakurai, T. (2000). Orexin-induced food intake involves neuropeptide Y pathway. *Brain Res.* **859,** 404–409.

Yamanaka, A., Beuckmann, C. T., Willie, J. T., Hara, J., Tsujino, N., Mieda, M., Tominaga, M., Yagami, K., Sugiyama, F., Goto, K., Yanagisawa, M., and Sakurai, T. (2003). Hypothalamic orexin neurons regulate arousal according to energy balance in mice. *Neuron* **38,** 701–713.

Zhu, Y., Miwa, Y., Yamanaka, A., Yada, T., Shibahara, M., Abe, Y., Sakurai, T., and Goto, K. (2003). Orexin receptor type-1 couples exclusively to pertussis toxin-insensitive G-proteins, while orexin receptor type-2 couples to both pertussis toxin-sensitive and -insensitive G-proteins. *J. Pharmacol. Sci.* **92,** 259–266.

CHAPTER THREE

Plasticity in Neurons Synthesizing Wake/Arousal Promoting Hormone Hypocretin/Orexin

Xiao-Bing Gao

Contents

Abstract

The hypothalamus is a critical brain structure regulating physiological functions essential to the survival of individuals and species. One of the striking characteristics of this brain region is the abundance of nerve cells (neurons) expressing a great numbers of neurotransmitters and neuromodulators, among which are hormones released into the blood stream through brain neuroendocrinological routes. The neurons in the lateral hypothalamus take part in intra- and extrahypothalamic circuits controlling basic physiological functions essential for the well being of animal bodies (such as cardiovascular function, respiratory function, immune responses, etc.), animal behaviors required for the maintenance of the survival of individuals (food foraging, flight,

Section of Comparative Medicine, Program in Integrative Cell Signaling and Neurobiology of Metabolism, Yale University School of Medicine, New Haven, Connecticut, USA

Vitamins and Hormones, Volume 89
ISSN 0083-6729, http://dx.doi.org/10.1016/B978-0-12-394623-2.00003-2

fight, etc.) and species (reproductive function), and higher brain functions (learning and memory, mental state, etc.). Hypocretin (also called orexin) comprises of two neuropeptides exclusively synthesized by neurons in the perifornical/lateral hypothalamus. Although hypocretin/orexin was initially found to enhance food intake, it is now clear that the functions mediated by hypocretin/orexin are well beyond what were originally proposed. Specifically, hypocretin/orexin is a crucial promoter of wakefulness; deficiency in the hypocretin/orexin system leads to diseases and disorders such as narcolepsy. It is clear that neurons synthesizing hypocretin/orexin are consistently under regulation originating from various parts of the brain and that the status of activity in hypocretin/orexin neurons is closely related with the nutritional and behavioral state of animals. Therefore, the demand to make adaptive changes in hypocretin/orexin neurons to accommodate the changes in the external environment and behavioral state of animals is expected. The latest developments in the studies of plasticity in hypocretin/orexin neurons under the challenges from environmental and behavioral factors have dramatically shaped the understanding of the roles of hypocretin/orexin neurons in the maintenance of the survival of animals. More importantly, the studies of plasticity in hypocretin/orexin neurons as the consequence of physiological, behavioral, and environmental challenges may shed new insight on the understanding and treatment of sleep disorders (such as insomnia).

I. Introduction

The study of the role of the hypothalamus in the regulation of sleep can be dated back to the early part of the twentieth century. A prominent researcher and neurologist in Vienna, Austria, Professor Constantine von Economo, discovered that the lesions (loss of neurons) to the posterior hypothalamus and the mesencephalic reticular formation in the brains of patients with encephalitis lethargica caused sleep coma and that the patients had never awakened from the coma (Von Economo, 1930). This is the first report of the role of the hypothalamus in regulating the sleep/wake cycle. The discovery of the neuropeptide hypocretin/orexin and its role in the promotion of wakefulness has led to a new avenue to decipher the mechanisms underlying the control of sleep/wake cycle and the behavioral state by the hypothalamus in animals (de Lecea *et al.*, 1998; Sakurai *et al.*, 1998).

It is now generally accepted that peptide hypocretin/orexin was discovered by two groups of researchers independently (de Lecea *et al.*, 1998; Sakurai *et al.*, 1998). As early as 1996, Gautvik and colleagues reported the identification of mRNA species only expressed in the hypothalamus in rats by using directional tag PCR subtraction (Gautvik *et al.*, 1996). A novel clone named "clone 35" was demonstrated to encode a preprohormone

2 years later and two novel peptide hormones named hypocretin 1 and 2 are cleaved from this preprohormone (de Lecea *et al.*, 1998). Hypocretin 1 and 2 are selectively synthesized in neurons in the perifornical and lateral hypothalamus (LH) and excitatory in nature (de Lecea *et al.*, 1998). At the same time, another research group identified two G-protein coupled receptors and their natural ligands exclusively expressed in the LH, which could promote food intake in animals and were named as orexins (orexin-a and orexin-b) (Sakurai *et al.*, 1998). Eventually, hypocretin and orexin were demonstrated to be the same peptide hormone. As an indispensible component of the brain circuitry governing basic animal behaviors and higher functions, hypocretin/orexin neurons possess many unique characteristics, which undergo substantial changes in response to physiological and environmental factors. The most recent results from others and us demonstrate that the physiological and behavioral consequences resulting from these changes (plasticity) may have significant impacts on the behavior and survival of animals and pathological processes in humans.

II. Assessment of Neural Plasticity in Hypocretin/Orexin Neurons

Despite their critical functions in animals and humans, the neurons selectively synthesizing hypocretin/orexin were difficult to access to perform cellular studies on live neurons previously due to several technical limitations. First, the number of hypocretin/orexin neurons is small with an estimate of a few thousand in rodents and 50–90 thousand in humans (Peyron *et al.*, 1998; Sutcliffe and de Lecea, 2002; Thannickal *et al.*, 2000). Second, these cells are scattered diffusively in the perifornical and LH area and embedded within local and passing nerve fibers (Sawchenko, 1998). The latter includes the medial forebrain bundle, which plays a substantial role in the reward-seeking behaviors mediated by the LH area and supplies critical excitatory and inhibitory inputs onto hypocretin/orexin neurons (Henny and Jones, 2006a). Third, hypocretin/orexin cells do not form a clearly defined cluster in the perifornical/LH area but rather intermingle with other types of neurons nearby, such as melanin-concentrating hormone (MCH)- or leptin receptor-containing neurons (Louis *et al.*, 2010; Peyron *et al.*, 1998). To overcome these difficulties, Sakurai and colleagues developed a transgenic mouse line with the expression of green fluorescent protein (GFP) exclusively in hypocretin/orexin neurons (Li *et al.*, 2002; Yamanaka *et al.*, 2003), in which the examination of cellular physiology (including neural plasticity) of hypocretin/orexin neurons was performed.

A. Electrophysiological approaches

Although there are reports of direct examination of neuronal functions with electrophysiological approaches in the brain of live animals (*in vivo* patch clamp recording), in most cases, the regulation of central neurons, specifically, the determination of neuronal plasticity in central neurons, is performed in neurons in primary cell cultures or freshly prepared brain slices. The use of GFP-labeled mice facilitates the experimentation on hypocretin/orexin neurons, since the recorded neurons will have to be verified after the completion of experiments with selective antibodies without the prelabeling of hypocretin/orexin cells. The determination of changes in the properties (neural plasticity) of hypocretin/orexin neurons can be achieved by measuring basic membrane and synaptic properties, since the experience-dependent neuronal plasticity occurs at both synapses on neurons and cell bodies of neurons. The measurement of properties at cell bodies includes the measurement of intrinsic membrane properties such as resting membrane potential, input resistance, membrane capacitance, action potential threshold, and action potential frequency, etc., with whole-cell patch clamp recording (Li *et al.*, 2002; Liu and Gao, 2007; Yamanaka *et al.*, 2003). These parameters, which are usually measured in the presence of the antagonists of excitatory and inhibitory neurotransmitters to remove the influence of synaptic transmission on the cell body, represent the excitability of tested neurons and are critical to the generation of action potentials (Li *et al.*, 2002; Liu and Gao, 2007). Although the electrical signals are collected by microelectrodes made of glass filled with intracellular solutions containing ions and molecules resembling cytosolic content found in neurons, the latest reports demonstrate that the maintenance of intactness of intracellular content is critical in examining the membrane properties of hypocretin/orexin neurons, since the generation of action potentials in hypocretin/orexin neurons is sensitive to the energy status of the cells (Liu *et al.*, 2011; Parsons and Hirasawa, 2010).

The assessment of synaptic properties of hypocretin/orexin neurons is usually performed through examining postsynaptic currents/potentials with whole-cell patch clamp recording (Horvath and Gao, 2005; Li *et al.*, 2002; Rao *et al.*, 2007, 2008). It has been well established that spontaneous electrical signals recorded in neurons in the presence of blockers of action potentials (sometimes plus voltage-gated calcium channel blockers) represent synaptic events originating from spontaneous exocytosis of neurotransmitters from presynaptic terminals. The neurotransmission under this condition is quantized, which was originally reported by Katz and colleagues in neuromuscular junctions (Katz, 1969) and adopted in the studies of synapses on central neurons (Regehr and Stevens, 2001). The frequency and amplitude of these events (called miniature postsynaptic currents/potentials (mPSCs/mPSPs)) are parameters representing pre- and postsynaptic properties, respectively. Changes in the frequency of mPSCs/mPSPs represent plasticity occurring at the presynaptic site, while changes in the amplitude of mPSCs/mPSPs indicate modifications at the postsynaptic components (Regehr and Stevens, 2001). Therefore, by measuring the frequency and amplitude of mPSCs/mPSPs, the synaptic efficacy can be examined. This approach has been widely used in the studies on synaptic plasticity in central neurons including hypocretin/orexin neurons (Horvath and Gao, 2005; Rao *et al.*, 2007, 2008). The other parameters that are widely used to examine synaptic properties are the release probability and the ratio between AMPA-type and NMDA-type glutamate receptor-carried postsynaptic currents (AMPAR/NMDAR ratio). Both parameters have been demonstrated to be elevated at glutamatergic synapses undergoing long-term potentiation (LTP) at pre- and postsynaptic sites, respectively (Hessler *et al.*, 1993; Perkel and Nicoll, 1993; Rosenmund *et al.*, 1993). We have employed the measurement of AMPAR/NMDAR ratio to determine changes in synaptic efficacy of glutamatergic synapses on hypocretin/orexin neurons (Rao *et al.*, 2007, 2008). In addition, the examination of changes in the composition of postsynaptic AMPA receptors, particularly the expression of GluR2, can also be used to examine changes at the postsynaptic site (Man, 2011). AMPA receptors lacking the subunit GluR2 have specific channel-gating properties, that is, the rectification of electrical currents carried by GluR2-lacking receptors. GluR2-lacking AMPA receptors are calcium-permeable and critical to the triggering of activity/experience-dependent synaptic plasticity in central neurons (Man, 2011; Plant *et al.*, 2006).

B. Alternative approaches

In addition to the direct measurement of changes in the synaptic strength of glutamatergic synapses on hypocretin/orexin neurons with electrophysiological methods summarized above, molecular, morphological, and imaging approaches can also be used to examine changes in the expression and function of pre- and postsynaptic proteins relevant to the synaptic transmission and plasticity in central neurons. For instance, by using FM1-43, a styryl dye that emits fluorescence when it enters cytoplasma membrane, the trafficking of vesicles containing glutamate within the presynaptic terminals can be visualized and determined (Bamford *et al.*, 2004; Murthy and Stevens, 1998; Murthy *et al.*, 1997; Pyle *et al.*, 1999; Ryan *et al.*, 1997; Winterer *et al.*, 2006). With this approach that was initially used in cultured neurons the changes in synaptic efficacy at the presynaptic component was examined after the development of synaptic plasticity (Bamford *et al.*, 2004; Murthy and Stevens, 1998; Murthy *et al.*, 1997; Pyle *et al.*, 1999; Ryan *et al.*, 1997). This approach has been effectively applied in studies on freshly prepared brain slices from animals undergoing changes in presynaptic release of glutamate as well (Bamford *et al.*, 2004; Pyle *et al.*, 1999; Winterer *et al.*, 2006). By using molecular and biochemical methods, the expression, trafficking, and modification (such as phosphorylation) of glutamatergic receptor proteins in postsynaptic neurons following the development of synaptic plasticity can be determined (Barria *et al.*, 1997; Nayak *et al.*, 1998; Shi *et al.*, 1999). In addition, the ultrastructural analysis of synapses with electron microscopy is a powerful method in identifying morphological changes following the development of synaptic plasticity (Fiala *et al.*, 2002; Horvath and Gao, 2005; Pinto *et al.*, 2004; Sorra and Harris, 1998). All these non-electrophysiological approaches have been well established and widely used in the studies of synaptic plasticity in the hippocampus, cortex, and cerebellum and the application of these approaches in the studies on synaptic plasticity in hypocretin/orexin neurons are emerging (Appelbaum *et al.*, 2010; Horvath and Gao, 2005). The most recent progress along this direction is reported in an elegant study by Mayford's group at the Scripps Institute. The ectopic expression of the GluR1 subunit fused to an enhanced GFP (EGFP-tagged GluR1) is under the control of the c-fos promoter in a transgenic mouse line developed by these authors (Matsuo *et al.*, 2008). Since the expression of EGFP-tagged GluR1 proteins is activity/experience-dependent, fear conditioning significantly induced expression of EGFP-tagged GluR1 subunits in learning relevant circuitry (the hippocampus) in the brain, which is easily detected and quantitated with the readout of fluorescence from EGFP (Matsuo *et al.*, 2008). With this approach, the trafficking of newly synthesized glutamate receptors to the postsynaptic membrane during the development of synaptic plasticity can be evaluated. This strain of transgenic mice will be a powerful tool to aid the investigation of synaptic plasticity in hypocretin/orexin neurons. As the improvement of methods designed to be used in cultured neuronal systems and innovation of new techniques, the study of synaptic plasticity in hypocretin/orexin neurons *in vivo* in animals challenged by environmental and behavioral factors will be greatly advanced.

III. The Expression of Experience-Dependent Plasticity in Hypocretin/Orexin Neurons

A. Basic properties of hypocretin/orexin neurons

The neurons exclusively synthesizing hypocretin/orexin are localized in the perifornical and lateral hypothalamic area, while the nerve fibers containing hypocretin/orexin are identified all over the brain and in the spinal cord as well (Peyron *et al.*, 1998; van den Pol, 1999). The loss of hypocretin/orexin neurons leads to narcolepsy in humans, dogs, and rodents (Chemelli *et al.*, 1999; Lin *et al.*, 1999; Nishino *et al.*, 2000). A well-established body of evidence demonstrates that the hypocretin/orexin system is a critical arousal promoter in animals (Bonnavion and de Lecea, 2010; Kilduff and Peyron, 2000; Sakurai *et al.*, 2010; Saper *et al.*, 2001). By using whole-cell patch clamp recordings in hypocretin/orexin neurons in brain slices, it is revealed that the frequency of miniature excitatory postsynaptic currents (mEPSCs) recorded at the soma of these cells is about 10-fold higher than that of miniature inhibitory postsynaptic currents (mIPSCs) (Horvath and Gao 2005; Xie *et al.* 2006). In the same study, it is reported based on the ultrastructural evidence that there are more asymmetric (putatively stimulating) synapses than symmetric (putatively inhibitory) synapses on cell bodies of hypocretin/orexin neurons (Horvath and Gao 2005; Fig.3.1). Therefore, these results strongly demonstrate that the cell bodies of hypocretin/orexin neurons are predominately innervated by excitatory (glutamatergic) but not inhibitory (GABAergic) synapses, which is drastically different from other long projection neurons such as the pyramidal neurons of the neocortex, in which only inhibitory (GABAergic) synapses are found on the somata (Douglas *et al.*, 2004). It has been previously shown that the inhibition of ionotropic glutamatergic transmission onto hypocretin/orexin neurons by selective antagonists for NMDA and AMPA receptors significantly attenuates the generation of action potentials while the inhibition of GABAergic tone with GABA-A receptor antagonists has no significant effects on spontaneous action potential firings in hypocretin/orexin neurons (Li *et al.*, 2002; Xie *et al.*, 2006). The unique organization of excitatory and inhibitory synapses on hypocretin/orexin neurons summarized above provides a neurobiological basis for the critical roles of glutamatergic synapses in the activation of the hypocretin/orexin system (Horvath and Gao, 2005; Li *et al.*, 2002). The origin of the nerve fibers forming synapses on hypocretin/orexin neurons is not clear, but they may originate from neurons both within and beyond the LH as shown in recent studies (Henny and Jones, 2006a,b; Li *et al.*, 2002; Yoshida *et al.*, 2006).

At glutamatergic synapses on hypocretin/orexin neurons, we have shown that the AMPAR-mediated postsynaptic currents are significantly higher (greater than twofold) than that mediated by NMDARs under the baseline condition, which leads to the AMPAR/NMDAR ratio larger than 1.0 (Rao *et al.*, 2007, 2008). This is in drastic contrast to results that the relative contribution of AMPA receptor to the EPSCs is smaller than that mediated by NMDA receptor (AMPAR/NMDAR ratio smaller than 1.0) in CA1 pyramidal neurons in the hippocampus (Isaac *et al.*, 1995; Perkel and Nicoll, 1993). Since the small AMPAR/NMDAR ratio (less than 1.0) suggests the existence of "silent" synapses on neurons in the hippocampus, in which only NMDA receptors are expressed at the postsynaptic site (Isaac *et al.*, 1995), the results from hypocretin/orexin neurons suggest that there may not be many "silent" synapses on these neurons (Rao *et al.*, 2007,

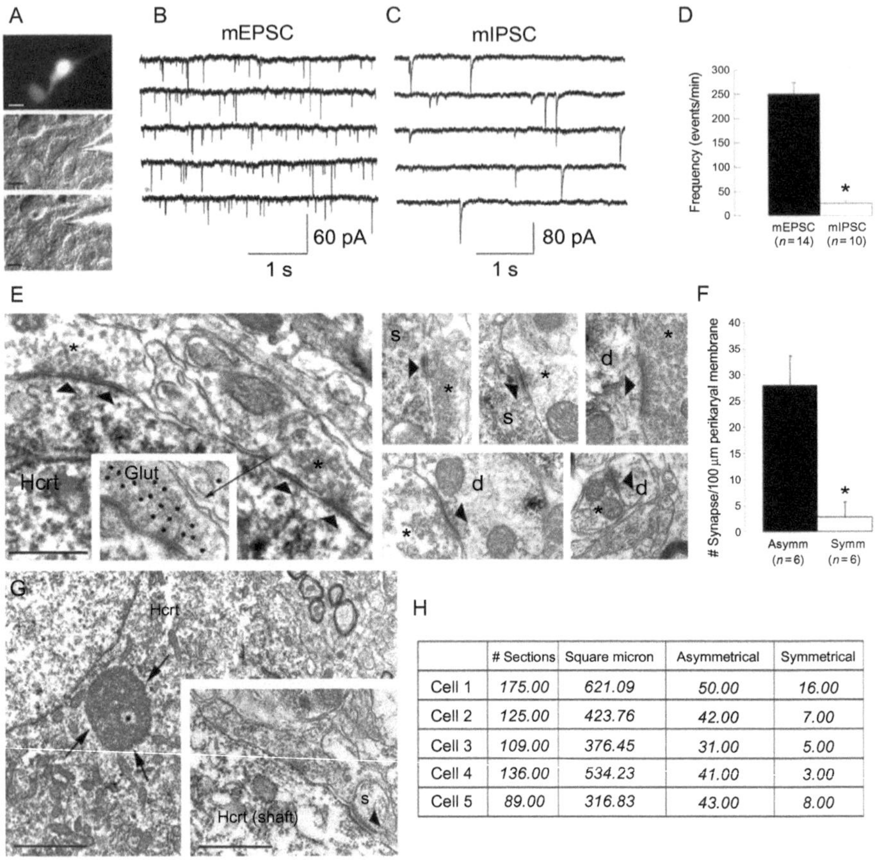

	# Sections	Square micron	Asymmetrical	Symmetrical
Cell 1	*175.00*	*621.09*	*50.00*	*16.00*
Cell 2	*125.00*	*423.76*	*42.00*	*7.00*
Cell 3	*109.00*	*376.45*	*31.00*	*5.00*
Cell 4	*136.00*	*534.23*	*41.00*	*3.00*
Cell 5	*89.00*	*316.83*	*43.00*	*8.00*

Figure 3.1 Hypocretin/orexin-containing cell bodies are dominantly innervated by excitatory glutamatergic synapses. (A–D) Whole-cell patch clamp recording in hypocretin/orexin neurons (A) in mice revealed that the frequency of mEPSCs mediated by glutamate ((B), (D)) was about 10-fold of that of mIPSCs mediated by GABA (C and D). (A) Hypocretin/orexin neurons were identified with the expression of GFP under the control of a selective hypocretin/orexin promoter. Scale bar = 10 μm. (E–H) Electron microscopic studies showed that asymmetric (putative excitatory) axon terminals (E) dominated symmetric (inhibitory) contacts on hypocretin/orexin-containing perikarya. (E) Asymmetric contacts (indicated by arrowheads) on somata (s) and dendrites (d) of hypocretin/orexin neurons were clearly shown. Bar scale = 1 μm. (G) An asymmetric contact between a hypocretin/orexin dendritic shaft and an unidentified dendritic spine (s). Bar scales represent 3 μm (main panel) and 1 μm (insert). (H) A table showing results of 3D reconstruction of five randomly selected hypocretin/orexin-immunopositive neurons from mice ($n = 5$). From Horvath and Gao (2005) with permission from *Cell Metabolism* (Elsevier).

2008). The exact physiological significance of the absence of silent synapses on hypocretin/orexin neurons is not clear. However, it is expected that glutamatergic transmission onto hypocretin/orexin neurons may be more efficient without silent synapses, since silent synapses containing only NMDA receptors require a substantial depolarization to relieve the blockade of NMDA receptors by Mg^{2+} to conduct glutamatergic transmission (Isaac *et al.*, 1995). Moreover, since the NMDA receptor-mediated calcium influx is critical to synaptic plasticity in central neurons, the AMPAR/NMDAR ratio in hypocretin/orexin neurons implies a distinctive machinery underlying the development of synaptic plasticity in these cells as compared to pyramidal neurons in the CA1 area of the hippocampus. Our most recent results on the existence of calcium permeable AMPA receptors in hypocretin/orexin neurons provide additional evidence along this direction (Gan, G. and Gao, X. B., unpublished observations). Nevertheless, the unique glutamatergic and GABAergic synaptic organization on soma of hypocretin/orexin neurons and composition of glutamate receptors on hypocretin/orexin cells provide a functional basis for the role of these cells in the regulation of the sleep/wake cycle, energy homeostasis, addiction, and reward seeking in animals; that is, the overwhelming existence of excitatory inputs at cell bodies of hypocretin/orexin neurons and the high efficiency of glutamatergic transmission may make it easier for this system to be excited and help it undergo adaptive changes when animals are challenged by environmental stimuli such as deficiency in food or lack of sleep (Horvath and Gao 2005; Rao *et al.*, 2007).

B. Food restriction induces reorganization of synapses on hypocretin/orexin neurons

When hypocretin/orexin was initially discovered, an appetite-enhancing effect of hypocretin/orexin was observed in animals (which leads to the naming of "orexin" for this neuropeptide by the investigators) (Sakurai *et al.*, 1998). Later, it is reported that food deprivation induced expression of c-Fos in hypocretin/orexin neurons and increased the mRNA level of hypocretin/orexin in animals (Diano *et al.*, 2003). Consistent with these results, food deprivation does not induce wakefulness in mice with deficiency in hypocretin/orexin (Yamanaka *et al.*, 2003), suggesting that hypocretin/orexin neurons are activated during the course of food deprivation and that it may contribute to arousal/wakefulness induced by hunger, a well-established phenomenon in animals (Borbely, 1977; Jacobs and McGinty 1971). Our study on the experience-dependent synaptic plasticity in hypocretin/orexin neurons induced by food deficiency has shed new light on the role of hypocretin/orexin in the association between energy homeostasis and arousal regulation (Horvath and Gao, 2005). In hypothalamic slices from C57/B6 mice undergoing one episode of overnight fasting, the frequency of mEPSCs recorded in hypocretin/orexin neurons significantly increased as compared with the fed littermates, while the frequency of mIPSCs recorded in these neurons was comparable between fasted and fed groups (Horvath and Gao, 2005; Fig. 3.2). Consistent with these findings from electrophysiological recordings, the number of asymmetric (putatively excitatory) but not symmetric (inhibitory) synapses on hypocretin/orexin-containing cell bodies elevated significantly in mice with one episode of food deprivation as compared with fed controls (Horvath and Gao, 2005; Fig. 3.2). Since in fasting animals the levels of leptin are low, which may serve as a cue for food deficiency in animals, it is plausible to examine whether the lowered level of leptin triggers changes in fasting animals. If it is true, the leptin replacement during food deprivation may compensate for the effects triggered by fasting. Both electrophysiological and ultrastructural data showed that leptin administration (i.p.) abolished the effects of fasting on glutamatergic synapses on hypocretin/orexin neurons in fasted mice. The frequency of mEPSCs was comparable in hypocretin/orexin neurons from fasted mice simultaneously treated with leptin and fed controls. The number of asymmetric synapses on hypocretinergic cell bodies was similar between these two groups as well (Horvath and Gao, 2005). Consistent with the effect of leptin replacement on fasting-triggered synaptic plasticity in hypocretin/orexin neurons, electrophysiological and ultrastructural studies also showed that the frequency of mEPSCs and the number of asymmetric synapses on these cells were not significantly different between control mice and fasted mice undergoing subsequent refeeding (Horvath and Gao, 2005).

It has already been demonstrated that food deprivation increased wakefulness and decreased sleep in animals (Borbely, 1977; Jacobs and McGinty, 1971), which is abolished in mice lacking hypocretin/orexin neurons (Yamanaka *et al.*, 2003). More importantly, a significant enhancement of c-fos expression in hypocretin/orexin neurons induced by food deprivation indicates an intensive activation of these cells during this process (Diano *et al.*, 2003). Therefore, although it has not been directly demonstrated, it is worth hypothesizing that a strong activation of neuronal circuitry centered on hypocretin/orexin neurons during food deprivation contributes to synaptic plasticity in these neurons and that synaptic plasticity in hypocretin/orexin neurons is activity/experience-dependent in nature. The hypocretin/orexin system may be one of the loci (if it is not the only one) where the crosstalk between energy homeostasis regulation and sleep/wake regulation occurs. From an evolutionary point of view, synaptic plasticity in hypocretin/orexin neurons may be a critical mechanism contributing to the determination of behavioral status by energy status in animals.

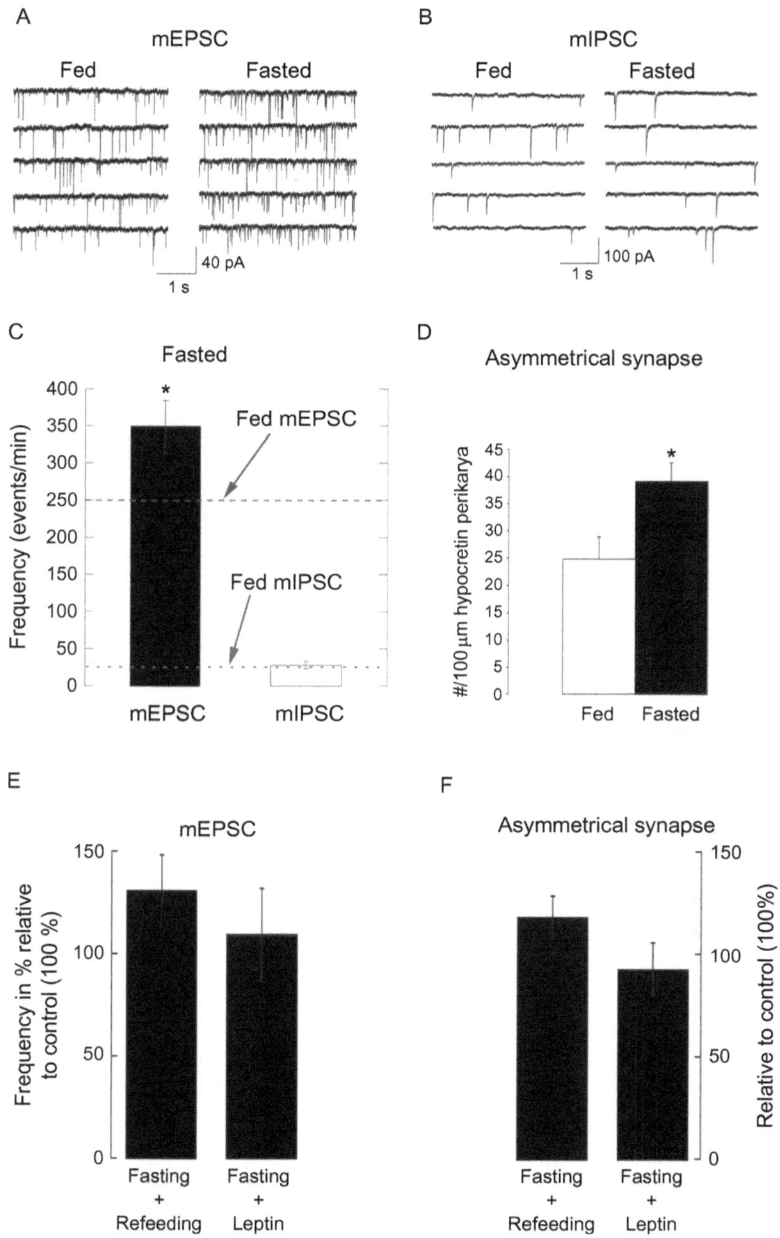

Figure 3.2 Food deprivation potentiates excitatory (glutamatergic) but not inhibitory (GABAergic) synapses on hypocretin/orexin neurons. (A–D) Electrophysiological and electron microscopic studies show that fasting enhanced the frequency of mEPSCs (A and C) and the number of asymmetric (excitatory) synapses (D) on hypocretin/orexin neurons. The frequency of mIPSCs (B and C) in hypocretin/orexin neurons in fasted animals did not change as compared with the fed controls. The effects of fasting on mEPSC frequency and the number of asymmetric (excitatory) synapses on hypocretin/orexin neurons were eliminated by refeeding following fasting (left panels, E and F) and replacement of leptin during fasting (right panels, E and F). From Horvath and Gao (2005) with permission from *Cell Metabolism* (Elsevier).

C. Prolonged wakefulness induces synaptic plasticity in hypocretin/orexin neurons

Consistent with the idea that the hypocretin/orexin system is required to promote wakefulness and arousal, the activity levels of hypocretin/orexin neurons are high during wakefulness and low during sleep (Estabrooke *et al.*, 2001; Lee *et al.*, 2005; Mileykovskiy *et al.*, 2005). To maintain a prolonged (voluntary or forced) wakefulness in animals, a long-term activation of hypocretin/orexin neurons is required. According to the Hebbian theory (Hebb, 1949), the synchronized activation of hypocretin/orexin neurons and other neurons innervating hypocretin/orexin cells to convey information encoding environmental cues inducing prolonged wakefulness will lead to an enhanced efficacy of glutamatergic synapses on hypocretin/orexin neurons. Therefore, the prolonged wakefulness may be able to induce experience-dependent (Hebbian) synaptic potentiation in hypocretin/orexin neurons (Rao *et al.*, 2007).

In the study of sleep/wake regulation, animals can be kept in a state of prolonged wakefulness by both chemical and physical approaches. The chemical method includes the application of psychostimulants (such as modafinil) to animals during the rest (sleep) phase. Modafinil, diphenyl-methyl-sulfonyl-2-acetamide, is an FDA-approved drug for the treatment of narcolepsy and other conditions (Ballon and Feifel, 2006). The administration of modafinil significantly enhances wakefulness in humans and animals through the activation of dopamine (DA)-dependent pathways and hypocretin/orexin neurons are among the targets activated by modafinil (Korotkova *et al.*, 2007; Scammell *et al.*, 2000; Wisor *et al.*, 2001). One of the physical methods is sleep deprivation by gentle handling, in which rodents are kept awake by being gently touched with a small paintbrush upon the closure of their eyes by an experimenter. Activation of hypocretin/orexin neurons by examination of c-fos expression has been reported in animals being sleep-deprived with this method (Modirrousta *et al.*, 2005). The effects of both methods on synaptic efficacy in hypocretin/orexin neurons have been examined. Behaviorally, an acute application of a single dose of modafinil induces long-lasting (>2 h) wakefulness in mice during the light (sleep) phase. The efficacy of glutamatergic synapses on hypocretin/orexin neurons from control (with normal sleep) and modafinil-treated mice were analyzed. Synaptic efficacy was significantly potentiated 1 and 2 h after the administration of modafinil (Fig. 3.3). Synaptic potentiation occurred at both pre- and postsynaptic sites of glutamatergic synapses on hypocretin/orexin neurons in modafinil-treated mice as compared to saline-treated controls since the frequency and amplitude of mEPSCs were potentiated (Rao *et al.*, 2007). Consistent with these results, a 4-h sleep deprivation through gentle handling induced a similar potentiation of glutamatergic synapses on hypocretin/orexin neurons at pre- and

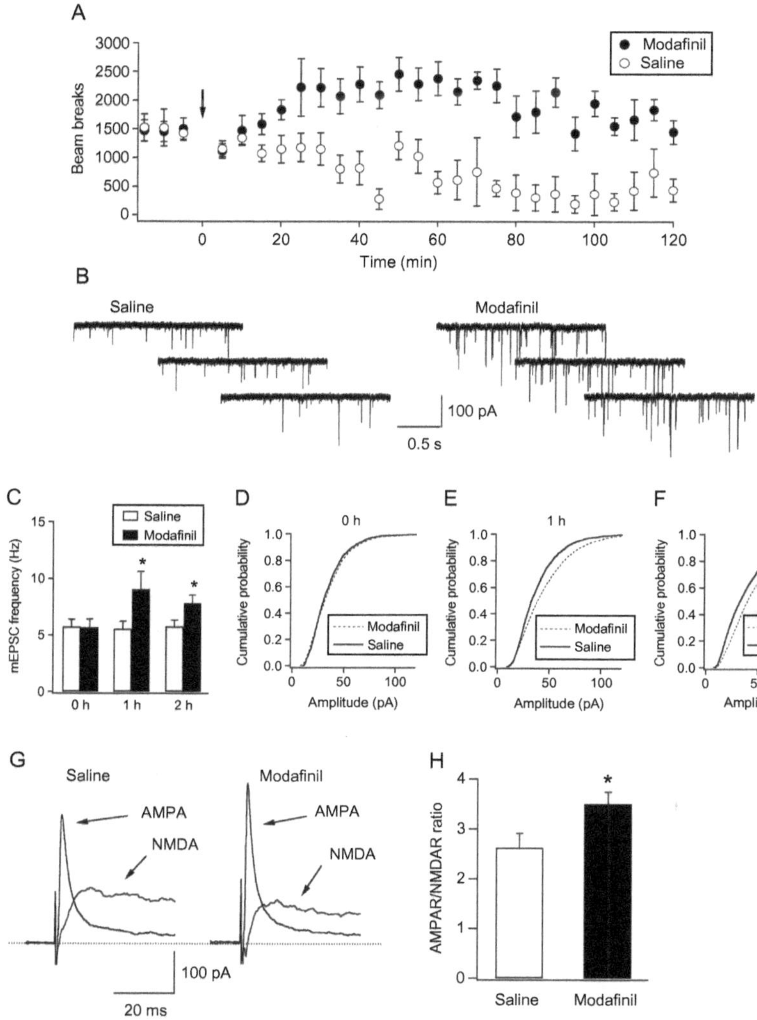

Figure 3.3 Prolonged wakefulness induces long-term potentiation of glutamatergic synapses on hypocretin/orexin neurons. A single dose of modafinil induced a long-lasting wakefulness during the light phase in mice (A). The efficacy of glutamatergic synapses on hypocretin/orexin neurons was examined at different time points (0, 1, and 2 h) following the treatment of modafinil (B–F). Electrophysiological studies revealed that the frequency and amplitude of mEPSCs (representative traces shown in (B)) were significantly enhanced 1 and 2 h after the treatment of modafinil (C–F). The AMPAR/NMDAR ratio of evoked EPSCs (representative traces shown in (G)) was significantly increased 1 h after the treatment of modafinil in hypocretin/orexin neurons from modafinil-treated mice as compared to controls (H). From Rao *et al.* (2007) with permission from American Society for Clinical Investigation.

postsynaptic sites as well (Rao *et al.*, 2007). Further, the repeated exposure to prolonged wakefulness (once daily for a week) significantly elevated the number of asymmetric (excitatory) synapses on hypocretin/orexin neurons as compared with control animals in addition to the enhancement in the frequency and amplitude of mEPSCs, suggesting that chronic sleep loss resulting from prolonged wakefulness may initiate long-term effects on the wake-promoting circuitry centered on hypocretin/orexin neurons (Rao *et al.*, 2007). The synaptic plasticity induced by prolonged wakefulness does not occur in non-hypocretin/orexin neurons, demonstrating the specificity of the effects of prolonged wakefulness (Rao *et al.*, 2007).

It has been reported that the action of modafinil depends on the blockade of DA transporters in the brain, which has been suggested as one of the cellular functions of modafinil (Ballon and Feifel, 2006). DA receptor-mediated pathways modulate activity in hypocretin/orexin neurons (Alberto *et al.*, 2006; Bubser *et al.*, 2005). The application of D1 DA receptor antagonists before the administration of modafinil abolished modafinil-induced wake-promoting effects and the potentiation of presynaptic glutamate release in animals, demonstrating the requirement of DA-mediated pathways in this process (Rao *et al.*, 2007). It is reported previously that activation of protein kinase A (PKA) by forskolin induces LTP (forskolin-LTP) in hippocampal neurons and that forskolin-LTP occludes the induction of LTP triggered by other stimuli (such as high-frequency stimulation) at the same synapses (Frey *et al.*, 1993; Huang and Kandel, 1995; Otmakhov *et al.*, 2004a,b). These results suggest that forskolin-LTP shares the same pathways with LTP induced by high-frequency stimulation in the hippocampus. The same strategy was adopted in the study of mechanisms underlying synaptic plasticity in hypocretin/orexin neurons. Forskolin-LTP was induced at glutamatergic synapses on hypocretin/orexin neurons both pre- and postsynaptically. As expected, the induction of forskolin-LTP was significantly occluded in hypocretin/orexin neurons in mice acutely or repeatedly exposed to modafinil, indicating that synaptic plasticity induced by modafinil treatment shares common pathways (e.g., PKA-mediated pathways) with forskolin-LTP in these cells (Rao *et al.*, 2007). Since the PKA activation usually leads to the activation of CREB-mediated responses in neurons, it is very likely that epigenetic processes downstream to the PKA-CREB activation may occur in hypocretin/orexin neurons following prolonged wakefulness, which is not yet examined such far.

In summary, an emerging body of evidence demonstrates that the basic synaptic properties of glutamatergic synapses on hypocretin/orexin neurons are well evolved to accommodate the role of these neurons as a critical arousal promoter. Physiological, behavioral, and environmental factors leading to adaptations in animals in response to changes in the internal and external environments may result in changes in the efficacy of glutamatergic synapses (synaptic plasticity) on hypocretin/orexin neurons. It is now clear that the hypocretin/orexin system is at the center of a complex network of modulations mediated by neurotransmitters and neuromodulators encoding physiological, behavioral, and environmental cues critical to the survival of animals at both the individual and species levels (Bonnavion and de Lecea, 2010; Burt *et al.*, 2011; de Lecea, 2010; Elias *et al.*, 1998; Henny and Jones, 2006a,b; Sakurai *et al.*, 2005). Therefore, it is expected that this network of modulations will inevitably shape the development of synaptic plasticity in hypocretin/orexin neurons.

IV. Factors Modifying the Plasticity in Hypocretin/Orexin Neurons

The hypocretin/orexin system is under a complex network of modulations in terms of both morphological and functional aspects. First, it is now clear that hypocretin/orexin neurons receive afferent innervations from many critical brain areas controlling energy balance, sleep/wake homeostasis, reward seeking, and stress response (Elias *et al.*, 1998; Henny and Jones, 2006a,b; Sakurai *et al.*, 2005). Second, it is well established that a wide array of neurotransmitters, neuromodulators, hormones, and bioactive substances modulate activity in hypocretin/orexin neurons via regulating synaptic transmission onto these neurons and capacity of action potential firing in these cells (Li *et al.*, 2002; Yamanaka *et al.*, 2003; see reviews by Bonnavion and de Lecea, 2010; Burt *et al.*, 2011; de Lecea, 2010). To be consistent with the main topic of this volume, we will discuss how the substances regulating the sleep/wake cycle modulate synaptic plasticity in hypocretin/orexin neurons.

Adenosine is a well-established neurotransmitter serving as a potent sleep-promoter in animals (Basheer *et al.*, 2004; Huang *et al.*, 2011; Porkka-Heiskanen and Kalinchuk, 2011). Adenosine is released from neurons as the result of degradation of ATP (use of ATP as "fuel" in animal cells) during the long period of activity, which is considered a homeostatic regulator of sleep (Basheer *et al.*, 2004; Huang *et al.*, 2011; Porkka-Heiskanen and Kalinchuk, 2011). Generally, adenosine inhibits neuronal activity in many regions of the brain (Arrigoni *et al.*, 2006; Haas and Greene, 1984; Lupica *et al.*, 1992; Prince and Stevens, 1992; Scanziani *et al.*, 1992; Thakkar *et al.*, 2003). In hypothalamic slices, the application of adenosine inhibits action potential generation in hypocretin/orexin neurons (Liu and Gao, 2007). This inhibitory effect is due to the inhibition of glutamatergic transmission onto hypocretin/orexin neurons (e.g., reduction of glutamate release from presynaptic terminals and decrease in the response of postsynaptic glutamate receptors) mediated by A1 adenosine receptor (Liu and Gao, 2007). Although adenosine does not directly inhibit hypocretin/orexin neurons through hyperpolarization of membrane potential at soma as seen in hippocampal and basal forebrain neurons (Arrigoni *et al.*, 2006; Haas and Greene, 1984), it significantly inhibits voltage-dependent calcium channels at soma (Liu and Gao, 2007). Consistent with the inhibitory role of adenosine in regulating activity in hypocretin/orexin neurons, a recent report demonstrates that endogenously released adenosine is able to modulate glutamatergic synapses on hypocretin/orexin neurons in the LH area (Xia *et al.*, 2009). The role of adenosine in the regulation of synaptic plasticity in hypocretin/orexin neurons was demonstrated in two lines of evidence. First, when a train of electrical stimulation at a low frequency (10 Hz) applied to the LH area, a long-lasting depression of glutamatergic transmission onto hypocretin/orexin neurons was observed. The presence of a selective A1 adenosine receptor antagonist 8-cyclopentyltheophylline (CPT) partially attenuated the long-lasting synaptic depression in hypocretin/orexin neurons (Xia *et al.*, 2009). In a parallel experiment, a train of high-frequency (100 Hz) electrical stimulation induced the LTP of glutamatergic synapses on hypocretin/orexin neurons and the application of CPT facilitated the induction of LTP. Altogether, these results indicate that the endogenously released adenosine may attenuate or inhibit activity/experience-dependent synaptic potentiation in hypocretin/orexin neurons.

The other case of modulation of synaptic plasticity in hypocretin/orexin neurons occurs in the interaction between the hypocretin/orexin neurons and neighboring nerve cells selectively synthesizing the neuropeptide MCH. MCH is another important neuropeptide that is exclusively synthesized in the perifornical/LH area and that participates in many critical brain functions such as food intake, sleep regulation, and immune response (Adamantidis and de Lecea, 2009; Bittencourt *et al.*, 1992; Elias *et al.*, 1998; Griffond and Risold, 2009; Lakaye *et al.*, 2009; Peyron *et al.*, 2009). We have previously showed that MCH is inhibitory at the cellular level in the hypothalamus (Gao and van den Pol, 2001, 2002), which has been verified in many other brain areas (Sears *et al.*, 2010; Wu *et al.*, 2009). Neurons containing hypocretin/orexin and MCH do not overlap in the perifornial/LH area and reciprocally innervates each other (Elias *et al.*, 1998; Guan *et al.*, 2002; van den Pol *et al.*, 2004). In hypothalamic slices, we have shown that MCH attenuates an enhanced activity in hypocretin/orexin neurons without altering basal activity level (Rao *et al.*, 2008). In mice with deficiency in receptors for MCH (MCH receptor 1, MCHR-1), the synaptic efficacy of glutamatergic transmission onto hypocretin/orexin neurons was upregulated and the generation of action potential triggered by excitatory inputs was facilitated (Rao *et al.*, 2008). We further showed that MCHR-1 KO mice were sensitive to arousal-promoting agent modafinil, suggesting that the arousal threshold may be lowered in KO mice as compared to wild-type (WT) littermates (Rao *et al.*, 2008). Consistent with our findings at the cellular and behavioral levels, the MCHR-1 KO was reported to be hyperactive, lean with higher basal metabolic rate than WT littermates, and sensitive to the novel environment (Marsh *et al.*, 2002). Therefore, it is plausible to propose that MCH may antagonize the activity in hypocretin/orexin neurons to prevent the development of synaptic plasticity (likely synaptic potentiation), since the removal of MCHR-1-mediated pathway induces an upregulated synaptic efficacy in hypocretin/orexin neurons (Rao *et al.*, 2008).

Both adenosine and MCH serve as important factors in the regulation of the sleep/wake cycle (Huang *et al.*, 2011; Peyron *et al.*, 2009; Porkka-Heiskanen and Kalinchuk, 2011). The release of adenosine is activity dependent and the accumulation of adenosine in the extracellular space usually represents sleep pressure (Huang *et al.*, 2011; Porkka-Heiskanen and Kalinchuk, 2011). MCH neurons are activated following the sleep deprivation and during the recovery sleep (Peyron *et al.*, 2009). The antagonism of the expression of synaptic potentiation in hypocretin/orexin neurons by adenosine and MCH underscores the crucial role of neural plasticity in the hypocretin/orexin system in the maintenance of arousal/wakefulness. It is both intriguing and essential to ask whether the process of plasticity in hypocretin/orexin neurons is required to maintain a prolonged wakefulness in animals under physiological conditions. More importantly, it is critical to ask whether the synaptic plasticity in hypocretin/orexin neurons as the consequence of the adaptation of the brain to certain physiological and behavioral status (e.g., the "recent history") of animals leads to altered arousal/wake threshold and impaired sleep/wake regulation.

V. Conclusions and Future Directions

The experience-dependent synaptic plasticity in hypocretin/orexin neurons is an adaptive response of these nerve cells to the brain in the course of accommodating changes in the internal and external environments and/or behavioral and energy state of the animals. Currently, the mechanisms underlying synaptic plasticity in hypocretin/orexin neurons and the physiological significance of synaptic plasticity in these cells are not yet clear. Through studies by others and our group, the signaling pathways mediated by protein kinases (such as PKA) and neurotransmitters/neuromodulators (such as leptin, MCH, and adenosine) are demonstrated to participate in this process (Horvath and Gao, 2005; Rao *et al.*, 2007, 2008; Xia *et al.*, 2009). We propose that experience-dependent plasticity induced by environmental and/or behavioral factors may include both early and late changes in hypocretin/orexin neurons (Fig. 3.4). The early changes comprise of functional potentiation of glutamatergic synapses on hypocretin/orexin neurons at pre- and postsynaptic sites, such as that occurs within hours after the exposure to an acute episode of prolonged

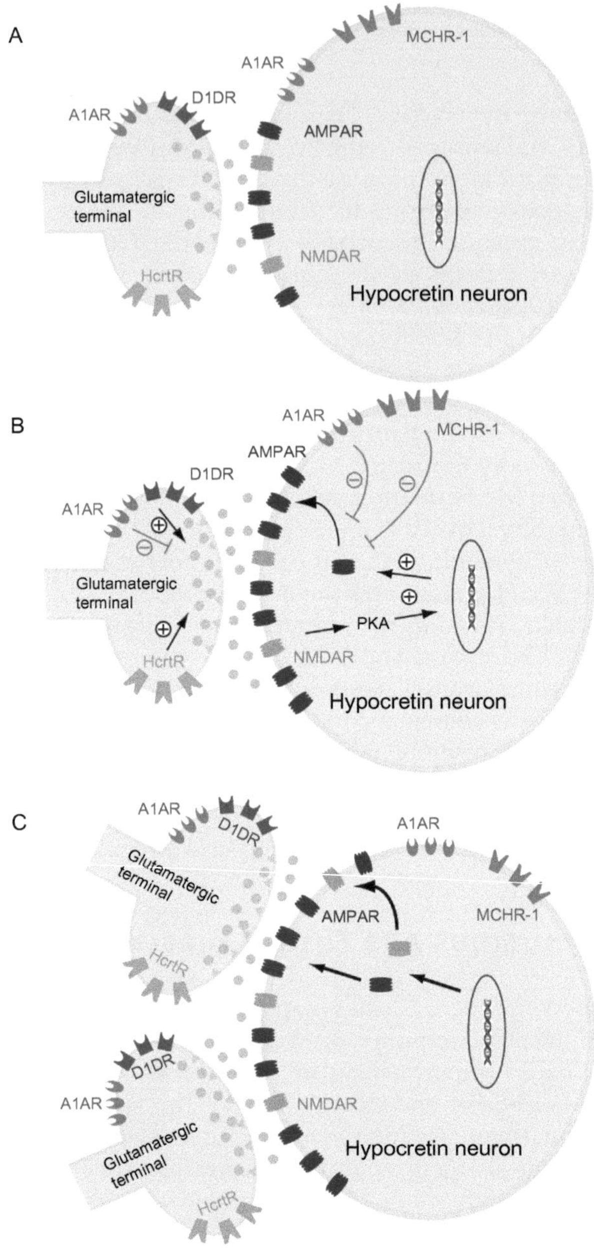

Figure 3.4 Experience-dependent synaptic plasticity in hypocretin/orexin neurons. (A) Glutamatergic synapses on hypocretin/orexin neurons before synaptic potentiation. (B) Synaptic potentiation of glutamatergic synapses on hypocretin/orexin neurons triggered by an acute exposure to environmental factors (food deficiency or sleep restriction) occurs in an activity/experience-dependent manner as reported in the expression of LTP. Synaptic potentiation may occur at both pre- and postsynaptic sites, for example, enhanced release of glutamate from presynaptic terminals and upregulation of glutamate receptors in hypocretin/orexin neurons. (C) Repeated exposure to environmental factors leads to reorganization of synaptic architecture in hypocretin/orexin neurons, including the increased number of excitatory (glutamatergic) synapses on hypocretin/orexin neurons. AMPAR, AMPA receptor; NMDAR, NMDA receptor; D1DR, D1 dopamine receptor; HcrtR, hypocretin/orexin receptor; MCHR-1, MCH receptor-1; A1AR, A1 adenosine receptor; PKA, protein kinase A. (See Color Insert.)

wakefulness (the modafinil-mediated effect) or sleep loss (sleep restriction by gentle handling) (Fig. 3.4B). The presynaptic changes may include the increase in the release of glutamate from presynaptic terminals depending on the synthesis and transportation of new proteins from neuronal soma along neuritis to nerve terminals (Blundon and Zakharenko, 2008; Lisman *et al.*, 2007). The postsynaptic changes may include trafficking of AMPA-type glutamate receptors (specifically the GluR2-lacking, calcium permeable AMPA receptor) to postsynaptic neuronal membrane (Lisman and Raghavachari, 2006; Man, 2011) and expansion of dendritic spines as previously seen in other brain areas such as the hippocampus (Blundon and Zakharenko, 2008). The late changes induced by repeated exposure to environmental stimuli (such as prolonged wakefulness) may involve morphological changes in glutamatergic synapses (e.g., addition of new synapses) on hypocretin/orexin neurons (Fig. 3.4C). The late changes should be of particular importance, which may suggest that the projections from certain brain areas to hypocretin/orexin neurons have been strengthened and the brain circuitry centered on hypocretin/orexin neurons may be "rewired" as the consequence of certain experience or the recent "history" of animals. Future studies on the molecular and epigenetic mechanisms underlying experience-dependent plasticity in hypocretin/orexin neurons induced by physiological, behavioral, and environmental factors are expected.

The consequences of experience-dependent plasticity in hypocretin/orexin neurons are not yet clear but emerging. Since prolonged wakefulness induces synaptic potentiation in hypocretin/orexin neurons, it is reasonable to postulate that the enhanced synaptic efficacy is the consequence of the prolonged wakefulness. More importantly, synaptic potentiation may be required in the process of maintaining the prolonged wakefulness and the development of synaptic plasticity in hypocretin/orexin neurons may be a process through which the arousal threshold is regulated to accommodate the behavioral state of animals (Gao and Wang, 2010). Future studies along this direction should include the investigations on whether neural plasticity in hypocretin/orexin neurons underlies biological processes leading to a resetting of arousal threshold and whether plasticity in hypocretin/orexin neurons contributes to the pathological processes in diseases and conditions relevant to impaired sleep/wake regulation (such as insomnia) (Ruoff *et al.*, 2011; Scammell and Winrow, 2011). Results from these studies may lead to new concepts on the understanding of sleep/wake regulation and sleep disorders.

ACKNOWLEDGMENTS

The author's work has been supported by NIH grants DK 61478, DK070723, American Heart Association (AHA) Scientist Development Grant, and Foundation For Prader-Willi Syndrome Research (FPWR) grant. The author would like to thank Ms. Susan Andranovich for help with the chapter.

REFERENCES

Adamantidis, A., and de Lecea, L. (2009). A role for melanin-concentrating hormone in learning and memory. *Peptides* **30,** 2066–2070.

Alberto, C. O., Trask, R. B., Quinlan, M. E., and Hirasawa, M. (2006). Bidirectional dopaminergic modulation of excitatory synaptic transmission in orexin neurons. *J. Neurosci.* **26,** 10043–10050.

Appelbaum, L., Wang, G., Yokogawa, T., Skariah, G. M., Smith, S. J., Mourrain, P., and Mignot, E. (2010). Circadian and homeostatic regulation of structural synaptic plasticity in hypocretin neurons. *Neuron* **68,** 87–98.

Arrigoni, E., Chamberlin, N. L., Saper, C. B., and McCarley, R. W. (2006). Adenosine inhibits basal forebrain cholinergic and noncholinergic neurons *in vitro*. *Neuroscience* **140,** 403–413.

Ballon, J. S., and Feifel, D. (2006). A systematic review of modafinil: Potential clinical uses and mechanisms of action. *J. Clin. Psychiatry* **67,** 554–566.

Bamford, N. S., Robinson, S., Palmiter, R. D., Joyce, J. A., Moore, C., and Meshul, C. K. (2004). Dopamine modulates release from corticostriatal terminals. *J. Neurosci.* **24,** 9541–9552.

Barria, A., Muller, D., Derkach, V., Griffith, L. C., and Soderling, T. R. (1997). Regulatory phosphorylation of AMPA-type glutamate receptors by CaM-KII during long-term potentiation. *Science* **276,** 2042–2045.

Basheer, R., Strecker, R. E., Thakkar, M. M., and McCarley, R. W. (2004). Adenosine and sleep-wake regulation. *Prog. Neurobiol.* **73,** 379–396.

Bittencourt, J. C., Presse, F., Arias, C., Peto, C., Vaughan, J., Nahon, J. L., Vale, W., and Sawchenko, P. E. (1992). The melanin-concentrating hormone system of the rat brain: An immuno- and hybridization histochemical characterization. *J. Comp. Neurol.* **319,** 218–245.

Blundon, J. A., and Zakharenko, S. S. (2008). Dissecting the components of long-term potentiation. *Neuroscientist* **14,** 598–608.

Bonnavion, P., and de Lecea, L. (2010). Hypocretins in the control of sleep and wakefulness. *Curr. Neurol. Neurosci. Rep.* **10,** 174–179.

Borbely, A. A. (1977). Sleep in the rat during food deprivation and subsequent restitution of food. *Brain Res.* **124,** 457–471.

Bubser, M., Fadel, J. R., Jackson, L. L., Meador-Woodruff, J. H., Jing, D., and Deutch, A. Y. (2005). Dopaminergic regulation of orexin neurons. *Eur. J. Neurosci.* **21,** 2993–3001.

Burt, J., Alberto, C. O., Parsons, M. P., and Hirasawa, M. (2011). Local network regulation of orexin neurons in the lateral hypothalamus. *Am. J. Physiol. Regul. Integr. Comp. Physiol.* **301,** R572–R580.

Chemelli, R. M., Willie, J. T., Sinton, C. M., Elmquist, J. K., Scammell, T., Lee, C., Richardson, J. A., Williams, S. C., Xiong, Y., Kisanuki, Y., Fitch, T. E., Nakazato, M., *et al.* (1999). Narcolepsy in orexin knockout mice: Molecular genetics of sleep regulation. *Cell* **98,** 437–451.

de Lecea, L. (2010). A decade of hypocretins: Past, present and future of the neurobiology of arousal. *Acta Physiol (Oxf.)* **198,** 203–208.

De Lecea, L., Kilduff, T. S., Peyron, C., Gao, X. B., Foye, P. E., Danielson, P. E., Fukuhara, C., Battenberg, E. L. F., Gautvik, V. T., Bartlett, F. S., Frankel, W. N., van den Pol, A. N., *et al.* (1998). The hypocretins: Hypothalamus-specific peptides with neuroexcitatory activity. *Proc. Natl. Acad. Sci. U.S.A.* **95,** 322–327.

Diano, S., Horvath, B., Urbanski, H. F., Sotonyi, P., and Horvath, T. L. (2003). Fasting activates the nonhuman primate hypocretin (orexin) system and its postsynaptic targets. *Endocrinology* **144,** 3774–3778.

Douglas, R., Markram, H., and Martin, K. (2004). Neocortex. *In* "The Synaptic Organization of the Brain," (G. M. Shepherd, Ed.), pp. 499–558. Oxford University Press, New York.

Elias, C. F., Saper, C. B., Maratos-Flier, E., Tritos, N. A., Lee, C., Kelly, J., Tatro, J. B., Hoffman, G. E., Ollmann, M. M., Barsh, G. S., Sakurai, T., Yanagisawa, M., *et al.* (1998). Chemically defined projections linking the mediobasal hypothalamus and the lateral hypothalamic area. *J. Comp. Neurol.* **402,** 442–459.

Estabrooke, I. V., McCarthy, M. T., Ko, E., Chou, T. C., Chemelli, R. M., Yanagisawa, M., Saper, C. B., and Scammell, T. E. (2001). Fos expression in orexin neurons varies with behavioral state. *J. Neurosci.* **21,** 1656–1662.

Fiala, J. C., Allwardt, B., and Harris, K. M. (2002). Dendritic spines do not split during hippocampal LTP or maturation. *Nat. Neurosci.* **5,** 297–298.

Frey, U., Huang, Y. Y., and Kandel, E. R. (1993). Effects of cAMP simulate a late stage of LTP in hippocampal CA1 neurons. *Science* **260,** 1661–1664.

Gao, X. B., and Wang, A. H. (2010). Experience-dependent plasticity in hypocretin/orexin neurones: Re-setting arousal threshold. *Acta Physiol (Oxf.)* **198,** 251–262.

Gao, X. B., and van den Pol, A. N. (2001). Melanin concentrating hormone depresses synaptic activity of glutamate and GABA neurons from rat lateral hypothalamus. *J. Physiol.* **533,** 237–252.

Gao, X. B., and van den Pol, A. N. (2002). Melanin-concentrating hormone depresses L-, N-, and P/Q-type voltage-dependent calcium channels in rat lateral hypothalamic neurons. *J. Physiol.* **542,** 273–286.

Gautvik, K. M., de Lecea, L., Gautvik, V. T., Danielson, P. E., Tranque, P., Dopazo, A., Bloom, F. E., and Sutcliffe, J. G. (1996). Overview of the most prevalent hypothalamus-specific mRNAs, as identified by directional tag PCR subtraction. *Proc. Natl. Acad. Sci. U.S.A.* **93,** 8733–8738.

Griffond, B., and Risold, P. Y. (2009). MCH and feeding behavior-interaction with peptidic network. *Peptides* **30,** 2045–2051.

Guan, J. L., Uehara, K., Lu, S., Wang, Q. P., Funahashi, H., Sakurai, T., Yanagizawa, M., and Shioda, S. (2002). Reciprocal synaptic relationships between orexin- and melanin-concentrating hormone-containing neurons in the rat lateral hypothalamus: A novel circuit implicated in feeding regulation. *Int. J. Obes. Relat. Metab. Disord.* **26,** 1523–1532.

Haas, H. L., and Greene, R. W. (1984). Adenosine enhances afterhyperpolarization and accommodation in hippocampal pyramidal cells. *Pflugers Arch.* **402,** 244–247.

Hebb, D. O. (1949). The Organization of Behavior. Wiley & Sons, New York.

Henny, P., and Jones, B. E. (2006a). Innervation of orexin/hypocretin neurons by GABAergic, glutamatergic or cholinergic basal forebrain terminals evidenced by immunostaining for presynaptic vesicular transporter and postsynaptic scaffolding proteins. *J. Comp. Neurol.* **499,** 645–661.

Henny, P., and Jones, B. E. (2006b). Vesicular glutamate (VGlut), GABA (VGAT), and acetylcholine (VACht) transporters in basal forebrain axon terminals innervating the lateral hypothalamus. *J. Comp. Neurol.* **496,** 453–467.

Hessler, N. A., Shirke, A. M., and Malinow, R. (1993). The probability of transmitter release at a mammalian central synapse. *Nature* **366,** 569–572.

Horvath, T. L., and Gao, X. B. (2005). Input organization and plasticity of hypocretin neurons: Possible clues to obesity's association with insomnia. *Cell Metab.* **1,** 279–286.

Huang, Y. Y., and Kandel, E. R. (1995). D1/D5 Receptor agonists induce a protein synthesis-dependent late potentiation in the CA1 region of the hippocampus. *Proc. Natl. Acad. Sci. U.S.A.* **92,** 2446–2450.

Huang, Z. L., Urade, Y., and Hayaishi, O. (2011). The role of adenosine in the regulation of sleep. *Curr. Top. Med. Chem.* **11,** 1047–1057.

Isaac, J. T., Nicoll, R. A., and Malenka, R. C. (1995). Evidence for silent synapses: Implications for the expression of LTP. *Neuron* **15,** 427–434.

Jacobs, B. L., and McGinty, D. J. (1971). Effects of food deprivation on sleep and wakefulness in the rat. *Exp. Neurol.* **30,** 212–222.

Katz, B. (1969). The Release of Neural Transmitter Substances. Liverpool University Press, Liverpool.

Kilduff, T. S., and Peyron, C. (2000). The hypocretin/orexin ligand-receptor system: Implications for sleep and sleep disorders. *Trends Neurosci.* **23,** 359–365.

Korotkova, T. M., Klyuch, B. P., Ponomarenko, A. A., Lin, J. S., Haas, H. L., and Sergeeva, O. A. (2007). Modafinil inhibits rat midbrain dopaminergic neurons through D2-like receptors. *Neuropharmacology* **52,** 626–633.

Lakaye, B., Coumans, B., Harray, S., and Grisar, T. (2009). Melanin-concentrating hormone and immune function. *Peptides* **30,** 2076–2080.

Lee, M. G., Hassani, O. K., and Jones, B. E. (2005). Discharge of identified orexin/hypocretin neurons across the sleep-waking cycle. *J. Neurosci.* **25,** 6716–6720.

Li, Y., Gao, X. B., Sakurai, T., and van den Pol, A. N. (2002). Hypocretin/orexin excites hypocretin neurons via a local glutamate neuron—A potential mechanism for orchestrating the hypothalamic arousal system. *Neuron* **36,** 1169–1181.

Lin, L., Faraco, J., Li, R., Kadotani, H., Rogers, W., Lin, X., Qiu, X., de Jong, P. J., Nishino, S., and Mignot, E. (1999). The sleep disorder canine narcolepsy is caused by a mutation in the hypocretin (orexin) receptor 2 gene. *Cell* **98,** 365–376.

Lisman, J., and Raghavachari, S. (2006). A unified model of the presynaptic and postsynaptic changes during LTP at CA1 synapses. *Sci. STKE* **2006,** re11.

Lisman, J. E., Raghavachari, S., and Tsien, R. W. (2007). The sequence of events that underlie quantal transmission at central glutamatergic synapses. *Nat. Rev. Neurosci.* **8,** 597–609.

Liu, Z. W., Gan, G., Suyama, S., and Gao, X. B. (2011). Intracellular energy status regulates activity in hypocretin/orexin neurones: A link between energy and behavioral states. *J Physiol* **589,** 4157–4166.

Liu, Z. W., and Gao, X. B. (2007). Adenosine inhibits activity of hypocretin/orexin neurons by the A1 receptor in the lateral hypothalamus: A possible sleep-promoting effect. *J. Neurophysiol.* **97,** 837–848.

Louis, G. W., Leinninger, G. M., Rhodes, C. J., and Myers, M. G., Jr. (2010). Direct innervation and modulation of orexin neurons by lateral hypothalamic LepRb neurons. *J. Neurosci.* **30,** 11278–11287.

Lupica, C. R., Proctor, W. R., and Dunwiddie, T. V. (1992). Presynaptic inhibition of excitatory synaptic transmission by adenosine in rat hippocampus: Analysis of unitary EPSP variance measured by whole-cell recording. *J. Neurosci.* **12,** 3753–3764.

Man, H. Y. (2011). GluA2-Lacking, calcium-permeable AMPA receptors—Inducers of plasticity? *Curr. Opin. Neurobiol.* **21,** 291–298.

Marsh, D. J., Weingarth, D. T., Novi, D. E., Chen, H. Y., Trumbauer, M. E., Chen, A. S., Guan, X. M., Jiang, M. M., Feng, Y., Camacho, R. E., Shen, Z., Frazier, E. G., *et al.* (2002). Melanin-concentrating hormone 1 receptor-deficient mice are lean, hyperactive, and hyperphagic and have altered metabolism. *Proc. Natl. Acad. Sci. U.S.A.* **99,** 3240–3245.

Matsuo, N., Reijmers, L., and Mayford, M. (2008). Spine-type-specific recruitment of newly synthesized AMPA receptors with learning. *Science* **319,** 1104–1107.

Mileykovskiy, B. Y., Kiyashchenko, L. I., and Siegel, J. M. (2005). Behavioral correlates of activity in identified hypocretin/orexin neurons. *Neuron* **46,** 787–798.

Modirrousta, M., Mainville, L., and Jones, B. E. (2005). Orexin and MCH neurons express c-Fos differently after sleep deprivation vs. recovery and bear different adrenergic receptors. *Eur. J. Neurosci.* **21,** 2807–2816.

Murthy, V. N., and Stevens, C. F. (1998). Synaptic vesicles retain their identity through the endocytic cycle. *Nature* **392,** 497–501.

Murthy, V. N., Sejnowski, T. J., and Stevens, C. F. (1997). Heterogeneous release properties of visualized individual hippocampal synapses. *Neuron* **18,** 599–612.

Nayak, A., Zastrow, D. J., Lickteig, R., Zahniser, N. R., and Browning, M. D. (1998). Maintenance of late-phase LTP is accompanied by PKA-dependent increase in AMPA receptor synthesis. *Nature* **394,** 680–683.

Nishino, S., Ripley, B., Overeem, S., Lammers, G. J., and Mignot, E. (2000). Hypocretin (orexin) deficiency in human narcolepsy. *Lancet* **355,** 39–40.

Otmakhov, N., Khibnik, L., Otmakhova, N., Carpenter, S., Riahi, S., Asrican, B., and Lisman, J. (2004a). Forskolin-induced LTP in the CA1 hippocampal region is NMDA receptor dependent. *J. Neurophysiol.* **91,** 1955–1962.

Otmakhov, N., Tao-Cheng, J. H., Carpenter, S., Asrican, B., Dosemeci, A., Reese, T. S., and Lisman, J. (2004b). Persistent accumulation of calcium/calmodulin-dependent protein kinase II in dendritic spines after induction of NMDA receptor-dependent chemical long-term potentiation. *J. Neurosci.* **24,** 9324–9331.

Parsons, M. P., and Hirasawa, M. (2010). ATP-sensitive potassium channel-mediated lactate effect on orexin neurons: Implications for brain energetics during arousal. *J. Neurosci.* **30,** 8061–8070.

Perkel, D. J., and Nicoll, R. A. (1993). Evidence for all-or-none regulation of neurotransmitter release: Implications for long-term potentiation. *J. Physiol.* **471,** 481–500.

Peyron, C., Tighe, D. K., van den Pol, A. N., de Lecea, L., Heller, H. C., Sutcliffe, J. G., and Kilduff, T. S. (1998). Neurons containing hypocretin (orexin) project to multiple neuronal systems. *J. Neurosci.* **18,** 9996–10015.

Peyron, C., Sapin, E., Leger, L., Luppi, P. H., and Fort, P. (2009). Role of the melanin-concentrating hormone neuropeptide in sleep regulation. *Peptides* **30,** 2052–2059.

Pinto, S., Roseberry, A. G., Liu, H., Diano, S., Shanabrough, M., Cai, X., Friedman, J. M., and Horvath, T. L. (2004). Rapid rewiring of arcuate nucleus feeding circuits by leptin. *Science* **304,** 110–115.

Plant, K., Pelkey, K. A., Bortolotto, Z. A., Morita, D., Terashima, A., McBain, C. J., Collingridge, G. L., and Isaac, J. T. (2006). Transient incorporation of native GluR2-lacking AMPA receptors during hippocampal long-term potentiation. *Nat. Neurosci.* **9,** 602–604.

Porkka-Heiskanen, T., and Kalinchuk, A. V. (2011). Adenosine, energy metabolism and sleep homeostasis. *Sleep Med. Rev.* **15,** 123–135.

Prince, D. A., and Stevens, C. F. (1992). Adenosine decreases neurotransmitter release at central synapses. *Proc. Natl. Acad. Sci. U.S.A.* **89,** 8586–8590.

Pyle, J. L., Kavalali, E. T., Choi, S., and Tsien, R. W. (1999). Visualization of synaptic activity in hippocampal slices with FM1-43 enabled by fluorescence quenching. *Neuron* **24,** 803–808.

Rao, Y., Liu, Z. W., Borok, E., Rabenstein, R. L., Shanabrough, M., Lu, M., Picciotto, M. R., Horvath, T. L., and Gao, X. B. (2007). Prolonged wakefulness induces experience-dependent synaptic plasticity in mouse hypocretin/orexin neurons. *J. Clin. Invest.* **117,** 4022–4033.

Rao, Y., Lu, M., Ge, F., Marsh, D. J., Qian, S., Wang, A. H., Picciotto, M. R., and Gao, X. B. (2008). Regulation of synaptic efficacy in hypocretin/orexin-containing neurons by melanin concentrating hormone in the lateral hypothalamus. *J. Neurosci.* **28,** 9101–9110.

Regehr, W. G., and Stevens, C. F. (2001). Physiology of synaptic transmission and short-term plasticity. *In* "Synapses," (W. M. Cowan, T. C. Südhof, and C. F. Stevens, Eds.), pp. 135–176. Johns Hopkins University Press, Baltimore.

Rosenmund, C., Clements, J. D., and Westbrook, G. L. (1993). Nonuniform probability of glutamate release at a hippocampal synapse. *Science* **262,** 754–757.

Ruoff, C., Cao, M., and Guilleminault, C. (2011). Hypocretin antagonists in insomnia treatment and beyond. *Curr. Pharm. Des.* **17,** 1476–1482.

Ryan, T. A., Reuter, H., and Smith, S. J. (1997). Optical detection of a quantal presynaptic membrane turnover. *Nature* **388,** 478–482.

Sakurai, T., Amemiya, A., Ishii, M., Matsuzaki, I., Chemelli, R. M., Tanaka, H., Williams, S. C., Richarson, J. A., Kozlowski, G. P., Wilson, S., Arch, J. R., Buckingham, R. E., *et al.* (1998). Orexins and orexin receptors: A family of hypothalamic neuropeptides and G protein-coupled receptors that regulate feeding behavior. *Cell* **92,** 573–585.

Sakurai, T., Mieda, M., and Tsujino, N. (2010). The orexin system: Roles in sleep/wake regulation. *Ann. N. Y. Acad. Sci.* **1200,** 149–161.

Sakurai, T., Nagata, R., Yamanaka, A., Kawamura, H., Tsujino, N., Muraki, Y., Kageyama, H., Kunita, S., Takahashi, S., Goto, K., Koyama, Y., Shioda, S., *et al.* (2005). Input of orexin/hypocretin neurons revealed by a genetically encoded tracer in mice. *Neuron* **46,** 297–308.

Saper, C. B., Chou, T. C., and Scammell, T. E. (2001). The sleep switch: Hypothalamic control of sleep and wakefulness. *Trends Neurosci.* **24,** 726–731.

Sawchenko, P. E. (1998). Toward a new neurobiology of energy balance, appetite, and obesity: The anatomists weigh in. *J. Comp. Neurol.* **402,** 435–441.

Scammell, T. E., Estabrooke, I. V., McCarthy, M. T., Chemelli, R. M., Yanagisawa, M., Miller, M. S., and Saper, C. B. (2000). Hypothalamic arousal regions are activated during modafinil-induced wakefulness. *J. Neurosci.* **20,** 8620–8628.

Scammell, T. E., and Winrow, C. J. (2011). Orexin receptors: Pharmacology and therapeutic opportunities. *Annu. Rev. Pharmacol. Toxicol.* **51,** 243–266.

Scanziani, M., Capogna, M., Gahwiler, B. H., and Thompson, S. M. (1992). Presynaptic inhibition of miniature excitatory synaptic currents by baclofen and adenosine in the hippocampus. *Neuron* **9,** 919–927.

Sears, R. M., Liu, R. J., Narayanan, N. S., Sharf, R., Yeckel, M. F., Laubach, M., Aghajanian, G. K., and DiLeone, R. J. (2010). Regulation of nucleus accumbens activity by the hypothalamic neuropeptide melanin-concentrating hormone. *J. Neurosci.* **30,** 8263–8273.

Shi, S. H., Hayashi, Y., Petralia, R. S., Zaman, S. H., Wenthold, R. J., Svoboda, K., and Malinow, R. (1999). Rapid spine delivery and redistribution of AMPA receptors after synaptic NMDA receptor activation. *Science* **284,** 1811–1816.

Sorra, K. E., and Harris, K. M. (1998). Stability in synapse number and size at 2 Hr after long-term potentiation in hippocampal area CA1. *J. Neurosci.* **18,** 658–671.

Sutcliffe, J. G., and de Lecea, L. (2002). The hypocretins: Setting the arousal threshold. *Nat. Rev. Neurosci.* **3,** 339–349.

Thakkar, M. M., Delgiacco, R. A., Strecker, R. E., and McCarley, R. W. (2003). Adenosinergic inhibition of basal forebrain wakefulness-active neurons: A simultaneous unit recording and microdialysis study in freely behaving cats. *Neuroscience* **122,** 1107–1113.

Thannickal, T. C., Moore, R. Y., Nienhuis, R., Ramanathan, L., Gulyani, S., Aldrich, M., Cornford, M., and Siegel, J. M. (2000). Reduced number of hypocretin neurons in human narcolepsy. *Neuron* **27,** 469–474.

van den Pol, A. N., Acuna-Goycolea, C., Clark, K. R., and Ghosh, P. K. (2004). Physiological properties of hypothalamic MCH neurons identified with selective expression of reporter gene after recombinant virus infection. *Neuron* **42,** 635–652.

van den Pol, A. N. (1999). Hypothalamic hypocretin (orexin): Robust innervation of the spinal cord. *J. Neurosci.* **19,** 3171–3182.

von Economo, C. (1930). Sleep as a problem of localization. *J. Nerv. Ment. Dis.* **71,** 249–259.

Winterer, J., Stanton, P. K., and Muller, W. (2006). Direct monitoring of vesicular release and uptake in brain slices by multiphoton excitation of the styryl FM 1-43. *Biotechniques* **40,** 343–351.

Wisor, J. P., Nishino, S., Sora, I., Uhl, G. H., Mignot, E., and Edgar, D. M. (2001). Dopaminergic role in stimulant-induced wakefulness. *J. Neurosci.* **21,** 1787–1794.

Wu, M., Dumalska, I., Morozova, E., van den Pol, A., and Alreja, M. (2009). Melanin-concentrating hormone directly inhibits GnRH neurons and blocks kisspeptin activation, linking energy balance to reproduction. *Proc. Natl. Acad. Sci. U.S.A.* **106,** 17217–17222.

Xia, J., Chen, F., Ye, J., Yan, J., Wang, H., Duan, S., and Hu, Z. (2009). Activity-dependent release of adenosine inhibits the glutamatergic synaptic transmission and plasticity in the hypothalamic hypocretin/orexin neurons. *Neuroscience* **162,** 980–988.

Xie, X., Crowder, T. L., Yamanaka, A., Morairty, S. R., Lewinter, R. D., Sakurai, T., and Kilduff, T. S. (2006). GABA(B) receptor-mediated modulation of hypocretin/orexin neurones in mouse hypothalamus. *J. Physiol.* **574,** 399–414.

Yamanaka, A., Beuckmann, C. T., Willie, J. T., Hara, J., Tsujino, N., Mieda, M., Tominaga, M., Yagami, K., Sugiyama, F., Goto, K., Yanagisawa, M., and Sakurai, T. (2003). Hypothalamic orexin neurons regulate arousal according to energy balance in mice. *Neuron* **38,** 701–713.

Yoshida, K., McCormack, S., Espana, R. A., Crocker, A., and Scammell, T. E. (2006). Afferents to the orexin neurons of the rat brain. *J. Comp. Neurol.* **494,** 845–861.

CHAPTER FOUR

Expression of Orexin Receptors in the Pituitary

Tadeusz Kaminski *and* Nina Smolinska

Contents

Abstract

Orexin receptors type 1 (OX1R) and type 2 (OX2R) are G protein-coupled receptors whose structure is highly conserved in mammals. OX1R is selective for orexin A, and OX2R binds orexin A and orexin B with similar affinity. Orexin receptor expression was observed in human, rat, porcine, sheep as well as *Xenopus laevis* pituitaries, both in the adenohypophysis and in the neurohypophysis. The expression level is regulated by gonadal steroid hormones and GnRH. The majority of orexins reaching the pituitary originate from the lateral hypothalamus, but due to the presence of the receptors and the local production of orexins in the pituitary, orexins could deliver an auto/paracrine effect within the gland. Cumulative data indicate that orexins are involved in the regulation of LH, GH, PRL, ACTH, and TSH secretion by pituitary cells, pointing to orexins' effect on the functioning of the endocrine axes. Those hormones may also serve as a signal linking metabolic status with endocrine control of sleep, arousal, and reproduction processes. © 2012 Elsevier Inc.

Department of Animal Physiology, University of Warmia and Mazury in Olsztyn, Oczapowskiego 1A, Olsztyn-Kortowo, Poland

Vitamins and Hormones, Volume 89
ISSN 0083-6729, http://dx.doi.org/10.1016/B978-0-12-394623-2.00004-4

I. Introduction

Orexin A (OXA) and Orexin B (OXB) bind and activate two types of G protein-coupled receptors, the orexin-1 receptor (OX1R) and the orexin-2 receptor (OX2R), which display 64% homology in their amino acid sequence. Amino acid identities between the human- and rat-orexin receptors are 94% for OX1R and 95% for OX2R, suggesting that both receptors are highly conserved between the species. OX1R preferentially binds OXA (IC_{50} was 20 and 250 nM for human OXA and OXB, respectively, in a binding experiment involving CHO cells), while OX2R binds OXA and OXB with similarly high affinity (20 nM), suggesting that OX2R is nonselective for both orexins (Sakurai *et al.*, 1998). In mice, Chen and Randeva (2004) identified two C-terminus splice variants of OX2R, OX2αR (443 aa), and OX2βR (460 aa), although OXA and OXB showed no differences in binding characteristic between splice variants. The activation of either receptor results in a receptor-mediated Ca^{2+} influx and an increase in intracellular Ca^{2+} levels (Sakurai *et al.*, 1998). Depending on the system used, orexins affect the activity of different signal-transduction pathways, including phospholipase C, protein kinase C, adenylyl cyclase, phosphoinositide-3-kinase, extracellular signal-regulated kinase, and p39 mitogen-activated protein kinase (Ammoun *et al.*, 2006a,b; Chen and Randeva, 2004; Holmqvist *et al.*, 2005; Tang *et al.*, 2008; Urbanska *et al.*, 2012).

II. Expression of OX1R and OX2R mRNAs and Proteins

The expression of OX1R and OX2R was observed in the human pituitary in RT-PCR and immunohistochemical assays (Blanco *et al.*, 2001). Receptor expression was also noted in the porcine gland at both gene and protein level (Kaminski *et al.*, 2010). Pituitary mRNA expression of orexin receptors was determined in rats (Date *et al.*, 2000; Johren *et al.*, 2001, 2003) and sheep (Zhang *et al.*, 2005), whereas OX1R-like immunoreactivity was found in the pituitary of *Xenopus laevis* (Suzuki *et al.*, 2007). In humans and rats, orexin receptors were more abundant in the adenohypophysis (AP) than in the neurohypophysis (NP) (Blanco *et al.*, 2001; Date *et al.*, 2000). In rats, the signal intensity of OX1R mRNA in the intermediate lobe was equal to that of OX2R (Date *et al.*, 2000), while only OX2R expression was found in the human pituitary (Blanco *et al.*, 2001). In the porcine gland, protein expression of orexin receptors was enhanced in the anterior pituitary in comparison with the posterior part during the mid-luteal phase of the estrous cycle (OX1R) or throughout the cycle (OX2R) (Fig. 4.1A and B).

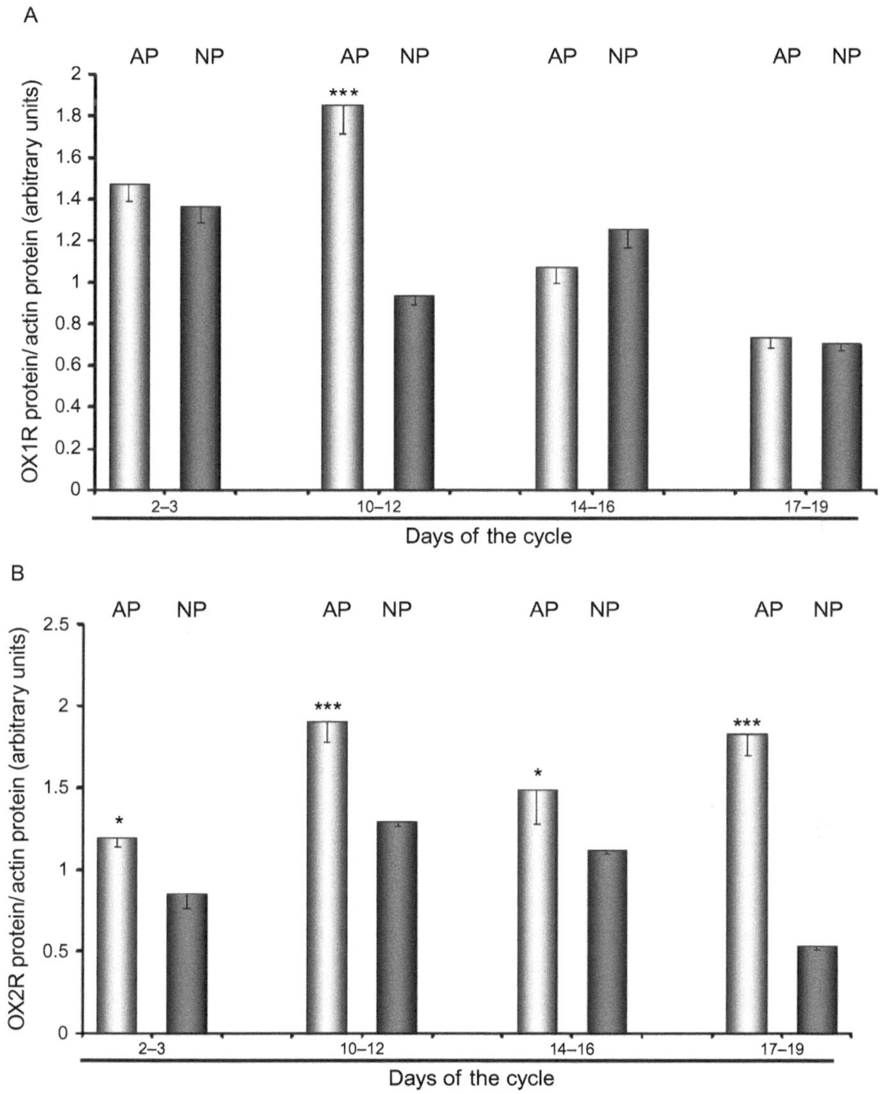

Figure 4.1 Comparison of orexin receptor 1 (OX1R) (A) and orexin receptor 2 (OX2R) (B) protein expression determined by Western blotting analysis between porcine anterior (AP) and posterior (NP) pituitary glands on days 2–3, 10–12, 14–16, and 17–19 of the estrous cycle. Values are expressed as means ± SEM in arbitrary optical density units ($n = 5$); $*p < 0.05$; $***p < 0.001$.

At gene level, this correlation was noted only with regard to OX1R during the early-luteal phase (Fig. 4.2) (Kaminski *et al.*, 2010). In studies of human pituitaries (Blanco *et al.*, 2001) and rat glands (Date *et al.*, 2000), OX1R-immunostained cells were much more numerous than the cells expressing

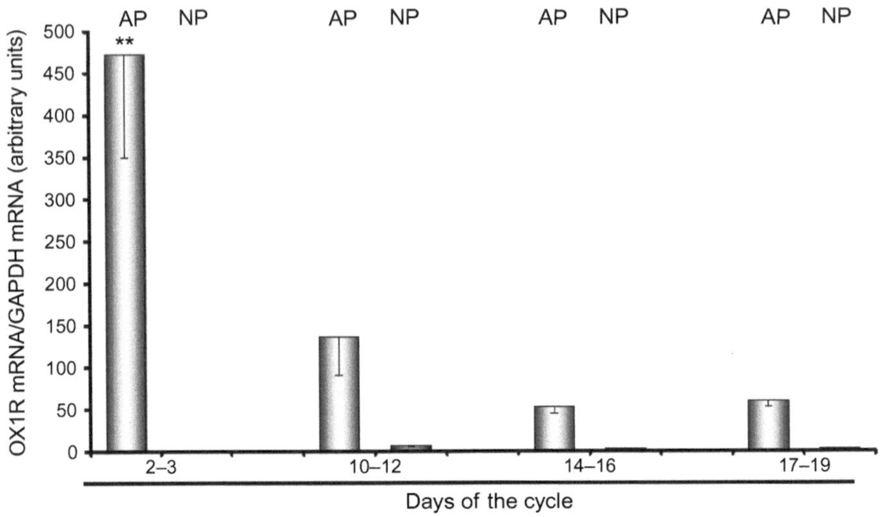

Figure 4.2 Comparison of orexin receptor 1 (OX1R) mRNA expression determined by quantitative real-time PCR between porcine anterior (AP) and posterior (NP) pituitary glands on days 2–3, 10–12, 14–16, and 17–19 of the estrous cycle. Results are means ± SEM ($n = 5$); $^{**}p < 0.01$.

OX2R. Histological and double immunofluorescence analyses revealed the presence of OX1R and OX2R in human somatotroph and corticotroph cells, respectively (Blanco *et al.*, 2001), and in the Xenopus pituitary, OX1R was expressed in PRL-containing cells (Suzuki *et al.*, 2007). The differences in the colocalization of cells between species can be probably attributed to the physiological status of each species.

Gene and protein expression of both types of orexin receptors was examined in gilt glands during four phases of the estrous cycle: days 2–3 (early-luteal phase), 10–12 (mid-luteal phase), 14–16 (late-luteal phase), and 17–19 (follicular phase). Using quantitative real-time PCR, statistically higher OX1R gene expression was detected in AP on days 2–3 relative to the remaining periods of the cycle. In NP, OX1R mRNA level was elevated on days 10–12 in comparison with other days (Fig. 4.3A). Expression of OX2R mRNA differed from that of OX1R. The highest OX2R mRNA level in AP was observed on days 17–19, and the lowest on days 10–12. In NP, markedly higher expression of the OX2R gene was observed on days 17–19 in comparison with the remaining phases (Fig. 4.3B). The expression pattern of receptor proteins differed from gene expression. The highest level of the OX1R protein was reported on days 10–12 in AP and on days 2–3 and 14–16 in NP. In both AP and NP, OX1R protein level was lowest during the follicular phase of the cycle (Fig. 4.4A). On days 2–3 and 14–16, OX2R protein expression in AP was lower than in the

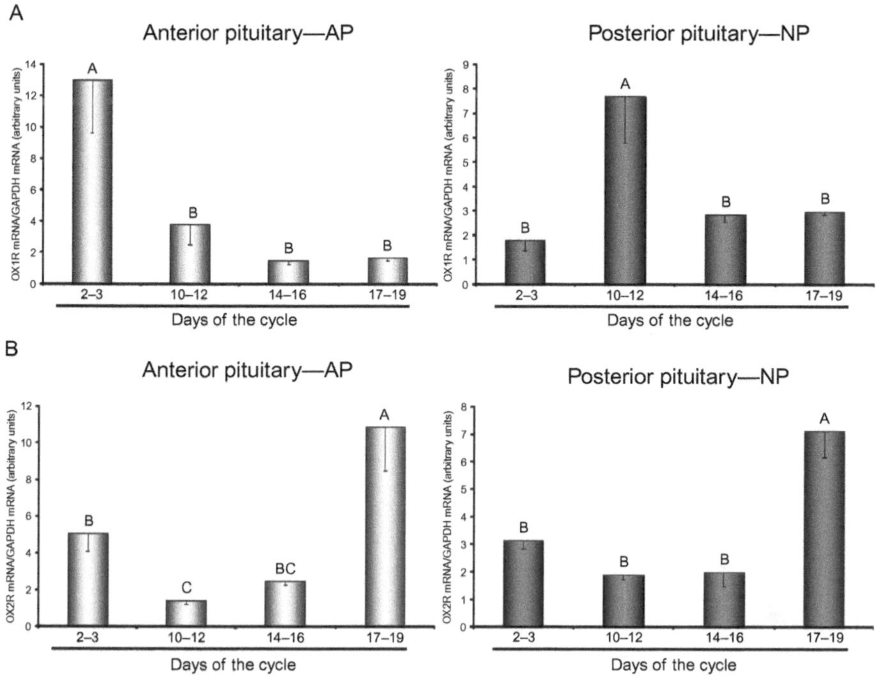

Figure 4.3 Comparison of orexin receptor 1 (OX1R) (A) and orexin receptor 2 (OX2R) (B) mRNA expression determined by quantitative real-time PCR in porcine anterior and posterior pituitary glands between days 2–3, 10–12, 14–16, and 17–19 of the estrous cycle. Results are means ± SEM ($n = 5$). Bars with different superscripts are significantly different. Capital letters indicate $p < 0.05$.

remaining phases. In NP, the lowest expression of OX2R protein was determined on days 17–19 and the highest on days 10–12 (Fig. 4.4B) (Kaminski *et al.*, 2010).

III. Regulation of Orexin Receptor Expression

The observed cycle-related changes in the expression of orexin receptors seem to be related to the hormonal status of pigs, implying that ovarian steroid hormones are involved in the control of receptor expression. Enhanced OX1R mRNA concentrations in the gland during the luteal phase and higher OX2R mRNA levels in the follicular phase of the cycle suggest that OX1R gene expression is stimulated by progesterone and OX2R gene expression—by estradiol. Similar conclusions concerning estradiol's involvement in regulating receptor expression can be drawn

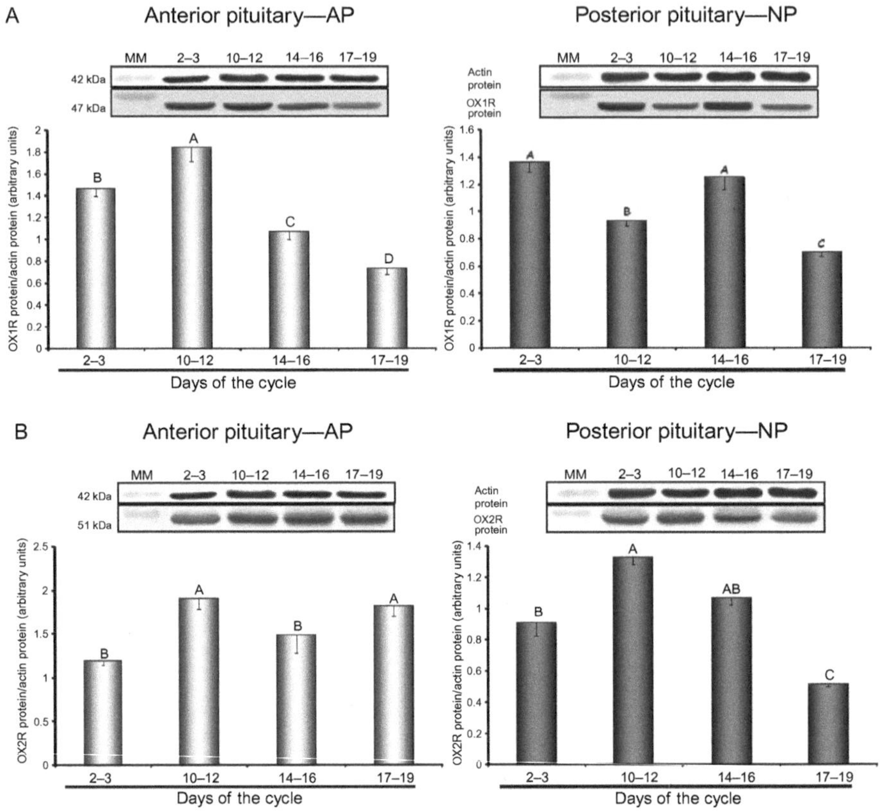

Figure 4.4 Comparison of orexin receptor 1 (OX1R) (A) and orexin receptor 2 (OX2R) (B) protein expression determined by Western blotting analysis in porcine anterior and posterior pituitary glands between days 2–3, 10–12, 14–16, and 17–19 of the estrous cycle. Upper panels: representative immunoblots (MM, molecular marker); lower panels: densitometric analysis of orexin receptor 1 and 2 proteins relative to actin protein. Values are expressed as means $\pm$ SEM in arbitrary optical density units ($n = 5$). Bars with different superscripts are significantly different. Capital letters indicate $p < 0.05$.

based on the work of Johren *et al.* (2001, 2003). The above authors found much higher OX1R mRNA levels in the male than in the female pituitary, pointing to sexually dimorphic expression of the receptor in the pituitary as well as a gender-specific role of orexins in the control of endocrine functions. In comparison with sham-operated animals, ovariectomized and orchidectomized rats demonstrated a manyfold increase in OX1R mRNA concentration in the pituitary. The effects of gonadectomy were suppressed by treatment with estradiol and testosterone in females and males, respectively. Thus, it seems that sex steroid hormones may differently regulate the expression of pituitary orexin receptors. On the other hand, the increase in OX1R and OX2R mRNA levels in anterior pituitaries of proestrous rats observed by Silveyra *et al.* (2007a) calls into question the inhibitory effect of estradiol. Priming with Cetrorelix, a synthetic antagonist of GnRH receptors, or pentobarbital, a drug blocking GnRH release, prevented an increase in OX1R and OX2R mRNA expression levels. Interestingly, orexin receptor expression was not affected in the anterior hypothalamus, mediobasal hypothalamus, and frontoparietal cortex of proestrous rats pretreated with Cetrorelix or pentobarbital, suggesting that receptor expression is regulated by two different mechanisms in the brain and the pituitary. Additionally, the inhibition of increased receptor expression in the AP of proestrous animals administered either of the above drugs implies that GnRH plays an important role as a regulator of receptor expression. The involvement of other hormones, such as progesterone and prolactin, in the regulation of orexin receptor expression cannot be ruled out; their preovulatory increases were also abolished by Cetrorelix and pentobarbital administration. Summarizing, the above suggests a clear correlation between the expression of orexin receptors and the hormonal milieu in mammal pituitaries.

IV. The Role of the Orexin System in the Pituitary

Orexin receptors are present in the pituitary, and orexins directly influence gland functions. This effect may be achieved by both classical endocrine action and auto/paracrine action. Classical endocrine action is probably enabled by orexin-producing neurons in the lateral hypothalamus that project to the median eminence (Date *et al.*, 2000). Orexins may reach AP via the long portal vessels of the hypothalamohypophysial vasculature. Alternatively, since axons staining positive for orexins are found in the posterior pituitary (Date *et al.*, 2000), the hormones may also access the AP through the short-portal vessels connecting both parts of the gland. Local production of peptides in the pituitary (Blanco *et al.*, 2003; Date *et al.*, 2000; Suzuki *et al.*, 2007) also contributes to the latter action. In humans, OXA was localized in 33% of pituitary cells, mainly lactotroph cells (82%), whereas OXB was found in nearly all corticotroph cells of the AP (Blanco *et al.*, 2003).

Considerable evidence has accumulated to implicate the involvement of orexins in the control of pituitary hormone production and the control of the pituitary branch of several endocrine axes. There is no doubt that the hypothalamic–pituitary–gonadal axis is one of the axes affected by orexins. Although OXA and OXB failed to modify basal and GnRH-induced LH secretion by pituitary cells harvested from male rats and random-cycle female rats (Samson and Taylor, 2001), OXA dose dependently inhibited GnRH-stimulated LH release in cultures of pituitary cells from proestrous rats (Russell *et al.*, 2001). In turn, OXB increased basal LH secretion in a dose-dependent manner, and when combined with GnRH, it potentiated the output of this gonadotropin from pig pituitary cells *in vitro* (Barb and Matteri, 2005). In addition to orexins' direct effect on pituitary cells, those peptides can modulate GnRH release that affects LH production. Hypothalamic GnRH neurons express orexin receptors, and 85% and 30% neurons were found to have direct synaptic contacts with orexin fibers in rats (Campbell *et al.*, 2003) and pigs (Su *et al.*, 2008), respectively. OXA enhanced GnRH release from cultured rat hypothalamic explants collected from male rats and proestrous female rats. This action was not observed in explants obtained at estrous and metestrous (Russell *et al.*, 2001). The *in vivo* effect of orexin varied subject to the site of administration. It had a stimulatory effect in the rostral preoptic area and an inhibitory effect in the medial preoptic area and the median eminence of the hypothalamus (Small *et al.*, 2003). Finally, OXA stimulated GnRH transcription and the release of this neuropeptide from immortalized GT1-7 hypothalamic GnRH neurons (Sasson *et al.*, 2006). Intracerebroventricularly administrated orexins had a dual effect on LH secretion. The discussed peptides were able to stimulate LH secretion in a dose- and time-dependent fashion in ovariectomized rats primed with estradiol and progesterone, but they inhibited gonadotropin release in untreated animals (Furuta *et al.*, 2002; Irahara *et al.*, 2001; Iwasa *et al.*, 2007; Pu *et al.*, 1998; Tamura *et al.*, 1999). The above findings support the hypothesis that the regulation of orexin receptors is steroid based. The involvement of orexins in the control of preovulatory LH and PRL surges in rats was also confirmed by Kohsaka *et al.* (2001). The above authors observed that the release of LH and PRL was inhibited by fasting and the recovery of hormonal surges after intracerebroventricular (i.c.v.) administration of OXA. They also noted that anti-OXA antisera given to normally fed female rats completely inhibited the surges of LH and PRL. It appeared that both orexin receptors are engaged in the control of gonadotropin release. In a rat model, OX1R and OX2R antagonists, administered on the proestrous afternoon, suppressed proestrous FSH and LH secretion (Silveyra *et al.*, 2007b). To our knowledge, the only study investigating orexins' influence on FSH secretion has been carried out by Silveyra *et al.* Pulsatile LH secretion (but not FSH) was found to be suppressed in orexin-deficient narcoleptic men (Kok *et al.*, 2004). The orexin system seems to create a link connecting metabolic status with endocrine control of reproduction and the sleep–wake cycle.

The role of orexins in the regulation of growth hormone (GH) production is unclear due to an apparent dichotomy which probably results from differences across species. In a study of primary cultured ovine somatotrophs, OXB alone potentiated GH output in a dose-dependent manner, but the potency of OXB was much weaker than the effect of GHRH.

OXA alone did not enhance GH secretion, but the combined administration of OXA and GHRH synergistically stimulated GH release *in vitro* (Chen and Xu, 2003; Xu *et al.*, 2002). It seems that the release of GH from ovine pituitaries may be related to the length of day. OXA augmented GH secretion by *in vitro* cultured pituitaries harvested from sheep on a long day, whereas in the cultures from ovine glands collected on a short day orexin inhibited GH secretion (Molik *et al.*, 2008). When combined with GHRH, OXB supressed GH secretion by pig pituitary cells compared to GHRH alone. Basal GH release was unaffected by the peptide (Barb and Matteri, 2005). In contrast to the data relating to *in vitro* cultured ovine and porcine pituitary cells, neither OXA nor OXB was able to affect basal or GHRH-induced secretion of GH by cultured anterior pituitary cells harvested from intact male or random-cycle female rat donors (Ferguson and Samson, 2003; Samson and Taylor, 2001). However, i.c.v. administration of OXA led to a decrease in spontaneous GH release in comparison with vehicle-primed male rats. OXA failed to modify *in vivo* GH responses to GHRH, although it significantly inhibited GH responses to ghrelin (Seoane *et al.*, 2004). In keeping with this, in a study by Hagan *et al.* (1999), i.c.v. administration of OXA caused a dose-dependent decrease in plasma GH levels in male rats. In several studies, attempts were made to explain the mechanism of orexin's action in relation to GH secretion (Chen and Xu, 2003; Xu *et al.*, 2002). It was shown that OXA and OXB markedly, dose dependently, and reversibly augmented the nifedipine-sensitive L-type Ca^{2+} current in ovine somatotroph cells. The increase in the L current by orexins was blunted by inhibitors of protein kinase C, but not blockers of protein kinase A. The combined administration of OXA and GHRH had an additive effect on the L current. It was, therefore, suggested that orexins may play an important role in the regulation of GHRH-stimulated GH secretion via an increase in the L-type Ca^{2+} current and protein kinase C-mediated signaling pathways.

The hypothalamic–pituitary–adrenal axis is yet another endocrine axis controlled by orexins. The presence of orexin receptors has been demonstrated at all levels of this axis (reviewed in Lopez *et al.*, 2009), including pituitary corticotroph cells (Blanco *et al.*, 2001). It seems, however, that the main site of orexin action is the hypothalamus. It was found that i.c.v. administration of OXA or OXB to rats resulted in a dose-dependent increase in plasma ACTH and corticosterone levels (Chang *et al.*, 2007; Kuru *et al.*, 2000; Russell *et al.*, 2001). OX2R mRNA is predominant in the paraventricular hypothalamic nucleus region (Marcus *et al.*, 2001; Trivedi *et al.*, 1998), and orexins probably exert their effect mainly via OX2R. At the pituitary level, orexins neither altered basal ACTH secretion by rat pituitary cells *in vitro* (Samson and Taylor 2001) nor affected proopiomelanocortin mRNA concentrations in the pituitary (Al-Barazanji *et al.*, 2001). While not affecting basal ACTH release, orexins markedly suppressed the response of corticotroph cells to stimulatory doses of CRH (Samson and

Taylor, 2001). According to the authors, the observed effect of the peptides was mediated by OX1R and the protein kinase C pathway.

Orexins' influence on PRL secretion and the lactotroph axis is controversial. Published studies indicate both the presence of pituitary cells' response to orexins (Molik *et al.*, 2008) and the lack thereof (Samson and Taylor, 2001). The former study demonstrated orexins' bimodal action on cultured ovine pituitaries, subject to the length of day. The administration of OXA on a long day enhanced PRL secretion in comparison with controls, whereas in cultures harvested during a short day, the hormone inhibited PRL release. In the latter study, OXA and OXB had no significant effect on basal- and TRH-stimulated secretion of PRL by rat pituitary cells *in vitro* over a log molar dose range of 0.1 pM to 100 nM. Although orexin receptors are expressed in rat (Date *et al.*, 2000; Johren *et al.*, 2003), human (Blanco *et al.*, 2001), and porcine (Kaminski *et al.*, 2010) pituitaries, orexins seem to influence PRL release mainly at the hypothalamus level. I.c.v. administration of OXA decreased plasma PRL concentrations in male rats by 71% at 20 min after the injection and in female rats by 83% at 90 min after the injection (Russell *et al.*, 2000). Similar data were presented by Hagan *et al.* (1999). Plasma PRL suppression was partly achieved through a pathway independent of the dopaminergic system (Russell *et al.*, 2000).

Among the different types of pituitary cells exposed to orexins, it seems that only thyrotrophs are free from the influence of these peptides. Such a conclusion can be drawn based on studies indicating an absence of orexins' effect on TSH release from pituitaries (Hagan *et al.*, 1999; Mitsuma *et al.*, 1999; Samson and Taylor, 2001).

V. Conclusions and Follow-up Research

Orexin receptors are present in the pituitary gland at both gene and protein levels. Their expression is modulated during the estrous cycle and by the steroid milieu. There is much evidence to suggest that the orexin system participates in the control of nearly all endocrine axes, creating an integrative link between homeostasis, reproduction, and the inner biological clock. Future work is required to clarify the relationship between orexins and other known and unknown systems involved in these processes.

Acknowledgments

The data presented in this chapter were acquired with partial support of the Polish Ministry of Science and Higher Education (Project Nos. NN308122134 and 528-0206.0805).

REFERENCES

Al-Barazanji, K. A., Wilson, S., Baker, J., Jessop, D. S., and Harbuz, M. S. (2001). Central orexin-A activates hypothalamic-pituitary-adrenal axis and stimulates hypothalamic corticotropin releasing factor and arginine vasopressin neurones in conscious rats. *J. Neuroendocrinol.* **13**(5), 421–424.

Ammoun, S., Lindholm, D., Wootz, H., Akerman, K. E., and Kukkonen, J. P. (2006a). G-protein-coupled OX1 orexin/hcrtr-1 hypocretin receptors induce caspase-dependent and -independent cell death through p38 mitogen-/stress-activated protein kinase. *J. Biol. Chem.* **281**(2), 834–842.

Ammoun, S., Johansson, L., Ekholm, M. E., Holmqvist, T., Danis, A. S., Korhonen, L., Sergeeva, O. A., Haas, H. L., Akerman, K. E., and Kukkonen, J. P. (2006b). OX1 orexin receptors activate extracellular signal-regulated kinase in Chinese hamster ovary cells via multiple mechanisms: The role of Ca2+ influx in OX1 receptor signaling. *Mol. Endocrinol.* **20**(1), 80–99.

Barb, C. R., and Matteri, R. L. (2005). Orexin-B modulates luteinizing hormone and growth hormone secretion from porcine pituitary cells in culture. *Domest. Anim. Endocrinol.* **28**(3), 331–337.

Blanco, M., López, M., García-Caballero, T., Gallego, R., Vázquez-Boquete, A., Morel, G., Señarís, R., Casanueva, F., Diéguez, C., and Beiras, A. (2001). Cellular localization of orexin receptors in human pituitary. *J. Clin. Endocrinol. Metab.* **86**(4), 1616–1619.

Blanco, M., Gallego, R., García-Caballero, T., Diéguez, C., and Beiras, A. (2003). Cellular localization of orexins in human anterior pituitary. *Histochem. Cell Biol.* **120**(4), 259–264.

Campbell, R. E., Grove, K. L., and Smith, M. S. (2003). Gonadotropin-releasing hormone neurons coexpress orexin 1 receptor immunoreactivity and receive direct contacts by orexin fibers. *Endocrinology* **144**(4), 1542–1548.

Chang, H., Saito, T., Ohiwa, N., Tateoka, M., Deocaris, C. C., Fujikawa, T., and Soya, H. (2007). Inhibitory effects of an orexin-2 receptor antagonist on orexin A- and stress-induced ACTH responses in conscious rats. *Neurosci. Res.* **57**(3), 462–466.

Chen, J., and Randeva, H. S. (2004). Genomic organization of mouse orexin receptors: Characterization of two novel tissue-specific splice variants. *Mol. Endocrinol.* **18**(11), 2790–2804.

Chen, C., and Xu, R. (2003). The in vitro regulation of growth hormone secretion by orexins. *Endocrine* **22**(1), 57–66.

Date, Y., Mondal, M. S., Matsukura, S., Ueta, Y., Yamashita, H., Kaiya, H., Kangawa, K., and Nakazato, M. (2000). Distribution of orexin/hypocretin in the rat median eminence and pituitary. *Brain Res. Mol. Brain Res.* **76**(1), 1–6.

Ferguson, A. V., and Samson, W. K. (2003). The orexin/hypocretin system: A critical regulator of neuroendocrine and autonomic function. *Front. Neuroendocrinol.* **24**(3), 141–150.

Furuta, M., Funabashi, T., and Kimura, F. (2002). Suppressive action of orexin A on pulsatile luteinizing hormone secretion is potentiated by a low dose of estrogen in ovariectomized rats. *Neuroendocrinology* **75**(3), 151–157.

Hagan, J. J., Leslie, R. A., Patel, S., Evans, M. L., Wattam, T. A., Holmes, S., Benham, C. D., Taylor, S. G., Routledge, C., Hemmati, P., Munton, R. P., Ashmeade, T. E., *et al.* (1999). Orexin A activates locus coeruleus cell firing and increases arousal in the rat. *Proc. Natl. Acad. Sci U. S. A.* **96**(19), 10911–10916.

Holmqvist, T., Johansson, L., Ostman, M., Ammoun, S., Akerman, K. E., and Kukkonen, J. P. (2005). OX1 orexin receptors couple to adenylyl cyclase regulation via multiple mechanisms. *J. Biol. Chem.* **280**(8), 6570–6579.

Irahara, M., Tamura, T., Matuzaki, T., Saito, S., Yasui, T., Yamano, S., Kamada, M., and Aono, T. (2001). Orexin-A suppresses the pulsatile secretion of luteinizing hormone via beta-endorphin. *Biochem. Biophys. Res. Commun.* **281**(1), 232–236.

Iwasa, T., Matsuzaki, T., Kiyokawa, M., Shimizu, F., Minakuchi, M., Kuwahara, A., Maegawa, M., Yasui, T., and Irahara, M. (2007). The type 2 corticotrophin-releasing hormone receptor mediates orexin A-induced luteinising hormone suppression in ovariectomised rats. *J. Neuroendocrinol.* **19**(9), 732–738.

Johren, O., Neidert, S. J., Kummer, M., Dendorfer, A., and Dominiak, P. (2001). Prepro-orexin and orexin receptor mRNAs are differentially expressed in peripheral tissues of male and female rats. *Endocrinology* **142**(8), 3324–3331.

Johren, O., Brüggemann, N., Dendorfer, A., and Dominiak, P. (2003). Gonadal steroids differentially regulate the messenger ribonucleic acid expression of pituitary orexin type 1 receptors and adrenal orexin type 2 receptors. *Endocrinology* **144**(4), 1219–1225.

Kaminski, T., Smolinska, N., Nitkiewicz, A., and Przala, J. (2010). Expression of orexin receptors 1 (OX1R) and 2 (OX2R) in the porcine pituitary during the oestrous cycle. *Anim. Reprod. Sci.* **117**(1–2), 111–118.

Kohsaka, A., Watanobe, H., Kakizaki, Y., Suda, T., and Schiöth, H. B. (2001). A significant participation of orexin-A, a potent orexigenic peptide, in the preovulatory luteinizing hormone and prolactin surges in the rat. *Brain Res.* **898**(1), 166–170.

Kok, S. W., Roelfsema, F., Overeem, S., Lammers, G. J., Frölich, M., Meinders, A. E., and Pijl, H. (2004). Pulsatile LH release is diminished, whereas FSH secretion is normal, in hypocretin-deficient narcoleptic men. *Am. J. Physiol. Endocrinol. Metab.* **287**(4), E630–E636.

Kuru, M., Ueta, Y., Serino, R., Nakazato, M., Yamamoto, Y., Shibuya, I., and Yamashita, H. (2000). Centrally administered orexin/hypocretin activates HPA axis in rats. *Neuroreport* **11**(9), 1977–1980.

Lopez, M., Tena-Sempere, M., and Diéguez, C. (2009). Cross-talk between orexins (hypocretins) and the neuroendocrine axes (hypothalamic-pituitary axes). *Front. Neuroendocrinol.* **31**(2), 113–127.

Marcus, J. N., Aschkenasi, C. J., Lee, C. E., Chemelli, R. M., Saper, C. B., Yanagisawa, M., and Elmquist, J. K. (2001). Differential expression of orexin receptors 1 and 2 in the rat brain. *J. Comp. Neurol.* **435**(1), 6–25.

Mitsuma, T., Hirooka, Y., Mori, Y., Kayama, M., Adachi, K., Rhue, N., Ping, J., and Nogimori, T. (1999). Effects of orexin A on thyrotropin-releasing hormone and thyrotropin secretion in rats. *Horm. Metab. Res.* **31**(11), 606–609.

Molik, E., Zieba, D. A., Misztal, T., Romanowicz, K., Wszola, M., Wierzchos, E., and Nowakowski, M. (2008). The role of orexin A in the control of prolactin and growth hormone secretions in sheep—In vitro study. *J. Physiol. Pharmacol.* **59**(Suppl. 9), 91–100.

Pu, S., Jain, M. R., Kalra, P. S., and Kalra, S. P. (1998). Orexins, a novel family of hypothalamic neuropeptides, modulate pituitary luteinizing hormone secretion in an ovarian steroid-dependent manner. *Regul. Pept.* **78**(1–3), 133–136.

Russell, S. H., Kim, M. S., Small, C. J., Abbott, C. R., Morgan, D. G., Taheri, S., Murphy, K. G., Todd, J. F., Ghatei, M. A., and Bloom, S. R. (2000). Central administration of orexin A suppresses basal and domperidone stimulated plasma prolactin. *J. Neuroendocrinol.* **12**(12), 1213–1218.

Russell, S. H., Small, C. J., Dakin, C. L., Abbott, C. R., Morgan, D. G., Ghatei, M. A., and Bloom, S. R. (2001). The central effects of orexin-A in the hypothalamic-pituitary-adrenal axis in vivo and in vitro in male rats. *J. Neuroendocrinol.* **13**(6), 561–566.

Sakurai, T., Amemiya, A., Ishii, M., Matsuzaki, I., Chemelli, R. M., Tanaka, H., Williams, S. C., Richardson, J. A., Kozlowski, G. P., Wilson, S., Arch, J. R., Buckingham, R. E., *et al.* (1998). Orexins and orexin receptors: A family of hypothalamic neuropeptides and G protein-coupled receptors that regulate feeding behavior. *Cell* **92** (4), 573–585.

Samson, W. K., and Taylor, M. M. (2001). Hypocretin/orexin suppresses corticotroph responsiveness in vitro. *Am. J. Physiol. Regul. Integr. Comp. Physiol.* **281**(4), R1140–R1145.

Sasson, R., Dearth, R. K., White, R. S., Chappell, P. E., and Mellon, P. L. (2006). Orexin A induces GnRH gene expression and secretion from GT1-7 hypothalamic GnRH neurons. *Neuroendocrinology* **84**(6), 353–363.

Seoane, L. M., Tovar, S. A., Perez, D., Mallo, F., Lopez, M., Señaris, R., Casanueva, F. F., and Dieguez, C. (2004). Orexin A suppresses in vivo GH secretion. *Eur. J. Neurosci.* **19** (8), 2080–2088.

Silveyra, P., Catalano, P. N., Lux-Lantos, V., and Libertun, C. (2007a). Impact of proestrous milieu on expression of orexin receptors and prepro-orexin in rat hypothalamus and hypophysis: Actions of Cetrorelix and Nembutal. *Am. J. Physiol. Endocrinol. Metab.* **292** (3), E820–E828.

Silveyra, P., Lux-Lantos, V., and Libertun, C. (2007b). Both orexin receptors are expressed in rat ovaries and fluctuate with the estrous cycle: Effects of orexin receptor antagonists on gonadotropins and ovulation. *Am. J. Physiol. Endocrinol. Metab.* **293**(4), E977–E985.

Small, C. J., Goubillon, M. L., Murray, J. F., Siddiqui, A., Grimshaw, S. E., Young, H., Sivanesan, V., Kalamatianos, T., Kennedy, A. R., Coen, C. W., Bloom, S. R., and Wilson, C. A. (2003). Central orexin A has site-specific effects on luteinizing hormone release in female rats. *Endocrinology* **144**(7), 3225–3236.

Su, J., Lei, Z., Zhang, W., Ning, H., and Ping, J. (2008). Distribution of orexin B and its relationship with GnRH in the pig hypothalamus. *Res. Vet. Sci.* **85**(2), 315–323.

Suzuki, H., Takemoto, Y., and Yamamoto, T. (2007). Differential distribution of orexin-A-like and orexin receptor 1 (OX1R)-like immunoreactivities in the Xenopus pituitary. *Tissue Cell* **39**(6), 423–430.

Tamura, T., Irahara, M., Tezuka, M., Kiyokawa, M., and Aono, T. (1999). Orexins, orexigenic hypothalamic neuropeptides, suppress the pulsatile secretion of luteinizing hormone in ovariectomized female rats. *Biochem. Biophys. Res. Commun.* **264**(3), 759–762.

Tang, J., Chen, J., Ramanjaneya, M., Punn, A., Conner, A. C., and Randeva, H. S. (2008). The signalling profile of recombinant human orexin-2 receptor. *Cell. Signal.* **20**(9), 1651–1661.

Trivedi, P., Yu, H., MacNeil, D. J., Van der Ploeg, L. H., and Guan, X. M. (1998). Distribution of orexin receptor mRNA in the rat brain. *FEBS Lett.* **438**(1–2), 71–75.

Urbanska, A., Sokolowska, P., Woldan-Tambor, A., Bieganska, K., Brix, B., Jöhren, O., Namiecinska, M., and Zawilska, J. B. (2012). Orexins/hypocretins acting at G(i) protein-coupled OX (2) receptors inhibit cyclic AMP synthesis in the primary neuronal cultures. *J. Mol. Neurosci.* **46**(1), 10–17.

Xu, R., Wang, Q., Yan, M., Hernandez, M., Gong, C., Boon, W. C., Murata, Y., Ueta, Y., and Chen, C. (2002). Orexin-A augments voltage-gated $Ca2+$ currents and synergistically increases growth hormone (GH) secretion with GH-releasing hormone in primary cultured ovine somatotropes. *Endocrinology* **143**(12), 4609–4619.

Zhang, S., Blache, D., Vercoe, P. E., Adam, C. L., Blackberry, M. A., Findlay, P. A., Eidne, K. A., and Martin, G. B. (2005). Expression of orexin receptors in the brain and peripheral tissues of the male sheep. *Regul. Pept.* **124**(1–3), 81–87.

CHAPTER FIVE

Transcriptional Regulation of the Hypocretin/Orexin Gene

Susumu Tanaka

Contents

Abstract

The hypocretin (also known as orexin) system reacts to environmental changes in the internal milieu (pH, glucose, and various hormones) and the external environment (activity, fasting, and sleep deprivation) and regulates various physiological functions. Several feedback mechanisms, such as those listed above, have been reported to regulate the hypocretin system even at the transcriptional level. In addition, some transcription factors, such as forkhead box A2; nuclear receptor

Department of Psychiatry and Behavioral Science, Tokyo Metropolitan Institute of Medical Science, Kamikitazawa 2-1-6, Setagaya-ku, Tokyo, Japan

Vitamins and Hormones, Volume 89
ISSN 0083-6729, http://dx.doi.org/10.1016/B978-0-12-394623-2.00005-6

subfamily 6, group A, member 1; and early B-cell factor 2, were determined to be regulators of the preprohypocretin gene. However, little is known concerning the specific components that react to environmental changes and the determinants of spatial expression of the hypocretin gene within the lateral hypothalamus. This review focuses on the recent findings of transcription factors that regulate preprohypocretin transcription in addition to discussing the future prospects for transcriptional regulation of the hypocretin gene.

I. Introduction

Hypocretin, a hypothalamic neuropeptide also known as orexin, is involved in the regulation of various physiological processes, such as arousal, sleep, food intake, energy expenditure, and reward processing (de Lecea and Sutcliffe, 2005; Sakurai, 2007). The hypocretin locus encodes two neuropeptides, hypocretin-1 (also known as orexin-A) and hypocretin-2 (orexin-B), produced from the same precursor (preprohypocretin). The transcription of preprohypocretin is exclusively localized in the perifornical area of the lateral hypothalamus (Moriguchi *et al.*, 2002). Expression of preprohypocretin in the hypothalamus has been found to increase with food restriction or other physiological changes that maintain the vigilance state; however, little is known regarding the molecular mechanisms involved in its transcription.

The symptoms and pathophysiology of a chronic hypersomnia, namely, narcolepsy, are reported to be caused by hypocretin deficiency (Chemelli *et al.*, 1999; Lin *et al.*, 1999; Peyron *et al.*, 2000; Thannickal *et al.*, 2000). Patients with narcolepsy have shown a marked decrease in hypocretin neurons (Peyron *et al.*, 2000; Thannickal *et al.*, 2000). However, it has not been clarified whether the decrease is caused by cell defects alone, disruption of the hypocretin mRNA transcription, failure of the translation in hypocretin neurons, or by other reasons. Therefore, careful investigation is required to further understand the mechanism of preprohypocretin transcription.

II. Hypocretin/Orexin Regulatory Elements

In transgenic mice, the 3.2-kb 5′-flanking region of the human preprohypocretin gene is sufficient for its specific expression in murine hypothalamic hypocretin neurons (Sakurai *et al.*, 1999). Two physiologically conserved promoter regions, that is, orexin regulatory element 1 and 2 (OE1 and OE2), were subsequently identified within a 3.2-kb fragment located upstream of the human preprohypocretin gene and were found to target the specific expression of the hypocretin within the lateral hypothalamus (Moriguchi *et al.*, 2002). Using deletion reporter mutants, the core region (57 base pairs (bp)) of OE1 was identified as the critical region for the spatial expression of lateral hypothalamic hypocretin mRNA, suggesting that OE1 contains crucial *cis*-acting elements that specifically regulate hypocretin transcription in the lateral hypothalamus.

III. Colocalization with STAT3 in Hypocretin Neurons

As evidence for the relationship to ingestive behavior by the leptin system through hypocretin action, leptin receptor immunoreactivity was shown to occur in most hypocretin neurons (Hakansson *et al.*, 1999). The transcription factor, signal transducer and activator of transcription 3 (STAT3), which is generally activated by leptin, is also observed in hypocretin neurons. The colocalization of leptin receptor and STAT3 with hypocretin neurons in the lateral hypothalamus suggests that leptin directly regulates hypocretin neurons. However, there is no direct evidence that STAT3 binds to the 5′-promoter region of the preprohypocretin gene.

STAT3 is also activated through tyrosine phosphorylation in response to cell surface cytokine receptors, such as the interleukin-6 signal transducer (also known as gp130) (Levy and Darnell, 2002) or the granulocyte colony-stimulating factor receptor gene (CSF3R) (Numata *et al.*, 2005). Some narcolepsy patients show a close association with immunological aspects (Cvetkovic-Lopes *et al.*, 2010; Dauvilliers, 2006; Dauvilliers *et al.*, 2010; Hallmayer *et al.*, 2009; Kawashima *et al.*, 2010; Kornum *et al.*, 2011; Mignot *et al.*, 2001; Toyoda *et al.*, 2010), this is primarily due to hypocretin cell loss (Peyron *et al.*, 2000; Thannickal *et al.*, 2000). Indeed, narcolepsy patients exhibit a significant elevation of TNF-alpha, IL-6, and p75 in their blood (Himmerich *et al.*, 2006; Okun *et al.*, 2004). To disclose the direct immunological involvement of hypocretin expression in this disorder, it is necessary to (1) examine more cytokines in detail, (2) confirm the colocalization with gp130 or CSF3R in hypothalamic hypocretin neurons, and (3) clarify the direct effect of STAT3, or the indirect effect via STAT3-inducible proteins (Snyder *et al.*, 2008), on the 5′-upstream region of the preprohypocretin gene. A recent finding showed that preprohypocretin mRNA levels were elevated in 2 hours and decreased in 4–6 h after lipopolysaccharide administration to rats (Novikova *et al.*, 2011), suggesting an immunological involvement in hypocretin transcriptional regulation.

IV. Interferon-Alpha Regulates Hypocretin-Promoter Activity *In Vitro*

Whether OE1, OE2, or other regions also serve as transcriptional modulators for preprohypocretin expression in response to changes in internal or external environmental conditions remains unknown. Interferon

(IFN)-alpha, a cytokine involved in the defense against viral infections, modulates the expression of preprohypocretin *in vitro*, an effect that is likely to be mediated through its binding to an IFN-stimulated regulatory element in the 5′-upstream region of the preprohypocretin gene (Waleh *et al.*, 2001). However, it remains to be clarified how IFN reaches the hypothalamic hypocretin neurons under physiological conditions. Waleh *et al.* discussed that other STAT members, that is, STAT1 and STAT2, also had an effect on hypocretin gene expression in SH-SY5Y cells (human neuroblastoma). Further *in vivo* studies are required to clarify this observation.

V. Hypocretin Expression in the Postnatal Period

de Lecea *et al.* (1998) first showed that the transcription of hypocretin mRNA began from postnatal day 5 by using Northern blot analysis in the rat hypothalamus. *In situ* hybridization analysis revealed that hypocretin mRNA could be detected at postnatal day 0 in the rat hypothalamus, followed by a marked increase between postnatal days 15 and 20 (Yamamoto *et al.*, 2000), which was also observed in northern blot analysis (de Lecea *et al.*, 1998). Further, in our previous study (Tanaka *et al.*, 2010), different hypocretin cell counts were observed in the murine hypothalamus on postnatal day 1 (~1000 cells) as compared with those in the adult lateral hypothalamus (~3500 cells) (Honda *et al.*, 2009); this suggests the presence of individual regulatory mechanisms that affect hypocretin transcription before and after maturation. These results also suggest that markedly renewed chromatin modifications occur within the preprohypocretin-promoter region during the postnatal stage (Ito, 2003; Ito *et al.*, 2000).

VI. Embryonic Hypocretin Expression

A. Initiation of hypocretin expression

Pregnant rats were given 5-bromo-2-deoxyuridine (BrdU), and analysis was performed to detect BrdU and hypocretin in the developing ventral diencephalon, including the embryonic hypothalamus (Amiot *et al.*, 2005). The generation of hypocretin neurons produced one sharp peak at embryonic day 12 in the rat hypothalamus. In C57/Black6J mice, prepro-hypocretin transcription could first be detected on embryonic day 10 using RT-PCR (Fig. 5.1). Unlike *in utero* electroporation with the GFP gene on embryonic days 13 and 14 (on electroporation days, GFP signals showed slight movement and no colocalization with hypocretin signals after birth), *in utero* electroporation on embryonic day 12 showed that some hypocretin neurons were colocalized with GFP (Tanaka *et al.*, 2010). These signals

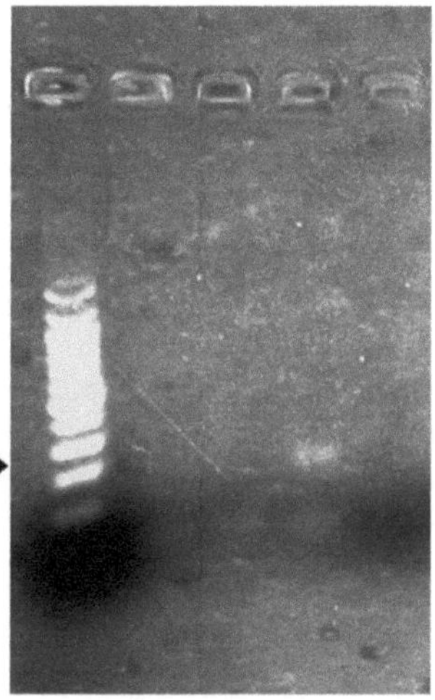

Figure 5.1 Onset of hypocretin expression in the embryonic murine brain. M: DNA marker; E8, 9, and 10: RT-PCR analysis conducted on brain cDNA of embryonic days 8, 9, and 10, respectively; W: water used as template for RT-PCR.

suggest that some hypocretin neurons originate from progenitor cells of the third ventricular zone between embryonic days 10 and 12. After migration to the designated area, these cells probably differentiate into hypocretin-producing cells by some factors such as sonic hedgehog, which is essential for anterior hypothalamic patterning (Shimogori *et al.*, 2010).

B. Coexpression factors in the embryo

Shimogori *et al.* conducted a comprehensive gene expression analysis based on microarrays at 12 different developmental stages along with *in situ* hybridization of 1045 genes (Shimogori *et al.*, 2010). Consistent with previous findings, the expression of hypocretin peaked during the postnatal period. Coexpression with the LIM homeobox 9 (Lhx9), which is essential for gonad development via the *Sf1* promoter (Birk *et al.*, 2000; Wilhelm and Englert, 2002), was observed in a subset of developmental hypocretin-positive cells in the lateral and dorsomedial hypothalamus (Shimogori *et al.*, 2010). Further functional studies are required to demonstrate the physiological relationship between Lhx9 and developmental hypocretin expression.

C. In zebrafish

Hypocretin is also conserved in fish. Initial hypocretin expression in zebrafish was observed at 22 h postfertilization, either unilaterally or bilaterally in loose clusters in the lateral ventral diencephalon corresponding to the developing hypothalamus (Faraco *et al.*, 2006). A well-conserved region of 13 bp in the zebrafish hypocretin promoter is essential for fish promoter activity. In the zebrafish experiment, activity of the 3.2 kb upstream region of the human preprohypocretin gene is undetectable, and there is no similarity between the 13 bp in zebrafish and the OE1/OE2 elements of the human promoter. The sets of transcription factors that determine hypocretin expression might be somewhat different because the hypocretin effect itself is different against sleep/consciousness (Yokogawa *et al.*, 2007). The intraventricular administration of hypocretin-1 increases locomotion in mammals (Fujiki *et al.*, 2003; Hagan *et al.*, 1999; Piper *et al.*, 2000), whereas in zebrafish, it promotes sleep in the dark (Yokogawa *et al.*, 2007). Moreover, the basal promoters themselves are different between mammals and fish (Faraco *et al.*, 2006).

VII. FOXA2 Regulates Hypocretin Expression

Hypocretin neurons are inhibited in response to feeding signals and are activated during fasting. Preprohypocretin mRNA is higher in fasted mice than in fed mice. A recent study showed that the forkhead box transcription factor 2 (FOXA2) translocates into the nucleus, binds to the hypocretin promoter, and stimulates the expression of preprohypocretin in the lateral hypothalamus during fasting (Silva *et al.*, 2009). Intriguingly, FOXA2 localized to the nucleus in the presence of glucose without insulin and was detected in the cytoplasm at low levels of glucose with insulin; however, *Foxa2* mRNA levels were not changed in all conditions. Chromatin immunoprecipitation (Chip) showed that FOXA2 binds to DNA containing three putative Foxa2-binding sites in the hypocretin promoter only in fasted mice. Because these FOXA2-binding sites differed from OE1/OE2 elements, FOXA2 might function as a specific enhancer for insulin signaling through the downstream basal TATA box promoter on the expression of hypocretin in the hypothalamus. During eating, insulin/PI3K/Akt signaling enhances FOXA2 phosphorylation; this leads to deprivation of FOXA2 transcriptional activation through its removal from the nucleus.

VIII. Is There Diurnal Variation in Hypocretin Expression?

Taheri *et al.* (2000) first reported a fluctuation of preprohypocretin mRNA in the rat (Taheri *et al.*, 2000). Although the release of hypocretin exhibits a clear diurnal fluctuation, no changes in the expression of the preprohypocretin gene have been reported across 24 h, including unpublished data from several laboratories (Terao *et al.*, 2000). Although the quantification of preprohypocretin mRNA has already been demonstrated by northern hybridization using the % oligo dT method (Taheri *et al.*, 2000), this may not be the most suitable method to quantify mRNA; therefore, it is desirable to confirm the reproducibility of the results by a different method. To increase the stringency of relative preprohypocretin mRNA measurements, we used multiple housekeeping genes identified by geNorm analysis (Vandesompele *et al.*, 2002) as a normalization factor for quantitative real-time PCR analysis instead of using a single housekeeping gene.

IX. IGFBP3 Modulates Hypocretin Expression Levels

To clarify the physiology of hypocretin neurons, we identified transcripts that are dysregulated in the human narcoleptic hypothalamus and in hypocretin/ataxin-3 hemizygous transgenic mice (Honda *et al.*, 2009), in which animals, most hypocretin neurons are impaired (Hara *et al.*, 2001). Insulin-like growth factor binding protein 3 (IGFBP3) was downregulated in both humans and transgenic mice and coexpressed in hypocretin neurons. An analysis of IGFBP3 transgenic mice (Modric *et al.*, 2001) found no hypocretin cell defects or decreases in cell number; however, a significant decrease in the hypothalamic preprohypocretin mRNA was found (Honda *et al.*, 2009). To determine whether IGFBP3 modulates the transcription of preprohypocretin, we conducted an *in vitro* luciferase reporter assay in the presence of IGFBP3. Reduction in preprohypocretin-promoter activity (3.2 kb) by IGFBP3 was found only in the neural cell line SH-SY5Y, suggesting the need for neural-specific cofactors to function as transcriptional modulators.

X. Does Nur77 Affect the Activity of the Preprohypocretin Promoter? (Tanaka *et al.*, 2009)

IGFBP3 is mainly produced and secreted by the liver and is a carrier of IGF1 and IGF2 in the blood. IGF–IGFBP3 complexes are reinternalized through IGF receptor 1 (Lee *et al.*, 2004) or by endocytic pathways (Lee *et al.*, 2004) into the cytoplasm. After internalization, IGFBP3 is translocated into the nucleus. The translocation was conducted by a nuclear localization signal included in IGFBP3 amino acid sequence and importin-β (Firth and Baxter, 2002). Once in the nucleus, it displaces the binding partner Nur77 (also called nuclear receptor subfamily 4, group A, member 1) of the retinoid-X-receptor-alpha (RXRA) (Stark *et al.*, 2011). In the presence of IGFBP3, the target transcriptional activities of Nur77 and RXRA are capable of being modulated. Nur77 is characterized by its ability to bind the nuclear receptor subfamily response element (NurRE) and to modulate the promoter activity through NurRE. We found one putative RXR-binding motif, AGGTCC, using Genomatix Software GmbH (http://www.genomatix.de). The AGGTCC motif is an noncanonical hexanucleotide motif, and perturbations in this variant motif disrupted RXRA hexamer binding to a 30 bp retinoid response element in the mouse tissue transglutaminase gene promoter (Nagy *et al.*, 1996).

We next explored whether Nur77 shares a similar domain of expression with preprohypocretin within the hypothalamus by using the NeuroBlast program of the Allen Brain Atlas database (Lein *et al.*, 2007), an *in situ* hybridization database of the C57BL/6J mice brain. In this database, we found that the Nur77 gene showed a similar local expression pattern as that of the preprohypocretin gene ($r=0.556717$). Using double immunohistochemical staining with anti-hypocretin and anti-Nur77 antibodies, we showed that Nur77 protein colocalizes in approximately half of the identified murine hypocretin-positive cells (Fig. 5.2D) and that Nur77 expression (Fig. 5.2C)

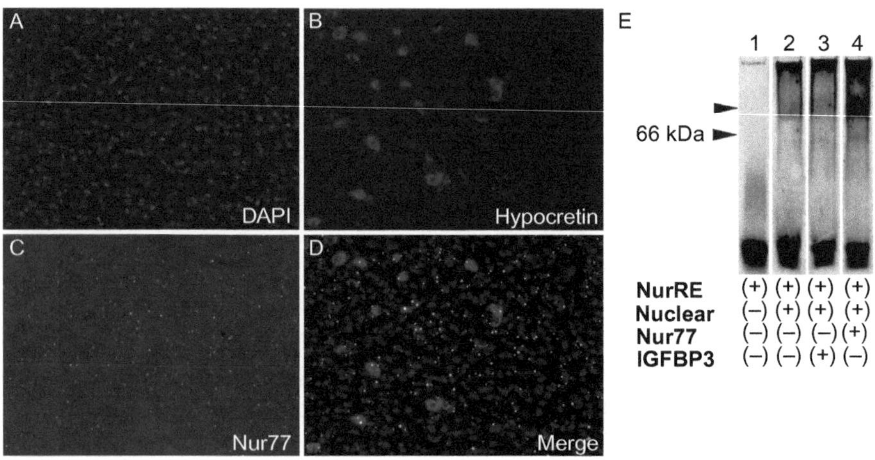

Figure 5.2 Colocalization of hypocretin with Nur77 in murine hypothalamic hypocretin neurons, and an electromobility shift assay with nuclear receptor subfamily response elements. (A) DAPI-labeled nuclei (blue); (B) hypocretin (red) visualized using Alexa-594; (C) Nur77 (green) visualized using Alexa-488; (D) Merged image of A, B, and C immunofluorescence; (E) electromobility shift assay using HeLa nuclear extract. Triplet NurRE oligonucleotides were subjected to nondenatured 4% PAGE after incubation with nuclear extracts from HeLa cells transfected with pCMVTNT vector (mock) (lane 2), with IGFBP3/TNT expression vector (lane 3), or with Nur77/TNT expression vector (lane 4). No protein was applied to lane 1, so triplet NurRE oligonucleotides maintained their original molecular weights. (See Color Insert.)

is more widespread than hypocretin expression (Fig. 5.2B). Of note, Nur77-immunoreactivity clearly localized within the nucleus in some cells, while in other cases, cytoplasmic localization was observed. NeuroBlast program searches revealed not only Nur77 but also two other Nur members, that is, nuclear receptor subfamily 1, group H, member 3 (Willy *et al.*, 1995) and nuclear receptor subfamily 2, group F, member 6 (Miyajima *et al.*, 1988; Warnecke *et al.*, 2005), as possible genes that colocalize with hypocretin neurons. Even so, these factors are not known to interact with a similar NurRE sequence, and additional studies are required to evaluate whether these two other proteins also modulate preprohypocretin expression.

A weak and a strong shift in NurRE signals was generated in the presence of HeLa cell nuclear extracts transfected with a Nur77 expression vector (Fig. 5.2E, lane 4) during an electromobility shift assay (EMSA). The molecular weight of the strongly shifted triplet NurRE sequence was much larger (100–120 kDa; Fig. 5.2E, upper arrow) than the estimated molecular weight of the Nur77 protein (~70 kDa; Fig. 5.2E, lower arrow). Additional HeLa cell nuclear extracts transfected with two other vectors (pCMVTNT or IGFBP3/TNT) did not elicit such a weak and strong shift (Fig. 5.2E, lane 2 and 3), suggesting that NurRE oligonucleotides bind to the large protein complex via Nur77 as an anchor protein for complex formation and that IGFBP3 may therefore affect preprohypocretin-promoter activity through Nur77. Unfortunately, however, no effect of Nur77 was found on the 3.2-kb 5′-flanking region of the human preprohypocretin gene when using an *in vitro* luciferase reporter assay (data not shown). Nur77 is involved in mitochondrial accumulation-induced apoptosis (Lee *et al.*, 2005). Therefore, the contribution of Nur77 to the pathophysiology of narcolepsy, where Hcrt cell loss occurs, should be investigated.

XI. Transcriptional Regulation of the Hypocretin/Orexin Gene by NR6A1

Downregulated genes, including *Nr6a1* and several other genes known to be colocalized with hypocretin neurons in hypocretin/ataxin-3 mice, have been described in our previous study (Honda *et al.*, 2009). NR6A1 binds to the DR0 element (AGGTCA) and represses transcriptional activities of downstream target genes (Chen *et al.*, 1994; Cooney *et al.*, 1998; Fuhrmann *et al.*, 2001; Yan *et al.*, 1997). The DR0 element and NurRE, a DR0-like motif (AGGTCC), were identified at positions −1350/−1345 and −544/−537, respectively, relative to the translation start site of the preprohypocretin gene. We examined whether NR6A1 modulates hypocretin transcription through these motifs. NR6A1 overexpression in SH-SY5Y cells modulated hypocretin-promoter activity.

Because of the lack of NurRE, the NR6A1 effect was contradicted, although all of the other deletion mutants, including the ΔDR0 deletion mutant, showed responsiveness against NR6A1. Indeed, a study using Chip–PCR revealed that endogenous NR6A1 binds to DNA containing the NurRE within the 3.2-kb 5′-flanking region of the human preprohypocretin gene. To demonstrate the functional connection to hypocretin neurons, colocalization with NR6A1 was shown in almost all hypocretin cells. Further, mice overexpressing *Nr6a1* in one side of the hypothalamus were generated using *in utero* electroporation according to a previously reported method (Shimogori and Ogawa, 2008). The results of the analysis using electroporated mice suggested that NR6A1 is a relatively specific regulator for hypocretin expression in the murine lateral hypothalamus (Tanaka *et al.*, 2010). Considering the proven function of NR6A1 in neuronal differentiation (Akamatsu *et al.*, 2009), further *in vivo* studies using cross-hybridization with Nr6a1tm3Coo mice (Lan *et al.*, 2003) and hypocretin-promoter Cre-mice (Matsuki *et al.*, 2009) are required to clarify whether hypocretin transcription is directly affected by NR6A1 or indirectly affected through other cells.

XII. Transcription Factors Downregulated in Hypocretin/Ataxin-3 Transgenic Mice

Besides NR6A1, some transcription factors are also downregulated in the hypocretin neuron-ablated mice (Honda *et al.*, 2009). To identify the master regulator for these downregulated genes, an *in silico* search was performed against the 0.5 kb upstream or 0.5 kb downstream regions of each transcriptional start site using a SABiosciences' proprietary database known as DECODE (http://www.sabiosciences.com/chipqpcr.php). Each transcription factor binding site is located within 1 kb of other genes (Fig. 5.3); this suggests that some transcription factors are reciprocally regulated. Of note, a divergent POU domain, class 2, transcription factor 1 (Pou2f1)-binding site is included in the OE1 II-4 sequence (Moriguchi *et al.*, 2002). However, the participation of Pou2f1 in OE1-binding could not be verified, because the OE1-binding factor complex could not be disturbed by the consensus octamer motif (ATGCAAAT) in EMSA (Moriguchi *et al.*, 2002). Moreover, De la Herran-Arita *et al.* found that narcolepsy–cataplexy syndrome occurs in early B-cell factor 2 (Ebf2)-null mice (De la Herran-Arita *et al.*, 2011). It was suggested that the narcoleptic syndrome is induced depending on the pronounced reduction of hypocretin neurons in the lateral hypothalamus (~1500 cells in wild mice and 300 cells in EBf2-null mice). To clarify the involvement of Ebf2 in hypocretin transcriptional regulation, two conserved putative

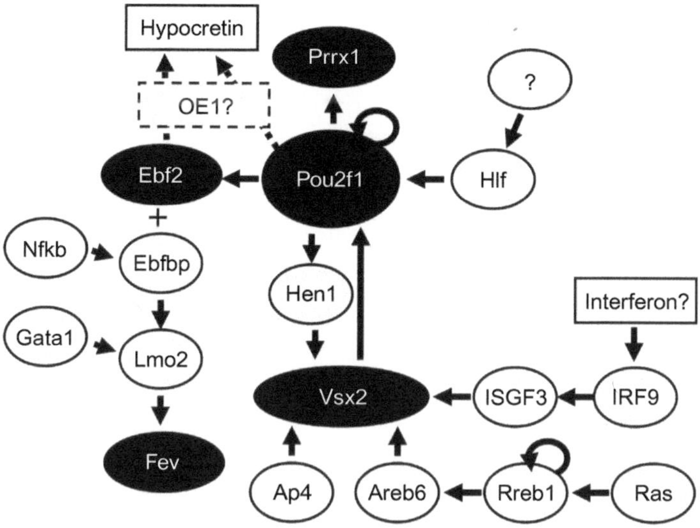

Figure 5.3 Reciprocal regulation among transcription factors is dysregulated in hypocretin/ataxin-3 transgenic mice. Black circles: Transcription factors listed as down-regulated genes in hypocretin/ataxin-3 mice (Honda et al., 2009). White circles: Binding motifs of transcription factors identified in SABiosciences DECODE database within 0.5 kb up- and downstream of the target gene (http://www.sabiosciences.com/chipqpcr.php). Arrow: Putative effect on target expression through binding motif. Cross: Known interaction between two proteins.

Ebf2-responsive sequences were identified within the promoter regions of the preprohypocretin gene. One of the putative Ebf2-binding sites is located within the OE-1 II-2 elements. The functional relevance of this will need to be proven in further studies.

XIII. Conclusions and Future Directions

The hypocretin system regulates various physiological functions, most notably sleep and wakefulness. Interestingly, the activity of the hypocretin system is known to react to environmental changes in the internal milieu (pH, glucose, and various hormones), as well as in the external environment (activity, fasting, and sleep deprivation) (de Lecea and Sutcliffe, 2005; Sakurai, 2007). Although several feedback loops have been reported to regulate the hypocretin system, including at the transcriptional level, little is known about the specific transcriptional units regulating the preprohypocretin gene. As shown in Foxa2 analysis and Ebf2-null mice, transcriptional regulation of the hypocretin gene via transcription factors could be essential in the regulation of adaptive behavior and the sleep–wake cycle. To further understand the physiological relationships with transcription factors involved in hypocretin transcriptional regulation, it is necessary to perform functional studies on transcription factors that are downregulated in the hypothalamus of hypocretin/ataxin-3 transgenic mice (paired-related homeobox gene 1, Prrx1 (Grueneberg *et al.*, 1992); fifth ewing sarcoma variant, Fev (Fyodorov *et al.*, 1998); visual system homeobox gene 2, Vsx2 (Reichman *et al.*, 2010)). Further, it is necessary to determine OE1-binding factor, which could help to clearly define the characteristics of hypocretin and its more precise localization in the lateral hypothalamus.

ACKNOWLEDGMENTS

This material is based upon work supported by Grants-in-Aid for Scientific Research (No. 20790868 and No. 17700362) from the Ministry of Education, Science and Culture of Japan, Mitsubishi Pharma Research Foundation, Nakayama Foundation for Human Science, and Takeda Science Foundation.

REFERENCES

Akamatsu, W., DeVeale, B., Okano, H., Cooney, A. J., and van der Kooy, D. (2009). Suppression of Oct4 by germ cell nuclear factor restricts pluripotency and promotes neural stem cell development in the early neural lineage. *J. Neurosci.* **29,** 2113–2124.

Amiot, C., Brischoux, F., Colard, C., La Roche, A., Fellmann, D., and Risold, P. Y. (2005). Hypocretin/orexin-containing neurons are produced in one sharp peak in the developing ventral diencephalon. *Eur. J. Neurosci.* **22,** 531–534.

Birk, O. S., Casiano, D. E., Wassif, C. A., Cogliati, T., Zhao, L., Zhao, Y., Grinberg, A., Huang, S., Kreidberg, J. A., Parker, K. L., Porter, F. D., and Westphal, H. (2000). The LIM homeobox gene Lhx9 is essential for mouse gonad formation. *Nature* **403,** 909–913.

Chemelli, R. M., Willie, J. T., Sinton, C. M., Elmquist, J. K., Scammell, T., Lee, C., Richardson, J. A., Williams, S. C., Xiong, Y., Kisanuki, Y., Fitch, T. E., Nakazato, M., *et al.* (1999). Narcolepsy in orexin knockout mice: Molecular genetics of sleep regulation. *Cell* **98,** 437–451.

Chen, F., Cooney, A. J., Wang, Y., Law, S. W., and O'Malley, B. W. (1994). Cloning of a novel orphan receptor (GCNF) expressed during germ cell development. *Mol. Endocrinol.* **8,** 1434–1444.

Cooney, A. J., Hummelke, G. C., Herman, T., Chen, F., and Jackson, K. J. (1998). Germ cell nuclear factor is a response element-specific repressor of transcription. *Biochem. Biophys. Res. Commun.* **245,** 94–100.

Cvetkovic-Lopes, V., Bayer, L., Dorsaz, S., Maret, S., Pradervand, S., Dauvilliers, Y., Lecendreux, M., Lammers, G. J., Donjacour, C. E., Du Pasquier, R. A., Pfister, C., Petit, B., *et al.* (2010). Elevated Tribbles homolog 2-specific antibody levels in narcolepsy patients. *J. Clin. Invest.* **120,** 713–719.

Dauvilliers, Y. (2006). Follow-up of four narcolepsy patients treated with intravenous immunoglobulins. *Ann. Neurol.* **60,** 153.

Dauvilliers, Y., Montplaisir, J., Cochen, V., Desautels, A., Einen, M., Lin, L., Kawashima, M., Bayard, S., Monaca, C., Tiberge, M., Filipini, D., Tripathy, A., *et al.* (2010). Post-H1N1 narcolepsy-cataplexy. *Sleep* **33,** 1428–1430.

De la Herran-Arita, A. K., Zomosa-Signoret, V. C., Millan-Aldaco, D. A., Palomero-Rivero, M., Guerra-Crespo, M., Drucker-Colin, R., and Vidaltamayo, R. (2011). Aspects of the Narcolepsy-Cataplexy syndrome in O/E3 (Ebf2)-null mutant mice. *Neuroscience* **183,** 134–143.

de Lecea, L., and Sutcliffe, J. G. (2005). The hypocretins and sleep. *FEBS J.* **272,** 5675–5688.

de Lecea, L., Kilduff, T. S., Peyron, C., Gao, X., Foye, P. E., Danielson, P. E., Fukuhara, C., Battenberg, E. L., Gautvik, V. T., Bartlett, F. S., 2nd, Frankel, W. N., van den Pol, A. N., *et al.* (1998). The hypocretins: Hypothalamus-specific peptides with neuroexcitatory activity. *Proc. Natl. Acad. Sci. U. S. A.* **95,** 322–327.

Faraco, J. H., Appelbaum, L., Marin, W., Gaus, S. E., Mourrain, P., and Mignot, E. (2006). Regulation of hypocretin (orexin) expression in embryonic zebrafish. *J. Biol. Chem.* **281,** 29753–29761.

Firth, S. M., and Baxter, R. C. (2002). Cellular actions of the insulin-like growth factor binding proteins. *Endocr. Rev.* **23,** 824–854.

Fuhrmann, G., Chung, A. C., Jackson, K. J., Hummelke, G., Baniahmad, A., Sutter, J., Sylvester, I., Scholer, H. R., and Cooney, A. J. (2001). Mouse germline restriction of Oct4 expression by germ cell nuclear factor. *Dev. Cell* **1,** 377–387.

Fujiki, N., Yoshida, Y., Ripley, B., Mignot, E., and Nishino, S. (2003). Effects of IV and ICV hypocretin-1 (orexin A) in hypocretin receptor-2 gene mutated narcoleptic dogs and IV hypocretin-1 replacement therapy in a hypocretin-ligand-deficient narcoleptic dog. *Sleep* **26,** 953–959.

Fyodorov, D., Nelson, T., and Deneris, E. (1998). Pet-1, a novel ETS domain factor that can activate neuronal nAchR gene transcription. *J. Neurobiol.* **34,** 151–163.

Grueneberg, D. A., Natesan, S., Alexandre, C., and Gilman, M. Z. (1992). Human and Drosophila homeodomain proteins that enhance the DNA-binding activity of serum response factor. *Science* **257,** 1089–1095.

Hagan, J. J., Leslie, R. A., Patel, S., Evans, M. L., Wattam, T. A., Holmes, S., Benham, C. D., Taylor, S. G., Routledge, C., Hemmati, P., Munton, R. P., Ashmeade, T. E., *et al.* (1999). Orexin A activates locus coeruleus cell firing and increases arousal in the rat. *Proc. Natl. Acad. Sci. U. S. A.* **96,** 10911–10916.

Hakansson, M., de Lecea, L., Sutcliffe, J. G., Yanagisawa, M., and Meister, B. (1999). Leptin receptor- and STAT3-immunoreactivities in hypocretin/orexin neurones of the lateral hypothalamus. *J. Neuroendocrinol.* **11,** 653–663.

Hallmayer, J., Faraco, J., Lin, L., Hesselson, S., Winkelmann, J., Kawashima, M., Mayer, G., Plazzi, G., Nevsimalova, S., Bourgin, P., Hong, S. C., Honda, Y., *et al.* (2009). Narcolepsy is strongly associated with the T-cell receptor alpha locus. *Nat. Genet.* **41,** 708–711.

Hara, J., Beuckmann, C. T., Nambu, T., Willie, J. T., Chemelli, R. M., Sinton, C. M., Sugiyama, F., Yagami, K., Goto, K., Yanagisawa, M., and Sakurai, T. (2001). Genetic ablation of orexin neurons in mice results in narcolepsy, hypophagia, and obesity. *Neuron* **30,** 345–354.

Himmerich, H., Beitinger, P. A., Fulda, S., Wehrle, R., Linseisen, J., Wolfram, G., Himmerich, S., Gedrich, K., Wetter, T. C., and Pollmacher, T. (2006). Plasma levels of tumor necrosis factor alpha and soluble tumor necrosis factor receptors in patients with narcolepsy. *Arch. Intern. Med.* **166,** 1739–1743.

Honda, M., Eriksson, K. S., Zhang, S., Tanaka, S., Lin, L., Salehi, A., Hesla, P. E., Maehlen, J., Gaus, S. E., Yanagisawa, M., Sakurai, T., Taheri, S., *et al.* (2009). IGFBP3 colocalizes with and regulates hypocretin (orexin). *PLoS One* **4,** e4254.

Ito, T. (2003). Nucleosome assembly and remodeling. *Curr. Top. Microbiol. Immunol.* **274,** 1–22.

Ito, T., Ikehara, T., Nakagawa, T., Kraus, W. L., and Muramatsu, M. (2000). p300-mediated acetylation facilitates the transfer of histone H2A-H2B dimers from nucleosomes to a histone chaperone. *Genes Dev.* **14,** 1899–1907.

Kawashima, M., Lin, L., Tanaka, S., Jennum, P., Knudsen, S., Nevsimalova, S., Plazzi, G., and Mignot, E. (2010). Anti-Tribbles homolog 2 (TRIB2) autoantibodies in narcolepsy are associated with recent onset of cataplexy. *Sleep* **33,** 869–874.

Kornum, B. R., Kawashima, M., Faraco, J., Lin, L., Rico, T. J., Hesselson, S., Axtell, R. C., Kuipers, H., Weiner, K., Hamacher, A., Kassack, M. U., Han, F., *et al.* (2011). Common variants in P2RY11 are associated with narcolepsy. *Nat. Genet.* **43,** 66–71.

Lan, Z. J., Gu, P., Xu, X., Jackson, K. J., DeMayo, F. J., O'Malley, B. W., and Cooney, A. J. (2003). GCNF-dependent repression of BMP-15 and GDF-9 mediates gamete regulation of female fertility. *EMBO J.* **22,** 4070–4081.

Lee, K. W., Liu, B., Ma, L., Li, H., Bang, P., Koeffler, H. P., and Cohen, P. (2004). Cellular internalization of insulin-like growth factor binding protein-3: Distinct endocytic pathways facilitate re-uptake and nuclear localization. *J. Biol. Chem.* **279,** 469–476.

Lee, K. W., Ma, L., Yan, X., Liu, B., Zhang, X. K., and Cohen, P. (2005). Rapid apoptosis induction by IGFBP-3 involves an insulin-like growth factor-independent nucleomitochondrial translocation of RXRalpha/Nur77. *J. Biol. Chem.* **280,** 16942–16948.

Lein, E. S., Hawrylycz, M. J., Ao, N., Ayres, M., Bensinger, A., Bernard, A., Boe, A. F., Boguski, M. S., Brockway, K. S., Byrnes, E. J., Chen, L., Chen, L., *et al.* (2007). Genome-wide atlas of gene expression in the adult mouse brain. *Nature* **445,** 168–176.

Levy, D. E., and Darnell, J. E., Jr. (2002). Stats: Transcriptional control and biological impact. *Nat. Rev. Mol. Cell Biol.* **3,** 651–662.

Lin, L., Faraco, J., Li, R., Kadotani, H., Rogers, W., Lin, X., Qiu, X., de Jong, P. J., Nishino, S., and Mignot, E. (1999). The sleep disorder canine narcolepsy is caused by a mutation in the hypocretin (orexin) receptor 2 gene. *Cell* **98,** 365–376.

Matsuki, T., Nomiyama, M., Takahira, H., Hirashima, N., Kunita, S., Takahashi, S., Yagami, K., Kilduff, T. S., Bettler, B., Yanagisawa, M., and Sakurai, T. (2009). Selective loss of GABA(B) receptors in orexin-producing neurons results in disrupted sleep/wakefulness architecture. *Proc. Natl. Acad. Sci. U. S. A.* **106,** 4459–4464.

Mignot, E., Lin, L., Rogers, W., Honda, Y., Qiu, X., Lin, X., Okun, M., Hohjoh, H., Miki, T., Hsu, S., Leffell, M., Grumet, F., *et al.* (2001). Complex HLA-DR and -DQ interactions confer risk of narcolepsy-cataplexy in three ethnic groups. *Am. J. Hum. Genet.* **68,** 686–699.

Miyajima, N., Kadowaki, Y., Fukushige, S., Shimizu, S., Semba, K., Yamanashi, Y., Matsubara, K., Toyoshima, K., and Yamamoto, T. (1988). Identification of two novel members of erbA superfamily by molecular cloning: The gene products of the two are highly related to each other. *Nucleic Acids Res.* **16,** 11057–11074.

Modric, T., Silha, J. V., Shi, Z., Gui, Y., Suwanichkul, A., Durham, S. K., Powell, D. R., and Murphy, L. J. (2001). Phenotypic manifestations of insulin-like growth factor-binding protein-3 overexpression in transgenic mice. *Endocrinology* **142,** 1958–1967.

Moriguchi, T., Sakurai, T., Takahashi, S., Goto, K., and Yamamoto, M. (2002). The human prepro-orexin gene regulatory region that activates gene expression in the lateral region and represses it in the medial regions of the hypothalamus. *J. Biol. Chem.* **277,** 16985–16992.

Nagy, L., Saydak, M., Shipley, N., Lu, S., Basilion, J. P., Yan, Z. H., Syka, P., Chandraratna, R. A., Stein, J. P., Heyman, R. A., and Davies, P. J. (1996). Identification and characterization of a versatile retinoid response element (retinoic acid receptor response element-retinoid X receptor response element) in the mouse tissue transglutaminase gene promoter. *J. Biol. Chem.* **271,** 4355–4365.

Novikova, N. S., Perekrest, S. V., Shainidze, K. Z., and Korneva, E. A. (2011). Hypothalamic orexin-containing neurons in the hypothalamus on exposure to antigenic and non-antigenic stimuli. *Neurosci. Behav. Physiol.* **41,** 188–197.

Numata, A., Shimoda, K., Kamezaki, K., Haro, T., Kakumitsu, H., Shide, K., Kato, K., Miyamoto, T., Yamashita, Y., Oshima, Y., Nakajima, H., Iwama, A., *et al.* (2005). Signal transducers and activators of transcription 3 augments the transcriptional activity of CCAAT/enhancer-binding protein alpha in granulocyte colony-stimulating factor signaling pathway. *J. Biol. Chem.* **280,** 12621–12629.

Okun, M. L., Giese, S., Lin, L., Einen, M., Mignot, E., and Coussons-Read, M. E. (2004). Exploring the cytokine and endocrine involvement in narcolepsy. *Brain Behav. Immun.* **18,** 326–332.

Peyron, C., Faraco, J., Rogers, W., Ripley, B., Overeem, S., Charnay, Y., Nevsimalova, S., Aldrich, M., Reynolds, D., Albin, R., Li, R., Hungs, M., *et al.* (2000). A mutation in a case of early onset narcolepsy and a generalized absence of hypocretin peptides in human narcoleptic brains. *Nat. Med.* **6,** 991–997.

Piper, D. C., Upton, N., Smith, M. I., and Hunter, A. J. (2000). The novel brain neuropeptide, orexin-A, modulates the sleep-wake cycle of rats. *Eur. J. Neurosci.* **12,** 726–730.

Reichman, S., Kalathur, R. K., Lambard, S., Ait-Ali, N., Yang, Y., Lardenois, A., Ripp, R., Poch, O., Zack, D. J., Sahel, J. A., and Leveillard, T. (2010). The homeobox gene CHX10/VSX2 regulates RdCVF promoter activity in the inner retina. *Hum. Mol. Genet.* **19,** 250–261.

Sakurai, T. (2007). The neural circuit of orexin (hypocretin): Maintaining sleep and wakefulness. *Nat. Rev. Neurosci.* **8,** 171–181.

Sakurai, T., Moriguchi, T., Furuya, K., Kajiwara, N., Nakamura, T., Yanagisawa, M., and Goto, K. (1999). Structure and function of human prepro-orexin gene. *J. Biol. Chem.* **274,** 17771–17776.

Shimogori, T., and Ogawa, M. (2008). Gene application with in utero electroporation in mouse embryonic brain. *Dev. Growth Differ.* **50,** 499–506.

Shimogori, T., Lee, D. A., Miranda-Angulo, A., Yang, Y., Wang, H., Jiang, L., Yoshida, A. C., Kataoka, A., Mashiko, H., Avetisyan, M., Qi, L., Qian, J., *et al.* (2010). A genomic atlas of mouse hypothalamic development. *Nat. Neurosci.* **13,** 767–775.

Silva, J. P., von Meyenn, F., Howell, J., Thorens, B., Wolfrum, C., and Stoffel, M. (2009). Regulation of adaptive behaviour during fasting by hypothalamic Foxa2. *Nature* **462,** 646–650.

Snyder, M., Huang, X. Y., and Zhang, J. J. (2008). Identification of novel direct Stat3 target genes for control of growth and differentiation. *J. Biol. Chem.* **283,** 3791–3798.

Stark, C., Breitkreutz, B. J., Chatr-Aryamontri, A., Boucher, L., Oughtred, R., Livstone, M. S., Nixon, J., Van Auken, K., Wang, X., Shi, X., Reguly, T., Rust, J. M., *et al.* (2011). The BioGRID Interaction Database: 2011 update. *Nucleic Acids Res.* **39,** D698–D704.

Taheri, S., Sunter, D., Dakin, C., Moyes, S., Seal, L., Gardiner, J., Rossi, M., Ghatei, M., and Bloom, S. (2000). Diurnal variation in orexin A immunoreactivity and prepro-orexin mRNA in the rat central nervous system. *Neurosci. Lett.* **279,** 109–112.

Tanaka, S., Honda, M., and Mignot, E. (2009). Novel candidate gene for narcolepsy to regulate orexin expression by comprehensive expression profile. *Annu. Rep. Pharmacopsychiatry Res. Found.* **41,** 97–108Japanese.

Tanaka, S., Kodama, T., Nonaka, T., Toyoda, H., Arai, M., Fukazawa, M., Honda, Y., Honda, M., and Mignot, E. (2010). Transcriptional regulation of the hypocretin/orexin gene by NR6A1. *Biochem. Biophys. Res. Commun.* **403,** 178–183.

Terao, A., Peyron, C., Ding, J., Wurts, S. W., Edgar, D. M., Heller, H. C., and Kilduff, T. S. (2000). Prepro-hypocretin (prepro-orexin) expression is unaffected by short-term sleep deprivation in rats and mice. *Sleep* **23,** 867–874.

Thannickal, T. C., Moore, R. Y., Nienhuis, R., Ramanathan, L., Gulyani, S., Aldrich, M., Cornford, M., and Siegel, J. M. (2000). Reduced number of hypocretin neurons in human narcolepsy. *Neuron* **27,** 469–474.

Toyoda, H., Tanaka, S., Miyagawa, T., Honda, Y., Tokunaga, K., and Honda, M. (2010). Anti-Tribbles homolog 2 autoantibodies in Japanese patients with narcolepsy. *Sleep* **33,** 875–878.

Vandesompele, J., De Preter, K., Pattyn, F., Poppe, B., Van Roy, N., De Paepe, A., and Speleman, F. (2002). Accurate normalization of real-time quantitative RT-PCR data by geometric averaging of multiple internal control genes. *Genome Biol.* **3**RESEARCH0034.

Waleh, N. S., Apte-Deshpande, A., Terao, A., Ding, J., and Kilduff, T. S. (2001). Modulation of the promoter region of prepro-hypocretin by alpha-interferon. *Gene* **262,** 123–128.

Warnecke, M., Oster, H., Revelli, J. P., Alvarez-Bolado, G., and Eichele, G. (2005). Abnormal development of the locus coeruleus in Ear2(Nr2f6)-deficient mice impairs the functionality of the forebrain clock and affects nociception. *Genes Dev.* **19,** 614–625.

Wilhelm, D., and Englert, C. (2002). The Wilms tumor suppressor WT1 regulates early gonad development by activation of Sf1. *Genes Dev.* **16,** 1839–1851.

Willy, P. J., Umesono, K., Ong, E. S., Evans, R. M., Heyman, R. A., and Mangelsdorf, D. J. (1995). LXR, a nuclear receptor that defines a distinct retinoid response pathway. *Genes Dev.* **9,** 1033–1045.

Yamamoto, Y., Ueta, Y., Hara, Y., Serino, R., Nomura, M., Shibuya, I., Shirahata, A., and Yamashita, H. (2000). Postnatal development of orexin/hypocretin in rats. *Brain Res. Mol. Brain Res.* **78,** 108–119.

Yan, Z. H., Medvedev, A., Hirose, T., Gotoh, H., and Jetten, A. M. (1997). Characterization of the response element and DNA binding properties of the nuclear orphan receptor germ cell nuclear factor/retinoid receptor-related testis-associated receptor. *J. Biol. Chem.* **272,** 10565–10572.

Yokogawa, T., Marin, W., Faraco, J., Pezeron, G., Appelbaum, L., Zhang, J., Rosa, F., Mourrain, P., and Mignot, E. (2007). Characterization of sleep in zebrafish and insomnia in hypocretin receptor mutants. *PLoS Biol.* **5,** e277.

CHAPTER SIX

Energy Expenditure: Role of Orexin

Jennifer A. Teske*,† *and* Vijayakumar Mavanji‡

Contents

Abstract

The orexins/hypocretins are endogenous, modulatory and multifunctional neuropeptides with prominent influence on several physiological processes. The influence of orexins on energy expenditure is highlighted with focus on orexin action on individual components of energy expenditure. As orexin stabilizes and maintains normal states of arousal and the sleep/wake cycle, we also highlight orexin mediation of sleep and how sleep interacts with energy expenditure.

I. Introduction

The hypocretins (hypocretin 1 and 2) are neuropeptides with significant amino acid homology to the secretin/incretin protein family that were described first by de Lecea *et al.* (1998) after their earlier report documented isolation of its precursor, preprohypocretin (Gautvik *et al.*, 1996). One month later, Sakurai *et al.* reported identification of the same neuropeptide and associated their two G-protein-coupled receptors, however, referred to the neuropeptides as orexins (orexin A and B, OXA and OXB) due to their

* Department of Nutritional Sciences, University of Arizona and Southern Arizona VA Health Care System, Tucson, Arizona, USA
† Department of Food Science and Nutrition, University of Minnesota, Saint Paul, Minnesota, USA
‡ Minnesota Obesity Prevention Training Program, School of Public Health, University of Minnesota and Minneapolis VA Health Care System, Minneapolis, Minnesota, USA

Vitamins and Hormones, Volume 89
ISSN 0083-6729, http://dx.doi.org/10.1016/B978-0-12-394623-2.00006-8

observation of hyperphagia after central administration (Sakurai *et al.*, 1998). Unlike other neuropeptides, synthesis of the precursor protein, preprohypocretin or prepro-orexin, is confined to discrete regions in the lateral and lateral/perifornical hypothalamus (Gautvik *et al.*, 1996). However, orexin protein is ubiquitously expressed in several brain nuclei, in all levels of the central nervous system and within discrete peripheral locations (Chen *et al.*, 1999; Cutler *et al.*, 1999; Date *et al.*, 2000; Nambu *et al.*, 1999; Peyron *et al.*, 1998). Like orexin protein distribution, orexin receptors (orexin receptor 1 and 2, OX1R and OX2R) are ubiquitously distributed centrally and in discrete peripheral locations (Cluderay *et al.*, 2002; Hervieu *et al.*, 2001; Johren *et al.*, 2001; Marcus *et al.*, 2001; Trivedi *et al.*, 1998). Of particular note, orexin receptors have been identified in human adipose tissue, and thus targeting orexin receptor-expressing adipose tissue may be an attractive therapeutic tool for metabolism-related pathologies including obesity and diabetes (Digby *et al.*, 2006). Despite the near concurrent location of orexin terminals and receptors, OX1R and OX2R are unequally distributed within central and peripheral sites (Cluderay *et al.*, 2002; Digby *et al.*, 2006; Hervieu *et al.*, 2001; Marcus *et al.*, 2001; Trivedi *et al.*, 1998). For instance, within discrete brain sites such as the locus coeruleus, OX1R is abundantly expressed while OX2R is relatively void. In contrast, OX2R is highly expressed in the hypothalamic paraventricular nucleus despite null expression of OX1R.

Unlike the expression patterns of prepro-orexin, orexin terminals, and their receptors, less is known regarding the mechanism of action or the intracellular signaling cascades following orexin receptor activation. Regarding the mechanism of action, it is clear that OX1R and OX2R have dissimilar affinity to OXA and OXB such that OX1R has 10-fold greater affinity for OXA relative to OXB, while OX2R appears to have equal affinity for OXA and OXB (Sakurai *et al.*, 1998). Although the significance of the dissimilar binding affinity is not readily apparent, the disparate behavioral effects of orexins on energy expenditure-related processes may uncover this physiological relevance. It is also clear that orexin receptor binding can activate various G-alpha subunit proteins including G_q, G_s, and $G_{i/o}$, which increases the complexity of understanding their signaling cascades (Bernard *et al.*, 2006; Holmqvist *et al.*, 2005; Karteris *et al.*, 2001, 2005; Randeva *et al.*, 2001). An early report documented that orexin receptor stimulation increased extracellular calcium influx (Ammoun *et al.*, 2003; van den Pol *et al.*, 1998). Further, neuronal excitation results from activation of L-type calcium channels (Kohlmeier *et al.*, 2004), T-type calcium channels (Zhang *et al.*, 2009), transient receptor potential cation channel subtypes C1 and C3 (Larsson *et al.*, 2005), nonselective cation channels (Yang and Ferguson, 2003), sodium–calcium exchange channel transporter (Burdakov *et al.*, 2003; Eriksson *et al.*, 2001), as well as the suppression of potassium conductance through G-protein inwardly rectifying potassium channels (Hoang *et al.*, 2003; Ivanov and Aston-Jones, 2000). Moreover, orexin stimulates release of glutamate and GABA (van den Pol *et al.*, 1998), and stimulation of orexin receptors by OXA and OXB activates p38 mitogen-activated phosphate kinase and extracellular signal-regulated kinases (ERK1/2) (Ammoun *et al.*, 2006; Tang *et al.*, 2008) by way of multiple signaling mechanisms. Moreover, orexin neurons are energy sensors sensitive to ATP levels (Liu *et al.*, 2011) and lactate (Parsons and Hirasawa, 2010) and have been differentially described based on synaptic input and their behavioral, morphological, and electrophysiological profile (Harris *et al.*, 2005; Horvath and Gao, 2005). A recent review suggests that orexin neurons function within a local network comprising both coexpressing neurotransmitters within orexin neurons (dynorphin, glutamate, nociceptin/orphanin FQ) as well as neurons devoid of orexin in the lateral hypothalamus that express melanin concentrating hormone, thyrotropin-releasing hormone, corticotropin-releasing hormone, neurotensin, galanin, and GABA (Burt *et al.*, 2011). Based on the mirrored distribution between orexin fibers and receptors, the multisynaptic input to the lateral hypothalamus and the local network within orexin neurons, it is not surprising that orexins mediate multiple physiological processes and their role as a physiological integrator could not be made more clear (de Lecea *et al.*, 1998; Sakurai *et al.*, 1998; Sutcliffe and de Lecea, 2000; Willie *et al.*, 2001).

A. Components of energy expenditure

Total energy expenditure can be partitioned into several components (D'Alessio *et al.*, 1988; Donahoo *et al.*, 2004; Joosen and Westerterp, 2006; Ravussin and Bogardus, 1992; Ravussin *et al.*, 1986). However, the relative contribution of each component to total energy expenditure is largely dependent upon the interindividual variability of each component. For example, energy expenditure from physical activity is the most variable (Ravussin *et al.*, 1986). The primary component of total energy expenditure comprising 60–70%, basal metabolism, is defined by the *Webster's Medical Dictionary* as "the turnover of energy in a fasting and resting organism using energy solely to maintain vital cellular activity, respiration, and circulation as measured by the basal metabolic rate" (BMR). Diet-induced thermogenesis, comprising 10–15% of total energy expenditure, is due to the energy required to digest, absorb, and store food. Adaptive thermogenesis or the energy required to thermoregulate and respond to changes in the environmental temperature comprises 10–15% of total energy expenditure. The final and most variable component of total energy expenditure, comprising 6–10%, is due to physical activity thermogenesis or the work derived from all forms of physical activity, postural maintenance, and muscular contraction. This includes both physical activity due to exercise and all other types of physical activity excluding exercise (e.g., spontaneous physical activity or nonexercise activity) (Levine *et al.*, 1999; Ravussin *et al.*, 1986).

B. Methodological considerations: Energy expenditure and sleep measurements in rodents in the context of obesity research

Orexin modulates food intake, BMR, physical activity, arousal, the sleep/wake cycle, and hormone regulation and thus has profound influences on energy expenditure. Therefore, it is important to reflect upon common methods currently used to measure energy expenditure, indirect calorimetry. With this method, rodents are placed in a calorimetry chamber and "reference" air of a known percentage of oxygen and carbon dioxide flows into the chamber. The rodent within the calorimetry chamber consumes oxygen and expires carbon dioxide, which combines with the air flowing into the chamber. Through periodic sampling, energy expenditure is calculated based on the difference between the percentage of oxygen and carbon dioxide between the reference and sampled air. Although indirect calorimetry is used to measure total energy expenditure, the method and analysis of energy expenditure are problematic when comparing energy expenditure in rodents within the context of obesity research (Arch *et al.*, 2006; Butler and Kozak, 2010; Rauh *et al.*, 1990). First, it is currently impossible to partition total energy expenditure into its relative components since an instantaneous change in basal metabolism, physical activity, temperature, or diet-induced thermogenesis cannot be detected in real time. Instead, BMR is commonly considered to be the lowest metabolic rate during the resting phase or derived from a series of metabolic rates with the lowest standard deviation during the resting phase for the animal. Adaptive thermogenesis is considered to be negligible at thermoneutral, which seems germane to consider when comparing energy expenditure between animals of varying body mass, surface area, and volume. Laboratory rodents are commonly housed at temperatures below their thermoneutral (Overton, 2010). Therefore, adaptive thermogenesis and BMR would be greater in rodents with smaller surfaces area to volume ratios. Thus, the derived or calculated BMR may overestimate the true BMR for small animals housed below thermoneutral in an indirect calorimeter, since the calculated BMR will include the energy required for adaptive thermogenesis. Also, while it is possible to measure physical activity and energy expenditure concurrently, physical activity-induced energy expenditure cannot be directly measured. Finally, the metabolic rate during sleep is reported infrequently in indirect calorimetry studies possibly due to the technical difficulties associated with quantifying and measuring sleep directly. Sleep can be classified broadly into rapid eye movement (REM) sleep and non-rapid eye movement (NREM or slow wave sleep (SWS)) sleep and each has distinct electrographic waveforms in electroencephalogram (EEG) and electromyogram (EMG) signals (Greene and Siegel, 2004). Quantification of sleep and wake first requires continuous recordings of EEG and EMG signals and then requires the EEG/EMG waveforms to be scored and classified as REM sleep, SWS, or wake. Pairing methodology to concurrently time stamp and differentiate sleep and wake states by EEG/EMG recordings and energy expenditure with indirect calorimetry would be an improvement over methods that estimate sleeping metabolic rate. Despite that pairing methodologies are imperfect, as mentioned previously, comparing patterns of sleep, wake, and energy expenditure in parallel will lead to a more accurate estimation of sleeping metabolic rate. This has physiological significance for human obesity given the effect of sleep deprivation on energy expenditure and body mass. Therefore, we focus on orexin modulation of total energy expenditure in addition to the components of energy expenditure including sympathetic outflow, thermoregulation, physical activity, and sleep; yet acknowledge that many neurotransmitter systems and neuropeptides contribute to the regulation of energy expenditure.

C. Total energy expenditure and metabolic rate

The earliest report of orexin modulation of total energy expenditure was reported shortly after their discovery (Lubkin and Stricker-Krongrad, 1998) and confirmed in later studies (Asakawa *et al.*, 2002; Semjonous *et al.*, 2009; Wang *et al.*, 2001). Mice with cannule directed toward the third ventricle were infused with a single dose of OXA in the light or dark phase among food-deprived or *ad libitum*-fed mice (Lubkin and Stricker-Krongrad, 1998). Interestingly, OXA stimulated metabolic rate and the duration of action was longer after the dark phase injection, suggesting that other components of energy expenditure may have been influenced. It is plausible that energy expenditure due to increased physical activity or sympathetic activity but not diet-induced thermogenesis contributed to the prolonged increase in BMR, since OXA stimulates both physical activity and sympathetic activity and the control-treated mice had greater food intake than the OXA-treated mice. As the site of action for an injectate infused into the brain ventricles is largely unknown, others tested the effects of OXA after infusion into specific brain sites to identify potential sites of action. Wang *et al.* found OXA stimulated whole body oxygen consumption in anesthetized rats after infusion into the arcuate nucleus only (Wang *et al.*, 2003). There was no increase after infusion into the locus coeruleus, paraventricular nucleus of thalamus or several hypothalamic nuclei including the medial preoptic area, paraventricular, dorsomedial, ventromedial, and the lateral hypothalamic area. In contrast, in awake freely moving rats, OXA increased whole body energy expenditure after infusion into the hypothalamic paraventricular nucleus (Kiwaki *et al.*, 2004; Novak *et al.*, 2006) and the lateral hypothalamus (Teske *et al.*, 2006). As physical activity would be absent in anesthetized rats, it is plausible that the positive effect of OXA on energy expenditure after infusion in the hypothalamic paraventricular nucleus and lateral hypothalamus in the latter studies may be due in part to increased energy expenditure associated with physical activity.

D. Components of total energy expenditure

1. Sympathetic outflow and thermoregulation

Orexin stimulates thermoregulatory and cardiovascular systems (Ferguson and Samson, 2003; Samson *et al.*, 2005; Shirasaka *et al.*, 2002; Szekely *et al.*, 2002), which would contribute to the increase in basal metabolism following central orexin noted previously. Orexin is largely sympathoexcitatory. Studies in rodents document orexin-stimulated elevations in blood pressure and heart rate (Chen *et al.*, 2000; Monda *et al.*, 2001; Samson *et al.*, 1999; Shirasaka *et al.*, 1999; Wang *et al.*, 2001) and sympathetic outflow indicated by increased renal sympathetic nerve activity, plasma epinephrine, noradrenaline release, and firing rate of sympathetic nerves (Hirota *et al.*, 2001; Matsumura *et al.*, 2001; Monda *et al.*, 2001, 2003, 2004; Shirasaka *et al.*, 1999). Despite that peripheral orexin receptors have been identified intravenous orexin infusion failed to increase heart rate (Chen *et al.*, 2000), which suggests that central sites of action such as the rostral ventrolateral medulla (Chen *et al.*, 2000), nucleus of the solitary tract (de Oliveira and Ciriello, 2003; Smith *et al.*, 2002), arcuate nucleus (Wang *et al.*, 2003), hypothalamic paraventricular nucleus (Sato-Suzuki *et al.*, 2002), and the diagonal band of Broca (Monda *et al.*, 2004) may be largely responsible for the tachycardic response since OXA readily transverses the blood–brain barrier (Kastin and Akerstrom, 1999). However, interestingly, both heart rate and blood pressure are increased after infusion into the rostral ventrolateral medulla (Chen *et al.*, 2000) and nucleus of the solitary tract (de Oliveira and Ciriello, 2003; Smith *et al.*, 2002). In contrast, OXA has been shown to have negative effects as OXA in the nucleus ambiguous (de Oliveira and Ciriello, 2003) and the subfornical organ reduced heart rate (Smith *et al.*, 2007), and OXA in the nucleus ambiguous (de Oliveira and Ciriello, 2003) had no effect on blood pressure but intra-subfornical organ OXA (Smith *et al.*, 2007) reduced blood pressure. The significance of the brain site of infusion is underscored by comparing the pressor and tachycardic response to OXA across brain sites.

Orexins role in thermoregulation is exemplified by the stimulatory effect of OXA on the interscapular brown adipose tissue (iBAT), a thermosensitive organ rich in uncoupling protein one, which is largely responsible for adaptive thermogenesis in rodents. Despite that iBAT is lacking in adult humans, the relevance of brown adipose tissue to human thermogenesis has been hotly debated and recent studies suggest relevance to human obesity (Sellayah *et al.*, 2011). Increased uncoupling protein one activity favors heat production rather than ATP production by shuttling protons across the inner mitochondrial membrane to dissipate the proton-motive force driving oxidative phosphorylation. Stimulation of sympathetic nerves innervating the iBAT stimulates colonic temperature, and cold exposure stimulates iBAT activity, which directly contrasts the effect of housing rodents above thermoneutral, which reduces iBAT activity. An early study demonstrated that OXA increased firing rate of sympathetic nerves innervating the iBAT (Monda *et al.*, 2001) and iBAT temperature (Monda *et al.*, 2001), both of which would be expected to increase thermogenesis and is consistent with OXA stimulation of colonic temperature (Monda *et al.*, 2001, 2004; Wang *et al.*, 2003; Zheng *et al.*, 2005). Recently, Morrison and colleagues proposed a neuroanatomical basis for OXA modulation of thermoregulation through the rostral raphe pallidus and lateral parapyramidal area, which are sites of BAT sympathetic premotor neurons. Orexin A injection into the rostral raphe pallidus and lateral parapyramidal area robustly increased iBAT sympathetic outflow, expired carbon dioxide and both core and iBAT temperature in anesthetized rats (Tupone *et al.*, 2011). Although this suggests that OXA-modulation of temperature does in fact increase energy expenditure, heart rate was also increased. Contrary to the stimulatory effect of OXA on thermoregulation, OXA failed to increase temperature after chronic infusion (Haynes *et al.*, 1999); however, it is plausible that the structural stability of OXA at body temperature may underlie this discrepancy. Thus, the cardiovascular, sympathetic, and thermoregulatory action of orexins support the stimulatory action of orexins on basal metabolism and total energy expenditure.

2. Physical activity

Physical activity contributes to energy expenditure and the promotion of physical activity by OXA is an irrefutable effect. Irrespective of the central site of microinfusion, OXA stimulates physical activity including locomotion, rearing, grooming, and burrowing behaviors after ventricular (Hagan *et al.*, 1999; Ida *et al.*, 1999) or intraparenchymal infusion. Further, a dose-dependent increase in physical activity is paralleled by elevated energy expenditure (Kiwaki *et al.*, 2004). While the magnitude of OXA-induced physical activity varies with respect to the location of the microinjection (Kotz *et al.*, 2008), the overall stimulatory effect remains consistent. Thus far, OXA infusion into the following brain sites has been shown to reliably stimulate physical activity: lateral hypothalamus, hypothalamic paraventricular nucleus, substantia nigra, tuberomammillary nucleus, dorsal raphe, nucleus accumbens, medial preoptic area, and locus coeruleus (Espana *et al.*, 2001; Kiwaki *et al.*, 2004; Kotz *et al.*, 2002, 2006, 2008; Novak and Levine, 2009; Novak *et al.*, 2006; Teske *et al.*, 2006, 2010; Thorpe and Kotz, 2005). Likewise, OXA infused into the medial preoptic area and medial septum elicits grooming (Espana *et al.*, 2001). Moreover, direct increases in muscle tone or EMG activity in specific muscles, which would be indicative of muscle tone, was observed following OXA microinfusion into the locus coeruleus (Kiyashchenko *et al.*, 2001), the alpha gigantocellular reticular nucleus in the medioventral medullary region (Mileykovskiy *et al.*, 2002), trigeminal motor nucleus, and hypoglossal motor nucleus (Peever *et al.*, 2003). Interestingly, orexin into the pontine inhibitory area (Kiyashchenko *et al.*, 2001) and the ventral gigantocellular reticular nucleus in the medioventral medullary region inhibited hindlimb muscle tone (Mileykovskiy *et al.*, 2002). Despite that inhibition of hindlimb muscle tone would seem to contraindicate the increases in physical activity after OXA, parallel activation and suppression of muscles in opposition are required for movement, which would be essential for normal locomotion.

3. Sleep

The role of orexin in sleep/wake regulation and subsequent influence on energy expenditure is exemplified in the pathological sleep condition narcolepsy due to the loss of orexin-containing neurons or orexin receptors in humans and animal models (Chemelli *et al.*, 1999; Lin *et al.*, 1999; Nishino *et al.*, 2000; Siegel, 1999). The symptomatology of narcolepsy, characterized by the inability to consolidate sleep or wake into long bouts, results in sleep fragmentation and sleep behavioral state instability (Mochizuki *et al.*, 2004; Nishino *et al.*, 2000; Sakurai, 2005; Willie *et al.*, 2003). These symptoms are dampened by exogenous OXA in narcoleptic animals (Mieda *et al.*, 2004), which highlights the importance of orexin in the maintenance and stabilization of sleep behavior.

Electrophysiological and molecular studies further support a role for orexin in the maintenance and stability of normal sleep and wakefulness. Orexin neurons display phasic firing patterns during wakefulness yet are silent during SWS (Lee *et al.*, 2005; Mileykovskiy *et al.*, 2005). In parallel, orexin levels display circadian rhythmicity and gradually increase in anticipation of the active phase and decrease prior to and during the rest phase (Fujiki *et al.*, 2001; Lee *et al.*, 2005; Yoshida *et al.*, 2001). Not surprisingly, orexin levels also increase following sleep deprivation (Allard *et al.*, 2007; Pedrazzoli *et al.*, 2004; Wu *et al.*, 2002). Orexin neuron activity during wakefulness is also modulated by the ascending arousal network including the sleep/wake regulating monoamines and acetylcholine (Li *et al.*, 2002; Saper *et al.*, 2010; Yamanaka *et al.*, 2003) such that aminergic and cholinergic arousal circuits sustain orexin cells during wake (Estabrooke *et al.*, 2001; Takahashi *et al.*, 2008). These circuits in turn send inhibitory input to the ventrolateral preoptic area sleep-active neurons of the hypothalamus, and thereby further maintain wakefulness (Gallopin *et al.*, 2000). Interestingly, orexin neurons also promote wake by actively hindering REM sleep by inhibiting the oral pontine reticular nucleus, a structure involved in the generation of REM sleep (Nunez *et al.*, 2006). Thus, the absence of orexin results in reduced activity throughout the arousal network and culminates in an inappropriately low threshold for the transition into sleep from wake, which results in narcolepsy characterized by behavioral instability.

Orexins essential role in maintaining and stabilizing wake is consistent with previously mentioned actions of orexins, including the stimulation of total energy expenditure by promoting elevations in physical activity, body temperature, and sympathetic outflow. One of the earliest investigations on sleep found that between SWS and REM sleep, oxygen consumption was lowest during SWS and highest during REM sleep (Brebbia and Altshuler, 1965). Interestingly, studies in narcoleptic animals and humans suggest that narcolepsy-associated weight gain may be primarily due to reduced availability of orexin and behavioral instability, rather than hypersomnia (excessive active period sleep), as patients with idiopathic hypersomnia had a lower body weight (Kok *et al.*, 2003). Like humans, mice lacking orexin weighed more than wild-type mice, yet they had reduced energy intake and physical activity (Hara *et al.*, 2001). Thus, reduced metabolic rate and energy expenditure resulting from the absence of long wake bouts likely contributes to the increased body weight in orexin-deficient humans and animals. Furthermore, behavioral studies show that orexin antagonism increases sleep fragmentation (Beuckmann *et al.*, 2004; Brisbare-Roch *et al.*, 2007; Chen *et al.*, 2006; Gerashchenko *et al.*, 2001, 2003; Llewellyn-Smith *et al.*, 2003; Thakkar *et al.*, 1999) while central administration of OXA increases arousal and wakefulness and reduces both NREM and REM sleep (Bourgin *et al.*, 2000; Espana *et al.*, 2001; Hagan *et al.*, 1999; John *et al.*, 2000; Methippara *et al.*, 2000; Piper *et al.*, 2000; Rodgers *et al.*, 2002; Xi *et al.*, 2001), which is blunted by preinfusion with the OX1R antagonist SB 334867 (Smith *et al.*, 2003). In a parallel manner, optogenetic silencing of orexin neurons induces SWS (Tsunematsu *et al.*, 2011), while optogenetic activation of orexin neurons prompts mice to wake from sleep (Adamantidis *et al.*, 2007; Carter *et al.*, 2009). Thus, several studies highlight the importance of orexin in sleep/wake and observations from persons with narcolepsy and animals models of narcolepsy underscore its physiological significance.

Apart from the stimulating energy expenditure by promoting wake and activity, orexin modulates body temperature during sleep (Mochizuki *et al.*, 2006). Orexin may have indirect effects on sleep and thermoregulation as OXA-induced physical activity during the day may increase body temperature and the accumulation of metabolic end products that promote sleep and heat loss in a circadian manner (Alam *et al.*, 1996; McGinty and Szymusiak, 2001). At the neural level, orexin neurons reciprocally innervate the preoptic area, which promotes sleep and heat loss (Alam *et al.*, 1995;

Kumar, 2004) and thermal stimuli to the preoptic area strongly modulates sleep propensity and EEG delta activity (Kumar, 2004). Orexin terminals project to critical thermoregulatory brain sites including the tuberomammillary neurons, locus coeruleus, basal forebrain, pontine inhibitory area dorsomedial hypothalamus, ventromedial hypothalamus, posterior hypothalamus, periaqueductal gray, dorsal raphe nucleus, and intermediolateral column of the spinal cord (Kornum *et al.*, 2011; Mochizuki *et al.*, 2006). Thus, orexins are neuroanatomically positioned to modulate thermoregulation and contribute to heat loss during sleep (Ohno and Sakurai, 2008).

Overall heat loss, due to reduced production and increased loss, is an essential aspect of sleep (Mochizuki *et al.*, 2006), which underscores the energy conservation function proposed for sleep. Circadian modulation of body temperature may also alter sleep propensity (Kumar, 2004), which would be expected to have energetic consequences. In parallel, a moderate fall in body temperature may be necessary for good-quality sleep (Gilbert *et al.*, 2004). When compared to persons with normal sleep quality, the normal decline in body temperature is blunted in individuals with poor sleep quality (Lushington *et al.*, 2000; Pierangeli *et al.*, 2001; Zepelin and McDonald, 1987). Thus, it is feasible that altered thermoregulation also contributes to sleep fragmentation in narcolepsy (Mochizuki *et al.*, 2006). Indeed, Mochizuki *et al.* showed parallel 24 h rhythms of physical activity, wake and body temperature in wild-type mice (Mochizuki *et al.*, 2006). This demonstrates an association between vigilance states and energy expenditure, which was less prominent in orexin knockout mice. Importantly, while both wild-type and orexin knockout mice exhibited declines in body temperature during sleep, temperature declined to a lesser extent during sleep in orexin knockout mice. Likewise, elevations in body temperature during active wake were minor in orexin knockout mice compared the elevations in wild-type mice. Hence, the blunted decline in body temperature may be due to the intermittent awakenings during sleep (Mochizuki *et al.*, 2006) while the dampened increase in body temperature may be due to shorter wake bouts and physical activity during wake in the orexin knockout mice (Mochizuki *et al.*, 2004). In sum, these data reiterate a role for orexin in heat loss during sleep, possibly through sleep stabilization (Mochizuki *et al.*, 2006).

It is plausible that orexin effects on sleep/wake are also modulated by the autonomic nervous system. During wake, orexin inhibits the heat loss-inducing parasympathetic nervous system (Dergacheva *et al.*, 2005) and promotes sympathetic nervous system activity. In contrast, during sleep, orexin neuron activity and orexin levels are low while parasympathetic activity predominates (Kuo *et al.*, 2008). As noted above, exogenous orexin activates the sympathetic nervous system and orexin injection into the raphe pallidus increases sympathetic outflow to the brown adipose tissue, which increases thermogenesis (Morrison and Nakamura, 2011; Tupone *et al.*, 2011). Conversely, mice lacking orexin have impaired brown adipose tissue thermogenesis (Sellayah *et al.*, 2011; Vijgen *et al.*, 2011). Thus, these data imply that orexin potently enhances energy expenditure, via stimulation of sympathetic activation and suppression of parasympathetic activity.

II. Conclusion

Orexins provide a crucial link between energy balance and arousal. The orexin neurons functionally interact with neural pathways for physical activity pathways and sleep and cardiovascular and temperature regulatory centers in the brain, which positions orexin neurons to coordinate energy expenditure and the sleep–wake cycle. Corollary to this, obesity in humans and animal models is associated with altered sleep, reduced physical activity, and plasma and hypothalamic levels of orexin, whereas weight loss is associated with increased orexin levels in the plasma and improved sleep quality. These studies suggest that reduced component-specific energy expenditure due to lack of physical activity may culminate in weight gain in narcoleptic and obese humans as well as in orexin-deficient animals. Thus, the orexin system may act as a sensor for metabolism and send signals to intra- and extrahypothalamic targets to modify behavioral outputs based on energy needs.

References

Adamantidis, A. R., Zhang, F., Aravanis, A. M., Deisseroth, K., and de Lecea, L. (2007). Neural substrates of awakening probed with optogenetic control of hypocretin neurons. *Nature* **450,** 420–424.

Alam, M. N., McGinty, D., and Szymusiak, R. (1995). Neuronal discharge of preoptic/anterior hypothalamic thermosensitive neurons: Relation to NREM sleep. *Am. J. Physiol.* **269,** R1240–R1249.

Alam, M. N., McGinty, D., and Szymusiak, R. (1996). Preoptic/anterior hypothalamic neurons: Thermosensitivity in wakefulness and non rapid eye movement sleep. *Brain Res.* **718,** 76–82.

Allard, J. S., Tizabi, Y., Shaffery, J. P., and Manaye, K. (2007). Effects of rapid eye movement sleep deprivation on hypocretin neurons in the hypothalamus of a rat model of depression. *Neuropeptides* **41,** 329–337.

Ammoun, S., Holmqvist, T., Shariatmadari, R., Oonk, H. B., Detheux, M., Parmentier, M., Akerman, K. E., and Kukkonen, J. P. (2003). Distinct recognition of OX1 and OX2 receptors by orexin peptides. *J. Pharmacol. Exp. Ther.* **305,** 507–514.

Ammoun, S., Lindholm, D., Wootz, H., Akerman, K. E., and Kukkonen, J. P. (2006). G-protein-coupled OX1 orexin/hcrtr-1 hypocretin receptors induce caspase-dependent and -independent cell death through p38 mitogen-/stress-activated protein kinase. *J. Biol. Chem.* **281,** 834–842.

Arch, J. R., Hislop, D., Wang, S. J., and Speakman, J. R. (2006). Some mathematical and technical issues in the measurement and interpretation of open-circuit indirect calorimetry in small animals. *Int. J. Obes. (Lond.)* **30,** 1322–1331.

Asakawa, A., Inui, A., Goto, K., Yuzuriha, H., Takimoto, Y., Inui, T., Katsuura, G., Fujino, M. A., Meguid, M. M., and Kasuga, M. (2002). Effects of agouti-related protein, orexin and melanin-concentrating hormone on oxygen consumption in mice. *Int. J. Mol. Med.* **10,** 523–525.

Bernard, R., Lydic, R., and Baghdoyan, H. A. (2006). Hypocretin (orexin) receptor subtypes differentially enhance acetylcholine release and activate g protein subtypes in rat pontine reticular formation. *J. Pharmacol. Exp. Ther.* **317,** 163–171.

Beuckmann, C. T., Sinton, C. M., Williams, S. C., Richardson, J. A., Hammer, R. E., Sakurai, T., and Yanagisawa, M. (2004). Expression of a poly-glutamine-ataxin-3 transgene in orexin neurons induces narcolepsy-cataplexy in the rat. *J. Neurosci.* **24,** 4469–4477.

Bourgin, P., Huitron-Resendiz, S., Spier, A. D., Fabre, V., Morte, B., Criado, J. R., Sutcliffe, J. G., Henriksen, S. J., and de Lecea, L. (2000). Hypocretin-1 modulates rapid eye movement sleep through activation of locus coeruleus neurons. *J. Neurosci.* **20,** 7760–7765.

Brebbia, D. R., and Altshuler, K. Z. (1965). Oxygen consumption rate and electroencephalographic stage of sleep. *Science* **150,** 1621–1623.

Brisbare-Roch, C., Dingemanse, J., Koberstein, R., Hoever, P., Aissaoui, H., Flores, S., Mueller, C., Nayler, O., van Gerven, J., de Haas, S. L., Hess, P., Qiu, C., *et al.* (2007). Promotion of sleep by targeting the orexin system in rats, dogs and humans. *Nat. Med.* **13,** 150–155.

Burdakov, D., Liss, B., and Ashcroft, F. M. (2003). Orexin excites GABAergic neurons of the arcuate nucleus by activating the sodium–calcium exchanger. *J. Neurosci.* **23,** 4951–4957.

Burt, J., Alberto, C. O., Parsons, M. P., and Hirasawa, M. (2011). Local network regulation of orexin neurons in the lateral hypothalamus. *Am. J. Physiol. Regul. Integr. Comp. Physiol.* **301,** R572–R580.

Butler, A. A., and Kozak, L. P. (2010). A recurring problem with the analysis of energy expenditure in genetic models expressing lean and obese phenotypes. *Diabetes* **59,** 323–329.

Carter, M. E., Adamantidis, A., Ohtsu, H., Deisseroth, K., and de Lecea, L. (2009). Sleep homeostasis modulates hypocretin-mediated sleep-to-wake transitions. *J. Neurosci.* **29,** 10939–10949.

Chemelli, R. M., Willie, J. T., Sinton, C. M., Elmquist, J. K., Scammell, T., Lee, C., Richardson, J. A., Williams, S. C., Xiong, Y., Kisanuki, Y., Fitch, T. E., Nakazato, M., *et al.* (1999). Narcolepsy in orexin knockout mice: Molecular genetics of sleep regulation. *Cell* **98,** 437–451.

Chen, C. T., Dun, S. L., Kwok, E. H., Dun, N. J., and Chang, J. K. (1999). Orexin A-like immunoreactivity in the rat brain. *Neurosci. Lett.* **260,** 161–164.

Chen, C. T., Hwang, L. L., Chang, J. K., and Dun, N. J. (2000). Pressor effects of orexins injected intracisternally and to rostral ventrolateral medulla of anesthetized rats. *Am. J. Physiol. Regul. Integr. Comp. Physiol.* **278,** R692–R697.

Chen, L., Thakkar, M. M., Winston, S., Bolortuya, Y., Basheer, R., and McCarley, R. W. (2006). REM sleep changes in rats induced by siRNA-mediated orexin knockdown. *Eur. J. Neurosci.* **24,** 2039–2048.

Cluderay, J. E., Harrison, D. C., and Hervieu, G. J. (2002). Protein distribution of the orexin-2 receptor in the rat central nervous system. *Regul. Pept.* **104,** 131–144.

Cutler, D. J., Morris, R., Sheridhar, V., Wattam, T. A., Holmes, S., Patel, S., Arch, J. R., Wilson, S., Buckingham, R. E., Evans, M. L., Leslie, R. A., and Williams, G. (1999). Differential distribution of orexin-A and orexin-B immunoreactivity in the rat brain and spinal cord. *Peptides* **20,** 1455–1470.

D'Alessio, D. A., Kavle, E. C., Mozzoli, M. A., Smalley, K. J., Polansky, M., Kendrick, Z. V., Owen, L. R., Bushman, M. C., Boden, G., and Owen, O. E. (1988). Thermic effect of food in lean and obese men. *J. Clin. Invest.* **81,** 1781–1789.

Date, Y., Mondal, M. S., Matsukura, S., and Nakazato, M. (2000). Distribution of orexin-A and orexin-B (hypocretins) in the rat spinal cord. *Neurosci. Lett.* **288,** 87–90.

de Lecea, L., Kilduff, T. S., Peyron, C., Gao, X., Foye, P. E., Danielson, P. E., Fukuhara, C., Battenberg, E. L., Gautvik, V. T., Bartlett, F. S., 2nd, Frankel, W. N., van den Pol, A. N., *et al.* (1998). The hypocretins: Hypothalamus-specific peptides with neuroexcitatory activity. *Proc. Natl. Acad. Sci. U. S. A.* **95,** 322–327.

de Oliveira, C. V., and Ciriello, J. (2003). Cardiovascular responses to hypocretin-1 in nucleus ambiguus of the ovariectomized female rat. *Brain Res.* **986,** 148–156.

Dergacheva, O., Wang, X., Huang, Z. G., Bouairi, E., Stephens, C., Gorini, C., and Mendelowitz, D. (2005). Hypocretin-1 (orexin-A) facilitates inhibitory and diminishes excitatory synaptic pathways to cardiac vagal neurons in the nucleus ambiguus. *J. Pharmacol. Exp. Ther.* **314,** 1322–1327.

Digby, J. E., Chen, J., Tang, J. Y., Lehnert, H., Matthews, R. N., and Randeva, H. S. (2006). Orexin receptor expression in human adipose tissue: Effects of orexin-A and orexin-B. *J. Endocrinol.* **191,** 129–136.

Donahoo, W. T., Levine, J. A., and Melanson, E. L. (2004). Variability in energy expenditure and its components. *Curr. Opin. Clin. Nutr. Metab. Care* **7,** 599–605.

Eriksson, K. S., Sergeeva, O., Brown, R. E., and Haas, H. L. (2001). Orexin/hypocretin excites the histaminergic neurons of the tuberomammillary nucleus. *J. Neurosci.* **21,** 9273–9279.

Espana, R. A., Baldo, B. A., Kelley, A. E., and Berridge, C. W. (2001). Wake-promoting and sleep-suppressing actions of hypocretin (orexin): Basal forebrain sites of action. *Neuroscience* **106,** 699–715.

Estabrooke, I. V., McCarthy, M. T., Ko, E., Chou, T. C., Chemelli, R. M., Yanagisawa, M., Saper, C. B., and Scammell, T. E. (2001). Fos expression in orexin neurons varies with behavioral state. *J. Neurosci.* **21,** 1656–1662.

Ferguson, A. V., and Samson, W. K. (2003). The orexin/hypocretin system: A critical regulator of neuroendocrine and autonomic function. *Front. Neuroendocrinol.* **24,** 141–150.

Fujiki, N., Yoshida, Y., Ripley, B., Honda, K., Mignot, E., and Nishino, S. (2001). Changes in CSF hypocretin-1 (orexin A) levels in rats across 24 hours and in response to food deprivation. *Neuroreport* **12,** 993–997.

Gallopin, T., Fort, P., Eggermann, E., Cauli, B., Luppi, P. H., Rossier, J., Audinat, E., Muhlethaler, M., and Serafin, M. (2000). Identification of sleep-promoting neurons in vitro. *Nature* **404,** 992–995.

Gautvik, K. M., de Lecea, L., Gautvik, V. T., Danielson, P. E., Tranque, P., Dopazo, A., Bloom, F. E., and Sutcliffe, J. G. (1996). Overview of the most prevalent hypothalamus-specific mRNAs, as identified by directional tag PCR subtraction. *Proc. Natl. Acad. Sci. U. S. A.* **93,** 8733–8738.

Gerashchenko, D., Kohls, M. D., Greco, M., Waleh, N. S., Salin-Pascual, R., Kilduff, T. S., Lappi, D. A., and Shiromani, P. J. (2001). Hypocretin-2-saporin lesions of the lateral hypothalamus produce narcoleptic-like sleep behavior in the rat. *J. Neurosci.* **21,** 7273–7283.

Gerashchenko, D., Blanco-Centurion, C., Greco, M. A., and Shiromani, P. J. (2003). Effects of lateral hypothalamic lesion with the neurotoxin hypocretin-2-saporin on sleep in Long-Evans rats. *Neuroscience* **116,** 223–235.

Gilbert, S. S., van den Heuvel, C. J., Ferguson, S. A., and Dawson, D. (2004). Thermoregulation as a sleep signalling system. *Sleep Med. Rev.* **8,** 81–93.

Greene, R., and Siegel, J. (2004). Sleep: A functional enigma. *Neuromolecular Med.* **5,** 59–68.

Hagan, J. J., Leslie, R. A., Patel, S., Evans, M. L., Wattam, T. A., Holmes, S., Benham, C. D., Taylor, S. G., Routledge, C., Hemmati, P., Munton, R. P., Ashmeade, T. E., *et al.* (1999). Orexin A activates locus coeruleus cell firing and increases arousal in the rat. *Proc. Natl. Acad. Sci. U. S. A.* **96,** 10911–10916.

Hara, J., Beuckmann, C. T., Nambu, T., Willie, J. T., Chemelli, R. M., Sinton, C. M., Sugiyama, F., Yagami, K., Goto, K., Yanagisawa, M., and Sakurai, T. (2001). Genetic ablation of orexin neurons in mice results in narcolepsy, hypophagia, and obesity. *Neuron* **30,** 345–354.

Harris, G. C., Wimmer, M., and Aston-Jones, G. (2005). A role for lateral hypothalamic orexin neurons in reward seeking. *Nature* **437,** 556–559.

Haynes, A. C., Jackson, B., Overend, P., Buckingham, R. E., Wilson, S., Tadayyon, M., and Arch, J. R. (1999). Effects of single and chronic intracerebroventricular administration of the orexins on feeding in the rat. *Peptides* **20,** 1099–1105.

Hervieu, G. J., Cluderay, J. E., Harrison, D. C., Roberts, J. C., and Leslie, R. A. (2001). Gene expression and protein distribution of the orexin-1 receptor in the rat brain and spinal cord. *Neuroscience* **103,** 777–797.

Hirota, K., Kushikata, T., Kudo, M., Kudo, T., Lambert, D. G., and Matsuki, A. (2001). Orexin A and B evoke noradrenaline release from rat cerebrocortical slices. *Br. J. Pharmacol.* **134,** 1461–1466.

Hoang, Q. V., Bajic, D., Yanagisawa, M., Nakajima, S., and Nakajima, Y. (2003). Effects of orexin (hypocretin) on GIRK channels. *J. Neurophysiol.* **90,** 693–702.

Holmqvist, T., Johansson, L., Ostman, M., Ammoun, S., Akerman, K. E., and Kukkonen, J. P. (2005). OX1 orexin receptors couple to adenylyl cyclase regulation via multiple mechanisms. *J. Biol. Chem.* **280,** 6570–6579.

Horvath, T. L., and Gao, X. B. (2005). Input organization and plasticity of hypocretin neurons: Possible clues to obesity's association with insomnia. *Cell Metab.* **1,** 279–286.

Ida, T., Nakahara, K., Katayama, T., Murakami, N., and Nakazato, M. (1999). Effect of lateral cerebroventricular injection of the appetite-stimulating neuropeptide, orexin and neuropeptide Y, on the various behavioral activities of rats. *Brain Res.* **821,** 526–529.

Ivanov, A., and Aston-Jones, G. (2000). Hypocretin/orexin depolarizes and decreases potassium conductance in locus coeruleus neurons. *Neuroreport* **11,** 1755–1758.

John, J., Wu, M. F., and Siegel, J. M. (2000). Systemic administration of hypocretin-1 reduces cataplexy and normalizes sleep and waking durations in narcoleptic dogs. *Sleep Res. Online* **3,** 23–28.

Johren, O., Neidert, S. J., Kummer, M., Dendorfer, A., and Dominiak, P. (2001). Prepro-orexin and orexin receptor mRNAs are differentially expressed in peripheral tissues of male and female rats. *Endocrinology* **142,** 3324–3331.

Joosen, A. M., and Westerterp, K. R. (2006). Energy expenditure during overfeeding. *Nutr. Metab.* **3,** 25.

Karteris, E., Randeva, H. S., Grammatopoulos, D. K., Jaffe, R. B., and Hillhouse, E. W. (2001). Expression and coupling characteristics of the CRH and orexin type 2 receptors in human fetal adrenals. *J. Clin. Endocrinol. Metab.* **86,** 4512–4519.

Karteris, E., Machado, R. J., Chen, J., Zervou, S., Hillhouse, E. W., and Randeva, H. S. (2005). Food deprivation differentially modulates orexin receptor expression and signaling in rat hypothalamus and adrenal cortex. *Am. J. Physiol. Endocrinol. Metab.* **288,** E1089–E1100.

Kastin, A. J., and Akerstrom, V. (1999). Orexin A but not orexin B rapidly enters brain from blood by simple diffusion. *J. Pharmacol. Exp. Ther.* **289,** 219–223.

Kiwaki, K., Kotz, C. M., Wang, C., Lanningham-Foster, L., and Levine, J. A. (2004). Orexin A (hypocretin 1) injected into hypothalamic paraventricular nucleus and spontaneous physical activity in rats. *Am. J. Physiol. Endocrinol. Metab.* **286,** E551–E559.

Kiyashchenko, L. I., Mileykovskiy, B. Y., Lai, Y. Y., and Siegel, J. M. (2001). Increased and decreased muscle tone with orexin (hypocretin) microinjections in the locus coeruleus and pontine inhibitory area. *J. Neurophysiol.* **85,** 2008–2016.

Kohlmeier, K. A., Inoue, T., and Leonard, C. S. (2004). Hypocretin/orexin peptide signaling in the ascending arousal system: Elevation of intracellular calcium in the mouse dorsal raphe and laterodorsal tegmentum. *J. Neurophysiol.* **92,** 221–235.

Kok, S. W., Overeem, S., Visscher, T. L., Lammers, G. J., Seidell, J. C., Pijl, H., and Meinders, A. E. (2003). Hypocretin deficiency in narcoleptic humans is associated with abdominal obesity. *Obes. Res.* **11,** 1147–1154.

Kornum, B. R., Faraco, J., and Mignot, E. (2011). Narcolepsy with hypocretin/orexin deficiency, infections and autoimmunity of the brain. *Curr. Opin. Neurobiol.* **21,** 897–903.

Kotz, C. M., Teske, J. A., Levine, J. A., and Wang, C. (2002). Feeding and activity induced by orexin A in the lateral hypothalamus in rats. *Regul. Pept.* **104,** 27–32.

Kotz, C. M., Wang, C., Teske, J. A., Thorpe, A. J., Novak, C. M., Kiwaki, K., and Levine, J. A. (2006). Orexin A mediation of time spent moving in rats: Neural mechanisms. *Neuroscience* **142,** 29–36.

Kotz, C. M., Teske, J. A., and Billington, C. J. (2008). Neuroregulation of nonexercise activity thermogenesis and obesity resistance. *Am. J. Physiol. Regul. Integr. Comp. Physiol.* **294,** R699–R710.

Kumar, V. M. (2004). Why the medial preoptic area is important for sleep regulation. *Indian J. Physiol. Pharmacol.* **48,** 137–149.

Kuo, T. B., Shaw, F. Z., Lai, C. J., and Yang, C. C. (2008). Asymmetry in sympathetic and vagal activities during sleep-wake transitions. *Sleep* **31,** 311–320.

Larsson, K. P., Peltonen, H. M., Bart, G., Louhivuori, L. M., Penttonen, A., Antikainen, M., Kukkonen, J. P., and Akerman, K. E. (2005). Orexin-A-induced Ca^{2+} entry: Evidence for involvement of trpc channels and protein kinase C regulation. *J. Biol. Chem.* **280,** 1771–1781.

Lee, M. G., Hassani, O. K., and Jones, B. E. (2005). Discharge of identified orexin/hypocretin neurons across the sleep-waking cycle. *J. Neurosci.* **25,** 6716–6720.

Levine, J. A., Eberhardt, N. L., and Jensen, M. D. (1999). Role of nonexercise activity thermogenesis in resistance to fat gain in humans. *Science* **283,** 212–214.

Li, Y., Gao, X. B., Sakurai, T., and van den Pol, A. N. (2002). Hypocretin/orexin excites hypocretin neurons via a local glutamate neuron-A potential mechanism for orchestrating the hypothalamic arousal system. *Neuron* **36,** 1169–1181.

Lin, L., Faraco, J., Li, R., Kadotani, H., Rogers, W., Lin, X., Qiu, X., de Jong, P. J., Nishino, S., and Mignot, E. (1999). The sleep disorder canine narcolepsy is caused by a mutation in the hypocretin (orexin) receptor 2 gene. *Cell* **98,** 365–376.

Liu, Z. W., Gan, G., Suyama, S., and Gao, X. B. (2011). Intracellular energy status regulates activity in hypocretin/orexin neurones: A link between energy and behavioural states. *J. Physiol.* **589,** 4157–4166.

Llewellyn-Smith, I. J., Martin, C. L., Marcus, J. N., Yanagisawa, M., Minson, J. B., and Scammell, T. E. (2003). Orexin-immunoreactive inputs to rat sympathetic preganglionic neurons. *Neurosci. Lett.* **351,** 115–119.

Lubkin, M., and Stricker-Krongrad, A. (1998). Independent feeding and metabolic actions of orexins in mice. *Biochem. Biophys. Res. Commun.* **253,** 241–245.

Lushington, K., Dawson, D., and Lack, L. (2000). Core body temperature is elevated during constant wakefulness in elderly poor sleepers. *Sleep* **23,** 504–510.

Marcus, J. N., Aschkenasi, C. J., Lee, C. E., Chemelli, R. M., Saper, C. B., Yanagisawa, M., and Elmquist, J. K. (2001). Differential expression of orexin receptors 1 and 2 in the rat brain. *J. Comp. Neurol.* **435,** 6–25.

Matsumura, K., Tsuchihashi, T., and Abe, I. (2001). Central orexin-A augments sympathoadrenal outflow in conscious rabbits. *Hypertension* **37,** 1382–1387.

McGinty, D., and Szymusiak, R. (2001). Brain structures and mechanisms involved in the generation of NREM sleep: Focus on the preoptic hypothalamus. *Sleep Med. Rev.* **5,** 323–342.

Methippara, M. M., Alam, M. N., Szymusiak, R., and McGinty, D. (2000). Effects of lateral preoptic area application of orexin-A on sleep-wakefulness. *Neuroreport* **11,** 3423–3426.

Mieda, M., Willie, J. T., Hara, J., Sinton, C. M., Sakurai, T., and Yanagisawa, M. (2004). Orexin peptides prevent cataplexy and improve wakefulness in an orexin neuron-ablated model of narcolepsy in mice. *Proc. Natl. Acad. Sci. U. S. A.* **101,** 4649–4654.

Mileykovskiy, B. Y., Kiyashchenko, L. I., and Siegel, J. M. (2002). Muscle tone facilitation and inhibition after orexin-a (hypocretin-1) microinjections into the medial medulla. *J. Neurophysiol.* **87,** 2480–2489.

Mileykovskiy, B. Y., Kiyashchenko, L. I., and Siegel, J. M. (2005). Behavioral correlates of activity in identified hypocretin/orexin neurons. *Neuron* **46,** 787–798.

Mochizuki, T., Crocker, A., McCormack, S., Yanagisawa, M., Sakurai, T., and Scammell, T. E. (2004). Behavioral state instability in orexin knock-out mice. *J. Neurosci.* **24,** 6291–6300.

Mochizuki, T., Klerman, E. B., Sakurai, T., and Scammell, T. E. (2006). Elevated body temperature during sleep in orexin knockout mice. *Am. J. Physiol. Regul. Integr. Comp. Physiol.* **291,** R533–R540.

Monda, M., Viggiano, A., Mondola, P., and De Luca, V. (2001). Inhibition of prostaglandin synthesis reduces hyperthermic reactions induced by hypocretin-1/orexin A. *Brain Res.* **909,** 68–74.

Monda, M., Viggiano, A., and De Luca, V. (2003). Paradoxical [correction of parodoxical] effect of orexin A: Hypophagia induced by hyperthermia. *Brain Res.* **961,** 220–228.

Monda, M., Viggiano, A., Viggiano, A., Fuccio, F., and De Luca, V. (2004). Injection of orexin A into the diagonal band of Broca induces sympathetic and hyperthermic reactions. *Brain Res.* **1018,** 265–271.

Morrison, S. F., and Nakamura, K. (2011). Central neural pathways for thermoregulation. *Front. Biosci.* **16,** 74–104.

Nambu, T., Sakurai, T., Mizukami, K., Hosoya, Y., Yanagisawa, M., and Goto, K. (1999). Distribution of orexin neurons in the adult rat brain. *Brain Res.* **827,** 243–260.

Nishino, S., Ripley, B., Overeem, S., Lammers, G. J., and Mignot, E. (2000). Hypocretin (orexin) deficiency in human narcolepsy. *Lancet* **355,** 39–40.

Novak, C. M., and Levine, J. A. (2009). Daily intraparaventricular orexin-A treatment induces weight loss in rats. *Obesity (Silver Spring)* **17,** 1493–1498.

Novak, C. M., Kotz, C. M., and Levine, J. A. (2006). Central orexin sensitivity, physical activity, and obesity in diet-induced obese and diet-resistant rats. *Am. J. Physiol. Endocrinol. Metab.* **290,** E396–E403.

Nunez, A., Moreno-Balandran, M. E., Rodrigo-Angulo, M. L., Garzon, M., and De Andres, I. (2006). Relationship between the perifornical hypothalamic area and oral pontine reticular nucleus in the rat. Possible implication of the hypocretinergic projection in the control of rapid eye movement sleep. *Eur. J. Neurosci.* **24,** 2834–2842.

Ohno, K., and Sakurai, T. (2008). Orexin neuronal circuitry: Role in the regulation of sleep and wakefulness. *Front. Neuroendocrinol.* **29,** 70–87.

Overton, J. M. (2010). Phenotyping small animals as models for the human metabolic syndrome: Thermoneutrality matters. *Int. J. Obes. (Lond.)* **34**(Suppl. 2), S53–S58.

Parsons, M. P., and Hirasawa, M. (2010). ATP-sensitive potassium channel-mediated lactate effect on orexin neurons: Implications for brain energetics during arousal. *J. Neurosci.* **30,** 8061–8070.

Pedrazzoli, M., D'Almeida, V., Martins, P. J., Machado, R. B., Ling, L., Nishino, S., Tufik, S., and Mignot, E. (2004). Increased hypocretin-1 levels in cerebrospinal fluid after REM sleep deprivation. *Brain Res.* **995,** 1–6.

Peever, J. H., Lai, Y. Y., and Siegel, J. M. (2003). Excitatory effects of hypocretin-1 (orexin-A) in the trigeminal motor nucleus are reversed by NMDA antagonism. *J. Neurophysiol.* **89,** 2591–2600.

Peyron, C., Tighe, D. K., van den Pol, A. N., de Lecea, L., Heller, H. C., Sutcliffe, J. G., and Kilduff, T. S. (1998). Neurons containing hypocretin (orexin) project to multiple neuronal systems. *J. Neurosci.* **18,** 9996–10015.

Pierangeli, G., Provini, F., Maltoni, P., Barletta, G., Contin, M., Lugaresi, E., Montagna, P., and Cortelli, P. (2001). Nocturnal body core temperature falls in Parkinson's disease but not in Multiple-System Atrophy. *Mov. Disord.* **16,** 226–232.

Piper, D. C., Upton, N., Smith, M. I., and Hunter, A. J. (2000). The novel brain neuropeptide, orexin-A, modulates the sleep-wake cycle of rats. *Eur. J. Neurosci.* **12,** 726–730.

Randeva, H. S., Karteris, E., Grammatopoulos, D., and Hillhouse, E. W. (2001). Expression of orexin-A and functional orexin type 2 receptors in the human adult adrenals: Implications for adrenal function and energy homeostasis. *J. Clin. Endocrinol. Metab.* **86,** 4808–4813.

Rauh, R. A., Senior, D. G., and Miller, W. P. (1990). Delayed complete heart block complicating percutaneous transluminal coronary angioplasty. *Am. Heart J.* **120,** 972–975.

Ravussin, E., and Bogardus, C. (1992). A brief overview of human energy metabolism and its relationship to essential obesity. *Am. J. Clin. Nutr.* **55,** 242S–245S.

Ravussin, E., Lillioja, S., Anderson, T. E., Christin, L., and Bogardus, C. (1986). Determinants of 24-hour energy expenditure in man. Methods and results using a respiratory chamber. *J. Clin. Invest.* **78,** 1568–1578.

Rodgers, R. J., Ishii, Y., Halford, J. C., and Blundell, J. E. (2002). Orexins and appetite regulation. *Neuropeptides* **36,** 303–325.

Sakurai, T. (2005). Reverse pharmacology of orexin: From an orphan GPCR to integrative physiology. *Regul. Pept.* **126,** 3–10.

Sakurai, T., Amemiya, A., Ishii, M., Matsuzaki, I., Chemelli, R. M., Tanaka, H., Williams, S. C., Richardson, J. A., Kozlowski, G. P., Wilson, S., Arch, J. R., Buckingham, R. E., *et al.* (1998). Orexins and orexin receptors: A family of hypothalamic neuropeptides and G protein-coupled receptors that regulate feeding behavior. *Cell* **92,** 573–585.

Samson, W. K., Gosnell, B., Chang, J. K., Resch, Z. T., and Murphy, T. C. (1999). Cardiovascular regulatory actions of the hypocretins in brain. *Brain Res.* **831,** 248–253.

Samson, W. K., Taylor, M. M., and Ferguson, A. V. (2005). Non-sleep effects of hypocretin/orexin. *Sleep Med. Rev.* **9,** 243–252.

Saper, C. B., Fuller, P. M., Pedersen, N. P., Lu, J., and Scammell, T. E. (2010). Sleep state switching. *Neuron* **68,** 1023–1042.

Sato-Suzuki, I., Kita, I., Seki, Y., Oguri, M., and Arita, H. (2002). Cortical arousal induced by microinjection of orexins into the paraventricular nucleus of the rat. *Behav. Brain Res.* **128,** 169–177.

Sellayah, D., Bharaj, P., and Sikder, D. (2011). Orexin is required for brown adipose tissue development, differentiation, and function. *Cell Metab.* **14,** 478–490.

Semjonous, N. M., Smith, K. L., Parkinson, J. R., Gunner, D. J., Liu, Y. L., Murphy, K. G., Ghatei, M. A., Bloom, S. R., and Small, C. J. (2009). Coordinated changes in energy intake and expenditure following hypothalamic administration of neuropeptides involved in energy balance. *Int. J. Obes. (Lond.)* **33,** 775–785.

Shirasaka, T., Nakazato, M., Matsukura, S., Takasaki, M., and Kannan, H. (1999). Sympathetic and cardiovascular actions of orexins in conscious rats. *Am. J. Physiol.* **277,** R1780–R1785.

Shirasaka, T., Kunitake, T., Takasaki, M., and Kannan, H. (2002). Neuronal effects of orexins: Relevant to sympathetic and cardiovascular functions. *Regul. Pept.* **104,** 91–95.

Siegel, J. M. (1999). Narcolepsy: A key role for hypocretins (orexins). *Cell* **98,** 409–412.

Smith, P. M., Connolly, B. C., and Ferguson, A. V. (2002). Microinjection of orexin into the rat nucleus tractus solitarius causes increases in blood pressure. *Brain Res.* **950,** 261–267.

Smith, M. I., Piper, D. C., Duxon, M. S., and Upton, N. (2003). Evidence implicating a role for orexin-1 receptor modulation of paradoxical sleep in the rat. *Neurosci. Lett.* **341,** 256–258.
Smith, P. M., Samson, W. K., and Ferguson, A. V. (2007). Cardiovascular actions of orexin-A in the rat subfornical organ. *J. Neuroendocrinol.* **19,** 7–13.
Sutcliffe, J. G., and de Lecea, L. (2000). The hypocretins: Excitatory neuromodulatory peptides for multiple homeostatic systems, including sleep and feeding. *J. Neurosci. Res.* **62,** 161–168.
Szekely, M., Petervari, E., Balasko, M., Hernadi, I., and Uzsoki, B. (2002). Effects of orexins on energy balance and thermoregulation. *Regul. Pept.* **104,** 47–53.
Takahashi, K., Lin, J. S., and Sakai, K. (2008). Neuronal activity of orexin and non-orexin waking-active neurons during wake-sleep states in the mouse. *Neuroscience* **153,** 860–870.
Tang, J., Chen, J., Ramanjaneya, M., Punn, A., Conner, A. C., and Randeva, H. S. (2008). The signalling profile of recombinant human orexin-2 receptor. *Cell. Signal.* **20,** 1651–1661.
Teske, J. A., Levine, A. S., Kuskowski, M., Levine, J. A., and Kotz, C. M. (2006). Elevated hypothalamic orexin signaling, sensitivity to orexin A, and spontaneous physical activity in obesity-resistant rats. *Am. J. Physiol. Regul. Integr. Comp. Physiol.* **291,** R889–R899.
Teske, J. A., Billington, C. J., and Kotz, C. M. (2010). Hypocretin/orexin and energy expenditure. *Acta Physiol. (Oxf.)* **198,** 303–312.
Thakkar, M. M., Ramesh, V., Cape, E. G., Winston, S., Strecker, R. E., and McCarley, R. W. (1999). REM sleep enhancement and behavioral cataplexy following orexin (hypocretin)-II receptor antisense perfusion in the pontine reticular formation. *Sleep Res. Online* **2,** 112–120.
Thorpe, A. J., and Kotz, C. M. (2005). Orexin A in the nucleus accumbens stimulates feeding and locomotor activity. *Brain Res.* **1050,** 156–162.
Trivedi, P., Yu, H., MacNeil, D. J., Van der Ploeg, L. H., and Guan, X. M. (1998). Distribution of orexin receptor mRNA in the rat brain. *FEBS Lett.* **438,** 71–75.
Tsunematsu, T., Kilduff, T. S., Boyden, E. S., Takahashi, S., Tominaga, M., and Yamanaka, A. (2011). Acute optogenetic silencing of orexin/hypocretin neurons induces slow-wave sleep in mice. *J. Neurosci.* **31,** 10529–10539.
Tupone, D., Madden, C. J., Cano, G., and Morrison, S. F. (2011). An orexinergic projection from perifornical hypothalamus to raphe pallidus increases rat brown adipose tissue thermogenesis. *J. Neurosci.* **31,** 15944–15955.
van den Pol, A. N., Gao, X. B., Obrietan, K., Kilduff, T. S., and Belousov, A. B. (1998). Presynaptic and postsynaptic actions and modulation of neuroendocrine neurons by a new hypothalamic peptide, hypocretin/orexin. *J. Neurosci.* **18,** 7962–7971.
Vijgen, G. H., Bouvy, N. D., Teule, G. J., Brans, B., Schrauwen, P., and van Marken Lichtenbelt, W. D. (2011). Brown adipose tissue in morbidly obese subjects. *PLoS One* **6,** e17247.
Wang, J., Osaka, T., and Inoue, S. (2001). Energy expenditure by intracerebroventricular administration of orexin to anesthetized rats. *Neurosci. Lett.* **315,** 49–52.
Wang, J., Osaka, T., and Inoue, S. (2003). Orexin-A-sensitive site for energy expenditure localized in the arcuate nucleus of the hypothalamus. *Brain Res.* **971,** 128–134.
Willie, J. T., Chemelli, R. M., Sinton, C. M., and Yanagisawa, M. (2001). To eat or to sleep? Orexin in the regulation of feeding and wakefulness. *Annu. Rev. Neurosci.* **24,** 429–458.
Willie, J. T., Chemelli, R. M., Sinton, C. M., Tokita, S., Williams, S. C., Kisanuki, Y. Y., Marcus, J. N., Lee, C., Elmquist, J. K., Kohlmeier, K. A., Leonard, C. S., Richardson, J. A., *et al.* (2003). Distinct narcolepsy syndromes in orexin receptor-2 and orexin null mice: Molecular genetic dissection of Non-REM and REM sleep regulatory processes. *Neuron* **38,** 715–730.

Wu, M. F., John, J., Maidment, N., Lam, H. A., and Siegel, J. M. (2002). Hypocretin release in normal and narcoleptic dogs after food and sleep deprivation, eating, and movement. *Am. J. Physiol. Regul. Integr. Comp. Physiol.* **283,** R1079–R1086.

Xi, M. C., Morales, F. R., and Chase, M. H. (2001). Effects on sleep and wakefulness of the injection of hypocretin-1 (orexin-A) into the laterodorsal tegmental nucleus of the cat. *Brain Res.* **901,** 259–264.

Yamanaka, A., Muraki, Y., Tsujino, N., Goto, K., and Sakurai, T. (2003). Regulation of orexin neurons by the monoaminergic and cholinergic systems. *Biochem. Biophys. Res. Commun.* **303,** 120–129.

Yang, B., and Ferguson, A. V. (2003). Orexin-A depolarizes nucleus tractus solitarius neurons through effects on nonselective cationic and K+ conductances. *J. Neurophysiol.* **89,** 2167–2175.

Yoshida, Y., Fujiki, N., Nakajima, T., Ripley, B., Matsumura, H., Yoneda, H., Mignot, E., and Nishino, S. (2001). Fluctuation of extracellular hypocretin-1 (orexin A) levels in the rat in relation to the light-dark cycle and sleep-wake activities. *Eur. J. Neurosci.* **14,** 1075–1081.

Zepelin, H., and McDonald, C. S. (1987). Age differences in autonomic variables during sleep. *J. Gerontol.* **42,** 142–146.

Zhang, L., Renaud, L. P., and Kolaj, M. (2009). Properties of a T-type Ca^{2+} channel-activated slow after hyperpolarization in thalamic paraventricular nucleus and other thalamic midline neurons. *J. Neurophysiol.* **101,** 2741–2750.

Zheng, H., Patterson, L. M., and Berthoud, H. R. (2005). Orexin-A projections to the caudal medulla and orexin-induced c-Fos expression, food intake, and autonomic function. *J. Comp. Neurol.* **485,** 127–142.

CHAPTER SEVEN

Orexins: Tissue Localization, Functions, and Its Relation to Insulin Secretion and Diabetes Mellitus

Ernest Adeghate

Contents

Department of Anatomy, Faculty of Medicine & Health Sciences, United Arab Emirates University, Al Ain, United Arab Emirates

Vitamins and Hormones, Volume 89
ISSN 0083-6729, http://dx.doi.org/10.1016/B978-0-12-394623-2.00007-X

Abstract

Orexins play a role in many biological functions include sleep, feeding, and energy balance. They also regulate circadian rhythms and the way that we feel pain. Orexins have been identified in a variety of tissues including the cerebrospinal fluid, blood, hypothalamus, spinal cord, sensory ganglion, enteric nervous system, pituitary, adrenal, salivary and lacrimal glands, testis, vestibular gland, and skin. Orexins play a role in a variety of biological functions including arousal, sleeping, food and fluid intake, pain, memory, perception of odor, and sexual activity. Orexins have also been implicated in the regulation of glucose metabolism. The expression of orexin is induced by hypoglycemia, low food, pregnancy, and hemodialysis. In contrast, factors that inhibit the expression of orexins include obstructive sleep apnea, aging, depression, obesity, traumatic brain injury, and inflammatory molecules such as liposaccharide. In conclusion, orexins are widely distributed and involved in a large variety of biological activities.

I. Introduction

Orexins play an important role in the regulation of a variety of biological functions including feeding behavior, sleep and arousal, and energy balance. Disturbance in sleep and arousal may lead to narcolepsy, which is associated with extreme tendency to sleep during the day, cataplexy, and nocturnal dyssomnia (Abad and Guilleminault, 2004). In addition, it has been reported that orexins can stimulate cognitive arousal and influence the function of the neuroendocrine system (Acuna-Goycolea and van den Pol, 2009). Orexins have also been implicated in the perception of odor because they affect the neural circuit of the olfactory bulb (Apelbaum *et al.*, 2005). The role of orexins in the perception of odor was confirmed when intranasal orexin A was given to restore olfactory dysfunction in narcolepsy patients (Baier *et al.*, 2008).

The role of orexin in feeding is supported by the fact that food intake is significantly increased when orexin is injected into the lateral ventricles or the nuclei of the forebrain (Baird *et al.*, 2009).

Recent reports have shown that orexin-positive neurons originating from the lateral hypothalamic nucleus may contribute to addiction and the process of reward. The reason for this phenomenon is because orexinergic fibers project into areas such as the ventral tegmental areas, which regulate the pattern of behavior (Aston-Jones *et al.*, 2010). In order to further widen the range of activities modulated by orexin, a recent report indicated that orexins decrease sexual preference when administered centrally (Bai *et al.*, 2009).

All of these examples show that orexins are involved in a large variety of functions. This review describes the localization of orexins in several body tissues and functions associated with it. It also examined the interaction of orexins with glucose metabolism and diabetes mellitus.

II. Origin of Orexins

It was postulated that orexins were previously a member of the incretin family of peptides. The gene that codes orexin probably evolved more than 650 million years ago in the early chordate era (Alvarez and Sutcliffe, 2002). Orexins later cleaved form the incretin family via genetic exchange of chromosomes. Orexin is first seen in neurons at embryonic days 11–14. The highest peak of synthesis is at day 12 (Amiot *et al.*, 2005).

III. Structure of Orexins

The amino acid (aa) number of preproorexin varies from 66 in sheep to 148 in chicken. Preproorexin is a 131 aa in humans and many other mammals (Table 7.1). Preproorexin splits into two chains, with chain A (orexin A) left with 33 aa and chain B (orexin B) 28 aa. The precursor (preproorexin) of orexins has been identified in nonmammalian species. For example, it was shown to be a 143 aa peptide in the hypothalamus of the Atlantic cod (*Gadus morhua*). Three distinct parts were associated with it, namely, a signal peptide with 38 aa, a 50 aa part designated as the orexin A peptide portion, and lastly a 29 aa segment referred to as orexin B part (Xu and Volkoff, 2007).

IV. Receptors of Orexins

Two types of receptors, orexin receptor 1 (OX1R) and 2 (OX2R), found in many organs and tissues respond to and translate the effects of orexins. The receptors are large polypeptides with several hundreds (445)

Table 7.1 Amino acid number and chromosome location of prepro-orexin

Species	Amino acid number	Chromosome; location
Human	131	17; q21
Chimpanzee	130	17
Monkey	131	16; 16
Pig	131	19
Dog	130	9; 9
Cattle	131	19; 19
Sheep	66	
Rat	130	10; q32.1
Mouse	130	11; 61.2 cM
Chicken	148	27; 27
Atlantic cod	143	
Zebrafish	129	3; 3

amino acids. Orexin B binds OX2R in the same way as orexin A but has a much lower affinity (10–100 times lower) for OX1R (Ammoun *et al.*, 2003). Several selective agonists of OX1R and OX2R including [Ala^{11}, D-Leu^{15}]orexin B have been developed to help in the elucidation of the effects of orexins (Asahi *et al.*, 2003). However, recent studies have shown that orexin receptor agonists show large variation, making interpretation of their binding difficult to interpret (Putula *et al.*, 2011).

In addition to the development of orexin receptor agonists, attention has also been drawn to the identification of antagonists of orexin. Some antagonists of orexin have been based on the addition of an *N*-methyl arm to the benzimidazole moiety of a proline bis-amide compound (Bergman *et al.*, 2008). Bergman *et al.* (2008) observed a central activity of the compound when given *in vivo*. Almorexant, a universal antagonist for orexin, can block the function of both orexins A and B (Malherbe *et al.*, 2009).

V. Tissue Distribution of Orexins

A. Cerebrospinal fluid

The cerebrospinal fluid (CSF) contains orexins, which has been used as a diagnostic tool in many conditions related to sleep and arousal (Abdo *et al.*, 2008). Reduction in CSF orexins has been reported in hypothalamus injury resulting from hemorrhage of subarachnoid aneurysm (Ang *et al.*, 2005). The normal level of orexin A in human CSF is 382–667 pg/ml with a mean of 521 pg/ml (Baumann *et al.*, 2004). This range is much higher than those measured in the blood. This observation showed that the quantity of orexins in the central nervous system outweighs those in the peripheral nervous system.

B. Serum

Orexin A has also been identified in serum, where the concentration is 0.28 mg/l in normal and healthy subjects (Abulaiti *et al.*, 2008). This appears to be very high compared to the value (1.9 pmol/l) obtained by Arihara *et al.* (2001).

C. Hypothalamus

Studies have shown that the posterior and lateral hypothalamic nuclei contain orexins. These orexin-positive neurons also contain glutamate (Abrahamson *et al.*, 2001). The presence of glutamate in the orexin-producing hypothalamic nuclei may indicate a modulatory role for glutamate in the regulation of orexin function. Glutamate may not be the only neurotransmitter modulating the action of orexins. It has been shown that GLP-1 agonists are capable of exciting orexin-containing hypothalamic nuclei possibly by input from the gut (Acuna-Goycolea and van den Pol, 2004).

The lateral hypothalamic region has also been shown to contain glucose-sensitive neurons. These neurons have been shown to be capable of secreting orexin types A and B alike (Aou *et al.*, 2003).

It thus appears that orexins do not exist in isolation in the central nervous system, they colocalize with a number of neurotransmitters and neuropeptides including melanin-concentrating hormone and GABA receptor alpha 3 (Backberg *et al.*, 2004), in addition to glutamate and GLP-1. This observation suggests that the function of orexins is probably modified by other bioactive agents.

Reports have also indicated that orexin receptors colocalize with oxytocin and vasopressin in the large neurons of the paraventricular and supraoptic nuclei of the hypothalamus (Backberg *et al.*, 2002).

1. Role of orexins in brain disorders

The number of orexin A-positive neurons in the lateral nuclei of the hypothalamus of patients suffering from Huntington disease is significantly lower than that of control (Aziz *et al.*, 2008). This observation suggests that orexins may play a role in the pathogenesis and/or clinical manifestation of Huntington disease. This observation is in contrast to that of Baumann *et al.* (2006a) who reported that the level of orexin A is normal in Huntington disease. Some investigators (Bjorkqvist *et al.*, 2006) warn that the level of orexins in the CSF should not be used as a diagnostic tool in the management of Huntington disease. The CSF level of orexins is also altered in

Parkinson disease. A significant loss of orexin A neurons were observed in the brains of patients with Parkinson disease (Fronczek *et al.*, 2007). Decreased level of CSF-orexin is common with a longer disease period and higher occurrence of sleep attack (Asai *et al.*, 2009). A low level of orexin A in the CSF was observed in a patient with multiple sclerosis (Kato *et al.*, 2003; Oka *et al.*, 2004). This particular patient was suffering from hypersomnia.

All of these observations indicate how important this peptide is in different disease conditions affecting the lateral hypothalamic and related regions.

D. Sensory ganglia

Orexins and their receptors have been identified in the nodose ganglion of the rat and human subjects (Burdyga *et al.*, 2003). In addition, orexin A and OX1R have been detected in the spinal ganglion of rats (Bingham *et al.*, 2001). This indicates that orexins may have a functional role in both the central and the peripheral nervous systems.

E. Pituitary gland

Orexins have been identified in the anterior pituitary of several animal species. Blanco *et al.* (2003) showed that orexins A and B are found in the anterior portion of the hypophysis. Other investigators, including Xu and Volkoff (2007) showed that orexins are present in the pituitary gland of nonvertebrate fish. The localization of orexins to the pituitary gland may suggest a role for orexins in the regulation of this important endocrine organ.

F. Adrenal medulla

OX1R and OX2R were identified in the rat adrenal medulla using RT-PCR and immunohistochemical methods (Lopez *et al.*, 1999). Some investigators indicated that the adrenal gland may belong to one of the circuits responsible for the function of the orexinergic system. Previous reports have shown that orexin can stimulate the sympathoadrenal system when administered centrally (Matsumura *et al.*, 2001).

G. The enteric nervous system and pancreas

Both orexins A and B have been identified in several organs of the enteric nervous system including the pancreas (Adeghate *et al.*, 2010) and the gut (Adam *et al.*, 2002). Orexin receptors are present in the nerves and endocrine cells of the pancreas of several rodents (Fig. 7.1), where they coexist

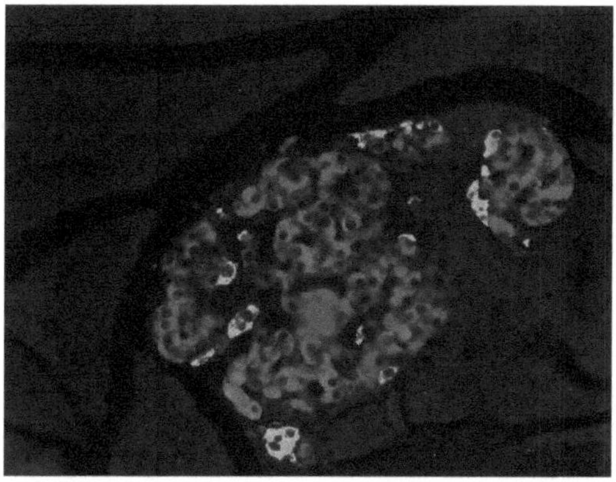

Figure 7.1 Light micrograph showing OX1R-positive cells (red) in pancreatic islet of cells of Goto-Kakizaki rats. Glucagon-immunopositive cells (green) are located in the periphery of pancreatic islet of Langerhans. Note the large number of islet cells containing OX1R in the central region of the islet. Magnification: 200×. (See Color Insert.)

with insulin in beta cells (Adeghate *et al.*, 2010). This indicates that orexins may have peripheral functions in addition to those they exert in the central nervous system.

Animal studies have shown that orexins stimulate gastric secretion and modulate gastrointestinal movement (Baccari, 2010; Bulbul *et al.*, 2010). Although orexins have been identified in the enteric neurons of mouse and rat (Baccari *et al.*, 2009; Ehrstrom *et al.*, 2005), horse (Dall'aglio *et al.*, 2009), and dog (Dall'aglio *et al.*, 2008), some investigators doubt whether enteric neurons are capable of producing orexins (Baumann *et al.*, 2008).

H. Kidney and urine

It has been shown that the human kidney contain orexins, which are located mainly in the convoluted tubules (Takahashi *et al.*, 2006) of the renal cortex. Takahashi *et al.* (2006) also reported that orexin A is present in human urine. The role of the kidney in the metabolism of orexins is explained by the fact that hemodialysis increases the plasma level of orexins (Sugimoto *et al.*, 2002). These observations emphasize the role of kidney in the metabolism of orexins and shows that they are excreted into urine.

I. Salivary glands

Orexins and their receptors are present in the parotid, submandibular as well as the sublingual glands of the pig (Dall'aglio *et al.*, 2011). The pattern of distribution of orexins varies between one gland and the other.

The submandibular gland appears to contain more prepro-orexin mRNA, compared to other salivary glands. Orexins A and B, coupled with their receptors, are abundant in the excretory ducts of the submandibular gland and appear to be absent in the duct of the sublingual and parotid glands. The localization of orexins to the ductal system agrees with the observation of Adeghate and Hameed (2005) in the lacrimal gland (Tables 7.2 and 7.3).

By virtue of their localization, orexins may take part in the secretory and other metabolic activities of the salivary ducts.

J. Lacrimal gland

Orexin B has been localized to the interacinar parts of the lacrimal gland of Wistar rats, while orexin receptor was observed in vascular nerves. It appears that the pattern of distribution of OX1R-positive nerves was not affected by diabetes mellitus (Adeghate and Hameed, 2005). Orexins may therefore play a role in the regulation of tear from the lacrimal gland.

K. Testis

Orexins and their receptors have been identified in the rat testes, where they were observed mostly in the Leydig cells and spermatocytes (Barreiro *et al.*, 2005). Orexin A is capable of stimulating the release of testosterone (Barreiro *et al.*, 2004). The localization of orexins in the testes will point to a role in the modulation of the male reproductive system.

L. Vestibular gland

Orexin A and OX1R have been identified in the vestibular glands (Pavone *et al.*, 2009) and urethroprostatic complex (Russo *et al.*, 2008) of cattle. This indicates that orexins may play a role in the function of both male and female genital organs.

M. Skin

Prepro-orexin and orexin receptors have been detected in Merkel cells of the skin of pig (Beiras-Fernandez *et al.*, 2004). Merkel cell are neuroendocrine in nature and can be found in the lower part of the epidermis. The localization of orexins and their receptors to the Merkel cells of the skin might suggest a functional role for orexins in the maintenance of epidermal function and/or integrity. It may also form a link between the metabolism of the skin and that of the central nervous system.

Table 7.2 Distribution of orexins and their receptors in vertebrate tissues

Tissue/cell	Type of orexin	Species	Method of localization	Authors (reference)
Hippocampus CA1 region	Orexin 1 receptor	Rat	Immunohistochemistry	Akbari *et al.* (2008)
Spinal cord	Orexins	Human Rat Mouse	Immunohistochemistry	Cutler *et al.* (1999); Van den Pol (1999)
Dentate gyrus	Orexin 1 receptor	Rat	Immunohistochemistry	Akbari *et al.* (2008)
Ventral tegmental area	Orexin	Rat	Immunohistochemistry	Balcita-Pedicino and Sesack (2007)
Zona incerta	Prepro-orexin mRNA	Sheep	*In situ* hybridization	Archer *et al.* (2002)
Neuroblastoma	Orexin	Human	Immunohistochemistry	Arihara *et al.* (2000)
Spinal ganglion	Orexin A, Orexin 1 receptor	Rat Mouse	Immunohistochemistry	Bingham *et al.* (2001)
Nodose ganglion	Orexin, Orexin receptors	Human	RT-PCR, Immunohistochemistry	Burdyga *et al.* (2003)
CSF	Orexin 1	Human	Enzyme immunoassay	Ang *et al.* (2005)
Kidney and urine	Orexin, Orexin receptors	Human	Immunohistochemistry	Takahashi *et al.* (2006)
Urethroprostatic complex	Orexin, Orexin receptors	Cattle	Immunohistochemistry	Russo *et al.* (2008)
Vestibular glands	Orexin, Orexin receptors	Cattle	Immunohistochemistry	Pavone *et al.* (2009)
Salivary glands	Orexin A and receptor	Pig	RT-PCR, Immunohistochemistry	Dall'aglio *et al.* (2011)
Lacrimal gland	Orexin B, Orexin 1 receptor	Rat	Immunohistochemistry	Adeghate and Hameed (2005)
Pancreas	Orexin B, Orexin 1 receptor	Rat	Immunohistochemistry	Adeghate *et al.* (2010)
Pituitary	Orexin	Human	Immunohistochemistry	Blanco *et al.* (2003)

(*Continued*)

Table 7.2 (*Continued*)

Tissue/cell	Type of orexin	Species	Method of localization	Authors (reference)
Adrenal medulla	Orexin receptors	Rat	RT-PCR, Immunohistochemistry	Lopez *et al.* (1999)
Stomach	Orexin 1 receptor	Mouse	Immunohistochemistry	Baccari *et al.* (2009)
Stomach and gut	Orexin A and receptor	Dog	Immunohistochemistry	Dall'aglio *et al.* (2008)
Stomach and gut	Orexin A and receptor	Horse	Immunohistochemistry	Dall'aglio *et al.* (2009)
Stomach	Orexin A and receptor	Rat	Immunohistochemistry	Ehrstrom *et al.* (2005)
Testis	Orexin A	Rat	Immunohistochemistry	Barreiro *et al.* (2005)
Skin (Merkel cells)	Prepro-orexin mRNA, Orexin receptors	Pig	Immunohistochemistry	Beiras-Fernandez *et al.* (2004)

Table 7.3 Distribution of orexins and their receptors in invertebrate tissues

Tissue/cell	Type of orexin	Species	Method of localization	Authors (reference)
Brain	Prepro-orexin cDNA	Fish (cod)	RT-PCR	Xu and Volkoff (2007)
Brain	Orexin	Fish	Immunohistochemistry	Amiya *et al.* (2007)
Brain	Orexin	Axolotls	Immunohistochemistry	Suzuki *et al.* (2008)
Brain	Orexins	Amphibians	Immunohistochemistry	Lopez *et al.* (2009)
Pituitary	Orexin	Human	Immunohistochemistry	Blanco *et al.* (2003)
Spleen	Prepro-orexin mRNA	Fish	RT-PCR	Xu and Volkoff (2007)
Kidney	Prepro-orexin mRNA	Fish	RT-PCR	Xu and Volkoff (2007)
Skin	Prepro-orexin mRNA	Fish	RT-PCR	Xu and Volkoff (2007)
Stomach	Prepro-orexin mRNA	Fish	RT-PCR	Xu and Volkoff (2007)
Gut	Prepro-orexin mRNA	Fish	RT-PCR	Xu and Volkoff (2007)

N. Tumor cells

Orexin A has been observed in neuroblastoma as well as ganglioneuroblastoma using immunohistochemical techniques (Arihara *et al.*, 2000). The role of orexins in neural cancer cells is unknown. However, it is possible that orexins may play a role in the transformation of normal to abnormal forms of neurons.

O. Inductors of orexin expression

The level of orexin A is elevated in the CSF of patients suffering from the restless leg syndrome (Allen *et al.*, 2002). This is highly significant at the beginning of the illness. Restless leg syndrome is also known as Willis-Ekbom disease. It is a neurological disease with an urge to swing the legs as a way of getting out of stress. Cai *et al.* (2001) showed that hypoglycemia induces the level of orexins. This is in agreement with the observation of Griffond *et al.* (1999), Xu and Volkoff (2007), and Zhao *et al.* (2005) that small diet induces increases in the level of orexin. Anukulkitch *et al.* (2010) observed that a lean weight is associated with an increase in the circulating level of orexins. It has also been shown that pregnancy increases the expression of prepro-orexin mRNA in the rat brain (Kanenishi *et al.*, 2004). It is not clear why pregnancy would stimulate the production of orexins, but it is possible that an increase in the level of orexin may play a role in the altered feeding pattern observed in pregnant women.

The level of plasma orexin A is high in patients undergoing hemodialysis (Sugimoto *et al.*, 2002). This suggests that the kidney may be involved in the clearance of orexins from the body (Table 7.4).

P. Inhibitors of orexin expression

It has been shown that aging is associated with a decrease in the level of orexin A in old rats (Akimoto-Takano *et al.*, 2005; Brownell and Conti, 2010; Kessler *et al.*, 2011). This is thought to be associated with a decrease in the number of viable neurons. However, it is worth noting that in a study involving a large cohort of 157 males and 115 females, aged 0–79 years old, there was no difference in the CSF level of orexins, when age was considered (Kanbayashi *et al.*, 2002). In addition to aging, people suffering from obstructive sleep apnea have been shown to have low plasma levels of orexins (Aksu *et al.*, 2009). Low level of orexin has also been associated with depression in Wistar Kyoto rats. Allard *et al.* (2004) showed that the number and size of orexin-positive neurons are significantly smaller compared to control. A more recent report showed that the CSF level of orexin was significantly lower in suicidal patients with severe depression (Brundin

Table 7.4 Factors that induce or reduce orexin expression

Inducers of orexin expression	Inhibitors of orexin expression	Factors with controversial effect
Small diet (Xu and Volkoff, 2007)	Obstructive sleep apnea (Aksu *et al.*, 2009)	Aging
Restless leg syndrome (Willis–Ekbom disease) (Allen *et al.*, 2002	Aging (Akimoto-Takano *et al.*, 2005; Brownell and Conti, 2010; Kessler *et al.*, 2011)	
Lean weight (Anukulkitch *et al.*, 2010)	Depression (Allard *et al.*, 2004)	
Hypoglycemia (Cai *et al.*, 2001; Griffond *et al.*, 1999; Zhao *et al.*, 2005)	Obesity (Anukulkitch *et al.*, 2010; Cai *et al.*, 2000)	
Pregnancy (Kanenishi *et al.*, 2004)	Traumatic brain injury (Baumann *et al.*, 2009)	
Hemodialysis (Sugimoto *et al.*, 2002)	Liposaccharide (Becskei *et al.*, 2008)	

et al., 2007). Trauma of the brain is an important factor that leads to a reduction in the number of orexin-positive neurons (Baumann *et al.*, 2009).

Studies have shown that liposaccharide, found in the cell wall of Gram-negative bacteria, inhibits the expression of orexin A in neurons that are located in the lower part of the lateral hypothalamic area (Becskei *et al.*, 2008).

Like many neuropeptides, the expression of orexin is influenced by a variety of factors, which allows orexins to maintain optimal tissue levels in order to preserve its functions (Table 7.4).

VI. Physiological Effects

A. Arousal

Studies examining the effect of orexins on arousal have shown that orexin agonist, [Ala^{11}]orexin B, can significantly extend the degree of wakefulness when injected into cerebral ventricles (Akanmu and Honda, 2005). They showed that while orexin B and its agonists have the ability to induce wakefulness, it is orexin A that has the stronger effect in the generation of wakefulness. This may be due to the fact that orexin A acts on both receptor types (OX1R and OX2R) and may therefore be able to recruit more receptors in the maintenance of arousal when compared to orexin B. It has been shown that deficiency of orexin A in the CSF causes cataplexy and excessive daytime sleepiness in human subjects (Baumann *et al.*, 2006b).

B. Pain

Orexins and their receptors have been localized to the spinal cord and the sensory spinal ganglia in rodents (Bingham *et al.*, 2001). They showed that orexin A causes analgesia more that the way morphine does. This study showed a strong evidence for the role of orexins in the alleviation of pain.

C. Food intake

Studies conducted by Akiyama *et al.* (2004) confirmed the role orexins in the induction of food anticipatory activity (FAA). They showed that FAA is significantly reduced in animals with ablated orexigenic neurons. Since food intake is related to metabolic diseases such as diabetes mellitus, regulation of food intake by orexins may have an impact on the pathogenesis of diabetes mellitus.

D. Water intake

Orexins, via OX1R, have been shown to mediate water intake. This is mediated by the influence of orexins on either histamine- or osmosis-induced increases in the amount of plasma vasopressin (Kis *et al.*, 2012). In fact, it appears that the increase in drinking caused by electrical stimulation of the lateral hypothalamus area observed by Mogenson and Stevenson (1967) as far back as 1967 before the discovery of orexins might have been due to the effect of orexins. In just a little more than three decades later, Kunii *et al.* (1999) showed that, drinking behavior is actually modulated by orexin-positive neurons, sitting in the lateral hypothalamic area, moreso when orexins are injected directly into cerebral ventricles.

E. Memory

Orexins and their receptors have been linked to memory. Akbari *et al.* (2008) showed that SB-334867-A an antagonist of OX1R inhibited memory when injected into CA1 region of the hippocampus.

VII. Mechanism of Orexin Action

Orexins colocalize with many neurotransmitters and neuropeptides (Backberg *et al.*, 2004). In addition, they also terminate on neurons that module a specific type of activity. For example, it has been shown that orexin-containing neurons of the lateral hypothalamic area terminate on GABA- and dopamine-positive neurons of the ventral tegmental area of the rat brain (Balcita-Pedicino and Sesack, 2007). Since the ventral tegmental area is involved in the modulation of motive behavior, it is possible that orexins exerts its influence by modulating the activities of neurons destined for a specific function.

It has also been shown that orexinergic neurons do indeed project into other important areas of the brain. Bisetti *et al.* (2006) showed that, orexin-containing neurons of the lateral hypothalamic area project into the central medial nucleus of the amygdala, considered to be a major output of the amygdale nucleus. Orexins from the lateral hypothalamic nucleus excite a group of neurons responsible for the initiation and regulation of how the body respond to stress, emotion, and fear (Bisetti *et al.*, 2006).

The initiation and maintenance of rapid eye movement sleep and narcolepsy attributed to orexins is said to be regulated via the locus coeruleus, located in the brain stem on the floor of the fourth ventricle. Bourgin *et al.* (2000) showed that administration of orexin A enhanced the activity of locus coeruleus neurons.

Orexins are also able to stimulate serotonergic neurons located in the nucleus raphe dorsalis of the brain stem (Brown *et al.*, 2001). This implies that orexins can also act via the serotonergic system, which is involved in a variety of psychiatric disorders including anxiety and depression. Evidence that orexins are found in the area postrema (Guan *et al.*, 2005), the vomiting center of the brain shows that orexins may take part in the regulation of a large variety of functions.

A. How does orexin trigger cellular signaling?

Orexins A and B trigger their responses by binding to and activating the G-protein-coupled receptors (GPCRs; Zhu *et al.*, 2003). Orexin A triggers OX1R mainly, while OX2R is used by both orexins A and B (Sakurai *et al.*, 1998). Activation of GPCR eventually leads to increase in intracellular calcium (Zhu *et al.*, 2003) resulting in the manifestation of hormonal effect.

However, Ammoun *et al.* (2006) showed that orexin receptor facilitates the influx of Ca^{2+} which allows the participation of other cell signaling pathways.

B. Orexin and glucose metabolism

Since the lateral hypothalamic area houses neurons that are excited by decreases in blood glucose, and inhibited in hyperglycemic conditions (Cai *et al.*, 1999, 2001; Griffond *et al.*, 1999), it is not surprising, therefore, that orexins play a role in glucose metabolism and subsequently in anomalies associated with it. Some studies have shown inverse correlation between glucose and orexin levels in the CSF (Doherty *et al.*, 2005). However, studies looking at the interaction of orexins and glucose at the level of the pancreas showed that glucose stimulated the release of orexin A from the pancreas (Ouedraogo *et al.*, 2003). The regulation of basal endogenous glucose generation coupled with peripheral insulin resistance is a function of the orexinergic neurons of the lateral hypothalamic area (Yi *et al.*, 2009). All of these clearly show that the regulation of glucose metabolism is controlled in part by orexins.

C. Orexin and obesity

The plasma level of orexin A is inversely proportional to body mass index, indicating that the plasma level of orexins are lower in severely obese patients (Adam *et al.*, 2002). This shows that the functions of orexins are not confined only to the central nervous system. There are large number of evidence pointing to the association of disorders in sleeping hormones and metabolic diseases, such as obesity and diabetes mellitus (Adamantidis and de Lecea, 2008).

Anukulkitch *et al.* (2009), through biological modeling, showed that the genes responsible for orexins are closely associated with alterations in the metabolic status of the animal. The level of orexin B is significantly increased in hypoglycemic conditions (Cai *et al.*, 1999, 2001).

The interaction between orexins and obesity is further substantiated by the fact that obesity has been shown to be common in patients with narcolepsy (Dahmen *et al.*, 2001). In addition, narcoleptic people with orexin A deficiency often develop abdominal obesity (Kok *et al.*, 2003).

D. Orexin, insulin, and diabetes mellitus

Since several studies have confirmed that orexins regulate the sleep/wake cycle and feeding behavior. It is therefore logical that orexins would have a role to play in metabolic disorders including obesity and diabetes mellitus. To this end, many investigators have searched and reported for the localization of orexins in the pancreas (Adeghate and Hameed, 2011; Adeghate *et al.*, 2010). It is well known that the exocrine as well as the endocrine pancreas play a role in the modulation of food metabolism and energy equilibrium. Adeghate *et al.* (2010) showed that OX1R is widely distributed in the islet cells of a variety of animals including Wistar, Goto-Kakizaki, and mice. They noted that the number of OX1R-containing cells and tissue level of OX1R increased significantly in the endocrine pancreas of rats with diabetes mellitus. These observations showed that orexins and their receptors may indeed play a major role in the pathogenesis of diabetes mellitus.

In contrast to the increase in the number of OX1R in the islets of rats with diabetes, it has been shown that the number of orexin B-positive cells decrease significantly after the onset of diabetes (Adeghate and Hameed, 2011). The interaction of orexins and diabetes mellitus is confirmed by the fact that orexin B stimulates insulin release from the *in vitro* rat pancreas (Adeghate and Hameed, 2011). In a study of the effect of orexins on normal pancreas, Nowak *et al.* (2000, 2005) showed that orexins A and B can stimulate insulin release in an *in vitro* setting. This indicates that orexins do have a direct role in peripheral regulation of glucose metabolism.

In an event that may eventually lead to diabetes, Tsuneki *et al.* (2008) demonstrated that orexin knockout mice are prone to developing age-related impaired glucose tolerance without obesity. Tsuneki *et al.* (2002) also reported that orexins reduced glucose level in experimental diabetic mice in the fasting phase, probably by increased utilization/uptake of glucose.

VIII. Conclusion and Future Perspectives

Orexins are found in many tissues including the hypothalamus, spinal cord, sensory ganglia, pancreas, pituitary, adrenal, salivary, and lacrimal glands. The level of orexins can be easily measured in blood, urine, and CSF. Orexins are involved in a variety of biological functions including arousal, sleeping, food and fluid intake, pain, and memory. Orexins have also been implicated in the regulation of glucose metabolism. Orexins appear to be ubiquitous with a large array of biological functions. Further studies will likely identify more functions for this relatively new neuropeptides. It could achieve therapeutic role in the near future.

ACKNOWLEDGMENTS

The study was supported by grants from the UAE University.

REFERENCES

Abad, V. C., and Guilleminault, C. (2004). Emerging drugs for narcolepsy. *Expert Opin. Emerg. Drugs* **9,** 281–291.

Abdo, W. F., Bloem, B. R., Kremer, H. P., Lammers, G. J., Verbeek, M. M., and Overeem, S. (2008). CSF hypocretin-1 levels are normal in multiple-system atrophy. *Parkinsonism Relat. Disord.* **14,** 342–344.

Abrahamson, E. E., Leak, R. K., and Moore, R. Y. (2001). The suprachiasmatic nucleus projects to posterior hypothalamic arousal systems. *Neuroreport* **12,** 435–440.

Abulaiti, A., Xu, P. R., and Duo, L. K. (2008). Diagnostic values of serum orexin-A levels in children with obstructive sleep apnea-hypoopnea syndrome. *Zhonghua Er. Ke. Za. Zhi* **46,** 291–296.

Acuna-Goycolea, C., and van den Pol, A. (2004). Glucagon-like peptide 1 excites hypocretin/orexin neurons by direct and indirect mechanisms: Implications for viscera-mediated arousal. *J. Neurosci.* **24,** 8141–8152.

Acuna-Goycolea, C., and van den Pol, A. N. (2009). Neuroendocrine proopiomelanocortin neurons are excited by hypocretin/orexin. *J. Neurosci.* **29,** 1503–1513.

Adam, J. A., Menheere, P. P., van Dielen, F. M., Soeters, P. B., Buurman, W. A., and Greve, J. W. (2002). Decreased plasma orexin-A levels in obese individuals. *Int. J. Obes. Relat. Metab. Disord.* **26,** 274–276.

Adamantidis, A., and de Lecea, L. (2008). Sleep and metabolism: Shared circuits, new connections. *Trends Endocrinol. Metab.* **19,** 362–370.

Adeghate, E., and Hameed, R. S. (2005). Immunohistochemical localization of orexin-B, orexin-1 receptor, ghrelin, GHS-R in the lacrimal gland of normal and diabetic rats. *Peptides* **26,** 2585–2589.

Adeghate, E., and Hameed, R. (2011). Mechanism of orexin B-stimulated insulin and glucagon release from the pancreas of normal and diabetic rats. *Pancreas* **40,** 131–136.

Adeghate, E., Fernandez-Cabezudo, M., Hameed, R., El-Hasasna, H., El Wasila, M., Abbas, T., and Al-Ramadi, B. (2010). Orexin-1 receptor co-localizes with pancreatic hormones in islet cells and modulates the outcome of streptozotocin-induced diabetes mellitus. *PLoS One* **5,** e8587.

Akanmu, M. A., and Honda, K. (2005). Selective stimulation of orexin receptor type 2 promotes wakefulness in freely behaving rats. *Brain Res.* **1048,** 138–145.

Akbari, E., Motamedi, F., Naghdi, N., and Noorbakhshnia, M. (2008). The effect of antagonization of orexin 1 receptors in CA1 and dentate gyrus regions on memory processing in passive avoidance task. *Behav. Brain Res.* **187,** 172–177.

Akimoto-Takano, S., Sakurai, C., Kanai, S., Hosoya, H., Ohta, M., and Miyasaka, K. (2005). Differences in the appetite-stimulating effect of orexin, neuropeptide Y and ghrelin among young, adult and old rats. *Neuroendocrinology* **82,** 256–263.

Akiyama, M., Yuasa, T., Hayasaka, N., Horikawa, K., Sakurai, T., and Shibata, S. (2004). Reduced food anticipatory activity in genetically orexin (hypocretin) neuron-ablated mice. *Eur. J. Neurosci.* **20,** 3054–3062.

Aksu, K., Firat Guven, S., Aksu, F., Ciftci, B., Ulukavak Ciftci, T., Aksaray, S., Sipit, T., and Peker, Y. (2009). Obstructive sleep apnoea, cigarette smoking and plasma orexin-A in a sleep clinic cohort. *J. Int. Med. Res.* **37,** 331–340.

Allard, J. S., Tizabi, Y., Shaffery, J. P., Trouth, C. O., and Manaye, K. (2004). Stereological analysis of the hypothalamic hypocretin/orexin neurons in an animal model of depression. *Neuropeptides* **38,** 311–315.

Allen, R. P., Mignot, E., Ripley, B., Nishino, S., and Earley, C. J. (2002). Increased CSF hypocretin-1 (orexin-A) in restless legs syndrome. *Neurology* **59,** 639–641.

Alvarez, C. E., and Sutcliffe, J. G. (2002). Hypocretin is an early member of the incretin gene family. *Neurosci. Lett.* **324,** 169–172.

Amiot, C., Brischoux, F., Colard, C., La Roche, A., Fellmann, D., and Risold, P. Y. (2005). Hypocretin/orexin-containing neurons are produced in one sharp peak in the developing ventral diencephalon. *Eur. J. Neurosci.* **22,** 531–534.

Amiya, N., Amano, M., Oka, Y., Iigo, M., Takahashi, A., and Yamamori, K. (2007). Immunohistochemical localization of orexin/hypocretin-like immunoreactive peptides and melanin-concentrating hormone in the brain and pituitary of medaka. *Neurosci. Lett.* **427,** 16–21.

Ammoun, S., Holmqvist, T., Shariatmadari, R., Oonk, H. B., Detheux, M., Parmentier, M., Akerman, K. E., and Kukkonen, J. P. (2003). Distinct recognition of OX1 and OX2 receptors by orexin peptides. *J. Pharmacol. Exp. Ther.* **305,** 507–514.

Ammoun, S., Johansson, L., Ekholm, M. E., Holmqvist, T., Danis, A. S., Korhonen, L., Sergeeva, O. A., Haas, H. L., Akerman, K. E., and Kukkonen, J. P. (2006). OX1 orexin receptors activate extracellular signal-regulated kinase in Chinese hamster ovary cells via multiple mechanisms: The role of Ca^{2+} influx in OX1 receptor signaling. *Mol. Endocrinol.* **20,** 80–99.

Ang, B. T., Tan, W. L., Lim, J., and Ng, I. (2005). Cerebrospinal fluid orexin in aneurysmal subarachnoid haemorrhage—A pilot study. *J. Clin. Neurosci.* **12,** 758–762.

Anukulkitch, C., Rao, A., Dunshea, F. R., and Clarke, I. J. (2009). A test of the lipostat theory in a seasonal (ovine) model under natural conditions reveals a close relationship between adiposity and melanin concentrating hormone expression. *Domest. Anim. Endocrinol.* **36,** 138–151.

Anukulkitch, C., Rao, A., Pereira, A., McEwan, J., and Clarke, I. J. (2010). Expression of genes for appetite-regulating peptides in the hypothalamus of genetically selected lean and fat sheep. *Neuroendocrinology* **91,** 223–238.

Aou, S., Li, X. L., Li, A. J., Oomura, Y., Shiraishi, T., Sasaki, K., Imamura, T., and Wayner, M. J. (2003). Orexin-A (hypocretin-1) impairs Morris water maze performance and CA1-Schaffer collateral long-term potentiation in rats. *Neuroscience* **119,** 1221–1228.

Apelbaum, A. F., Perrut, A., and Chaput, M. (2005). Orexin A effects on the olfactory bulb spontaneous activity and odor responsiveness in freely breathing rats. *Regul. Pept.* **129,** 49–61.

Archer, Z. A., Findlay, P. A., Rhind, S. M., Mercer, J. G., and Adam, C. L. (2002). Orexin gene expression and regulation by photoperiod in the sheep hypothalamus. *Regul. Pept.* **104,** 41–45.

Arihara, Z., Takahashi, K., Murakami, O., Totsune, K., Sone, M., Satoh, F., Ito, S., Hayashi, Y., Sasano, H., and Mouri, T. (2000). Orexin-A in the human brain and tumor tissues of ganglioneuroblastoma and neuroblastoma. *Peptides* **21,** 565–570.

Arihara, Z., Takahashi, K., Murakami, O., Totsune, K., Sone, M., Satoh, F., Ito, S., and Mouri, T. (2001). Immunoreactive orexin-A in human plasma. *Peptides* **22,** 139–142.

Asahi, S., Egashira, S., Matsuda, M., Iwaasa, H., Kanatani, A., Ohkubo, M., Ihara, M., and Morishima, H. (2003). Development of an orexin-2 receptor selective agonist, [Ala(11), D-Leu(15)]orexin-B. *Bioorg. Med. Chem. Lett.* **13,** 111–113.

Asai, H., Hirano, M., Furiya, Y., Udaka, F., Morikawa, M., Kanbayashi, T., Shimizu, T., and Ueno, S. (2009). Cerebrospinal fluid-orexin levels and sleep attacks in four patients with Parkinson's disease. *Clin. Neurol. Neurosurg.* **111,** 341–344.

Aston-Jones, G., Smith, R. J., Sartor, G. C., Moorman, D. E., Massi, L., Tahsili-Fahadan, P., and Richardson, K. A. (2010). Lateral hypothalamic orexin/hypocretin neurons: A role in reward-seeking and addiction. *Brain Res.* **1314,** 74–90.

Aziz, A., Fronczek, R., Maat-Schieman, M., Unmehopa, U., Roelandse, F., Overeem, S., van Duinen, S., Lammers, G. J., Swaab, D., and Roos, R. (2008). Hypocretin and melanin-concentrating hormone in patients with Huntington disease. *Brain Pathol.* **18,** 474–483.

Baccari, B. C. (2010). Orexins and gastrointestinal functions. *Curr. Protein Pept. Sci.* **11,** 148–155.

Baccari, M. C., Bani, D., and Calamai, F. (2009). Evidence for a modulatory role of orexin A on the nitrergic neurotransmission in the mouse gastric fundus. *Regul. Pept.* **154,** 54–59.

Backberg, M., Hervieu, G., Wilson, S., and Meister, B. (2002). Orexin receptor-1 (OX-R1) immunoreactivity in chemically identified neurons of the hypothalamus: Focus on orexin targets involved in control of food and water intake. *Eur. J. Neurosci.* **15,** 315–328.

Backberg, M., Ultenius, C., Fritschy, J. M., and Meister, B. (2004). Cellular localization of GABA receptor alpha subunit immunoreactivity in the rat hypothalamus: Relationship with neurones containing orexigenic or anorexigenic peptides. *J. Neuroendocrinol.* **16,** 589–604.

Bai, Y. J., Li, Y. H., Zheng, X. G., Han, J., Yang, X. Y., and Sui, N. (2009). Orexin A attenuates unconditioned sexual motivation in male rats. *Pharmacol. Biochem. Behav.* **91,** 581–589.

Baier, P. C., Weinhold, S. L., Huth, V., Gottwald, B., Ferstl, R., and Hinze-Selch, D. (2008). Olfactory dysfunction in patients with narcolepsy with cataplexy is restored by intranasal Orexin A (Hypocretin-1). *Brain* **131,** 2734–2741.

Baird, J. P., Choe, A., Loveland, J. L., Beck, J., Mahoney, C. E., Lord, J. S., and Grigg, L. A. (2009). Orexin-A hyperphagia: Hindbrain participation in consummatory feeding responses. *Endocrinology* **150,** 1202–1216.

Balcita-Pedicino, J. J., and Sesack, S. R. (2007). Orexin axons in the rat ventral tegmental area synapse infrequently onto dopamine and gamma-aminobutyric acid neurons. *J. Comp. Neurol.* **503,** 668–684.

Barreiro, M. L., Pineda, R., Navarro, V. M., Lopez, M., Suominen, J. S., Pinilla, L., Senaris, R., Toppari, J., Aguilar, E., Dieguez, C., and Tena-Sempere, M. (2004). Orexin 1 receptor messenger ribonucleic acid expression and stimulation of testosterone secretion by orexin-A in rat testis. *Endocrinology* **145,** 2297–2306.

Barreiro, M. L., Pineda, R., Gaytan, F., Archanco, M., Burrell, M. A., Castellano, J. M., Hakovirta, H., Nurmio, M., Pinilla, L., Aguilar, E., Toppari, J., Dieguez, C., *et al.* (2005). Pattern of orexin expression and direct biological actions of orexin-A in rat testis. *Endocrinology* **146,** 5164–5175.

Baumann, C. R., Dauvilliers, Y., Mignot, E., and Bassetti, C. L. (2004). Normal CSF hypocretin-1 (orexin A) levels in dementia with Lewy bodies associated with excessive daytime sleepiness. *Eur. Neurol.* **52,** 73–76.

Baumann, C. R., Hersberger, M., and Bassetti, C. L. (2006a). Hypocretin-1 (orexin A) levels are normal in Huntington's disease. *J. Neurol.* **253,** 1232–1233.

Baumann, C. R., Khatami, R., Werth, E., and Bassetti, C. L. (2006b). Hypocretin (orexin) deficiency predicts severe objective excessive daytime sleepiness in narcolepsy with cataplexy. *J. Neurol. Neurosurg. Psychiatry* **77,** 402–404.

Baumann, C. R., Clark, E. L., Pedersen, N. P., Hecht, J. L., and Scammell, T. E. (2008). Do enteric neurons make hypocretin? *Regul. Pept.* **147,** 1–3.

Baumann, C. R., Bassetti, C. L., Valko, P. O., Haybaeck, J., Keller, M., Clark, E., Stocker, R., Tolnay, M., and Scammell, T. E. (2009). Loss of hypocretin (orexin) neurons with traumatic brain injury. *Ann. Neurol.* **66,** 555–559.

Becskei, C., Riediger, T., Hernadfalvy, N., Arsenijevic, D., Lutz, T. A., and Langhans, W. (2008). Inhibitory effects of lipopolysaccharide on hypothalamic nuclei implicated in the control of food intake. *Brain Behav. Immun.* **22,** 56–64.

Beiras-Fernandez, A., Gallego, R., Blanco, M., Garcia-Caballero, T., Dieguez, C., and Beiras, A. (2004). Merkel cells, a new localization of prepro-orexin and orexin receptors. *J. Anat.* **204,** 117–122.

Bergman, J. M., Roecker, A. J., Mercer, S. P., Bednar, R. A., Reiss, D. R., Ransom, R. W., Meacham Harrell, C., Pettibone, D. J., Lemaire, W., Murphy, K. L., Li, C., Prueksaritanont, T., *et al.* (2008). Proline bis-amides as potent dual orexin receptor antagonists. *Bioorg. Med. Chem. Lett.* **18,** 1425–1430.

Bingham, S., Davey, P. T., Babbs, A. J., Irving, E. A., Sammons, M. J., Wyles, M., Jeffrey, P., Cutler, L., Riba, I., Johns, A., Porter, R. A., Upton, N., *et al.* (2001). Orexin-A, an hypothalamic peptide with analgesic properties. *Pain* **92,** 81–90.

Bisetti, A., Cvetkovic, V., Serafin, M., Bayer, L., Machard, D., Jones, B. E., and Muhlethaler, M. (2006). Excitatory action of hypocretin/orexin on neurons of the central medial amygdala. *Neuroscience* **142,** 999–1004.

Bjorkqvist, M., Petersen, A., Nielsen, J., Ecker, D., Mulder, H., Hayden, M. R., Landwehrmeyer, B., Brundin, P., and Leavitt, B. R. (2006). Cerebrospinal fluid levels of orexin-A are not a clinically useful biomarker for Huntington disease. *Clin. Genet.* **70,** 78–79.

Blanco, M., Gallego, R., Garcia-Caballero, T., Dieguez, C., and Beiras, A. (2003). Cellular localization of orexins in human anterior pituitary. *Histochem. Cell Biol.* **120,** 259–264.

Bourgin, P., Huitron-Resendiz, S., Spier, A. D., Fabre, V., Morte, B., Criado, J. R., Sutcliffe, J. G., Henriksen, S. J., and de Lecea, L. (2000). Hypocretin-1 modulates rapid eye movement sleep through activation of locus coeruleus neurons. *J. Neurosci.* **20,** 7760–7765.

Brown, R. E., Sergeeva, O., Eriksson, K. S., and Haas, H. L. (2001). Orexin A excites serotonergic neurons in the dorsal raphe nucleus of the rat. *Neuropharmacology* **40,** 457–459.

Brownell, S. E., and Conti, B. (2010). Age- and gender-specific changes of hypocretin immunopositive neurons in C57Bl/6 mice. *Neurosci. Lett.* **472,** 29–32.

Brundin, L., Bjorkqvist, M., Petersen, A., and Traskman-Bendz, L. (2007). Reduced orexin levels in the cerebrospinal fluid of suicidal patients with major depressive disorder. *Eur. Neuropsychopharmacol.* **17,** 573–579.

Bulbul, M., Babygirija, R., Ludwig, K., and Takahashi, T. (2010). Central orexin-A increases gastric motility in rats. *Peptides* **31,** 2118–2122.

Burdyga, G., Lal, S., Spiller, D., Jiang, W., Thompson, D., Attwood, S., Saeed, S., Grundy, D., Varro, A., Dimaline, R., and Dockray, G. J. (2003). Localization of orexin-1 receptors to vagal afferent neurons in the rat and humans. *Gastroenterology* **124,** 129–139.

Cai, X. J., Widdowson, P. S., Harrold, J., Wilson, S., Buckingham, R. E., Arch, J. R., Tadayyon, M., Clapham, J. C., Wilding, J., and Williams, G. (1999). Hypothalamic orexin expression: Modulation by blood glucose and feeding. *Diabetes* **48,** 2132–2137.

Cai, X. J., Lister, C. A., Buckingham, R. E., Pickavance, L., Wilding, J., Arch, J. R., Wilson, S., and Williams, G. (2000). Down-regulation of orexin gene expression by severe obesity in the rats: Studies in zucker fatty and zucker diabetic fatty rats and effects of rosiglitazone. *Brain Res. Mol. Brain Res.* **77,** 131–137.

Cai, X. J., Evans, M. L., Lister, C. A., Leslie, R. A., Arch, J. R., Wilson, S., and Williams, G. (2001). Hypoglycemia activates orexin neurons and selectively increases hypothalamic orexin-B levels: Responses inhibited by feeding and possibly mediated by the nucleus of the solitary tract. *Diabetes* **50,** 105–112.

Cutler, D. J., Morris, R., Sheridhar, V., Wattam, T. A., Holmes, S., Patel, S., Arch, J. R., Wilson, S., Buckingham, R. E., Evans, M. L., Leslie, R. A., and Williams, G. (1999). Differential distribution of orexin-A and orexin-B immunoreactivity in the rat brain and spinal cord. *Peptides* **20,** 1455–1470.

Dahmen, N., Bierbrauer, J., and Kasten, M. (2001). Increased prevalence of obesity in narcoleptic patients and relatives. *Eur. Arch. Psychiatry Clin. Neurosci.* **251,** 85–89.

Dall'Aglio, C., Pascucci, L., Mercati, F., Giontella, A., Pedini, V., Scocco, P., and Ceccarelli, P. (2008). Identification of orexin A- and orexin type 2 receptor-positive cells in the gastrointestinal tract of neonatal dogs. *Eur. J. Histochem.* **52,** 229–235.

Dall'aglio, C., Pascucci, L., Mercati, F., Giontella, A., Pedini, V., and Ceccarelli, P. (2009). Immunohistochemical identification and localization of orexin A and orexin type 2 receptor in the horse gastrointestinal tract. *Res. Vet. Sci.* **86,** 189–193.

Dall'aglio, C., Zannoni, A., Mercati, F., Forni, M., Bacci, M. L., and Boiti, C. (2011). Differential gene expression and immune localization of the orexin system in the major salivary glands of pigs. *Regul. Pept.* **172,** 51–57.

Doherty, M. J., Watson, N. F., Hallam, D. K., Chandler, W. L., and Longstreth, W. T., Jr. (2005). Ventricular cerebrospinal fluid hypocretin-1 inversely correlates with glucose levels in cerebrospinal fluid and serum from patients with neurological injuries. *Neurocrit. Care* **3,** 230–233.

Ehrstrom, M., Levin, F., Kirchgessner, A. L., Schmidt, P. T., Hilsted, L. M., Gryback, P., Jacobsson, H., Hellstrom, P. M., and Naslund, E. (2005). Stimulatory effect of endogenous orexin A on gastric emptying and acid secretion independent of gastrin. *Regul. Pept.* **132,** 9–16.

Fronczek, R., Overeem, S., Lee, S. Y., Hegeman, I. M., van Pelt, J., van Duinen, S. G., Lammers, G. J., and Swaab, D. F. (2007). Hypocretin (orexin) loss in Parkinson's disease. *Brain* **130,** 1577–1585.

Griffond, B., Risold, P. Y., Jacquemard, C., Colard, C., and Fellmann, D. (1999). Insulin-induced hypoglycemia increases preprohypocretin (orexin) mRNA in the rat lateral hypothalamic area. *Neurosci. Lett.* **262,** 77–80.

Guan, J. L., Wang, Q. P., Kageyama, H., Kita, T., Takenoya, F., Hori, T., and Shioda, S. (2005). Characterization of orexin A immunoreactivity in the rat area postrema. *Regul. Pept.* **129,** 17–23.

Kanbayashi, T., Yano, T., Ishiguro, H., Kawanishi, K., Chiba, S., Aizawa, R., Sawaishi, Y., Hirota, K., Nishino, S., and Shimizu, T. (2002). Hypocretin-1 (orexin-A) levels in human lumbar CSF in different age groups: Infants to elderly persons. *Sleep* **25,** 337–339.

Kanenishi, K., Ueno, M., Momose, S., Kuwabara, H., Tanaka, H., Sato, C., Kobayashi, T., Hino, O., Sakamoto, H., and Hata, T. (2004). Prepro-orexin mRNA expression in the rat brain is increased during pregnancy. *Neurosci. Lett.* **368,** 73–77.

Kato, T., Kanbayashi, T., Yamamoto, K., Nakano, T., Shimizu, T., Hashimoto, T., and Ikeda, S. (2003). Hypersomnia and low CSF hypocretin-1 (orexin-A) concentration in a patient with multiple sclerosis showing bilateral hypothalamic lesions. *Intern. Med.* **42,** 743–745.

Kessler, B. A., Stanley, E. M., Frederick-Duus, D., and Fadel, J. (2011). Age-related loss of orexin/hypocretin neurons. *Neuroscience* **178,** 82–88.

Kis, G., Molnár, A., Daruka, L., Gardi, J., Rákosi, K., László, F., László, F., and Varga, C. (2012). The osmotically and histamine-induced enhancement of the plasma vasopressin level is diminished by intracerebroventricularly administered orexin in rats. *Pflugers Arch.* **463,** 531–536.

Kok, S. W., Overeem, S., Visscher, T. L., Lammers, G. J., Seidell, J. C., Pijl, H., and Meinders, A. E. (2003). Hypocretin deficiency in narcoleptic humans is associated with abdominal obesity. *Obes. Res.* **11,** 1147–1154.

Kunii, K., Yamanaka, A., Nambu, T., Matsuzaki, I., Goto, K., and Sakurai, T. (1999). Orexins/hypocretins regulate drinking behaviour. *Brain Res.* **842,** 256–261.

Lopez, M., Senaris, R., Gallego, R., Garcia-Caballero, T., Lago, F., Seoane, L., Casanueva, F., and Dieguez, C. (1999). Orexin receptors are expressed in the adrenal medulla of the rat. *Endocrinology* **140,** 5991–5994.

Lopez, J. M., Dominguez, L., Moreno, N., and Gonzalez, A. (2009). Comparative immunohistochemical analysis of the distribution of orexins (hypocretins) in the brain of amphibians. *Peptides* **30,** 873–887.

Malherbe, P., Borroni, E., Pinard, E., Wettstein, J. G., and Knoflach, F. (2009). Biochemical and electrophysiological characterization of almorexant, a dual orexin 1 receptor (OX1)/orexin 2 receptor (OX2) antagonist: Comparison with selective OX1 and OX2 antagonists. *Mol. Pharmacol.* **76,** 618–631.

Matsumura, K., Tsuchihashi, T., and Abe, I. (2001). Central orexin-A augments sympathoadrenal outflow in conscious rabbits. *Hypertension* **37,** 1382–1387.

Mogenson, G. J., and Stevenson, J. A. (1967). Drinking induced by electrical stimulation of the lateral hypothalamus. *Exp. Neurol.* **17,** 119–127.

Nowak, K. W., Mackowiak, P., Switonska, M. M., Fabis, M., and Malendowicz, L. K. (2000). Acute orexin effects on insulin secretion in the rat: In vivo and in vitro studies. *Life Sci.* **66,** 449–454.

Nowak, K. W., Strowski, M. Z., Switonska, M. M., Kaczmarek, P., Singh, V., Fabis, M., Mackowiak, P., Nowak, M., and Malendowicz, L. K. (2005). Evidence that orexins A and B stimulate insulin secretion from rat pancreatic islets via both receptor subtypes. *Int. J. Mol. Med.* **15,** 969–972.

Oka, Y., Kanbayashi, T., Mezaki, T., Iseki, K., Matsubayashi, J., Murakami, G., Matsui, M., Shimizu, T., and Shibasaki, H. (2004). Low CSF hypocretin-1/orexin-A associated with hypersomnia secondary to hypothalamic lesion in a case of multiple sclerosis. *J. Neurol.* **251,** 885–886.

Ouedraogo, R., Naslund, E., and Kirchgessner, A. L. (2003). Glucose regulates the release of orexin-A from the endocrine pancreas. *Diabetes* **52,** 111–117.

Pavone, L. M., Tafuri, S., Avallone, L., Staiano, N., and Vittoria, A. (2009). Expression of orexin A and its receptor 1 in the vestibular glands of the cattle genital tract. *Anat. Rec. (Hoboken)* **292,** 202–206.

Putula, J., Turunen, P. M., Jantti, M. H., Ekholm, M. E., and Kukkonen, J. P. (2011). Agonist ligand discrimination by the two orexin receptors depends on the expression system. *Neurosci. Lett.* **494,** 57–60.

Russo, F., Pavone, L. M., Tafuri, S., Avallone, L., Staiano, N., and Vittoria, A. (2008). Expression of orexin A and its receptor 1 in the bovine urethroprostatic complex. *Anat. Rec. (Hoboken)* **291,** 169–174.

Sakurai, T., Amemiya, A., Ishii, M., Matsuzaki, I., Chemelli, R. M., Tanaka, H., Williams, S. C., Richardson, J. A., Kozlowski, G. P., Wilson, S., Arch, J. R., Buckingham, R. E., *et al.* (1998). Orexins and orexin receptors: A family of hypothalamic neuropeptides and G protein-coupled receptors that regulate feeding behavior. *Cell* **92,** 573–585.

Sugimoto, T., Nagake, Y., Sugimoto, S., Akagi, S., Ichikawa, H., Nakamura, Y., Ogawa, N., and Makino, H. (2002). Plasma orexin concentrations in patients on hemodialysis. *Nephron* **90,** 379–383.

Suzuki, H., Kubo, Y., and Yamamoto, T. (2008). Orexin-A immunoreactive cells and fibers in the central nervous system of the axolotl brain and their association with tyrosine hydroxylase and serotonin immunoreactive somata. *J. Chem. Neuroanat.* **35,** 295–305.

Takahashi, K., Arihara, Z., Suzuki, T., Sone, M., Kikuchi, K., Sasano, H., Murakami, O., and Totsune, K. (2006). Expression of orexin-A and orexin receptors in the kidney and the presence of orexin-A-like immunoreactivity in human urine. *Peptides* **27,** 871–877.

Tsuneki, H., Sugihara, Y., Honda, R., Wada, T., Sasaoka, T., and Kimura, I. (2002). Reduction of blood glucose level by orexins in fasting normal and streptozotocin-diabetic mice. *Eur. J. Pharmacol.* **448,** 245–252.

Tsuneki, H., Murata, S., Anzawa, Y., Soeda, Y., Tokai, E., Wada, T., Kimura, I., Yanagisawa, M., Sakurai, T., and Sasaoka, T. (2008). Age-related insulin resistance in hypothalamus and peripheral tissues of orexin knockout mice. *Diabetologia* **51,** 657–667.

van den Pol, A. N. (1999). Hypothalamic hypocretin (orexin): Robust innervation of the spinal cord. *J. Neurosci.* **19,** 3171–3182.

Xu, M., and Volkoff, H. (2007). Molecular characterization of prepro-orexin in Atlantic cod (Gadus morhua): Cloning, localization, developmental profile and role in food intake regulation. *Mol. Cell. Endocrinol.* **271,** 28–37.

Yi, C. X., Serlie, M. J., Ackermans, M. T., Foppen, E., Buijs, R. M., Sauerwein, H. P., Fliers, E., and Kalsbeek, A. (2009). A major role for perifornical orexin neurons in the control of glucose metabolism in rats. *Diabetes* **58,** 1998–2005.

Zhao, Y. Y., Guo, L., Du, J., and Liu, G. L. (2005). Effects of acute hypoglycemia on the orexin system in rat. *Chin. Med. Sci. J.* **20,** 55–58.

Zhu, Y., Miwa, Y., Yamanaka, A., Yada, T., Shibahara, M., Abe, Y., Sakurai, T., and Goto, K. (2003). Orexin receptor type-1 couples exclusively to pertussis toxin-insensitive G-proteins, while orexin receptor type-2 couples to both pertussis toxin sensitive and -insensitive G-proteins. *J. Pharmacol. Sci.* **92,** 259–266.

CHAPTER EIGHT

Orexin Neurons and Emotional Stress

Tomoyuki Kuwaki *and* Wei Zhang[1]

Contents

Department of Physiology, Kagoshima University Graduate School of Medical and Dental Sciences, Sakuragaoka 8-35-1, Kagoshima, Japan
[1] Present address: Department of Surgery, University of Alabama at Birmingham, Birmingham, Alabama, USA.

Vitamins and Hormones, Volume 89
ISSN 0083-6729, http://dx.doi.org/10.1016/B978-0-12-394623-2.00008-1

Abstract

Stress increases cardiac function, ventilation, and body temperature and induces analgesia. These changes, which result in an increase in metabolic rate, oxygen supply, and the conduction velocity of nerve impulses, prepare the body for a fight-or-flight response. A part of the hypothalamus called the defense area has long been known to play a key role in these responses, but the precise mechanisms are largely unknown. Our recent findings suggest that orexin (hypocretin) neurons act as a master switch of the fight-or-flight response. In addition, our results, as well as those from other researchers, suggest that orexin neurons do not modulate specific behaviors such as the fight-or-flight responses but rather integrate the autonomic functions and behaviors in a broad sense or in a vigilance state-dependent manner. The orexin system seems to be a pivotal link between the subconscious and the conscious brain functions.

I. Introduction

Research on the neural mechanisms underlying state-dependent adjustments of central autonomic regulation has been sparse, despite the importance of these adjustments from the perspective of the well-being of an organism. In addition to calm and resting states, our daily life involves many perturbations that induce active conditions, such as those involving locomotion, eating, and communication. During such active periods, cardiovascular, respiratory, and body temperature regulation needs to be adjusted according to situational demands, which differ from those during resting states, and this occurs through the modulation of or the resetting of homeostatic set points (Kumada *et al.*, 1990). One of the neural substrates that regulate these adjustments appears to be located in the hypothalamus because stimulation of the so-called defense area in the dorsal hypothalamus elicits behavioral rage along with the specific autonomic responses; this has been called the defense response (Hess, 1954).

Several neurotransmitters have been proposed to be involved in the modulation of the efferent pathways of the defense responses against stressors. For example, the activation of serotonin (5HT)-1A receptors in the medullary raphe reduces cardiovascular changes (Nalivaiko *et al.*, 2005), and the inhibition of 5HT-3 receptors in the nucleus tractus solitarius prevents the inhibition of baroreflex bradycardia during the defense response (Sévoz-Couche *et al.*, 2003). Microinjections of adenosine into the rostral ventrolateral medulla augment the increase in blood pressure that is induced by electrical stimulation of the hypothalamic defense area (Thomas and Spyer, 1996). The evidence of glutamate participation in the cardiovascular components of the defense response

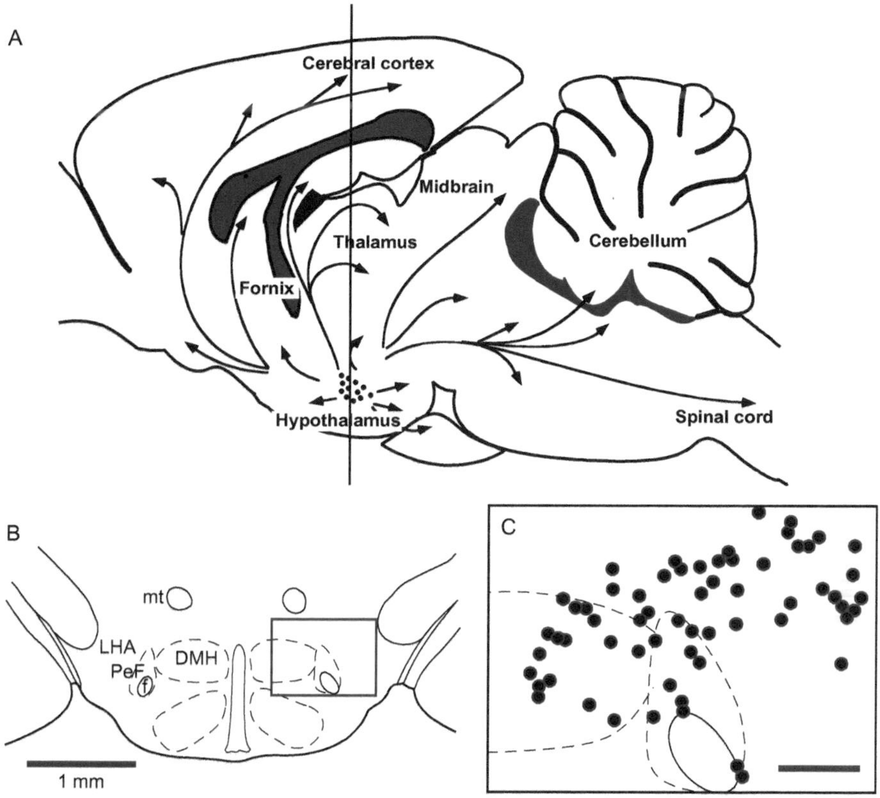

Figure 8.1 Distribution of orexin neurons in the brain. (A) Schematic drawing of a sagittal section of a rodent brain showing the restricted distribution of orexin-containing neuronal cell bodies (circles) in the hypothalamus and the wide distribution of their axons (arrows) throughout the brain. The vertical line indicates the plane in (B). Adapted from Nambu *et al.* (1999). (B) A coronal section through the hypothalamus. The rectangle denotes the area examined in (C). DMH, dorsomedial hypothalamus; f, fornix; LHA, lateral hypothalamic area; mt, mammillothalamic tract; PeF, perifornical area. (C) The distribution of the orexin-like immunoreactivity (circles) in a representative mouse brain. Bar, 200 μm in (C). Adapted from Zhang *et al.* (2010).

has been debated (Kiely and Gordon, 1994; Sun and Guyenet, 1986). However, there have been no reports on the molecular basis of the defense response that underlies the multifaceted nature of the simultaneous and coordinated changes in cardiovascular, respiratory, sensory, thermal, and behavioral parameters. Because orexin-containing cell bodies (Fig. 8.1) are located in the perifornical area (PFA) and the dorsomedial hypothalamus (DMH), which overlaps the defense area, we set out to investigate the possible role of orexin in the defense response against stressors.

II. Orexin Neurons

A. Orexin (hypocretin)

Orexins (orexin-A and orexin-B), which are also known as hypocretins (hypocretin 1 and hypocretin 2, respectively), are recently discovered hypothalamic neuropeptides (de Lecea *et al.*, 1998; Sakurai *et al.*, 1998). They are cleaved from a common precursor molecule, prepro-orexin (130 residues), to form orexin-A (33 amino acids) and orexin-B (28 amino acids) (Sakurai *et al.*, 1998; Willie *et al.*, 2001). Orexin-A binds with equal affinity to the orexin receptor-1 and receptor-2, whereas orexin-B selectively binds to orexin receptor-2 (Sakurai *et al.*, 1998; Willie *et al.*, 2001).

Although orexins were first described as hypothalamic neuropeptides that influence appetite (Sakurai *et al.*, 1998) and consciousness (Chemelli *et al.*, 1999), it was later found that orexins also modulate reward processes (Harris and Aston-Jones, 2006), pain processes (Watanabe *et al.*, 2005; Yamamoto *et al.*, 2002), and the autonomic regulation of the cardiovascular (Dun *et al.*, 2000; Shirasaka *et al.*, 1999; Zhang *et al.*, 2006b), respiratory (Young *et al.*, 2005; Zhang *et al.*, 2005), and neuroendocrine (Jászberényi *et al.*, 2000) systems.

B. Coexisting transmitter/modulators

Orexin neurons contain not only orexin but also other putative neurotransmitter/modulator candidates, such as glutamate (Abrahamson *et al.*, 2001; Rosin *et al.*, 2003; Torrealba *et al.*, 2003), dynorphin (Chou *et al.*, 2001), galanin (Hakansson *et al.*, 1999), and nitric oxide (Cheng *et al.*, 2003). Dynorphin and glutamate may act synergistically with orexin to promote wakefulness (Arrigoni *et al.*, 2010). However, the precise role (s) of the substances that are colocalized with orexin are largely unknown.

C. Anatomy of orexin-containing neurons

Orexin-containing cell bodies are restricted to the lateral hypothalamic area (LHA), the PFA, and the DMH (Fig. 8.1). Their distribution is rostrocaudally restricted within 1 mm in mice (Sunanaga *et al.*, 2009). Conversely, orexin-containing nerve terminals and receptors are widely distributed in the hypothalamus, thalamus, cerebral cortex, circumventricular organs, brain stem, cerebellum, and spinal cord, suggesting that the orexin neurons have widespread connections with other regions in the brain (Elias *et al.*, 1998; Marcus *et al.*, 2001; Nambu *et al.*, 1999). Specifically, the cardiorespiratory-related areas that receive orexinergic innervation are the nucleus tractus solitarius, the pre-Bötzinger complex, the periaqueductal gray, the

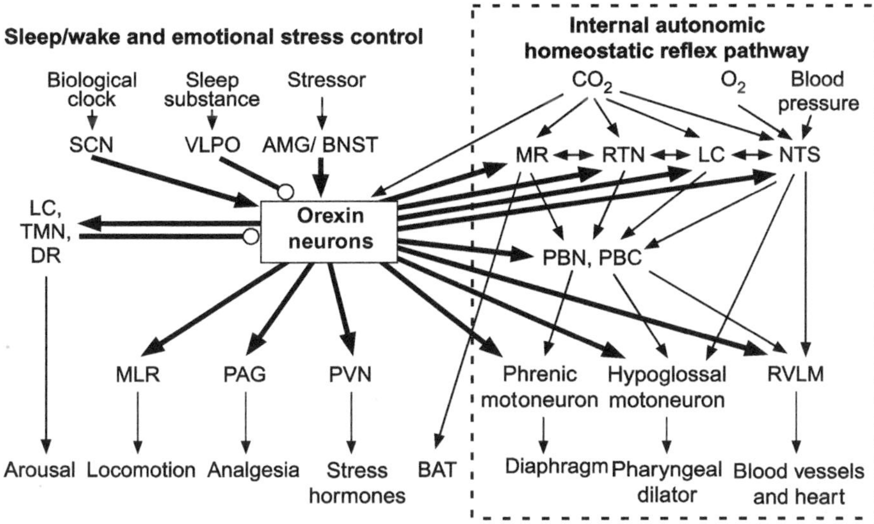

Figure 8.2 Pivotal role of orexin neurons in linking state-dependent behavioral regulatory systems and internal autonomic homeostatic reflex pathways. Among the known connections from/to orexin neurons in the hypothalamus, the thick lines indicate the selected brain nuclei that are relevant to our study. Many nuclei that are located at both input (MR, RTN, LC, and NTS) and output (cardiorespiratory motor neurons) interfaces in the internal homeostatic reflex pathway receive projections from the orexin neurons (right half). Simultaneously, orexinergic connections are engaged in sleep/wake regulation and emotional stress-induced behavioral changes (left half). Thus, orexin can modulate internal autonomic homeostasis in a state-dependent and feed-forward manner. Arrows indicate a probable excitatory connection, and circles indicate an inhibitory connection. Connections shown with thin lines are either direct or indirect. Abbreviations: AMG, amygdala; BAT, brown adipose tissue; BNST, bed nucleus of the stria terminalis; DR, dorsal raphe; LC, locus coeruleus; MLR, medullary locomotor region; MR, medullary raphe; NTS, nucleus tractus solitarius; PAG, periaqueductal gray; PBC, pre-Bötzinger complex; PBN, parabrachial nucleus; PVN, paraventricular nucleus; RTN, retrotrapezoid nucleus; RVLM, rostral ventrolateral medulla where sympathetic cardiovascular premotor neurons are located; SCN, suprachiasmatic nucleus; TMN, tuberomammillary nucleus; VLPO, ventrolateral preoptic nucleus. Adapted from Kuwaki and Zhang (2010).

rostral ventrolateral medulla, the intermediolateral cell column of the spinal cord, and the retrotrapezoid, hypoglossal, medullary raphe, parabrachial/Kölliker-Fuse, and phrenic nuclei (Fig. 8.2) (Antunes *et al.*, 2001; Berthoud *et al.*, 2005; Dergacheva *et al.*, 2005; Dun *et al.*, 2000; Fung *et al.*, 2001; Geerling *et al.*, 2003; Kuwaki, 2008; Kuwaki and Zhang, 2010; Marcus *et al.*, 2001; Peyron *et al.*, 1998; Rosin *et al.*, 2006; Smith *et al.*, 2002; Volgin *et al.*, 2002; Young *et al.*, 2005). Approximately 50% of the hypothalamic neurons that innervate both of the sympathetic efferent nuclei and of either the motor or the medial prefrontal cortex, which is implicated in mental stress, show orexin-like immunoreactivity (Krout *et al.*, 2003, 2005).

Moreover, orexin neurons receive inputs from the sites that regulate the circadian clock, the sleep/wake cycle, and emotional stress, including the ventrolateral preoptic area, the locus coeruleus, the dorsal raphe, the amygdala, the bed nucleus of stria terminalis (BNST), and the suprachiasmatic and tuberomammillary nuclei (Fig. 8.2) (Kuwaki and Zhang, 2010; Sakurai, 2007; Sakurai *et al.*, 2005; Saper *et al.*, 2005; Yoshida *et al.*, 2006; Zhang *et al.*, 2009). Numerous neurons in the amygdala, which is a putative center for biological value judgments (Pitkanen *et al.*, 1997), were retrogradely labeled after a cholera toxin B subunit was injected into the PFA (Yoshida *et al.*, 2006) and by the transsynaptic transport of tetanus toxin that was expressed by the orexin promoter (Sakurai *et al.*, 2005).

These anatomic features establish the basis for the hypothesis of the contribution of orexin to the link between the regulatory systems of consciousness (sleep/wake cycle or emotional stress) and unconscious homeostatic reflexes (Fig. 8.2; Kuwaki and Zhang, 2010).

D. Orexin and arousal

Orexins, which play a key role in the stabilization of wakefulness, are thought to be arousal-promoting peptides (Carter *et al.*, 2009). Diminished orexin function can result in a specific clinical syndrome, namely, narcolepsy, in animals and humans (Chemelli *et al.*, 1999; Thannickal *et al.*, 2000). Orexin neurons show state-dependent activity (Lee *et al.*, 2005; Mileykovskiy *et al.*, 2005; Takahashi *et al.*, 2008): orexin levels increase just before wakening, remain high during wakefulness, increase considerably during exercise and/or heightened alertness, decrease during non-rapid eye movement (NREM) sleep (also called slow-wave sleep), and again increase during rapid eye movement (REM) sleep. Orexin neurons receive dense projections from the suprachiasmatic nucleus, which is a circadian rhythm oscillator (Saper *et al.*, 2005), as well as from many other sites (see Fig. 8.2), and the release of orexins into the extracellular fluid in the hypothalamus is greater in the dark, that is, the active period, than in the light, that is, the resting period, in nocturnal rats (Yoshida *et al.*, 2001). Orexin neuron firing rates vary according to the state of vigilance, even within a circadian period (*vide supra*), and the direct activation of orexin neurons through the *in vivo* photostimulation of channelrhodopsin-2 elicits rapid awakening regardless of the circadian period (Carter *et al.*, 2009). The photoinactivation of orexin neurons expressing halorhodopsin induces NREM sleep only during the daytime when sleep pressure is high in mice (Tsunematsu *et al.*, 2011). Orexins, which are known to play an important role in circadian variations during cardiorespiratory control (Mortola, 2004; Stephenson, 2007), are likely to play a role in cardiorespiratory control relative to the state of vigilance within circadian periods.

E. Orexin-deficient mice—An animal model of human narcolepsy

Narcolepsy is a sleep disorder that is characterized by excessive daytime sleepiness, and patients with narcolepsy experience extreme fatigue and suddenly fall asleep at inappropriate times. Although the cause of narcolepsy was not determined for many years after its discovery, a strong link between narcolepsy and orexin was discovered a year after the discovery of orexin. The cause of narcolepsy in Doberman with hereditary narcolepsy is a mutation in the orexin receptor-2 gene (Lin *et al.*, 1999), and prepro-orexin-knockout (ORX-KO) mice exhibit a narcoleptic phenotype (Chemelli *et al.*, 1999). Indeed, the number of orexin neurons is reduced in humans with narcolepsy (Thannickal *et al.*, 2000).

At present, there are two genetically engineered mice models of orexin deficiency that are used to study the possible roles of intrinsic orexin in physiological functions, including sleep/wake regulation. One is the ORX-KO mouse that was developed by a conventional knockout technique (Chemelli *et al.*, 1999), and the other is the orexin neuron-ablated (ORX-AB) mouse (Hara *et al.*, 2001). The latter was developed using a transgenic technique that introduced a truncated Machado–Joseph disease gene product (ataxin-3) with an expanded polyglutamine stretch that was under the control of the orexin promoter. In these orexin/ataxin-3-transgenic mice, orexin-containing neurons selectively degenerate postnatally, and a loss of 99% or more of the neurons occurs by the age of 4 months (Hara *et al.*, 2001). Orexinergic neurons contain not only orexin but also other neuropeptides or modulatory factors (see Section II.B). In addition to orexin, these substances also disappear in the "orexin neurons" of ORX-AB mice.

In addition to these orexin-deficient mice models, orexin receptor-1- and -2-knockout mice (Mieda *et al.*, 2011), naturally occurring orexin receptor-2-mutant dogs (Lin *et al.*, 1999), and ORX-AB rats (Beuckmann *et al.*, 2004) are currently available for the study of the possible roles of orexin/orexin receptor systems *in vivo*. Although the cause of orexin/orexin receptor deficiency in these models is not the same as that in humans (which is presumably autoimmune) (Hallmayer *et al.*, 2009), all of these animals express a narcoleptic phenotype and, therefore, demonstrate the importance of the orexin signaling system in sleep/wake regulation.

III. Behavior-Associated Changes in Autonomic Functions

A. Emotional stress

Animals cope with stressors with two strategies (Korte *et al.*, 2005). An active coping strategy (fight-or-flight) is evoked if the stress is predictable, controllable, or escapable. A passive coping strategy (immobility or decreased responsiveness to the environment) is evoked if the stress is inescapable. The active strategy is associated with sympathoexcitation (hypertension, tachycardia), whereas the passive strategy is associated with sympathoinhibition and/or parasympathetic activation (hypotension, bradycardia). The passive strategy also helps to facilitate recovery and healing. The active strategy is called the fight-or-flight response from a behavioral point of view or the defense response from an autonomic point of view. The passive strategy is sometimes called playing dead or paradoxical fear. The distinct neural substrates that mediate active versus passive emotional coping have been identified within the brainstem (Bandler *et al.*, 2000; Nosaka, 1996).

B. Sleep and wake

It is well known that blood pressure, respiration, and body temperature fluctuate with an ~24-h rhythm (circadian rhythm) with nadirs occurring during nighttime in humans. In sharp contrast to humans, mice and rats sleep for a short duration (an episode of sleep lasts for 10–30 min) many times during both daytime and nighttime. These animals are called nocturnal because their total wake time is longer during the nighttime than the daytime and not because they are continuously awake during the nighttime as humans are during the daytime. In these fragmented sleepers, blood pressure, respiration, and body temperature decrease while they are sleeping regardless of the time of day. Therefore, the state of vigilance is a strong determinant of these autonomic parameters.

The reduced metabolic demand during sleep cannot explain the diminished blood pressure and minute ventilation that occurs at that time because the partial pressure of arterial CO_2 increases during sleep (Krieger, 2000). During NREM sleep, the rhythm and amplitude of the ventilation and heartbeats are stable and regular. Sleep-related neuronal mechanisms may actively suppress ventilation because minute ventilation decreases during sleep, even in a hypercapnic environment. During NREM sleep, the tonus of the upper airway muscles decreases so markedly that airway resistance increases considerably. At the same time, decreases in the contraction of the intercostal muscles and of the diaphragm are small (Krieger, 2000). Therefore, sleep affects the neurons that regulate the upper airway and those controlling the thorax differently. During REM sleep, there are remarkable surges and pauses in cardiorespiratory activity, although metabolic demands seem not to be remarkably changed. The general hypersensitivity of the nervous system during REM sleep can be ruled out since hypoxic and hypercapnic ventilatory responses are smaller during REM sleep than during NREM sleep. The pulmonary stretch receptor reflex and the irritant receptor reflex are also suppressed during sleep, and hence, cough develops only after arousal from sleep (Douglas, 2000). Although these phenomena are well known, their underlying mechanisms remain to be elucidated.

IV. Lessons from Orexin-Deficient Mice

Taking into account the background mentioned above, we hypothesized that orexin-containing neurons in the hypothalamus may be the missing link between arousal/active stress-coping behaviors and the associated bodily changes that are mainly governed by the autonomic nervous system. In fact, stressors activate orexin-containing neurons (Espana *et al.*, 2003; Ida *et al.*, 2000; Kuwaki *et al.*, 2007; Watanabe *et al.*, 2005; Winsky-Sommerer *et al.*, 2004; Zhang *et al.*, 2010; Zhu *et al.*, 2002). Anatomical (Fig. 8.2) and pharmacological (Section V) evidence supports our hypothesis. In order to test the hypothesis, we used ORX-KO and ORX-AB mice and observed their responses to direct stimulation of the hypothalamus and natural stressful stimuli.

A. Basal parameters

In both ORX-KO and ORX-AB mice, basal blood pressure was significantly lower by about 20 mmHg than that in their wild-type littermates in either anesthetized or conscious condition (Kayaba *et al.*, 2003; Zhang *et al.*, 2006a). The circadian fluctuation of blood pressure and heart rate was similar between ORX-KO and wild-type mice except that the blood pressure in ORX-KO mice was consistently lower during both dark and light phases. Drowsiness and lower activity in ORX-KO mice cannot explain the differences in blood pressure because these behavioral abnormalities were only apparent during dark phases (the active phase for nocturnal mice), while lower blood pressure was observed, even in the light phase, when the behavioral abnormalities were not significant. Alpha-adrenergic blockade with prazosin or ganglion blockade with hexamethonium eliminated the difference in basal blood pressure. Heart rate and cardiac contractile parameters determined by echocardiography did not differ from those in wild-type mice. These results indicate that there was lower sympathetic vasoconstrictor tone in orexin-deficient mice. It should be noted here that a similar baseline hypotension was reported in ORX-AB rats (Schwimmer *et al.*, 2010), while another group reported slight hypertension in ORX-AB mice (Bastianini *et al.*, 2011). We do not currently know the exact reason for the differences but possible differences in environmental stresses may explain the discrepancy because orexin neurons are deeply involved in stress-induced hypertension (see Section IV. B).

Basal ventilation (respiratory frequency and tidal volume) (Nakamura *et al.*, 2007) and basal body temperature (Zhang *et al.*, 2010) were not significantly altered in ORX-KO or ORX-AB mice.

B. Cardiorespiratory responses during stress

To date, three lines of evidence support our hypothesis of the contribution of orexin to the defense response. First, the stimulation of the PFA with the GABA-A receptor antagonist, bicuculline, resulted in an attenuated defense response in urethane-anesthetized ORX-KO and ORX-AB mice. Increases in arterial blood pressure, heart rate, respiratory frequency, and the β-band power of the electroencephalogram (an index of cortical arousal) were smaller and/or shorter in ORX-KO mice than in their wild-type littermates (Kayaba *et al.*, 2003). Similarly, increased blood pressure, heart rate, and respiratory minute volume and vascular dilatation in the skeletal muscle were attenuated in the ORX-AB mice (Zhang *et al.*, 2006a).

Second, the suppression of the baroreceptor reflex during the defense response was attenuated in ORX-AB mice, whereas characteristics of the baroreceptor reflex (gain and slope) at rest were normal in these mice (Zhang *et al.*, 2006a). During the defense response, the baroreceptor reflex is suppressed or reset to a higher-pressure range in order to allow a higher blood pressure than that in resting conditions (Kumada *et al.*, 1990; McDowall *et al.*, 2006). The suppression of the baroreflex is mediated by the DMH-medullary link (Sévoz-Couche *et al.*, 2003). Orexin appeared to contribute to the suppression of the baroreflex during defense responses, but not to the baroreflex during resting conditions.

Third, an attenuation of the defense response in the ORX-KO and ORX-AB mice was also observed in the mice during natural stimulation in unanesthetized and freely moving conditions (Fig. 8.3). We tested the defense response in conscious animals using the resident-intruder test or the air-jet stress paradigm in order to rule out the possibility that the observed differences between the orexin-deficient mice and their wild-type littermates resulted from differences in anesthetic susceptibilities. As expected, the emotional stressor-induced increases in blood pressure, heart rate, and locomotor activity were smaller in orexin-deficient mice (ORX-KO and ORX-AB) than in their wild-type littermates (Kayaba *et al.*, 2003; Zhang *et al.*, 2006a).

C. Stress-induced analgesia

Cardiorespiratory response is not the sole characteristic of the defense response. The defense response is characterized by a coordinated change in cardiovascular, respiratory, sensory, and motor functions (Fig. 8.4). One of

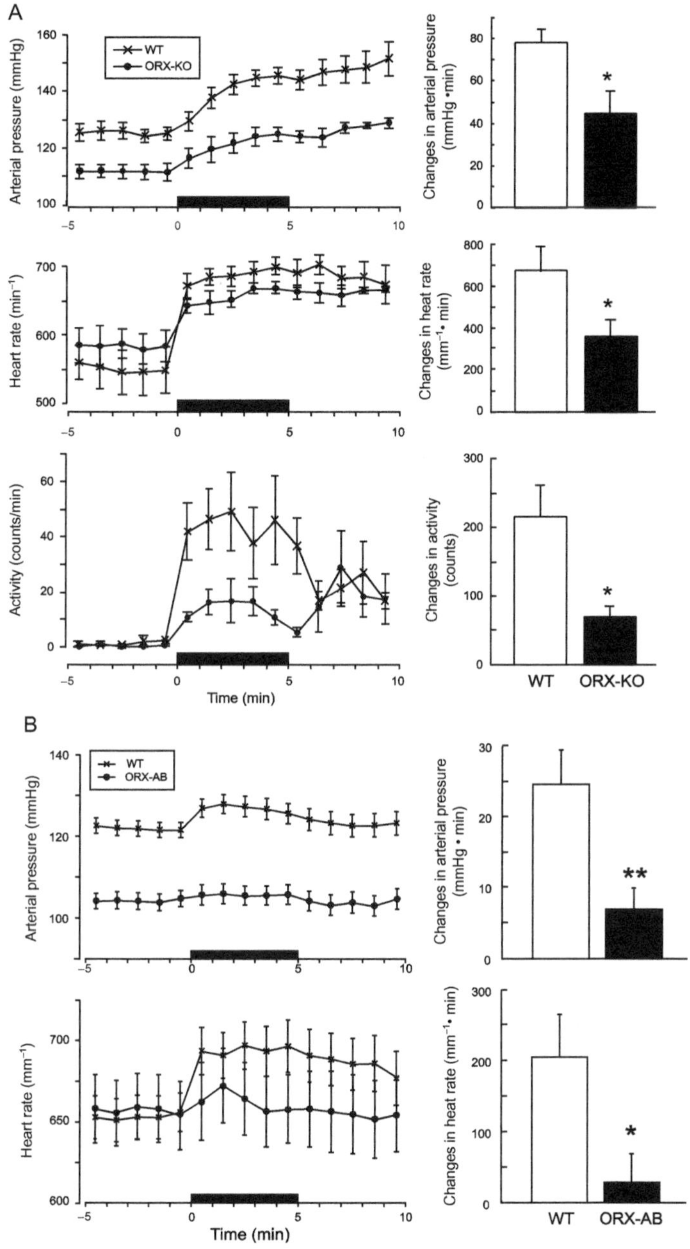

Figure 8.3 Cardiovascular and behavioral responses during natural stressful stimulation in conscious orexin-deficient and wild-type littermates. (A) A resident-intruder test was performed in radiotelemeter-indwelling freely moving wild-type (WT) and orexin-knockout (ORX-KO) mice. The horizontal solid bar indicates the presence of an intruder. The panels on the right side show the changes in blood pressure, heart rate, and activities that are expressed as area under the curve (AUC) during the 5 min when an intruder was present in the same cage. (B) Air-jet stress was applied to catheter-indwelling lightly restrained WT and orexin neuron-ablated (ORX-AB) mice. The horizontal solid bar indicates the duration of air-jet stress. The panels on the right side are the changes in arterial pressure and heart rate that are expressed as AUC during the 5 min of the stress. Data are presented as means ± standard error of the mean (SEM) of 6–8 mice in each genotype. *$P < 0.05$, **$P < 0.01$ versus WT mice. Adapted from Kuwaki and Zhang (2010).

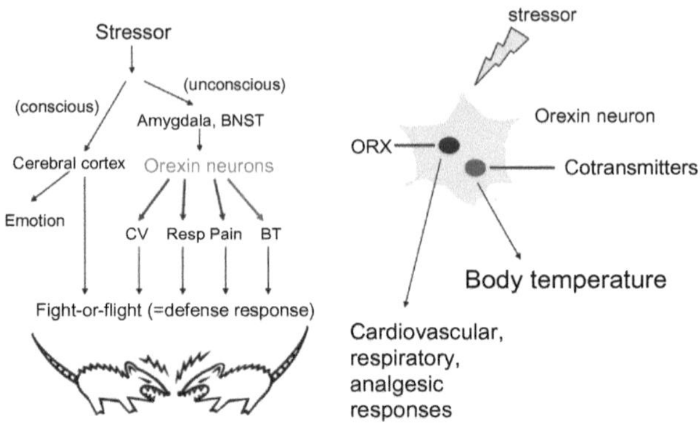

Figure 8.4 Hypothetical diagram showing the key role of orexin neurons in the fight-or-flight response. When animals confront a stressor, orexin neurons mediate cardiovascular (CV), respiratory (Resp), and analgesic (Pain) responses by using orexin as a transmitter. At the same time, orexin neurons regulate body temperature (BT) by using cotransmitters other than orexin. These responses are collectively called the defense response that prepares the body for the fight-or-flight behavior. Adapted from Kuwaki (2011). (See Color Insert.)

the multifaceted features of the defense response, stress-induced analgesia, was examined. In wild-type mice, foot shock induces long-lasting analgesia, as evidenced by increases in tail-flick latency from noxious hot water. Although ORX-KO mice showed moderate analgesia, the effect was significantly smaller than that shown by their wild-type littermates (Watanabe *et al.*, 2005).

D. Stress-induced hyperthermia

Because cardiorespiratory responses during stress (see Section IV.B) were equally attenuated in ORX-KO and ORX-AB mice and stress-induced analgesia was attenuated in ORX-KO mice (Section IV.C), we concluded at this point that orexin was the main contributor to these responses, and colocalized transmitter/modulator candidates had only a minor role, if any. In line with this notion, we hypothesized that stress-induced hyperthermia would also be influenced by orexin. On the contrary, we found that ORX-AB mice, and not ORX-KO mice, had blunted stress-induced hyperthermia (Zhang *et al.*, 2010) (Fig. 8.5A). The brown adipose tissue, which is a major thermogenic organ in rodents, did not respond to handling stress (Fig. 8.5B), although it did respond to direct pharmacologic stimulation (Fig. 8.5C). These abnormalities in ORX-AB mice were not observed in ORX-KO mice, in which the orexin peptide is deficient but the neurons are preserved. Therefore, the integrity (orexin and other coexisting neurotransmitter/modulators) of the orexin neurons is indispensable for the complete expression of multiple facets of the fight-or-flight response (Kuwaki, 2011; Kuwaki and Zhang, 2010) (Fig. 8.4).

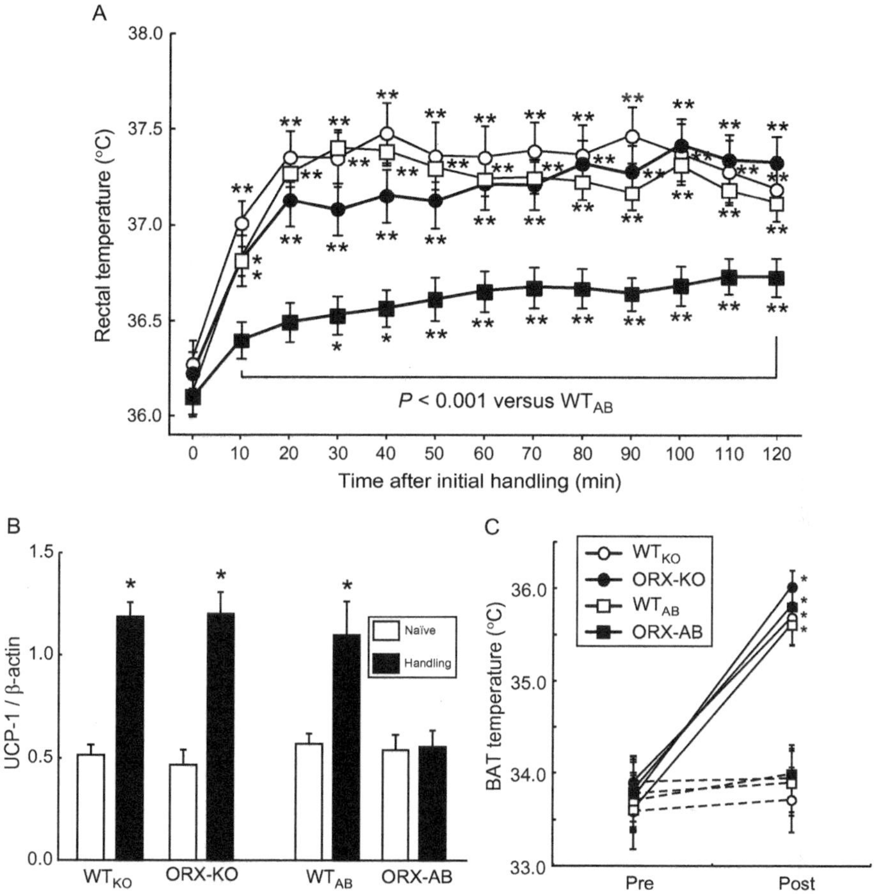

Figure 8.5 (A) Effect of repeated handling stress on the rectal temperature of mice of four genotypes. The temperature measurement (insertion of thermistor probe into the animal's rectum) itself was used as a stressor and repeatedly applied at 10-min intervals for 2 h. Data are presented as mean ± SEM of orexin-knockout mice (ORX-KO, $n=37$), orexin neuron-ablated mice (ORX-AB, $n=32$), and their corresponding wild-type littermates (WT_{KO}, $n=22$ and WT_{AB}, $n=21$). (B) Expression of uncoupling protein (UCP)-1 in the brown adipose tissue (BAT) of stressed or naïve mice. BAT was dissected from stressed mice (four rectal temperature measurements at 10-min intervals) and from naïve (unstressed) mice of the same genotypes. The total RNA extracted from the BAT and cDNA was reverse transcribed. UCP-1 mRNA was determined by quantitative real-time PCR in triplicate and normalized with β-actin mRNA. Data are presented as mean ± SEM of 7–9 animals. Note that handling stress increased the expression of UCP-1 in wild-type and ORX-KO mice but not in ORX-AB mice. $^{*}P<0.05$ versus naïve. (C) BAT function test. The change of BAT temperature in response to a β3-agonist, CL316243, was examined in chloralose- (75 mg/kg, ip) and urethane- (750 mg/kg, ip) anesthetized mice. The animals received intraperitoneal injections of saline (dashed line) or CL316243 (1 mg/kg, solid line). Data are presented as mean ± SEM of the peak values during the observation period of 120 min ($n=5$ for each group). $^{*}P<0.05$ versus pre-treatment value. These results indicate that blunted stress-induced hyperthermia in ORX-AB was caused by the loss of orexin neurons and abnormal BAT regulation and not due to an abnormality of BAT *per se*. Adapted from Zhang *et al*. (2010).

E. Afferent pathways to the orexin neurons

Disinhibition of the amygdala or the BNST by an injection of bicuculline in urethane-anesthetized ORX-AB mice scarcely caused the cardiorespiratory activation that was consistently observed in wild-type control mice (Zhang *et al.*, 2009). We concluded that orexin-containing neurons mediate at least part of the amygdala- and BNST-induced cardiorespiratory responses and act as a master switch for the activation of multiple efferent pathways of the defense response after stressor inputs (Fig. 8.4).

F. Vigilance state-dependent modulation

In both ORX-KO mice and wild-type control mice, the respiratory frequency [quiet wake (QW) $>$ NREM $\approx$ REM] and tidal volume (QW $>$ NREM $>$ REM) showed a clear sleep–wake dependency. Fragmentation of sleep episodes in the ORX-KO mice did not affect the relationship between the state of vigilance and minute ventilation (Nakamura *et al.*, 2007). Therefore, orexin does not appear to contribute to basal breathing when an animal is at rest and under normal air conditions.

The magnitudes of the hypercapnic- (5% CO_2–21% O_2 and 10% CO_2–21% O_2) and hypoxic- (15% O_2) ventilatory responses in both the ORX-KO and wild-type mice also showed a clear dependence on the state of vigilance (Nakamura *et al.*, 2007). That is, the order of the magnitudes of the changes in minute ventilation was QW $>$ NREM $>$ REM, irrespective of the stimulus or genotype (except for hypercapnic responses in ORX-KO mice: QW $\approx$ NREM). Unlike the general similarity between mutants and controls, the hypercapnic responses in the ORX-KO mice during QW were significantly attenuated to approximately half of that in wild-type mice when they were evaluated as an increase in minute ventilation (Fig. 8.6A). When evaluated as the slope of the hypercapnic chemoreflex, the hypercapnic ventilatory responses of the ORX-KO mice did not increase with arousal from sleep, although the SWS $>$ REM relationship was the same as that in the wild-type mice (Fig. 8.6B).

The above-mentioned respiratory abnormality in the ORX-KO mice was reproduced by the administration of the OX_1R-selective antagonist SB334867 (Smart *et al.*, 2001; Yamamoto *et al.*, 2002) to the wild-type mice without affecting the state of vigilance (Fig. 8.6C). In addition, supplementation with orexin-A or orexin-B partially restored the hypercapnic chemoreflex in the ORX-KO mice (Fig. 8.6D) (Deng *et al.*, 2007).

Based on these results, we previously proposed that the hypercapnic response during sleep periods relies on the unknown mechanisms that are independent of orexin and that the response is augmented by orexin during awake periods (Kuwaki, 2008). This proposal is consistent with the reports that state that the spontaneous activity of the orexin neurons is increased

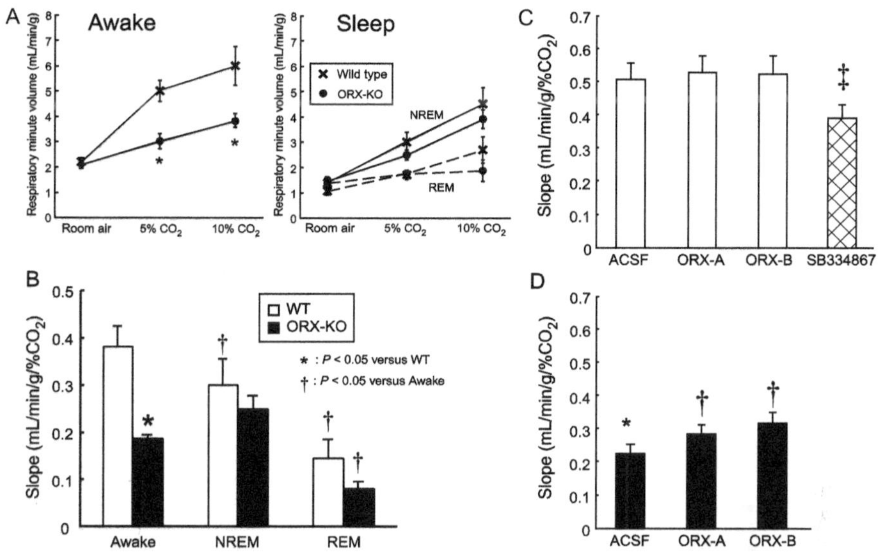

Figure 8.6 Abnormality of vigilance state-dependent changes in hypercapnic ventilatory responsiveness in prepro-orexin-knockout mice and partial restoration by exogenously administered orexin peptides. (A) Hypercapnic responses of respiratory minute volume in wild-type (WT) mice and prepro-orexin-knockout mice (ORX-KO) during quiet awake (upper left panel) and sleep (upper right panel) periods. (B) Hypercapnic responses are evaluated by calculating the slope of the relationship between inspired CO_2 concentration and respiratory minute volume. Data are presented as means $\pm$ SEM of five WT mice and five ORX-KO mice. Abbreviations: NREM, non-rapid eye movement sleep; REM, rapid eye movement sleep. (C, D) Wild-type mice ($n=6$–7 (C)) and ORX-KO mice ($n=9$ (D)) received artificial cerebrospinal fluid (ACSF, 2 μL), orexin-A (ORX-A, 3 nmol), orexin-B (ORX-B, 3 nmol), or the orexin receptor antagonist SB334667 (30 nmol), and their hypercapnic ventilatory responses were evaluated. Data are presented as means $\pm$ standard error of the mean (SEM). $\star P<0.05$ compared with ACSF-treated WT in (C). $\dagger P<0.05$ compared with ACSF-treated KO. $\ddagger P<0.05$ compared with ACSF- and vehicle-treated WT. Adapted from Kuwaki and Zhang (2010).

during wake periods and is decreased during sleep periods (Lee *et al.*, 2005; Mileykovskiy *et al.*, 2005). In addition, CO_2 is known to activate the orexin neurons in hypothalamic slice preparations (Williams *et al.*, 2007) and in mice *in vivo* (Sunanaga *et al.*, 2009). Wakefulness driving to respiration has been proposed to increase hypercapnic responsiveness (Phillipson, 1978), and the administration of orexin has been thought to increase ventilation through its awakening effect. However, ORX-KO mice do wake without orexin, and their hypercapnic responsiveness remains unchanged from the magnitude that is seen during sleep (Deng *et al.*, 2007), indicating that waking itself could not augment the hypercapnic responsiveness in the absence of orexin.

V. Relevant Data from Normal Rodents and Narcoleptic Humans

A. Exogenous administration of orexin and orexin receptor antagonists

The exogenous administration of orexin induces analgesia (Yamamoto *et al.*, 2002) and cardiovascular (Antunes *et al.*, 2001; Chen *et al.*, 2000; Machado *et al.*, 2002; Samson *et al.*, 1999; Shirasaka *et al.*, 1999; Zhang *et al.*, 2005) and respiratory (Dutschmann *et al.*, 2007; Young *et al.*, 2005; Zhang *et al.*, 2005) activation. As for the effect on body temperature, both hyperthermia (Monda *et al.*, 2003) and hypothermia (Székely *et al.*, 2002) were reported. These data are well in line with our hypothesis.

Nattie's group recently reported that the microdialysis of SB334867 into the medullary raphe nucleus of rats (Dias *et al.*, 2010) reduced the hypercapnic ventilatory response during wakefulness in the dark (active period) but not during wakefulness in the light (inactive period). Microdialysis of SB334867 into the retrotrapezoid nucleus (RTN) of rats (Dias *et al.*, 2009) reduced the hypercapnic ventilatory response predominantly during wakefulness in the light, which is the inactive period (it was not studied in the dark period). In fact, there are orexin-containing nerve terminals on the RTN neurons, and orexin excites them (Lazarenko *et al.*, 2011). These results suggest that either the medullary raphe or RTN may be the site responsible for the orexinergic modulation of hypercapnic chemostimulation and that the modulation depends on both the state of vigilance and the circadian period (Kuwaki *et al.*, 2010).

B. Functional neuroanatomy

We found that the exposure of awake and freely moving wild-type mice to a gas mixture of 10% CO_2, 21% O_2, and residual N_2 for 3 h significantly increased the expression of c-Fos in the orexin-containing cells that were located in the PFA/DMH ($15.8 \pm 1.6\%$ for room air vs. $28.4 \pm 2.7\%$ for CO_2, $P=0.011$) but not in the LHA ($12.3 \pm 1.2\%$ for room air vs. $12.4 \pm 3.0\%$ for CO_2) (Sunanaga *et al.*, 2009). Although this methodology cannot differentiate between a direct effect of CO_2 on the orexin-containing neurons and an indirect effect through other neurons, the inhalation of CO_2 was found to activate the orexin-containing neurons *in vivo*.

We also observed that numerous neurons with orexin-like immunoreactivity expressed c-Fos after foot shock stress (Kuwaki *et al.*, 2007; Watanabe *et al.*, 2005) and handling stress (Zhang *et al.*, 2010). Moreover, disinhibition of the amygdala or BNST induced significantly larger numbers of orexin-positive neurons that expressed c-Fos in the PFA/DMH ($58.2 \pm 6.4\%$ in the amygdala and $66.4 \pm 6.6\%$ in BNST) than did the vehicle (18.2±4.4% in the amygdala and 28.3±2.1% in BNST). Disinhibition of the BNST induced widespread expression of c-Fos in not only the orexin-containing neurons but also other neurons in the hypothalamus (Zhang *et al.*, 2009).

Transneuronal retrograde transport of a pseudorabies virus from the brown adipose tissue, which is a key structure in nonshivering thermogenesis, identified the caudal raphe neurons as a site of orexinergic innervation (Berthoud *et al.*, 2005) and orexin-containing neurons in the hypothalamus (Oldfield *et al.*, 2002).

The above-mentioned neuroanatomical data support our hypothesis of the state-dependent modulation of central cardiorespiratory regulation by orexin neurons.

C. Human narcolepsy

There are only a few reports describing autonomic regulation in narcoleptic patients. Sachs and Kaijser (1982) reported that unmedicated narcoleptic patients showed attenuated autonomic reflexes (changes in blood pressure and heart rate) in a handgrip test and Valsalva maneuver but not in face immersion or orthostatic tests. Because some, but not all, reflexes were disturbed, they proposed that peripheral nerves were intact and that the defect was localized to the central nervous system. Reports of basal blood pressure in narcoleptic patients are rather controversial. The same authors reported normal blood pressure and heart rate at rest before the autonomic testing (Sachs and Kaijser, 1982). However, Guilleminault (1993) reported that the withdrawal of medications containing amphetamine for 4 weeks significantly decreased blood pressure in narcoleptic patients, indicating that they have low blood pressure when not taking a central stimulant. Both sympathetic and parasympathetic basal activities seemed to be decreased because heart rate and blood pressure variabilities were significantly decreased in untreated narcoleptic patients (Fronczek *et al.*, 2008). As for the regulation of breathing, narcoleptic patients had more frequent sleep apneas compared to healthy controls (Chokroverty, 1986; Harsh *et al.*, 2000) or patients with idiopathic CNS hypersomnia (Baker *et al.*, 1986). A recent report showed that hypoxic, but not hypercapnic, responses were attenuated in human narcoleptic patients (Han *et al.*, 2010), but this report did not consider the possible effects of the circadian rhythm or the dependence on the state of vigilance.

VI. Conclusions

Orexin neurons probably contribute to multiple cardiorespiratory regulatory systems, such as the waking-associated augmentation of the hypercapnic chemoreflex, the determination of basal sympathetic nerve activity and blood pressure, and the simultaneous activation of multiple efferent pathways of the defense response. Orexin neurons do not seem to individually regulate the cardiovascular, respiratory, and body temperature systems but orchestrate them in a context-dependent manner. Although vigilance state-dependent responses and emotional stress-dependent responses may appear to be independent, we assume that the common features of these responses are state-dependent and feedforward adjustments of the central ventilatory and autonomic regulation in order to fit it to the situational demands that are associated with the behavioral and metabolic changes. An animal's arousal state or alertness is minimal during sleep, increases during quiet wakefulness, and further increases during active wakefulness that involves a number of activities, such as exercise, food seeking, stress, or panic. The level of this arousal activation by orexin is found to be greater in the dark (active period of the circadian cycle) than in the light (inactive period) in nocturnal mice. Apparently, the independent cardiorespiratory regulation in a specific state seems to be a different facet of a single control system in which orexin plays an important role. In line with this notion, orexin has recently been shown to play a key role in the cardiovascular and behavioral responses that are associated with panic attacks in both animal models and humans (Johnson *et al.*, 2010).

Diversity in the synaptic control of cardiovascular, respiratory, and thermoregulatory neurons appears to be necessary for the animals to adapt themselves to the constantly changing situations and behavioral states. The orexin and cotransmitter system is likely to function as one of the essential modulators for the orchestration of the circuits that control the autonomic functions and behavior.

ACKNOWLEDGMENTS

Part of the work was supported by a Grant-in Aid for Scientific Research from the Ministry of Education, Culture, Sports, Science and Technology, Japan.

REFERENCES

Abrahamson, E. E., Leak, R. K., and Moore, R. Y. (2001). The suprachiasmatic nucleus projects to posterior hypothalamic arousal systems. *Neuroreport* **12,** 435–440.

Antunes, V. R., Brailoiu, G. C., Kwok, E. H., Scruggs, P., and Dun, N. J. (2001). Orexins/hypocretins excite rat sympathetic preganglionic neurons in vivo and in vitro. *Am. J. Physiol. Regul. Integr. Comp. Physiol.* **281,** R1801–R1807.

Arrigoni, E., Mochizuki, T., and Scammell, T. E. (2010). Activation of the basal forebrain by the orexin/hypocretin neurons. *Acta Physiol (Oxf.)* **198,** 223–235.

Baker, T., Guilleminault, C., Nino-Murcia, G., and Dement, W. (1986). Comparative polysomnographic study of narcolepsy and idiopathic central nervous system hypersomnia. *Sleep* **9,** 232–242.

Bandler, R., Keay, K. A., Floyd, N., and Price, J. (2000). Central circuits mediating patterned autonomic activity during active vs. passive emotional coping. *Brain Res. Bull.* **53,** 95–104.

Bastianini, S., Silvani, A., Berteotti, C., Elghozi, J.-L., Franzini, C., Lenzi, P., Martire, V. L., and Zoccoli, G. (2011). Sleep related changes in blood pressure in hypocretin-deficient narcoleptic mice. *Sleep* **34,** 213–218.

Berthoud, H. R., Patterson, L. M., Sutton, G. M., Morrison, C., and Zheng, H. (2005). Orexin inputs to caudal raphe neurons involved in thermal, cardiovascular, and gastrointestinal regulation. *Histochem. Cell Biol.* **123,** 147–156.

Beuckmann, C. T., Sinton, C. M., Williams, S. C., Richardson, J. A., Hammer, R. E., Sakurai, T., and Yanagisawa, M. (2004). Expression of a poly-glutamine-ataxin-3 transgene in orexin neurons induces narcolepsy–cataplexy in the rat. *J. Neurosci.* **24,** 4469–4477.

Carter, M. E., Adamantidis, A., Ohtsu, H., Deisseroth, K., and de Lecea, L. (2009). Sleep homeostasis modulates hypocretin-mediated sleep-to-wake transitions. *J. Neurosci.* **29,** 10939–10949.

Chemelli, R. M., Willie, J. T., Sinton, C. M., Elmquist, J. K., Scammell, T. E., Lee, C., Richardson, J. A., Williams, S. C., Xiong, Y., Kisanuki, Y., Fitch, T. E., Nakazato, M., *et al.* (1999). Narcolepsy in orexin knockout mice: Molecular genetics of sleep regulation. *Cell* **98,** 437–451.

Chen, C. T., Hwang, L. L., Chang, J. K., and Dun, N. J. (2000). Pressor effects of orexins injected intracisternally and to rostral ventrolateral medulla of anesthetized rats. *Am. J. Physiol. Regul. Integr. Comp. Physiol.* **278,** R692–R697.

Cheng, S. B., Kuchiiwa, S., Gao, H. Z., Kuchiiwa, T., and Nakagawa, S. (2003). Morphological study of orexin neurons in the hypothalamus of the Long-Evans rat, with special reference to co-expression of orexin and NADPH-diaphorase or nitric oxide synthase activities. *Neurosci. Res.* **46,** 53–62.

Chokroverty, S. (1986). Sleep apnea in narcolepsy. *Sleep* **9,** 250–253.

Chou, T. C., Lee, C. E., Lu, J., Elmquist, J. K., Hara, J., Willie, J. T., Beuckmann, C. T., Chemelli, R. M., Sakurai, T., Yanagisawa, M., Saper, C. B., and Scammell, T. E. (2001). Orexin (hypocretin) neurons contain dynorphin. *J. Neurosci.* **21,** RC168, 1–6.

de Lecea, L., Kilduff, T., Peyron, C., Gao, X., Foye, P., Danielson, P., Fukuhara, C., Battenberg, E., Gautvik, V., Bartlett, F. S., 2nd, Frankel, W., van den Pol, A., *et al.* (1998). The hypocretins: Hypothalamus-specific peptides with neuroexcitatory activity. *Proc. Natl. Acad. Sci. U. S. A.* **95,** 322–327.

Deng, B.-S., Nakamura, A., Zhang, W., Yanagisawa, M., Fukuda, Y., and Kuwaki, T. (2007). Contribution of orexin in hypercapnic chemoreflex: Evidence from genetic and pharmacological disruption and supplementation studies in mice. *J. Appl. Physiol.* **103,** 1772–1779.

Dergacheva, O., Wang, X., Huang, Z. G., Bouairi, E., Stephens, C., Gorini, C., and Mendelowitz, D. (2005). Hypocretin-1 (orexin-A) facilitates inhibitory and diminishes excitatory synaptic pathways to cardiac vagal neurons in the nucleus ambiguus. *J. Pharmacol. Exp. Ther.* **314,** 1322–1327.

Dias, M., Li, A., and Nattie, E. (2009). Antagonism of orexin receptor-1 in the retrotrapezoid nucleus inhibits the ventilatory response to hypercapnia predominantly in wakefulness. *J. Physiol.* **587,** 2059–2067.

Dias, M. B., Li, A., and Nattie, E. E. (2010). The orexin receptor-1 (OX1R) in the rostral medullary raphe contributes to the hypercapnic chemoreflex in wakefulness, during the active period of the diurnal cycle. *Respir. Physiol. Neurobiol.* **170,** 96–102.

Douglas, N. J. (2000). Respiratory physiology: Control of ventilation. *In* "Principles and Practice of Sleep Medicine," (M. H. Kryger, T. Roth, and W. C. Dement, Eds.), pp. 221–228. W.B. Saunders, Philadelphia.

Dun, N. J., Le Dun, S., Chen, C. T., Hwang, L. L., Kwok, E. H., and Chang, J. K. (2000). Orexins: A role in medullary sympathetic outflow. *Regul. Pept.* **96,** 65–70.
Dutschmann, M., Kron, M., Mörschel, M., and Gestreau, C. (2007). Activation of Orexin B receptors in the pontine Kölliker-Fuse nucleus modulates pre-inspiratory hypoglossal motor activity in rat. *Respir. Physiol. Neurobiol.* **159,** 232–235.
Elias, C. F., Saper, C. B., Maratos-Flier, E., Tritos, N. A., Lee, C., Kelly, J., Tatro, J. B., Hoffman, G. E., Ollmann, M. M., Barsh, G. S., Sakurai, T., Yanagisawa, M., *et al.* (1998). Chemically defined projections linking the mediobasal hypothalamus and the lateral hypothalamic area. *J. Comp. Neurol.* **402,** 442–459.
Espana, R. A., Valentino, R. J., and Berridge, C. W. (2003). Fos immunoreactivity in hypocretin-synthesizing and hypocretin-1 receptor-expressing neurons: Effects of diurnal and nocturnal spontaneous waking, stress and hypocretin-1 administration. *Neuroscience* **121,** 201–217.
Fronczek, R., Overeem, S., Reijntjes, R., Lammers, G., van Dijk, J., and Pijl, H. (2008). Increased heart rate variability but normal resting metabolic rate in hypocretin/orexin-deficient human narcolepsy. *J. Clin. Sleep Med.* **4,** 248–254.
Fung, S. J., Yamuy, J., Sampogna, S., Morales, F. R., and Chase, M. H. (2001). Hypocretin (orexin) input to trigeminal and hypoglossal motoneurons in the cat: A double-labeling immunohistochemical study. *Brain Res.* **903,** 257–262.
Geerling, J. C., Mettenleiter, T. C., and Loewy, A. D. (2003). Orexin neurons project to diverse sympathetic outflow systems. *Neuroscience* **122,** 541–550.
Guilleminault, C. (1993). Amphetamines and narcolepsy: Use of the Stanford database. *Sleep* **16,** 199–201.
Hakansson, M., de Lecea, L., Sutcliffe, J. G., Yanagisawa, M., and Meister, B. (1999). Leptin receptor- and STAT3-immunoreactivities in hypocretin/orexin neurones of the lateral hypothalamus. *J. Neuroendocrinol.* **11,** 653–663.
Hallmayer, J., Faraco, J., Lin, L., Hesselson, S., Winkelmann, J., Kawashima, M., Mayer, G., Plazzi, G., Nevsimalova, S., Bourgin, P., Hong, S.-C., Honda, Y., *et al.* (2009). Narcolepsy is strongly associated with the T-cell receptor alpha locus. *Nat. Genet.* **41,** 708–711.
Han, F., Mignot, E., Wei, Y., Dong, S., Li, J., Lin, L., An, P., Wang, L., Wang, J., He, M., Gao, H., Li, M., *et al.* (2010). Ventilatory chemoresponsiveness, narcolepsy–cataplexy and human leukocyte antigen DQB1*0602 status. *Eur. Respir. J.* **36,** 577–583.
Hara, J., Beuckmann, C. T., Nambu, T., Willie, J. T., Chemelli, R. M., Sinton, C. M., Sugiyama, F., Yagami, K., Goto, K., Yanagisawa, M., and Sakurai, T. (2001). Genetic ablation of orexin neurons in mice results in narcolepsy, hypophagia, and obesity. *Neuron* **30,** 345–354.
Harris, G. C., and Aston-Jones, G. (2006). Arousal and reward: A dichotomy in orexin function. *Trends Neurosci.* **29,** 571–577.
Harsh, J., Peszka, J., Hartwig, G., and Mitler, M. (2000). Night-time sleep and daytime sleepiness in narcolepsy. *J. Sleep Res.* **9,** 309–316.
Hess, W. R. (1954). The Diencephalon: Autonomic and Extrapyramidal Functions. Grune & Stratton, New York.
Ida, T., Nakahara, K., Murakami, T., Hanada, R., Nakazato, M., and Murakami, N. (2000). Possible involvement of orexin in the stress reaction in rats. *Biochem. Biophys. Res. Commun.* **270,** 318–323.
Jászberényi, M., Bujdosó, E., Pataki, I., and Telegdy, G. (2000). Effects of orexins on the hypothalamic-pituitary-adrenal system. *J. Neuroendocrinol.* **12,** 1174–1178.
Johnson, P. L., Truitt, W., Fitz, S. D., Minick, P. E., Dietrich, A., Sanghani, S., Träskman-Bendz, L., Goddard, A. W., Brundin, L., and Shekhar, A. (2010). A key role for orexin in panic anxiety. *Nat. Med.* **16,** 111–115.
Kayaba, Y., Nakamura, A., Kasuya, Y., Ohuchi, T., Yanagisawa, M., Komuro, I., Fukuda, Y., and Kuwaki, T. (2003). Attenuated defense response and low basal blood

pressure in orexin knockout mice. *Am. J. Physiol. Regul. Integr. Comp. Physiol.* **285,** R581–R593.

Kiely, J. M., and Gordon, F. J. (1994). Role of rostral ventrolateral medulla in centrally mediated pressor responses. *Am. J. Physiol.* **267,** H1549–H1556.

Korte, S., Koolhaas, J., Wingfield, J., and McEwen, B. (2005). The Darwinian concept of stress: Benefits of allostasis and costs of allostatic load and the trade-offs in health and disease. *Neurosci. Biobehav. Rev.* **29,** 3–38.

Krieger, J. (2000). Respiratory physiology: Breathing in normal subjects. *In* "Principles and Practice of Sleep Medicine," (M. H. Kryger, T. Roth, and W. C. Dement, Eds.), pp. 229–241. W.B. Saunders, Philadelphia.

Krout, K. E., Mettenleiter, T. C., and Loewy, A. D. (2003). Single CNS neurons link both central motor and cardiosympathetic systems: A double-virus tracing study. *Neuroscience* **118,** 853–866.

Krout, K. E., Mettenleiter, T. C., Karpitskiy, V., Nguyen, X. V., and Loewy, A. D. (2005). CNS neurons with links to both mood-related cortex and sympathetic nervous system. *Brain Res.* **1050,** 199–202.

Kumada, M., Terui, N., and Kuwaki, T. (1990). Arterial baroreceptor reflex: Its central and peripheral neural mechanisms. *Prog. Neurobiol.* **35,** 331–361.

Kuwaki, T. (2008). Orexinergic modulation of breathing across vigilance states. *Respir. Physiol. Neurobiol.* **164,** 204–212.

Kuwaki, T. (2011). A key role of orexin (hypocretin) neurons in the fight-or-flight response. *Physiology News* **83,** 15–17.

Kuwaki, T., and Zhang, W. (2010). Orexin neurons as arousal-associated modulators of central cardiorespiratory regulation. *Respir. Physiol. Neurobiol.* **174,** 43–54.

Kuwaki, T., Zhang, W., and Nakamura, A. (2007). State-dependent adjustment of the central autonomic regulation: Role of orexin in emotional behavior and sleep/wake cycle. *In* "Central Mechanisms of Cardiovascular Regulation," (T. Kubo and T. Kuwaki, Eds.), pp. 57–73. Research Signport, Kerala (India).

Kuwaki, T., Li, A., and Nattie, E. E. (2010). State-dependent central chemoreception: A role of orexin. *Respir. Physiol. Neurobiol.* **173,** 223–229.

Lazarenko, R. M., Stornetta, R. L., Bayliss, D. A., and Guyenet, P. G. (2011). Orexin A activates retrotrapezoid neurons in mice. *Respir. Physiol. Neurobiol.* **175,** 283–287.

Lee, M., Hassani, O., and Jones, B. (2005). Discharge of identified orexin/hypocretin neurons across the sleep-waking cycle. *J. Neurosci.* **25,** 6716–6720.

Lin, L., Faraco, J., Li, R., Kadotani, H., Rogers, W., Lin, X., Qiu, X., de Jong, P. J., Nishino, S., and Mignot, E. (1999). The sleep disorder canine narcolepsy is caused by a mutation in the hypocretin (orexin) receptor 2 gene. *Cell* **98,** 365–376.

Machado, B. H., Bonagamba, L. G., Dun, S. L., Kwok, E. H., and Dun, N. J. (2002). Pressor response to microinjection of orexin/hypocretin into rostral ventrolateral medulla of awake rats. *Regul. Pept.* **104,** 75–81.

Marcus, J. N., Aschkenasi, C. J., Lee, C. E., Chemelli, R. M., Saper, C. B., Yanagisawa, M., and Elmquist, J. K. (2001). Differential expression of orexin receptors 1 and 2 in the rat brain. *J. Comp. Neurol.* **435,** 6–25.

McDowall, L. M., Horiuchi, J., Killinger, S., and Dampney, R. A. L. (2006). Modulation of the baroreceptor reflex by the dorsomedial hypothalamic nucleus and perifornical area. *Am. J. Physiol. Regul. Integr. Comp. Physiol.* **290,** R1020–R1026.

Mieda, M., Hasegawa, E., Kisanuki, Y. Y., Yanagisawa, C. M. S., and Sakurai, T. (2011). Differential roles of orexin receptor-1 and -2 in the regulation of non-REM and REM sleep. *J. Neurosci.* **31,** 6518–6526.

Mileykovskiy, B., Kiyashchenko, L., and Siegel, J. (2005). Behavioral correlates of activity in identified hypocretin/orexin neurons. *Neuron* **46,** 787–798.

Monda, M., Viggiano, A., and Luca, V. D. (2003). Paradoxical effect of orexin A: Hypophagia induced by hyperthermia. *Brain Res.* **961,** 220–228.

Mortola, J. P. (2004). Breathing around the clock: An overview of the circadian pattern of respiration. *Eur. J. Appl. Physiol.* **91,** 119–129.

Nakamura, A., Zhang, W., Yanagisawa, M., Fukuda, Y., and Kuwaki, T. (2007). Vigilance state-dependent attenuation of hypercapnic chemoreflex and exaggerated sleep apnea in orexin knockout mice. *J. Appl. Physiol.* **102,** 241–248.

Nalivaiko, E., Ootsuka, Y., and Blessing, W. W. (2005). Activation of 5-HT1A receptors in the medullary raphe reduces cardiovascular changes elicited by acute psychological and inflammatory stresses in rabbits. *Am. J. Physiol. Regul. Integr. Comp. Physiol.* **289,** R596–R604.

Nambu, T., Sakurai, T., Mizukami, K., Hosoya, Y., Yanagisawa, M., and Goto, K. (1999). Distribution of orexin neurons in the adult rat brain. *Brain Res.* **827,** 243–260.

Nosaka, S. (1996). Modifications of arterial baroreflexes: Obligatory roles in cardiovascular regulation in stress and poststress recovery. *Jpn. J. Physiol.* **46,** 271–288.

Oldfield, B. J., Giles, M. E., Watson, A., Anderson, C., Colvill, L. M., and McKinley, M. J. (2002). The neurochemical characterisation of hypothalamic pathways projecting polysynaptically to brown adipose tissue in the rat. *Neuroscience* **110,** 515–526.

Peyron, C., Tighe, D. K., van den Pol, A. N., de Lecea, L., Heller, H. C., Sutcliffe, J. G., and Kilduff, T. S. (1998). Neurons containing hypocretin (orexin) project to multiple neuronal systems. *J. Neurosci.* **18,** 9996–10015.

Phillipson, E. (1978). Control of breathing during sleep. *Am. Rev. Respir. Dis.* **118,** 909–939.

Pitkanen, A., Savander, V., and LeDoux, J. E. (1997). Organization of intra-amygdaloid circuitries in the rat: An emerging framework for understanding functions of the amygdala. *Trends Neurosci.* **20,** 517–523.

Rosin, D. L., Weston, M. C., Sevigny, C. P., Stornetta, R. L., and Guyenet, P. G. (2003). Hypothalamic orexin (hypocretin) neurons express vesicular glutamate transporters VGLUT1 or VGLUT2. *J. Comp. Neurol.* **465,** 593–603.

Rosin, D. L., Chang, D. A., and Guyenet, P. G. (2006). Afferent and efferent connections of the rat retrotrapezoid nucleus. *J. Comp. Neurol.* **499,** 64–89.

Sachs, C., and Kaijser, L. (1982). Autonomic regulation of cardiopulmonary functions in sleep apnea syndrome and narcolepsy. *Sleep* **5,** 227–238.

Sakurai, T. (2007). The neural circuit of orexin (hypocretin): Maintaining sleep and wakefulness. *Nat. Rev. Neurosci.* **8,** 171–181.

Sakurai, T., Amemiya, A., Ishii, M., Matsuzaki, I., Chemelli, R. M., Tanaka, H., Williams, S. C., Richarson, J. A., Kozlowski, G. P., Wilson, S., Arch, J. R., Buckingham, R. E., *et al.* (1998). Orexins and orexin receptors: A family of hypothalamic neuropeptides and G protein-coupled receptors that regulate feeding behavior. *Cell* **92,** 573–585.

Sakurai, T., Nagata, R., Yamanaka, A., Kawamura, H., Tsujino, N., Muraki, Y., Kageyama, H., Kunita, S., Takahashi, S., Goto, K., Koyama, Y., Shioda, S., *et al.* (2005). Input of orexin/hypocretin neurons revealed by a genetically encoded tracer in mice. *Neuron* **46,** 297–308.

Samson, W. K., Gosnell, B., Chang, J. K., Resch, Z. T., and Murphy, T. C. (1999). Cardiovascular regulatory actions of the hypocretins in brain. *Brain Res.* **831,** 248–253.

Saper, C. B., Scammell, T. E., and Lu, J. (2005). Hypothalamic regulation of sleep and circadian rhythms. *Nature* **437,** 1257–1263.

Schwimmer, H., Stauss, H. M., Abboud, F., Nishino, S., Mignot, E., and Zeitzer, J. M. (2010). Effects of sleep on the cardiovascular and thermoregulatory systems: A possible role for hypocretins. *J. Appl. Physiol.* **109,** 1053–1063.

Sévoz-Couche, C., Comet, M. A., Hamon, M., and Laguzzi, R. (2003). Role of nucleus tractus solitarius 5-HT3 receptors in the defense reaction-induced inhibition of the aortic baroreflex in rats. *J. Neurophysiol.* **90,** 2521–2530.

Shirasaka, T., Nakazato, M., Matsukura, S., Takasaki, M., and Kannan, H. (1999). Sympathetic and cardiovascular actions of orexins in conscious rats. *Am. J. Physiol.* **277,** R1780–R1785.

Smart, D., Sabido-David, C., Brough, S. J., Jewitt, F., Johns, A., Porter, R. A., and Jerman, J. C. (2001). SB-334867-A: The first selective orexin-1 receptor antagonist. *Br. J. Pharmacol.* **132,** 1179–1182.

Smith, B. N., Davis, S. F., Van Den Pol, A. N., and Xu, W. (2002). Selective enhancement of excitatory synaptic activity in the rat nucleus tractus solitarius by hypocretin 2. *Neuroscience* **115,** 707–714.

Stephenson, R. (2007). Circadian rhythms and sleep-related breathing disorders. *Sleep Med.* **8,** 681–687.

Sun, M. K., and Guyenet, P. G. (1986). Hypothalamic glutamatergic input to medullary sympathoexcitatory neurons in rats. *Am. J. Physiol.* **251,** R798–R810.

Sunanaga, J., Deng, B.-S., Zhang, W., Kanmura, Y., and Kuwaki, T. (2009). CO_2 activates orexin-containing neurons in mice. *Respir. Physiol. Neurobiol.* **166,** 184–186.

Székely, M., Pétervári, E., Balaskó, M., Hernádi, I., and Uzsoki, B. (2002). Effects of orexins on energy balance and thermoregulation. *Regul. Pept.* **104,** 47–53.

Takahashi, K., Lin, J. S., and Sakai, K. (2008). Neuronal activity of orexin and non-orexin waking-active neurons during wake–sleep states in the mouse. *Neuroscience* **153,** 860–870.

Thannickal, T. C., Moore, R. Y., Nienhuis, R., Ramanathan, L., Gulyani, S., Aldrich, M., Cornford, M., and Siegel, J. M. (2000). Reduced number of hypocretin neurons in human narcolepsy. *Neuron* **27,** 469–474.

Thomas, T., and Spyer, K. M. (1996). The role of adenosine receptors in the rostral ventrolateral medulla in the cardiovascular response to defence area stimulation in the rat. *Exp. Physiol.* **81,** 67–77.

Torrealba, F., Yanagisawa, M., and Saper, C. B. (2003). Colocalization of orexin A and glutamate immunoreactivity in axon terminals in the tuberomammillary nucleus in rats. *Neuroscience* **119,** 1033–1044.

Tsunematsu, T., Kilduff, T. S., Boyden, E. S., Takahashi, S., Tominaga, M., and Yamanaka, A. (2011). Acute optogenetic silencing of orexin/hypocretin neurons induces slow-wave sleep in mice. *J. Neurosci.* **31,** 10529–10539.

Volgin, D. V., Saghir, M., and Kubin, L. (2002). Developmental changes in the orexin 2 receptor mRNA in hypoglossal motoneurons. *Neuroreport* **13,** 433–436.

Watanabe, S., Kuwaki, T., Yanagisawa, M., Fukuda, Y., and Shimoyama, M. (2005). Persistent pain and stress activate pain-inhibitory orexin pathways. *Neuroreport* **16,** 5–8.

Williams, R. H., Jensen, L. T., Verkhratsky, A., Fugger, L., and Burdakov, D. (2007). Control of hypothalamic orexin neurons by acid and CO2. *Proc. Natl. Acad. Sci. U. S. A.* **104,** 10685–10690.

Willie, J. T., Chemelli, R. M., Sinton, C. M., and Yanagisawa, M. (2001). To eat or to sleep? Orexin in the regulation of feeding and wakefulness. *Annu. Rev. Neurosci.* **24,** 429–458.

Winsky-Sommerer, R., Yamanaka, A., Diano, S., Borok, E., Roberts, A. J., Sakurai, T., Kilduff, T. S., Horvath, T. L., and de Lecea, L. (2004). Interaction between the corticotropin-releasing factor system and hypocretins (orexins): A novel circuit mediating stress response. *J. Neurosci.* **24,** 11439–11448.

Yamamoto, T., Nozaki-Taguchi, N., and Chiba, T. (2002). Analgesic effect of intrathecally administered orexin-A in the rat formalin test and in the rat hot plate test. *Br. J. Pharmacol.* **137,** 170–176.

Yoshida, Y., Fujiki, N., Nakajima, T., Ripley, B., Matsumura, H., Yoneda, H., Mignot, E., and Nishino, S. (2001). Fluctuation of extracellular hypocretin-1 (orexin A) levels in the rat in relation to the light–dark cycle and sleep–wake activities. *Eur. J. Neurosci.* **14,** 1075–1081.

Yoshida, K., McCormack, S., Espana, R. A., Crocker, A., and Scammell, T. E. (2006). Afferents to the orexin neurons of the rat brain. *J. Comp. Neurol.* **494,** 845–861.

Young, J. K., Wu, M., Manaye, K. F., Kc, P., Allard, J. S., Mack, S. O., and Haxhiu, M. A. (2005). Orexin stimulates breathing via medullary and spinal pathways. *J. Appl. Physiol.* **98,** 1387–1395.

Zhang, W., Fukuda, Y., and Kuwaki, T. (2005). Respiratory and cardiovascular actions of orexin-A in mice. *Neurosci. Lett.* **385,** 131–136.

Zhang, W., Sakurai, T., Fukuda, Y., and Kuwaki, T. (2006a). Orexin neuron-mediated skeletal muscle vasodilation and shift of baroreflex during defense response in mice. *Am. J. Physiol. Regul. Integr. Comp. Physiol.* **290,** R1654–R1663.

Zhang, W., Shimoyama, M., Fukuda, Y., and Kuwaki, T. (2006b). Multiple components of the defense response depend on orexin: Evidence from orexin knockout mice and orexin neuron-ablated mice. *Auton. Neurosci.* **126–127,** 139–145.

Zhang, W., Zhang, N., Sakurai, T., and Kuwaki, T. (2009). Orexin neurons in the hypothalamus mediate cardiorespiratory responses induced by disinhibition of the amygdala and bed nucleus of the stria terminalis. *Brain Res.* **1262,** 25–37.

Zhang, W., Sunanaga, J., Takahashi, Y., Mori, T., Sakurai, T., Kanmura, Y., and Kuwaki, T. (2010). Orexin neurons are indispensable for stress-induced thermogenesis in mice. *J. Physiol.* **588,** 4117–4129.

Zhu, L., Onaka, T., Sakurai, T., and Yada, T. (2002). Activation of orexin neurones after noxious but not conditioned fear stimuli in rats. *Neuroreport* **13,** 1351–1353.

CHAPTER NINE

Orexin and Central Regulation of Cardiorespiratory System

Israt Z. Shahid,*,† Ahmed A. Rahman,*,† *and* Paul M. Pilowsky*

Contents

Abstract

The hypothalamic peptide orexin plays a role in many physiological systems including feeding behavior, sleep–wakefulness, reward system, stress, and nociception. In addition, it is now clear that orexin is involved in the central regulation of cardiorespiratory function. Here, we review the cardiorespiratory effects elicited by central orexin and consider the physiological role of this peptide in central cardiorespiratory control in normal and pathophysiological states. Orexin neurons are found exclusively in the hypothalamus but project to almost all brain regions including cardiorespiratory regulatory areas, where their receptors are also expressed. Administration of orexin into the nucleus tractus solitarius, rostral ventrolateral medulla, rostral ventromedial medulla, and spinal cord increases blood pressure, heart rate, and sympathetic nerve

* Australian School of Advanced Medicine, Macquarie University, Sydney, Australia
† Pharmacy Discipline, Life Science School, Khulna University, Khulna, Bangladesh

Vitamins and Hormones, Volume 89
ISSN 0083-6729, http://dx.doi.org/10.1016/B978-0-12-394623-2.00009-3

activity. Orexin neurons stimulate respiration and are sensitive to changes in pH. Orexin knockout mice have apnoeic episodes in sleep. Therefore, orexin may be a potentially important therapeutic target for the treatment of cardiorespiratory disorders.

I. Introduction

Since it was first identified only 13 years ago as ligands of two orphan G-protein-coupled receptors (GPCRs), orexins (also known as hypocretins) are implicated in a wide range of physiological processes including sleep–wakefulness, feeding, energy homeostasis, pain, metabolism, and hormonal secretion (de Lecea *et al.*, 1998; Sakurai *et al.*, 1998). A growing body of evidence suggests that orexins are involved in certain aspects of cardiovascular and respiratory functions. In this review, we will discuss the role of orexin on central autonomic function emphasizing on central regulation of cardiovascular and respiratory system, and consider the physiological role of orexin with respect to cardiorespiratory functioning in different physiological and pathophysiological states.

II. Orexins and Orexin Receptors

A. Orexins

Orexin A and orexin B (also called hypocretin 1 and hypocretin 2) were first identified in 1998 by two separate groups via two different approaches (Alexander *et al.*, 2011; de Lecea *et al.*, 1998; Sakurai *et al.*, 1998). In current review, we will use the term orexin, which is derived from the Greek word "*orexis*," meaning "appetite." Orexins were so named for their stimulatory role in feeding (Sakurai *et al.*, 1998). Both orexin A and orexin B are produced by proteolytic cleavage of the gene product prepro-orexin.

Mammalian (human, pig, dog, rat, mouse) prepro-orexin, composed of 130–131 amino acids, is highly conserved with 75% amino acid sequence identity (de Lecea *et al.*, 1998; Dyer *et al.*, 1999; Hungs *et al.*, 2001; Sakurai *et al.*, 1998). The human prepro-orexin gene is localized on chromosome 17q21 (Sakurai *et al.*, 1998). The mRNA of this precursor is abundantly and specifically expressed in the lateral hypothalamus and adjacent areas important in the central regulation of feeding behavior and energy homeostasis (Sakurai *et al.*, 1999).

Orexin A is a 33-amino acid peptide of 3562 Da. It consists of an N-terminal pyroglutamyl residue, two intramolecular disulfide bridges between Cys^6–Cys^{12} and Cys^7–Cys^{14}, and a C-terminal amidation. The primary structure of orexin A is completely conserved among several mammals (human, rat, mouse, dog, cow, sheep, and pig) (Fig. 9.1A). On the other hand, Orexin B is a 28-amino acid linear peptide of 2937 Da with a C-terminal amidation. Human orexin B differs by one amino acid from pig and dog orexin B and by two amino acids from rat and mouse orexin B (Fig. 9.1B). Orexin B shares 46% sequence identity with orexin A. The similarity in amino acid sequence lies mainly in the C-terminus, whereas the N-terminal half is more variable (Fig. 9.1A). The free N-terminal can be related to the rapid metabolism and shorter action of orexin B as compared to orexin A. In contrast, post-translational modifications of both termini and two intrachain disulfide bonds may render orexin A more stable and readily available in CSF. Orexin A also shows higher lipid solubility than orexin B which makes it more blood–brain barrier permeant (Kastin and Akerstrom, 1999).

B. Orexin receptors

HFGAN72, the orphan GPCR, was identified as an orexin receptor while orexin was discovered and was named orexin receptor 1 (OX_1R) (also called hypocretin 1 receptor). An extensive search for amino acid sequence identity

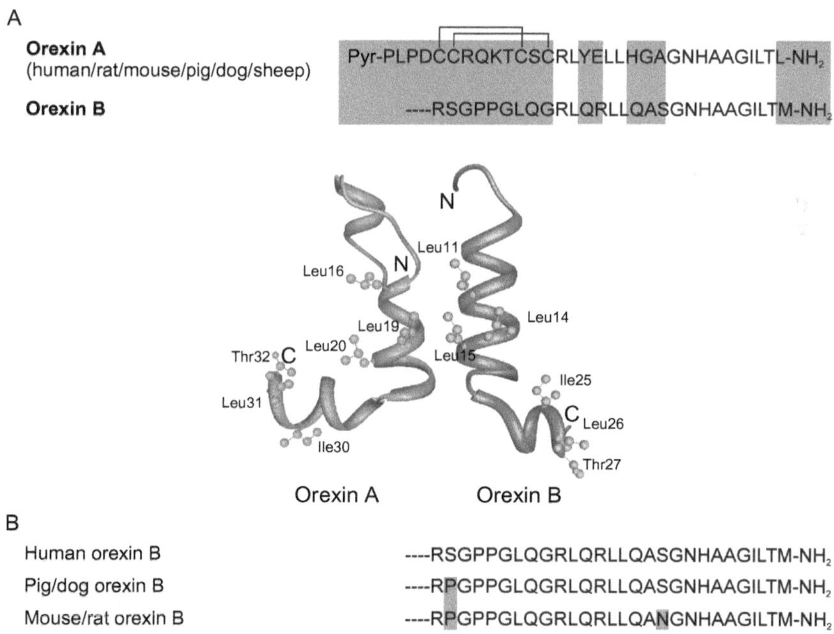

Figure 9.1 Structures of orexin A and orexin B and their sequences in different species (A, B). Gray boxes indicate dissimilar amino acids (as compared with human variants). Cystine bridges in orexin A are shown in (A) with black lines. Part of (A) adapted from Protein data bank (http://www.pdbj.org).

with OX_1R resulted in the discovery of a second receptor for orexin, another GPCR, named as orexin receptor 2 (OX_2R) (also known as hypocretin 2 receptor) (Alexander *et al.*, 2011; Sakurai *et al.*, 1998). Orexin receptors show only 20–28% structural similarity with the other GPCR neuropeptide receptors such as neuropeptide Y2 receptor, thyrotropin releasing hormone receptor, cholecystokinin type-A receptor, and neurokinin 2 receptor (Sakurai *et al.*, 1998).

Human OX_1R is a 425-amino acid long and OX_2R is a 444-amino acid long protein sharing 64% sequence identity with each other. OX_1R gene is localized on chromosome 1p33 and OX_2R gene on chromosome 6p11-q11 (de Lecea *et al.*, 1998; Sakurai *et al.*, 1998). Each of the receptors consists of seven putative transmembrane helices, several modifications (glycosylation and phosphorylation) of extracellular and intracellular loops, and is encoded by seven exons. In human OX_1R and OX_2R, all transmembrane segments, extracellular loops and intracellular loops I and II are highly conserved while the N-terminal extracellular domain, intracellular loop III, and the C-terminal tail exhibit great variability in amino acid sequence as well as length. The amino acid sequences of human OX_1R and OX_2R are 94% and 95% identical to their rat counterparts, respectively, indicating that both receptor genes are highly conserved among species (Peyron *et al.*, 2000).

Radioligand-binding studies have shown that OX_1R has one order of magnitude greater affinity for orexin A (IC_{50}: 20 nM) than for orexin B (IC_{50}: 420 nM), indicating that OX_1R is highly selective for orexin A. In contrast, tracer binding to OX_2R shows orexin A and orexin B bind with OX_2R with similar affinity indicating that OX_2R is nonselective receptor for both orexins (Okumura *et al.*, 2001; Sakurai *et al.*, 1998; Smart *et al.*, 2000). In recombinant systems, activation of either OX_1R or OX_2R, coupled to Gq G protein, results in the elevation of intracellular Ca^{2+} concentrations (Lund *et al.*, 2000; Smart *et al.*, 1999). In Chinese hamster ovary (CHO) cells, stimulation of OX_1R activates receptor-operated influx of extracellular Ca^{2+} that occurs via opening of N-/L-type voltage-gated Ca^{2+} channels. This influx of Ca^{2+} enhances Gq-mediated stimulation of phosphatidylinositol-specific phospholipase C leading to inositol triphosphate production and Ca^{2+} release from intracellular stores (Fig. 9.2) (Lund *et al.*, 2000; Smart *et al.*, 1999). In CHO cells, Smart *et al.* (1999) and Lund *et al.* (2000) have shown that Ca^{2+} elevation requires extracellular Ca^{2+}, and removal of extracellular Ca^{2+} causes a significant drop in the potency of orexin A for the OX_1R. The exact identity of the Ca^{2+} influx pathway, its activation mechanism by orexin receptors, and the relation between Ca^{2+} influx and Gq-mediated intracellular Ca^{2+} release remains unresolved; however, it can be suggested that in both neuronal and nonneuronal cells, orexin receptors activate both Ca^{2+} influx and the phosphatidylinositol-specific phospholipase C pathway (Fig. 9.2). Other studies have shown that orexin causes protein kinase C-mediated Ca^{2+} influx in hypothalamic cultures (van den Pol *et al.*, 1998), inhibits K^+

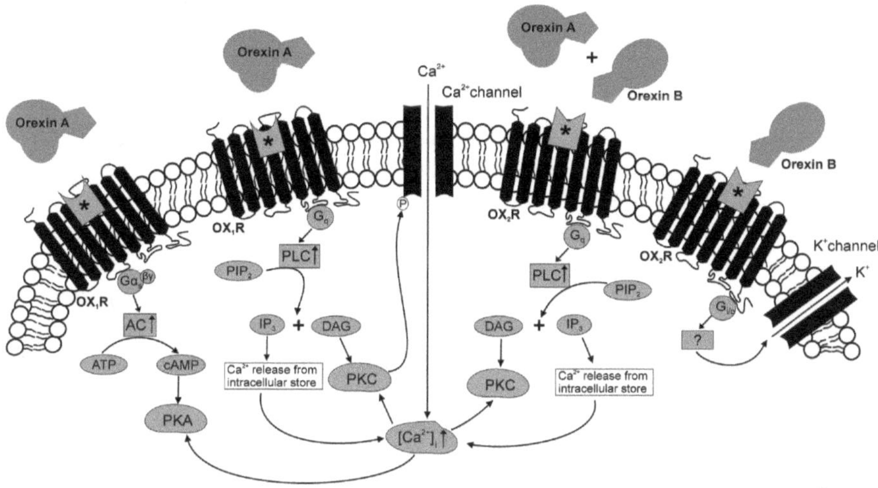

Figure 9.2 Schematic of the main signaling pathways of OX_1R and OX_2R upon the activation by orexin A and orexin A or orexin B, respectively. AC, adenylate cyclase; cAMP, cyclic adenosine monophosphate; DAG, diacylglycerol; G, G protein; IP_3, inositol triphosphate; P, phosphorylation site; PIP_2, phosphatidylinositol biphosphate; PKA, protein kinase A; PKC, protein kinase C; PLC, phospholipase C. Asterisks mark the orexin-recognizing sites of OX_1R and OX_2R. (See Color Insert.)

channels in rat locus coeruleus (LC) and in guinea pig ileal submucosal ganglia (Horvath *et al.*, 1999; Kirchgessner and Liu, 1999), and activates Ca^{2+}-sensitive K^+ channels in immune cells (Fig. 9.2) (Ichinose *et al.*, 1998).

C. Distribution in the CNS

Orexins and their precursor, prepro-orexin, have been identified in the CNS of mammals including human (Sakurai *et al.*, 1998), rat (Chen *et al.*, 1999; Mondal *et al.*, 1999; Nambu *et al.*, 1999), mouse, pig (Dyer *et al.*, 1999), cows (Sakurai *et al.*, 1999), as well as amphibians (Galas *et al.*, 2001; Shibahara *et al.*, 1999). Within the CNS, orexinergic cell bodies are localized solely in the hypothalamus, particularly in the perifornical nucleus, lateral hypothalamic area (LHA), and posterior hypothalamic area (Broberger *et al.*, 1998; Chen *et al.*, 1999; Cutler *et al.*, 1999; Date *et al.*, 1999; de Lecea *et al.*, 1998; Nambu *et al.*, 1999; Peyron *et al.*, 1998; Sakurai *et al.*, 1998). Occasionally, isolated orexinergic cell bodies have also been found in median eminence, dorsal and dorsomedial hypothalamus (DMH), and arcuate nucleus (Arc) and subincertal nucleus (Chen *et al.*, 1999; Cutler *et al.*, 1999; Peyron *et al.*, 1998). Orexin neurons are variable in size (diameter of cell body: 15–40 μm) and shape (spherical, fusiform, multipolar) (Chen *et al.*, 1999; Cutler *et al.*, 1999; Date *et al.*, 1999; Nambu *et al.*, 1999) and are believed to number 1100–3400, ~20,000 and 50,000–83,000 in rat, dog, and human brain, respectively (Harrison *et al.*, 1999; Peyron *et al.*, 1998; Ripley *et al.*, 2001; Thannickal *et al.*, 2000). While orexinergic cell bodies are restricted to the hypothalamus, orexin fibers project widely throughout the CNS. The most important areas receiving orexinergic projections include hypothalamus, cerebral cortex, thalamic nuclei, circumventricular organs, brainstem, and throughout all regions of the whole length of spinal cord (Table 9.1).

As with the orexin peptides, the distribution of orexin receptors in the CNS has been investigated in detail with molecular biological and immunological methods, mostly in rats. Orexin receptors are expressed in regions that have a high density of orexin projections, as stated above. OX_1R and OX_2R mRNAs show partially overlapping and partially distinct distribution patterns suggesting that they may play diverse physiological roles. Both OX_1R and OX_2R are expressed in many brain regions including, amygdala, hippocampus, thalamus, anterior hypothalamus, hypothalamic preoptic nucleus, Arc, paraventricular nucleus (PVN), ventromedial hypothalamus (VMH), supraoptic nucleus, dorsal tegmental nucleus, ventral tegmental area (VTA), dorsal raphe (DR), nucleus tractus solitarius (NTS), rostral ventromedial medulla (RVMM), nucleus ambiguus (NA), pre-Bötzinger complex, and spinal cord (Bingham *et al.*, 2001; Ciriello and de Oliveira, 2003; Cluderay *et al.*, 2002; Hervieu *et al.*, 2001; Marcus *et al.*, 2001; Trivedi *et al.*, 1998). On the other hand, OX_1R is prominent in prefrontal cortex, CA2 region of hippocampus, and LC while OX_2R is predominantly expressed in CA3 region of hippocampus, DMH, PVN of hypothalamus, tuberomammillary nucleus (TMN), and spinal trigeminal nucleus (Marcus

Table 9.1 Orexin distribution in rat central nervous system

Brain division	Orexin levels in subdivision
Forebrain	Olfactory nucleus, cerebral cortex, hippocampus, septal nucleus, BST, subfornical organ, amygdala, substantia nigra, subthalamic nucleus, PVN, preoptic area, supraoptic nucleus, zona incerta, VMH, DMH, Arc, posterior part of the paraventricular hypothalamic nucleus, TMN.
Brainstem	Dorsal raphe, median raphe, locus coeruleus, parabrachial nucleus, A1 noradrenergic cells, area postrema, NTS, RVMM, RVLM, NA, pre-Bötzinger complex, RTN, dorsal motor nucleus of the vagus, trigeminal motor nucleus, facial motor nucleus, hypoglossal nucleus, spinal trigeminal nucleus.
Spinal cord	Whole length of the spinal cord from cervical to lumbar segments.

Data are from Ciriello *et al.* (2003), Date *et al.* (1999), de Lecea *et al.* (1998), Machado *et al.* (2002), Nambu *et al.* (1999), Peyron *et al.* (1998), Young *et al.* (2005).

et al., 2001; Trivedi *et al.*, 1998). This differential distribution of the orexin receptors suggests that each may have a physiologically distinct role.

D. Distribution in the periphery

Orexin immunoreactivity or prepro-orexin mRNA has been found in a variety of peripheral organs, including both neurons and endocrine cells. Orexin immunoreactivity has been detected in the neurons (submucosal and myenteric plexi) and endocrine (enterochromaffin) cells of the gastrointestinal tract (rat, mouse, guinea pig, and human), extrinsic neurons in pancreatic ganglia and endocrine B cells of pancreas (rat, guinea pig), endocrine cells (anterior and intermediate lobe) of rat pituitary, rat testis and endocrine cells of rat pineal gland (Arihara *et al.*, 2000; Date *et al.*, 2000; Jöhren *et al.*, 2001; Kirchgessner and Liu, 1999; Nanmoku *et al.*, 2002; Näslund *et al.*, 2002). Orexin A has also been detected in human adult adrenals (Randeva *et al.*, 2001) and at very low levels in rat heart (Jöhren *et al.*, 2001). However, it still needs to be determined whether orexin A is released into plasma from the CNS and if so, to what extent peripheral and central orexin production sites contribute to the plasma levels of orexin.

As with orexins, orexin receptors are also expressed in the periphery and are mostly collocated with the same organs as the peptide proteins. The receptors might be expressed in endocrine, muscle, and nerve cells and the expression of receptor subtypes varies in different tissues. Immunoreactivity for both OX_1R and OX_2R has been found in the gastrointestinal tract, pancreas, pituitary, adrenals, medulla (including chromaffin cells), and cortex of mammals (human and rat) (Blanco *et al.*, 2001, 2002; Jöhren *et al.*, 2001; Kirchgessner and Liu, 1999; Lopez *et al.*, 1999; Malendowicz *et al.*, 2001a,b; Näslund *et al.*, 2002). Only OX_1R has been found in the kidney, thyroid, and testis (Jöhren *et al.*, 2001), while only OX_2R in the lung and pineal gland (Jöhren *et al.*, 2001; Mikkelsen *et al.*, 2001). Distribution of orexin and orexin receptors in the peripheral tissues suggest that orexins are involved in the regulation of many peripheral functions.

III. Connections of Orexins with Other Transmitters

Orexin neurons in the hypothalamus are innervated by a variety of upstream neuronal populations including those involved in feeding, reward system, sleep–wakefulness, and memory and emotional state regulation. Some of the important brain regions innervating orexin neurons include the basal forebrain (BF) cholinergic neurons, GABA-containing neurons in the ventrolateral preoptic area (VLPO), neurons in the dorsomedial/

posterior hypothalamus, VTA neurons, and serotonergic neurons in the raphe nuclei. Orexin neurons also receive inputs from the regions associated with energy homeostasis including neuropeptide Y (NPY)-, agouti-related peptide, and α-melanin-stimulating hormone-immunoreactive fibers presumably coming from Arc. Brain regions associated with emotion including amygdale, infralimbic cortex, shell region of nucleus accumbens (NAc), lateral septum (LS), and the bed nucleus of stria terminalis also innervate orexin neurons (Sakurai *et al.*, 2005; Yoshida *et al.*, 2006). Orexinergic neurons even make contact with other orexinergic neurons within the hypothalamus (Bäckberg *et al.*, 2002; Horvath *et al.*, 1999).

From the regions mentioned above, the neurons provide an input to orexin neurons and regulate orexin neuronal activity by secretion of neurotransmitters or neuromodulators. Orexin neurons are activated by glutamate, ghrelin, cholecystokinin, corticotrophin-releasing factor (CRF), neurotensin, vasopressin, oxytocins, and glucagon-like peptide (Acuna-Goycolea and van den Pol, 2004; Li *et al.*, 2002; Tsujino *et al.*, 2005; Winsky-Sommerer *et al.*, 2004; Yamanaka *et al.*, 2003a,b). On the other hand, GABA, noradrenaline, serotonin, dopamine, NPY, leptin, and adenosine inhibit the activity of orexin neurons (Fu *et al.*, 2004; Li *et al.*, 2002; Liu and Gao, 2007; Muraki *et al.*, 2004; Xie *et al.*, 2006; Yamanaka *et al.*, 2003a,b, 2006). The cholinergic agonist, carbachol, activates 27% and inhibits 6% of orexin neurons (Sakurai *et al.*, 2005; Yamanaka *et al.*, 2003b). Metabolic signals also contribute to the regulation of orexin neuron activity; hypoglycemia stimulates orexin neurons, whereas hyperglycemia inhibits them (Yamanaka *et al.*, 2003a). Orexin neurons are also affected by the physiological fluctuations in acid and CO_2 levels. Increased H^+ concentration or CO_2 level increases orexin neuronal excitability, whereas reduced level depresses it (Williams *et al.*, 2007).

Orexinergic nerves from the lateral hypothalamus also innervate, and regulate the activity of, various neuronal circuits that utilize many different neurotransmitters or neuromodulators, for instance, noradrenaline, glutamate, GABA, dopamine, serotonin, histamine, acetylcholine, vasopressin, vasoactive intestinal peptide (VIP), somatostatin, CRF, NPY, proopiomelanocortin (POMC), cocaine/amphetamine-regulated transcript, and melanin concentrating hormone (Bäckberg *et al.*, 2002; Cutler *et al.*, 1999; Date *et al.*, 1999; Nambu *et al.*, 1999; Peyron *et al.*, 1998).

IV. Systemic Effects of Orexin

A. In feeding behavior and energy homeostasis

There is a considerable body of evidence for the role of orexin in the regulation of feeding and energy homeostasis. Orexinergic cell bodies are located in the LHA that is a known feeding center. Orexin and orexin receptor immunoreactivity have also been found in the brain regions involved in food intake and energy homeostasis including Arc, VMH, DMH, and PVN suggesting a greater orexin contribution (Cutler *et al.*, 1999; Elias *et al.*, 1998; Marcus *et al.*, 2001; Nambu *et al.*, 1999; Peyron *et al.*, 1998; Sakurai *et al.*, 1998; Trivedi *et al.*, 1998). Intracerebroventricular (icv) and microinjection of orexin A into several hypothalamic nuclei, including PVN, DMH, LHA, and perifornical area, increase food intake (Dube *et al.*, 1999; Sakurai *et al.*, 1998; Sutcliffe and De Lecea, 2000; Willie *et al.*, 2001). Both prepro-orexin and orexin receptors are upregulated in fasted animals (Cai *et al.*, 1999; Lu *et al.*, 2000; Sakurai *et al.*, 1998). In addition, central administration of anti-orexin antibody or an OX_1R selective antagonist causes a profound inhibition of feeding in fasted rats as well as orexin A induced feeding (Haynes *et al.*, 2000; Rodgers *et al.*, 2001; Yamada *et al.*, 2000). Moreover, prepro-orexin knockout mice and transgenic mice lacking orexin neurons show less food intake than control wild-type mice (Hara *et al.*, 2001; Willie *et al.*, 2001). Taken together, these data provide strong pharmacological evidence for a physiological role of the endogenous orexin in the modulation of feeding behaviors.

Additional evidence for the role of orexin in feeding has been provided by the data from a wide range of studies. Orexin neurons in the LHA send dense projections to Arc and are innervated by POMC and NPY neurons in the Arc (Date *et al.*, 1999; Elias *et al.*, 1998; Peyron *et al.*, 1998; Yamanaka *et al.*, 2000). Icv injection of orexin increases *Fos* expression in NPY neurons of Arc (Yamanaka *et al.*, 2000), and electrophysiological data reveals that orexin directly or indirectly activates NPY neurons but inhibits POMC neurons (Li and van den Pol, 2006; Ma *et al.*, 2007; Muroya *et al.*, 2004; van den Top *et al.*, 2004). Furthermore, prior administration of NPY-Y1 receptor antagonist has been found to reduce orexin induced food intake (Yamanaka *et al.*, 2000). These experiments suggest that activation of NPY neurons are, at least in part, involved in orexin-stimulated food intake.

Recent studies have demonstrated that feeding behavior is increased following infusion of orexin A into the shell of NAc, an area involved in the regulation of limbic system (Thorpe and Kotz, 2005). Moreover, the administration of $GABA_A$ receptor agonist, muscimol, into the NAc shell causes a profound increase in food intake, and increases *Fos* expression, particularly, in orexin neurons (Baldo *et al.*, 2004). These findings indicate that interaction between orexin neurons and limbic systems also have a role in the regulation of feeding.

Orexin neurons also participate in the regulation of feeding and energy homeostasis via responding to several metabolic signals that reflect the state of energy resources. Increased extracellular glucose concentration, as well as leptin, inhibits firing of orexin neurons. Conversely, decreased glucose concentration activates and causes depolarization of the same neurons (Burdakov *et al.*, 2005; Yamanaka *et al.*, 2003a). In addition, prepro-orexin mRNA levels are increased after 48 h of fasting and by acute insulin induced hypoglycemia, suggesting activation of these neurons in hunger (Cai *et al.*, 1999; Mondal *et al.*, 1999; Sakurai *et al.*, 1998). However, hypothalamic prepro-orexin mRNA levels are not increased in rats with increased appetite due to insulin-deficient diabetes, or access to palatable foods, indicating that orexin neurons are not activated under all conditions of hunger (Cai *et al.*, 1999, 2000). Taken together, the findings suggest that low plasma glucose levels and/or absence of food from gut stimulates orexin neurons, and that orexins are involved in short-term regulation of feeding behavior.

B. In sleep–wakefulness

Regulation of sleep/wakefulness is the most well-demonstrated systemic effect of the orexinergic system. Anatomically, orexin neurons are placed between sleep-promoting neurons in the VLPO and wake-promoting neurons in the brain stem including neurons in the TMN, LC, and DR. VLPO neurons play a crucial role in initiation of non-rapid eye movement (NREM) sleep and maintenance of NREM and rapid eye movement (REM) sleep (Sherin *et al.*, 1998). These neurons fire rapidly at sleep, with attenuation of firing during waking period. Sleep-active neurons in the VLPO mostly contain GABA and/or galanin and inhibit wake-active monoaminergic and cholinergic neurons in the arousal regions including noradrenergic neurons of LC, serotonergic neurons of DR, and histaminergic neurons of TMN during sleep (Lu *et al.*, 2002; Sherin *et al.*, 1998). On the other hand, monoaminergic neurons in the TMN, LC, and DR play crucial roles for the maintenance of arousal. These neurons fire tonically during the awake state, less during NREM sleep, and are virtually silent during REM sleep (Vanni-Mercier *et al.*, 1984). These monoaminergic and cholinergic wake-promoting neurotransmitters inhibit sleep-active neurons in the VLPO during waking period (Gallopin *et al.*, 2000). These reciprocal interactions of inhibition between sleep-active and wake-active neurons are crucial for switching between the sleep/wake states.

In addition to the reciprocal connection between VLPO and sleep-active brainstem neurons, orexin neurons act as a link between these neurons and stabilize behavioral states by activating arousal regions during wakefulness and preventing undesirable transitions between wakefulness and sleep.

It is now well established that orexin neurons fire during active waking and virtually cease firing during sleep, including the NREM and REM periods (Lee *et al.*, 2005). Furthermore, monoaminergic neurons in the TMN, LC, and DR express both orexin receptors and are densely innervated by orexin neurons suggesting that these neurons might be activated during wakeful period, and that they exert excitatory influence on these wake-active neurons to sustain their activity. In fact, *in vitro* studies revealed that noradrenergic neurons of LC, dopaminergic cells of VTA, serotonergic neurons of DR, and histaminergic neurons of TMN are all activated by orexins (Brown *et al.*, 2002; Hagan *et al.*, 1999; Liu *et al.*, 2002; Nakamura *et al.*, 2000; Yamanaka *et al.*, 2002). On the other hand, noradrenergic and serotonergic neurons send inhibitory projections to orexin neurons (Muraki *et al.*, 2004; Sakurai, 2005; Yamanaka *et al.*, 2006). These connections between orexin neurons and wake-active neurons, and *in vitro* results suggest that orexin neurons activate monoaminergic neurons, which in turn inhibit orexin neurons during active waking. This small decrease in the activity of monoaminergic neurons results in decreased inhibitory influence on orexin neurons. Subsequently, orexin neurons are disinhibited and their excitatory influence on monoaminergic neurons to maintain their activity. Orexin neurons also receive dense projection from GABAergic neurons in the VLPO and are inhibited by them during sleep (Sakurai *et al.*, 2005; Xie *et al.*, 2006; Yamanaka *et al.*, 2003a; Yoshida *et al.*, 2006). Moreover, selective deletion of the $GABA_B$ receptor gene in orexin neurons causes highly unstable sleep/wake architecture in mice (Matsuki *et al.*, 2009). This pathway might be important to turn off orexin neurons during sleep. Orexin neurons are also reciprocally connected with cholinergic neurons of BF, which also play an important role in regulating arousal. Cholinergic neurons in the BF are activated by orexins, and in turn activate some population of these neurons, thereby playing a role in the stabilization of wakefulness (Eggermann *et al.*, 2001; Sakurai *et al.*, 2005).

Electrophysiological and knockout studies provide further evidence of the physiological role of orexins and/or orexin receptors in sleep–wakefulness. Icv injection of orexin during light period potently increases the awake period in rats. This effect is markedly attenuated by H_1 antagonists and is completely absent in histamine H_1-receptor-deficient mice suggesting that TMN-histaminergic pathway is an important effector site of orexin for sleep/wake regulation (Huang *et al.*, 2001; Yamanaka *et al.*, 2002). Prepro-orexin knockout mice and OX_1R/OX_2R-double knockout mice are severely affected by behaviorally abnormal attacks of NREM sleep and show a similar degree of disrupted wakefulness (Willie *et al.*, 2003). These findings suggest that the profound dysregulation of wakefulness in the narcolepsy syndrome is due to a loss of signaling through orexin and/or orexin receptor dependent pathways.

C. Other responses

1. Orexin and reward system

There is considerable evidence that orexins are involved in the modulation of reward function. Orexin neurons receive projections from the regions involved in reward system including the VTA, NAc, and LS (Yoshida *et al.*, 2006). In the LHA/PFA, dopamine has an inhibitory influence on reward pathways and inhibits orexin neurons (Yamanaka *et al.*, 2003b; Yang *et al.*,

1997). On the other hand, orexin neurons project to and directly activate dopaminergic neurons of VTA (Fadel and Deutch, 2002; Korotkova *et al.*, 2003; Nakamura *et al.*, 2000; Peyron *et al.*, 1998). These reciprocal interactions may constitute regulatory mechanisms of reward system. Injection of OX_1R antagonist into the VTA blocks the development of heroin-conditioned place preferences (Narita *et al.*, 2006). In addition, *in vivo* administration of OX_1R antagonist blocks locomotor sensitization to cocaine (Borgland *et al.*, 2006). Taken together, these findings suggest a role for orexin in the mechanism of reward system and drug addiction.

2. Neuroendocrine effects of orexin

The anatomical distribution of orexin as well as its receptors in Arc and PVN suggests that orexin systems are involved in the control of neuroendocrine function. Icv administration of orexins increases plasma levels of corticosterone in rats (Hagan *et al.*, 1999; Malendowicz *et al.*, 1999a). Orexins also stimulate the release of CRF, VIP, neurotensin, and luteinizing hormone-releasing hormone from the hypothalamic explants (Russell *et al.*, 2000). Orexin A also inhibits the plasma levels of prolactin via both dopamine -dependent and -independent mechanisms. Orexin A also inhibits the secretion of growth hormone by stimulating the release of somatostatin from the hypothalamus via a direct action on pituitary (Hagan *et al.*, 1999; Russell *et al.*, 2000).

3. Orexin and pain

Several studies suggest that orexins play a role in the transmission of nociceptive information. Orexin-A-immunoreactive fibers and orexin receptors, OX_1R in particular, are abundantly expressed throughout the spinal cord including lamina I, an area associated with nociception. OX_1R is also expressed in dorsal root ganglia. In addition, intravenous injection of orexin A is analgesic in mouse, and rat, models of nociception and hyperalgesia. This effect is mediated solely by OX_1R as the analgesic effect of orexin A was blocked by a selective OX_1R antagonist, SB334867, but not by the opioid antagonist, naloxone. Furthermore, SB334867 enhances hyperalgesia under certain inflammatory conditions suggesting a tonic inhibitory orexin input in these circumstances (Bingham *et al.*, 2001).

4. Peripheral effects of orexin

The presence of orexin, and orexin receptors, in different peripheral tissues suggests that orexins play an important role in the periphery along with its central function. Orexin A activates secretomotor neurons in the guinea pig submucosal plexus and regulates gut motility by increasing the velocity of propulsion in isolated guinea pig colon. Orexins have also been reported to inhibit fasting motility in rat duodenum (Yamanaka *et al.*, 2000). Orexins may affect glucose homeostasis by regulating the secretion of pancreatic hormones including insulin and glucagon. Both *in vivo* (subcutaneous injection of orexin A) and *in vitro* studies have revealed that orexin A stimulates insulin and glucagon secretion (Nowak *et al.*, 1999). Orexins may also activate adrenals independently of central mechanisms (via endocrine, paracrine, or neurocrine mechanisms) by binding with orexin receptors. Orexins stimulate corticosteroid secretion from rat and human adrenocortical cells (Malendowicz *et al.*, 1999b; Mazzocchi *et al.*, 2001). In addition, orexin A stimulates the release of adrenaline and noradrenaline from cultured porcine adrenal medullary cells and of aldosterone from cultured porcine adrenal cortex cells (Fujiki *et al.*, 2001).

V. Central Cardiovascular Effects of Orexin

The distribution of orexins, and orexin receptors, in the cardiovascular regulatory centers, as well as functional studies indicate a crucial role of orexin in the regulation of autonomic function. Orexin neurons in the hypothalamus project to PVN and to different brainstem nuclei involved in control of sympathetic and parasympathetic outflow including NTS, RVMM, RVLM, and NA and to the final relay center of sympathetic tone, that is, sympathetic preganglionic neurons of the spinal cord (Ciriello *et al.*, 2003; Cutler *et al.*, 1999; Date *et al.*, 1999; de Lecea *et al.*, 1998; Machado *et al.*, 2002; Nambu *et al.*, 1999; Peyron *et al.*, 1998; van den Pol, 1999). Orexin receptors are also expressed in these areas (Ciriello and de Oliveira, 2003; Cluderay *et al.*, 2002; Marcus *et al.*, 2001; Sunter *et al.*, 2001; Trivedi *et al.*, 1998; van den Top *et al.*, 2003). Recent study from our lab has also revealed that both OX_1R and OX_2R are expressed in the RVLM neurons including tyrosine hydroxylase immunoreactive (TH-ir) neurons (Shahid *et al.*, 2012).

In orexin knockout mice, the basal blood pressure (BP) is lower compared to their wild-type littermates (Kayaba *et al.*, 2003), suggesting that orexins physiologically stimulate sympathetic outflow. It has been demonstrated that icv injection of orexins increases BP and heart rate (HR), renal sympathetic nerve activity (RSNA) and plasma catecholamine in rat and rabbit (Matsumura *et al.*, 2001; Samson *et al.*, 1999; Shirasaka *et al.*, 1999). On the other hand, intravenous injection of orexin produces no cardiovascular effect (Matsumura *et al.*, 2001) suggesting that orexin mediated cardiovascular function is solely via central mechanisms. Furthermore, intrathecal (i.t.) injection of orexin A increases mean arterial pressure (MAP) and HR in urethane anesthetized rats and the effects are markedly attenuated by iv injection of α- or β-adrenoceptor antagonist (Antunes *et al.*, 2001). However, these workers injected orexin A at the level of thoracic 1–2 (T1–T2) a site that principally innervates the heart but not blood vessels. Recently, Shahid *et al.* (2011) demonstrated that i.t. orexin A injection at T6–T8, a site that innervates the splanchnic sympathetic bed, causes a profound increase in MAP, HR, and splanchnic SNA (sSNA), and that these effects are attenuated by SB334867 suggesting that orexin responses in the spinal cord are mediated by both OX_1R and OX_2R.

Direct microinjection of orexin A into the NA, an area involved in the parasympathetic control of HR, elicits a dose-related decrease in HR with little or no direct change in MAP and potentiates reflex bradycardia induced by the activation of arterial baroreflex. Whereas the effects of orexin A microinjection into the NTS is controversial and appears to depend on the doses administered. Low doses of orexin A (10 pM–10 nM) injected into the NTS dose-dependently increases MAP and HR (Smith *et al.*, 2002), whereas at high doses (25–250 μM), microinjection of orexin A into the NTS decreases MAP and HR in a dose-dependent manner, and potentiates reflex bradycardia induced by activation of baroreflex (De Oliveira *et al.*, 2003). On the contrary, Shih and Chuang (2007) showed that at a dose of 100 μM, orexin A injection into the NTS elicits slight decrease in MAP and HR while at higher doses of up to 4 mM, MAP and HR are decreased. Nitric oxide is suggested to be a neuromodulator responsible for the bidirectional activity of orexins. Low concentration of NO, synthesized by low dose of orexin, stimulates nitric oxide synthase (NOS) potentiating glutamatergic excitatory postsynaptic potentials, and thereby decreasing BP. On the other hand, high dose of orexin A stimulates the production of more NO that increases BP through potentiation of GABAergic inhibitory pathways (Shih and Chuang, 2007). Microinjection of orexin A into RVMM has also been shown to increase HR dose-dependently with a little or no change in MAP, and attenuate reflex bradycardia response (Ciriello *et al.*, 2003).

Orexin A has also been microinjected into the RVLM, a key nucleus for the tonic and reflex regulation of sympathetic tone, in both anesthetized and conscious rats. In both conditions, orexin A injection into RVLM increases MAP and HR (Chen *et al.*, 2000; Machado *et al.*, 2002). In addition, *in vitro* recordings of the RVLM neuronal activity showed that orexin dose-dependently depolarizes RVLM neurons and this depolarization is mediated predominantly via OX_2R (Huang *et al.*, 2010). On the other hand, Shahid *et al.* (2012) reported that both OX_1R and OX_2R are expressed in the RVLM and colocalize with TH-ir neurons. Furthermore, bilateral microinjection of orexin A into the RVLM elicits a dose-related increase in MAP, HR, and sSNA. These effects are attenuated by prior injection of SB334867 and reproduced by the injection of OX_2R agonist, [Ala_{11}, D-Leu_{15}]orexin B, into the RVLM (Shahid *et al.*, 2012). These latter findings suggest that both OX_1R and OX_2R mediate the autonomic effects of orexin A in the RVLM.

Recent studies reveal that orexins play an important role in the modulation of sympathetic reflexes including the somatosympathetic reflex, sympathetic baroreflex, and chemoreflex at the level of both RVLM and spinal cord. In the spinal cord, orexin A attenuates the somatosympathetic reflex while increasing baroreflex sensitivity. The pressor and sympathoexcitatory responses to brief hypoxia, a model to activate peripheral chemoreceptors, are also potentiated by i.t. orexin A (Shahid *et al.*, 2011). Similarly, in the RVLM, orexin A injection attenuates the somatosympathetic reflex but increases baroreflex sensitivity. Orexin A also increases or reduces the sympathoexcitation following activation of peripheral or central chemoreceptors in the RVLM respectively (Shahid *et al.*, 2012).

VI. Respiratory Effects of Orexin

The role of hypothalamic orexin system in the regulation of breathing is well recognized from both anatomical and functional evidence. Axons of orexin neurons project to respiratory-related nuclei including RVLM sympathoexcitatory neurons, pre-Bötzinger complex (part of respiratory rhythm generator), the NTS (area containing inspiratory cells responsive to sensory afferents), retrotrapezoid nucleus (RTN; central chemoreceptor), raphe nuclei (an area regulating respiratory long-term facilitation, LTF), and hypoglossal and phrenic nuclei (areas that control swallowing and diaphragm movements; Fung *et al.*, 2001; Krout *et al.*, 2003; Machado *et al.*, 2002; Rosin *et al.*, 2006; Volgin *et al.*, 2002; Young *et al.*, 2005). Orexin receptors are also expressed in all of these neurons (Cluderay *et al.*, 2002; Dias *et al.*, 2009; Marcus *et al.*, 2001; Shahid *et al.*, 2012; Sunter *et al.*, 2001; Trivedi *et al.*, 1998; Young *et al.*, 2005).

Physiological evidence indicates that orexins affect ventilation. Icv administration of orexin increases breathing frequency and tidal volume (Zhang *et al.*, 2005). In addition, microinjection of orexin A into the pre-Bötzinger complex and microperfusion into phrenic motoneurons results in the increase of diaphragm electromyographic activity (Young *et al.*, 2005). Furthermore, Shahid *et al.* (2012) looked at the direct effects on phrenic nerve activity (PNA) following microinjection of orexin A into the RVLM. Orexin A in the RVLM causes a long lasting increase of PNA, and the effect is attenuated by OX_1R antagonist and reproduced by OX_2R agonist (Shahid *et al.*, 2012). In addition, Toyama *et al.* (2009) showed that phrenic LTF is attenuated in orexin neuron-ablated mice. These results suggest that orexin stimulates respiration and play an important role in the development of respiratory LTF.

Further evidence linking orexin and breathing comes from studies on the response of orexin to changes in pH or extracellular CO_2 level. Orexin neurons themselves are chemosensitive both *in vivo* and *in vitro* (Sunanaga *et al.*, 2009; Williams *et al.*, 2007). Physiological levels of acidosis (low pH, high CO_2) depolarize orexin neurons and increase their firing, while alkalosis (high pH, low CO_2) causes hyperpolarization and an inhibition of firing (Williams *et al.*, 2007). Prepro-orexin deficient mice have a 50% decrease in the ventilatory CO_2 (hypercapnia) response during wakefulness but not sleep. Orexin knockout mice also display a markedly higher frequency of spontaneous apnoeic episodes during sleep (Nakamura *et al.*, 2007). Furthermore, icv administration of SB334867 decreases the respiratory chemoreflex in wild-type mice (Deng *et al.*, 2007) suggesting a role for orexin in modulation of chemoreflex. Moreover, antagonism of OX_1R in the RTN, which is a key chemosensory nucleus (Guyenet *et al.*, 2010; Stornetta *et al.*, 2009), or in medullary slices containing pre-Bötzinger complex and hypoglossal motornuclei blunts the response to hypercapnia (Corcoran *et al.*, 2010; Dias *et al.*, 2009). Additionally, orexin A microinjection into the RVLM markedly attenuates the respiratory response to hypoxia and hypercapnia (Shahid *et al.*, 2012). These findings suggest that orexin may modulate chemoreflex responses directly through the activation of orexin neurons or indirectly via an action in the RTN, pre-Bötzinger complex, hypoglossal motornuclei, or RVLM.

VII. Conclusion

Successful homeostatic regulation requires, *inter alia*, delicate interactions between neuroendocrine systems and central autonomic control pathways. Minor changes in any system will cause feedback changes in others. After more than a decade of research, orexin neurons have emerged as a crucial neurophysiological link between energy balance, emotion, reward systems, and arousal. Active waking causes increases in HR, MAP, respiration, and locomotor activity. However, the neural mechanisms and pathways that mediate the pressor, sympathoexcitatory, and tachycardic responses to arousal are poorly understood. Despite many studies, the physiological role of orexin in cardiovascular regulation is still not well understood. One reason for this is the lack of adequate agonists and antagonists to probe the function of orexin pathways in the anesthetized and awake animal. The presence of orexin immunoreactive fibers and orexin receptors in cardiovascular regulatory sites and the effects of OX-A on basal cardiovascular parameters and adaptive reflexes strongly suggest that OX receptor activation plays a key role in mediating the sympathoexcitatory responses to arousal, but further studies are needed (Fig. 9.3).

Similarly, little is known about the role of orexin in central respiratory regulation. *In vitro* studies have been conducted in the RTN, pre-Bötzinger complex, and hypoglossal motonuclei. *In vivo* studies have been conducted in the pre-Bötzinger complex, RVLM, and phrenic motonuclei. These studies suggest a critical role of orexin in breathing, at least during reflex

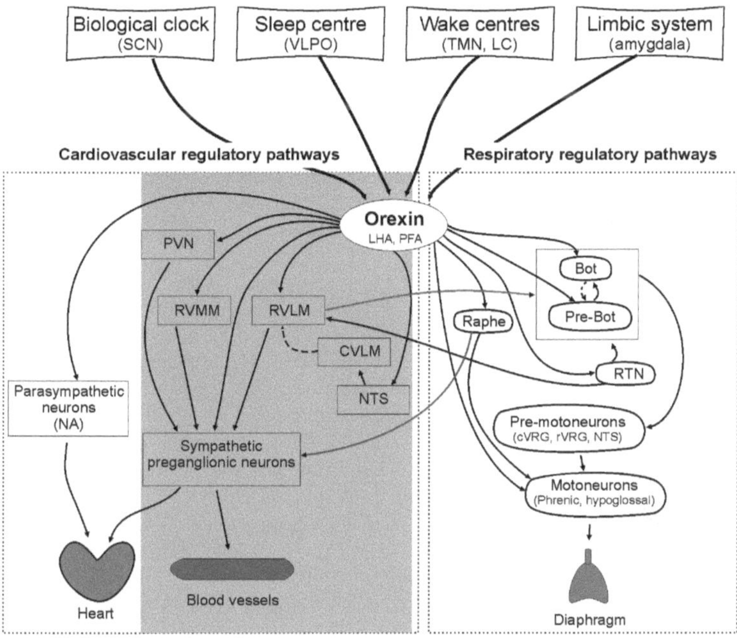

Figure 9.3 Schematic showing the role of orexin in the central regulation of cardiovascular and respiratory function. Orexin neurons receive projections from higher centers (thick lines). Orexin neurons play a complex role in the regulation of the cardiovascular system (left half) via projections to both sympathetic (shaded part) and parasympathetic neurons. Simultaneously orexin neurons project to respiratory regulatory centers (right half). Thus, orexin can modulate the cardiorespiratory system in a state-dependent manner. Arrows, excitatory projections; broken arrows, inhibitory projections. Bot, Bötzinger region; CVLM, caudal ventrolateral medulla; LC, locus coeruleus; NA, nucleus ambiguus, NTS, nucleus tractus solitarius; Pre-Bot, pre-Bötzinger region; PVN, paraventricular nucleus; RVLM, rostral ventrolateral medulla; RVMM, rostral ventromedial medulla; RTN, retrotrapezoid nucleus; SCN, suprachiasmatic nucleus; TMN, tuberomammillary nucleus; VLPO, ventrolateral preoptic area.

changes and homeostatic variations such as sleep/wake. Further *in vivo* studies that determine the role of orexins in the physiology and integration cardiorespiratory reflexes centrally are essential for a full understanding of this important neuropeptide in breathing in normal and pathophysiological states (Fig. 9.3).

ACKNOWLEDGMENTS

Work in the Authors' laboratory is supported by Grants from the National Health and Medical Research Council of Australia (1024489, 1030297, 9201100439, 604002), Australian Research Council (DP110102110, LP120100463), and Macquarie University. A. A. Rahman and I. Z. Shahid are supported by a Macquarie University Research Excellence Scholarship.

REFERENCES

Acuna-Goycolea, C., and van den Pol, A. (2004). Glucagon-like peptide 1 excites hypocretin/orexin neurons by direct and indirect mechanisms: Implications for viscera-mediated arousal. *J. Neurosci.* **24,** 8141–8152.

Alexander, S. P., Mathie, A., and Peters, J. A. (2011). Guide to receptors and channels (GRAC). *Br. J. Pharmacol.* **164,** S1–S324.

Antunes, V. R., Cristina Brailoiu, G., Kwok, E. H., Scruggs, P., and Dun, A. N. J. (2001). Orexins/hypocretins excite rat sympathetic preganglionic neurons in vivo and in vitro. *Am. J. Physiol.* **281,** R1801–R1807.

Arihara, Z., Takahashi, K., Murakami, O., Totsune, K., Sone, M., Satoh, F., Ito, S., Hayashi, Y., Sasano, H., and Mouri, T. (2000). Orexin-A in the human brain and tumor tissues of ganglioneuroblastoma and neuroblastoma. *Peptides* **21,** 565–570.

Bäckberg, M., Hervieu, G., Wilson, S., and Meister, B. (2002). Orexin receptor-1 (OX-R1) immunoreactivity in chemically identified neurons of the hypothalamus: Focus on orexin targets involved in control of food and water intake. *Eur. J. Neurosci.* **15,** 315–328.

Baldo, B. A., Gual-Bonilla, L., Sijapati, K., Daniel, R. A., Landry, C. F., and Kelley, A. E. (2004). Activation of a subpopulation of orexin/hypocretin-containing hypothalamic neurons by $GABA_A$ receptor-mediated inhibition of the nucleus accumbens shell, but not by exposure to a novel environment. *Eur. J. Neurosci.* **19,** 376–386.

Bingham, S., Davey, P. T., Babbs, A. J., Irving, E. A., Sammons, M. J., Wyles, M., Jeffrey, P., Cutler, L., Riba, I., Johns, A., Porter, R. A., Upton, N., *et al.* (2001). Orexin-A, an hypothalamic peptide with analgesic properties. *Pain* **92,** 81–90.

Blanco, M., García-Caballero, T., Fraga, M., Gallego, R., Cuevas, J., Forteza, J., Beiras, A., and Diéguez, C. (2002). Cellular localization of orexin receptors in human adrenal gland, adrenocortical adenomas and pheochromocytomas. *Regul. Pept.* **104,** 161–165.

Blanco, M., López, M., García-Caballero, T., Gallego, R., Vázquez-Boquete, A., Morel, G., Señarís, R., Casanueva, F., Diéguez, C., and Beiras, A. (2001). Cellular localization of orexin receptors in human pituitary. *J. Clin. Endocrinol. Metab.* **86,** 3444–3447.

Borgland, S. L., Taha, S. A., Sarti, F., Fields, H. L., and Bonci, A. (2006). Orexin A in the VTA is critical for the induction of synaptic plasticity and behavioral sensitization to cocaine. *Neuron* **49,** 589–601.

Broberger, C., De Lecea, L., Sutcliffe, J. G., and Hökfelt, T. (1998). Hypocretin/Orexin- and melanin-concentrating hormone-expressing cells form distinct populations in the rodent lateral hypothalamus: Relationship to the neuropeptide Y and agouti gene-related protein systems. *J. Comp. Neurol.* **402,** 460–474.

Brown, R. E., Sergeeva, O. A., Eriksson, K. S., and Haas, H. L. (2002). Convergent excitation of dorsal raphe serotonin neurons by multiple arousal systems (orexin/hypocretin, histamine and noradrenaline). *J. Neurosci.* **22,** 8850–8859.

Burdakov, D., Gerasimenko, O., and Verkhratsky, A. (2005). Physiological changes in glucose differentially modulate the excitability of hypothalamic melanin-concentrating hormone and orexin neurons in situ. *J. Neurosci.* **25,** 2429–2433.

Cai, X. J., Lister, C. A., Buckingham, R. E., Pickavance, L., Wilding, J., Arch, J. R. S., Wilson, S., and Williams, G. (2000). Down-regulation of orexin gene expression by severe obesity in the rats: Studies in Zucker fatty and Zucker diabetic fatty rats and effects of rosiglitazone. *Mol. Brain Res.* **77,** 131–137.

Cai, X. J., Widdowson, P. S., Harrold, J., Wilson, S., Buckingham, R. E., Arch, J. R., Tadayyon, M., Clapham, J. C., Wilding, J., and Williams, G. (1999). Hypothalamic orexin expression: Modulation by blood glucose and feeding. *Diabetes* **48,** 2132–2137.

Chen, C. T., Dun, S. L., Kwok, E. H., Dun, N. J., and Chang, J. K. (1999). Orexin A-like immunoreactivity in the rat brain. *Neurosci. Lett.* **260,** 161–164.

Chen, C. T., Hwang, L. L., Chang, J. K., and Dun, N. J. (2000). Pressor effects of orexins injected intracisternally and to rostral ventrolateral medulla of anesthetized rats. *Am. J. Physiol.* **278,** R692–R697.

Ciriello, J., and de Oliveira, C. V. (2003). Cardiac effects of hypocretin-1 in nucleus ambiguus. *Am. J. Physiol.* **284,** R1611–R1620.

Ciriello, J., Li, Z., and De Oliveira, C. V. R. (2003). Cardioacceleratory responses to hypocretin-1 injections into rostral ventromedial medulla. *Brain Res.* **991,** 84–95.

Cluderay, J. E., Harrison, D. C., and Hervieu, G. J. (2002). Protein distribution of the orexin-2 receptor in the rat central nervous system. *Regul. Pept.* **104,** 131–144.

Corcoran, A., Richerson, G., Harris, M., Homma, I., Fukuchi, Y., and Onimaru, H. (2010). Modulation of respiratory activity by hypocretin-1 (orexin A) in situ and *in vitro*. *Adv. Exp. Med. Biol.* **669,** 109–113.

Cutler, D. J., Morris, R., Sheridhar, V., Wattam, T. A. K., Holmes, S., Patel, S., Arch, J. R. S., Wilson, S., Buckingham, R. E., Evans, M. L., Leslie, R. A., and Williams, G. (1999). Differential distribution of orexin-A and orexin-B immunoreactivity in the rat brain and spinal cord. *Peptides* **20,** 1455–1470.

Date, Y., Mondal, M. S., Matsukura, S., and Nakazato, M. (2000). Distribution of orexin-A and orexin-B (hypocretins) in the rat spinal cord. *Neurosci. Lett.* **288,** 87–90.

Date, Y., Ueta, Y., Yamashita, H., Yamaguchi, H., Matsukura, S., Kangawa, K., Sakurai, T., Yanagisawa, M., and Nakazato, M. (1999). Orexins, orexigenic hypothalamic peptides, interact with autonomic, neuroendocrine and neuroregulatory systems. *Proc. Natl. Acad. Sci. U.S.A.* **96,** 748–753.

de Lecea, L., Kilduff, T. S., Peyron, C., Gao, X.-B., Foye, P. E., Danielson, P. E., Fukuhara, C., Battenberg, E. L. F., Gautvik, V. T., Bartlett, F. S., Frankel, W. N., van den Pol, A. N., *et al.* (1998). The hypocretins: Hypothalamus-specific peptides with neuroexcitatory activity. *Proc. Natl. Acad. Sci. U.S.A.* **95,** 322–327.

De Oliveira, C. V. R., Rosas-Arellano, M. P., Solano-Flores, L. P., and Ciriello, J. (2003). Cardiovascular effects of hypocretin-1 in nucleus of the solitary tract. *Am. J. Physiol.* **284,** H1369–H1377.

Deng, B. S., Nakamura, A., Zhang, W., Yanagisawa, M., Fukuda, Y., and Kuwaki, T. (2007). Contribution of orexin in hypercapnic chemoreflex: Evidence from genetic and pharmacological disruption and supplementation studies in mice. *J. Appl. Physiol.* **103,** 1772–1779.

Dias, M. B., Li, A., and Nattie, E. E. (2009). Antagonism of orexin receptor-1 in the retrotrapezoid nucleus inhibits the ventilatory response to hypercapnia predominantly in wakefulness. *J. Physiol.* **587,** 2059–2067.

Dube, M. G., Kalra, S. P., and Kalra, P. S. (1999). Food intake elicited by central administration of orexins/hypocretins: Identification of hypothalamic sites of action. *Brain Res.* **842,** 473–477.

Dyer, C. J., Touchette, K. J., Carroll, J. A., Allee, G. L., and Matteri, R. L. (1999). Cloning of porcine prepro-orexin cDNA and effects of an intramuscular injection of synthetic porcine orexin-B on feed intake in young pigs. *Domest. Anim. Endocrinol.* **16,** 145–148.

Eggermann, E., Serafin, M., Bayer, L., Machard, D., Saint-Mleux, B., Jones, B. E., and Muhlethaler, M. (2001). Orexins/hypocretins excite basal forebrain cholinergic neurones. *Neuroscience* **108,** 177–181.

Elias, C. F., Saper, C. B., Maratos-Flier, E., Tritos, N. A., Lee, C., Kelly, J., Tatro, J. B., Hoffman, G. E., Ollmann, M. M., Barsh, G. S., Sakurai, T., Yanagisawa, M., *et al.* (1998). Chemically defined projections linking the mediobasal hypothalamus and the lateral hypothalamic area. *J. Comp. Neurol.* **402,** 442–459.

Fadel, J., and Deutch, A. Y. (2002). Anatomical substrates of orexin-dopamine interactions: Lateral hypothalamic projections to the ventral tegmental area. *Neuroscience* **111,** 379–387.

Fu, L.-Y., Acuna-Goycolea, C., and van den Pol, A. N. (2004). Neuropeptide Y inhibits hypocretin/orexin neurons by multiple presynaptic and postsynaptic mechanisms: Tonic depression of the hypothalamic arousal system. *J. Neurosci.* **24,** 8741–8751.

Fujiki, N., Yoshida, Y., Ripley, B., Honda, K., Mignot, E., and Nishino, S. (2001). Changes in CSF hypocretin-1 (orexin A) levels in rats across 24 hours and in response to food deprivation. *Neuroreport* **12,** 993–997.

Fung, S. J., Yamuy, J., Sampogna, S., Morales, F. R., and Chase, M. H. (2001). Hypocretin (orexin) input to trigeminal and hypoglossal motoneurons in the cat: A double-labeling immunohistochemical study. *Brain Res.* **903,** 257–262.

Galas, L., Vaudry, H., Braun, B., Van Den Pol, A. N., De Lecea, L., Sutcliffe, J. G., and Chartrel, N. (2001). Immunohistochemical localization and biochemical characterization of hypocretin/orexin-related peptides in the central nervous system of the frog *Rana ridibunda*. *J. Comp. Neurol.* **429,** 242–252.

Gallopin, T., Fort, P., Eggermann, E., Cauli, B., Luppi, P.-H., Rossier, J., Audinat, E., Muhlethaler, M., and Serafin, M. (2000). Identification of sleep-promoting neurons *in vitro*. *Nature* **404,** 992–995.

Guyenet, P. G., Stornetta, R. L., Abbott, S. B. G., Depuy, S. D., Fortuna, M. G., and Kanbar, R. (2010). Central CO_2 chemoreception and integrated neural mechanisms of cardiovascular and respiratory control. *J. Appl. Physiol.* **108,** 995–1002.

Hagan, J. J., Leslie, R. A., Patel, S., Evans, M. L., Wattam, T. A., Holmes, S., Benham, C. D., Taylor, S. G., Routledge, C., Hemmati, P., Munton, R. P., Ashmeade, T. E., *et al.* (1999). Orexin A activates locus coeruleus cell firing and increases arousal in the rat. *Proc. Natl. Acad. Sci. U.S.A.* **96,** 10911–10916.

Hara, J., Beuckmann, C. T., Nambu, T., Willie, J. T., Chemelli, R. M., Sinton, C. M., Sugiyama, F., Yagami, K.-i., Goto, K., Yanagisawa, M., and Sakurai, T. (2001). Genetic ablation of orexin neurons in mice results in narcolepsy, hypophagia, and obesity. *Neuron* **30,** 345–354.

Harrison, T. A., Chen, C. T., Dun, N. J., and Chang, J. K. (1999). Hypothalamic orexin A-immunoreactive neurons project to the rat dorsal medulla. *Neurosci. Lett.* **273,** 17–20.

Haynes, A. C., Jackson, B., Chapman, H., Tadayyon, M., Johns, A., Porter, R. A., and Arch, J. R. S. (2000). A selective orexin-1 receptor antagonist reduces food consumption in male and female rats. *Regul. Pept.* **96,** 45–51.

Hervieu, G. J., Cluderay, J. E., Harrison, D. C., Roberts, J. C., and Leslie, R. A. (2001). Gene expression and protein distribution of the orexin-1 receptor in the rat brain and spinal cord. *Neuroscience* **103,** 777–797.

Horvath, T. L., Diano, S., and van den Pol, A. N. (1999). Synaptic interaction between hypocretin (orexin) and neuropeptide Y cells in the rodent and primate hypothalamus: A novel circuit implicated in metabolic and endocrine regulations. *J. Neurosci.* **19,** 1072–1087.

Huang, S.-C., Dai, Y.-W. E., Lee, Y.-H., Chiou, L.-C., and Hwang, L.-L. (2010). Orexins depolarize rostral ventrolateral medulla neurons and increase arterial pressure and heart rate in rats mainly via orexin 2 receptors. *J. Pharmacol. Exp. Ther.* **334,** 522–529.

Huang, Z.-L., Qu, W.-M., Li, W.-D., Mochizuki, T., Eguchi, N., Watanabe, T., Urade, Y., and Hayaishi, O. (2001). Arousal effect of orexin A depends on activation of the histaminergic system. *Proc. Natl. Acad. Sci. U.S.A.* **98,** 9965–9970.

Hungs, M., Fan, J., Lin, L., Lin, X., Maki, R. A., and Mignot, E. (2001). Identification and functional analysis of mutations in the hypocretin (orexin) genes of narcoleptic canines. *Genome Res.* **11,** 531–539.

Ichinose, M., Asai, M., Sawada, M., Sasaki, K., and Oomura, Y. (1998). Induction of outward current by orexin-B in mouse peritoneal macrophages. *FEBS Lett.* **440,** 51–54.

Jöhren, O., Neidert, S. J., Kummer, M., Dendorfer, A., and Dominiak, P. (2001). Prepro-orexin and orexin receptor mRNAs are differentially expressed in peripheral tissues of male and female rats. *Endocrinology* **142,** 3324–3331.

Kastin, A. J., and Akerstrom, V. (1999). Orexin A but not Orexin B rapidly enters brain from blood by simple diffusion. *J. Pharmacol. Exp. Ther.* **289,** 219–223.

Kayaba, Y., Nakamura, A., Kasuya, Y., Ohuchi, T., Yanagisawa, M., Komuro, I., Fukuda, Y., and Kuwaki, T. (2003). Attenuated defense response and low basal blood pressure in orexin knockout mice. *Am. J. Physiol.* **285,** R581–R593.

Kirchgessner, A. L., and Liu, M.-t. (1999). Orexin synthesis and response in the gut. *Neuron* **24,** 941–951.

Korotkova, T. M., Sergeeva, O. A., Eriksson, K. S., Haas, H. L., and Brown, R. E. (2003). Excitation of ventral tegmental area dopaminergic and nondopaminergic neurons by orexins/hypocretins. *J. Neurosci.* **23,** 7–11.

Krout, K. E., Mettenleiter, T. C., and Loewy, A. D. (2003). Single CNS neurons link both central motor and cardiosympathetic systems: A double-virus tracing study. *Neuroscience* **118,** 853–866.

Lee, M. G., Hassani, O. K., and Jones, B. E. (2005). Discharge of identified orexin/hypocretin neurons across the sleep-waking cycle. *J. Neurosci.* **25,** 6716–6720.

Li, Y., Gao, X. B., Sakurai, T., and Van den Pol, A. N. (2002). Hypocretin/orexin excites hypocretin neurons via a local glutamate neuron—A potential mechanism for orchestrating the hypothalamic arousal system. *Neuron* **36,** 1169–1181.

Li, Y., and van den Pol, A. N. (2006). Differential target-dependent actions of coexpressed inhibitory dynorphin and excitatory hypocretin/orexin neuropeptides. *J. Neurosci.* **26,** 13037–13047.

Liu, R.-J., van den Pol, A. N., and Aghajanian, G. K. (2002). Hypocretins (orexins) regulate serotonin neurons in the dorsal raphe nucleus by excitatory direct and inhibitory indirect actions. *J. Neurosci.* **22,** 9453–9464.

Liu, Z.-W., and Gao, X.-B. (2007). Adenosine inhibits activity of hypocretin/orexin neurons by the A1 receptor in the lateral hypothalamus: A possible sleep-promoting effect. *J. Neurophysiol.* **97,** 837–848.

Lopez, M., Senaris, R., Gallego, R., Garcia-Caballero, T., Lago, F., Seoane, L., Casanueva, F., and Dieguez, C. (1999). Orexin receptors are expressed in the adrenal medulla of the rat. *Endocrinology* **140,** 5991–5994.

Lu, J., Bjorkum, A. A., Xu, M., Gaus, S. E., Shiromani, P. J., and Saper, C. B. (2002). Selective activation of the extended ventrolateral preoptic nucleus during rapid eye movement sleep. *J. Neurosci.* **22,** 4568–4576.

Lu, X.-Y., Bagnol, D., Burke, S., Akil, H., and Watson, S. J. (2000). Differential distribution and regulation of OX1 and OX2 orexin/hypocretin receptor messenger RNA in the brain upon fasting. *Horm. Behav.* **37,** 335–344.

Lund, P.-E., Shariatmadari, R., Uustare, A., Detheux, M., Parmentier, M., Kukkonen, J. P., and Akerman, K. E. O. (2000). The orexin OX1 receptor activates a novel Ca^{2+} influx pathway necessary for coupling to phospholipase C. *J. Biol. Chem.* **275,** 30806–30812.

Ma, X., Zubcevic, L., Bruning, J. C., Ashcroft, F. M., and Burdakov, D. (2007). Electrical inhibition of identified anorexigenic POMC neurons by orexin/hypocretin. *J. Neurosci.* **27,** 1529–1533.

Machado, B. H., Bonagamba, L. G. H., Dun, S. L., Kwok, E. H., and Dun, N. J. (2002). Pressor response to microinjection of orexin/hypocretin into rostral ventrolateral medulla of awake rats. *Regul. Pept.* **104,** 75–81.

Malendowicz, L. K., Hochol, A., Ziolkowska, A., Nowak, M., Gottardo, L., and Nussdorfer, G. G. (2001a). Prolonged orexin administration stimulates steroid-hormone secretion, acting directly on the rat adrenal gland. *Int. J. Mol. Med.* **7,** 401–404.

Malendowicz, L. K., Jedrzejczak, N., Belloni, A. S., Trejter, M., Hochol, A., and Nussdorfer, G. G. (2001b). Effects of orexins A and B on the secretory and proliferative activity of immature and regenerating rat adrenal glands. *Histol. Histopathol.* **16,** 713–717.

Malendowicz, L. K., Tortorella, C., and Nussdorfer, G. G. (1999a). Acute effects of orexins A and B on the rat pituitary-adrenocortical axis. *Biomed. Res.* **20,** 301–304.

Malendowicz, L. K., Tortorella, C., and Nussdorfer, G. G. (1999b). Orexins stimulate corticosterone secretion of rat adrenocortical cells, through the activation of the adenylate cyclase-dependent signaling cascade. *J. Steroid Biochem. Mol. Biol.* **70,** 185–188.

Marcus, J. N., Aschkenasi, C. J., Lee, C. E., Chemelli, R. M., Saper, C. B., Yanagisawa, M., and Elmquist, J. K. (2001). Differential expression of orexin receptors 1 and 2 in the rat brain. *J. Comp. Neurol.* **435,** 6–25.

Matsuki, T., Nomiyama, M., Takahira, H., Hirashima, N., Kunita, S., Takahashi, S., Yagami, K. I., Kilduff, T. S., Bettler, B., Yanagisawa, M., and Sakurai, T. (2009). Selective loss of GABAB receptors in orexin-producing neurons results in disrupted sleep/wakefulness architecture. *Proc. Natl. Acad. Sci. U.S.A.* **106,** 4459–4464.

Matsumura, K., Tsuchihashi, T., and Abe, I. (2001). Central orexin-A augments sympathoadrenal outflow in conscious rabbits. *Hypertension* **37,** 1382–1387.

Mazzocchi, G., Malendowicz, L. K., Gottardo, L., Aragona, F., and Nussdorfer, G. G. (2001). Orexin A stimulates cortisol secretion from human adrenocortical cells through activation of the adenylate cyclase-dependent signaling cascade. *J. Clin. Endocrinol. Metab.* **86,** 778–782.

Mikkelsen, J. D., Hauser, F., DeLecea, L., Sutcliffe, J. G., Kilduff, T. S., Calgari, C., Pévet, P., and Simonneaux, V. (2001). Hypocretin (orexin) in the rat pineal gland: A central transmitter with effects on noradrenaline-induced release of melatonin. *Eur. J. Neurosci.* **14,** 419–425.

Mondal, M. S., Nakazato, M., Date, Y., Murakami, N., Yanagisawa, M., and Matsukura, S. (1999). Widespread distribution of orexin in rat brain and its regulation upon fasting. *Biochem. Biophys. Res. Commun.* **256,** 495–499.

Muraki, Y., Yamanaka, A., Tsujino, N., Kilduff, T. S., Goto, K., and Sakurai, T. (2004). Serotonergic regulation of the orexin/hypocretin neurons through the 5-HT1A receptor. *J. Neurosci.* **24,** 7159–7166.

Muroya, S., Funahashi, H., Yamanaka, A., Kohno, D., Uramura, K., Nambu, T., Shibahara, M., Kuramochi, M., Takigawa, M., Yanagisawa, M., Sakurai, T., Shioda, S., *et al.* (2004). Orexins (hypocretins) directly interact with neuropeptide Y, POMC and glucose-responsive neurons to regulate Ca^{2+} signaling in a reciprocal manner to leptin: Orexigenic neuronal pathways in the mediobasal hypothalamus. *Eur. J. Neurosci.* **19,** 1524–1534.

Nakamura, A., Zhang, W., Yanagisawa, M., Fukuda, Y., and Kuwaki, T. (2007). Vigilance state-dependent attenuation of hypercapnic chemoreflex and exaggerated sleep apnea in orexin knockout mice. *J. Appl. Physiol.* **102,** 241–248.

Nakamura, T., Uramura, K., Nambu, T., Yada, T., Goto, K., Yanagisawa, M., and Sakurai, T. (2000). Orexin-induced hyperlocomotion and stereotypy are mediated by the dopaminergic system. *Brain Res.* **873,** 181–187.

Nambu, T., Sakurai, T., Mizukami, K., Hosoya, Y., Yanagisawa, M., and Goto, K. (1999). Distribution of orexin neurons in the adult rat brain. *Brain Res.* **827,** 243–260.

Nanmoku, T., Isobe, K., Sakurai, T., Yamanaka, A., Takekoshi, K., Kawakami, Y., Goto, K., and Nakai, T. (2002). Effects of orexin on cultured porcine adrenal medullary and cortex cells. *Regul. Pept.* **104,** 125–130.

Narita, M., Nagumo, Y., Hashimoto, S., Narita, M., Khotib, J., Miyatake, M., Sakurai, T., Yanagisawa, M., Nakamachi, T., Shioda, S., and Suzuki, T. (2006). Direct involvement of orexinergic systems in the activation of the mesolimbic dopamine pathway and related behaviors induced by morphine. *J. Neurosci.* **26,** 398–405.

Näslund, E., Ehrström, M., Ma, J., Hellström, P. M., and Kirchgessner, A. L. (2002). Localization and effects of orexin on fasting motility in the rat duodenum. *Am. J. Physiol.* **282,** G470–G479.

Nowak, K. W., Mackowiak, P., Switonska, M. M., Fabis, M., and Malendowicz, L. K. (1999). Acute orexin effects on insulin secretion in the rat: *In vivo* and *in vitro* studies. *Life Sci.* **66,** 449–454.

Okumura, T., Takeuchi, S., Motomura, W., Yamada, H., Egashira, S.-i., Asahi, S., Kanatani, A., Ihara, M., and Kohgo, Y. (2001). Requirement of intact disulfide bonds in orexin-A-induced stimulation of gastric acid secretion that is mediated by OX1 receptor activation. *Biochem. Biophys. Res. Commun.* **280,** 976–981.

Peyron, C., Faraco, J., Rogers, W., Ripley, B., Overeem, S., Charnay, Y., Nevsimalova, S., Aldrich, M., Reynolds, D., Albin, R., Li, R., Hungs, M., *et al.* (2000). A mutation in a case of early onset narcolepsy and a generalized absence of hypocretin peptides in human narcoleptic brains. *Nat. Med.* **6,** 991–997.

Peyron, C., Tighe, D. K., van den Pol, A. N., de Lecea, L., Heller, H. C., Sutcliffe, J. G., and Kilduff, T. S. (1998). Neurons containing hypocretin (orexin) project to multiple neuronal systems. *J. Neurosci.* **18,** 9996–10015.

Randeva, H. S., Karteris, E., Grammatopoulos, D., and Hillhouse, E. W. (2001). Expression of orexin-A and functional orexin type 2 receptors in the human adult adrenals: Implications for adrenal function and energy homeostasis. *J. Clin. Endocrinol. Metab.* **86,** 4808–4813.

Ripley, B., Fujiki, N., Okura, M., Mignot, E., and Nishino, S. (2001). Hypocretin levels in sporadic and familial cases of canine narcolepsy. *Neurobiol. Dis.* **8,** 525–534.

Rodgers, R. J., Halford, J. C. G., Nunes de Souza, R. L., Canto de Souza, A. L., Piper, D. C., Arch, J. R. S., Upton, N., Porter, R. A., Johns, A., and Blundell, J. E. (2001). SB-334867, a selective orexin-1 receptor antagonist, enhances behavioural satiety and blocks the hyperphagic effect of orexin-A in rats. *Eur. J. Neurosci.* **13,** 1444–1452.

Rosin, D. L., Chang, D. A., and Guyenet, P. G. (2006). Afferent and efferent connections of the rat retrotrapezoid nucleus. *J. Comp. Neurol.* **499,** 64–89.

Russell, S. H., Kim, M. S., Small, C. J., Abbott, C. R., Morgan, D. G. A., Taheri, S., Murphy, K. G., Todd, J. F., Ghatei, M. A., and Bloom, S. R. (2000). Central administration of orexin A suppresses basal and domperidone stimulated plasma prolactin. *J. Neuroendocrinol.* **12,** 1213–1218.

Sakurai, T. (2005). Reverse pharmacology of orexin: From an orphan GPCR to integrative physiology. *Regul. Pept.* **126,** 3–10.

Sakurai, T., Amemiya, A., Ishii, M., Matsuzaki, I., Chemelli, R. M., Tanaka, H., Williams, S. C., Richarson, J. A., Kozlowski, G. P., Wilson, S., Arch, J. R., Buckingham, R. E., *et al.* (1998). Orexins and orexin receptors: A family of hypothalamic neuropeptides and G protein-coupled receptors that regulate feeding behavior. *Cell* **92,** 573–585.

Sakurai, T., Moriguchi, T., Furuya, K., Kajiwara, N., Nakamura, T., Yanagisawa, M., and Goto, K. (1999). Structure and function of human prepro-orexin gene. *J. Biol. Chem.* **274,** 17771–17776.

Sakurai, T., Nagata, R., Yamanaka, A., Kawamura, H., Tsujino, N., Muraki, Y., Kageyama, H., Kunita, S., Takahashi, S., Goto, K., Koyama, Y., Shioda, S., *et al.* (2005). Input of orexin/hypocretin neurons revealed by a genetically encoded tracer in mice. *Neuron* **46,** 297–308.

Samson, W. K., Gosnell, B., Chang, J. K., Resch, Z. T., and Murphy, T. C. (1999). Cardiovascular regulatory actions of the hypocretins in brain. *Brain Res.* **831,** 248–253.

Shahid, I. Z., Rahman, A. A., and Pilowsky, P. M. (2011). Intrathecal orexin A increases sympathetic outflow and respiratory drive, enhances baroreflex sensitivity and blocks the somato-sympathetic reflex. *Br. J. Pharmacol.* **162,** 961–973.

Shahid, I. Z., Rahman, A. A., and Pilowsky, P. M. (2012). Orexin A in rat rostral ventrolateral medulla is pressor, sympathoexcitatory, increases barosensitivity and attenuates the somatosympathetic reflex. *Br. J. Pharmacol.* **165,** 2292–2303.

Sherin, J. E., Elmquist, J. K., Torrealba, F., and Saper, C. B. (1998). Innervation of histaminergic tuberomammillary neurons by GABAergic and galaninergic neurons in the ventrolateral preoptic nucleus of the rat. *J. Neurosci.* **18,** 4705–4721.

Shibahara, M., Sakurai, T., Nambu, T., Takenouchi, T., Iwaasa, H., Egashira, S.-I., Ihara, M., and Goto, K. (1999). Structure, tissue distribution, and pharmacological characterization of Xenopus orexins. *Peptides* **20,** 1169–1176.

Shih, C. D., and Chuang, Y. C. (2007). Nitric oxide and GABA mediate bi-directional cardiovascular effects of orexin in the nucleus tractus solitarii of rats. *Neuroscience* **149,** 625–635.

Shirasaka, T., Nakazato, M., Matsukura, S., Takasaki, M., and Kannan, H. (1999). Sympathetic and cardiovascular actions of orexins in conscious rats. *Am. J. Physiol.* **277,** R1780–R1785.

Smart, D., Jerman, J. C., Brough, S. J., Neville, W. A., Jewitt, F., and Porter, R. A. (2000). The hypocretins are weak agonists at recombinant human orexin-1 and orexin-2 receptors. *Br. J. Pharmacol.* **129,** 1289–1291.

Smart, D., Jerman, J. C., Brough, S. J., Rushton, S. L., Murdock, P. R., Jewitt, F., Elshourbagy, N. A., Ellis, C. E., Middlemiss, D. N., and Brown, F. (1999). Characterization of recombinant human orexin receptor pharmacology in a Chinese hamster ovary cell-line using FLIPR. *Br. J. Pharmacol.* **128,** 1–3.

Smith, P. M., Connolly, B. C., and Ferguson, A. V. (2002). Microinjection of orexin into the rat nucleus tractus solitarius causes increases in blood pressure. *Brain Res.* **950,** 261–267.

Stornetta, R. L., Spirovski, D., Moreira, T. S., Takakura, A. C., West, G. H., Gwilt, J. M., Pilowsky, P. M., and Guyenet, P. G. (2009). Galanin is a selective marker of the retrotrapezoid nucleus in rats. *J. Comp. Neurol.* **512,** 373–383.

Sunanaga, J., Deng, B. S., Zhang, W., Kanmura, Y., and Kuwaki, T. (2009). CO_2 activates orexin-containing neurons in mice. *Respir. Physiol. Neurobiol.* **166,** 184–186.

Sunter, D., Morgan, I., Edwards, C. M. B., Dakin, C. L., Murphy, K. G., Gardiner, J., Taheri, S., Rayes, E., and Bloom, S. R. (2001). Orexins: Effects on behavior and localisation of orexin receptor 2 messenger ribonucleic acid in the rat brainstem. *Brain Res.* **907,** 27–34.

Sutcliffe, J. G., and De Lecea, L. (2000). The hypocretins: Excitatory neuromodulatory peptides for multiple homeostatic systems, including sleep and feeding. *J. Neurosci. Res.* **62,** 161–168.

Thannickal, T. C., Moore, R. Y., Nienhuis, R., Ramanathan, L., Gulyani, S., Aldrich, M., Cornford, M., and Siegel, J. M. (2000). Reduced number of hypocretin neurons in human narcolepsy. *Neuron* **27,** 469–474.

Thorpe, A. J., and Kotz, C. M. (2005). Orexin A in the nucleus accumbens stimulates feeding and locomotor activity. *Brain Res.* **1050,** 156–162.

Toyama, S., Sakurai, T., Tatsumi, K., and Kuwaki, T. (2009). Attenuated phrenic long-term facilitation in orexin neuron-ablated mice. *Respir. Physiol. Neurobiol.* **168,** 295–302.

Trivedi, P., Yu, H., MacNeil, D. J., Van Der Ploeg, L. H. T., and Guan, X. M. (1998). Distribution of orexin receptor mRNA in the rat brain. *FEBS Lett.* **438,** 71–75.

Tsujino, N., Yamanaka, A., Ichiki, K., Muraki, Y., Kilduff, T. S., Yagami, K.-i., Takahashi, S., Goto, K., and Sakurai, T. (2005). Cholecystokinin activates orexin/hypocretin neurons through the cholecystokinin a receptor. *J. Neurosci.* **25,** 7459–7469.

van den Pol, A. N. (1999). Hypothalamic hypocretin (orexin): Robust innervation of the spinal cord. *J. Neurosci.* **19,** 3171–3182.

van den Pol, A. N., Gao, X.-B., Obrietan, K., Kilduff, T. S., and Belousov, A. B. (1998). Presynaptic and postsynaptic actions and modulation of neuroendocrine neurons by a new hypothalamic peptide, hypocretin/orexin. *J. Neurosci.* **18,** 7962–7971.

van den Top, M., Lee, K., Whyment, A. D., Blanks, A. M., and Spanswick, D. (2004). Orexigen-sensitive NPY/AgRP pacemaker neurons in the hypothalamic arcuate nucleus. *Nat. Neurosci.* **7,** 493–494.

van den Top, M., Nolan, M. F., Lee, K., Richardson, P. J., Buijs, R. M., Davies, C. H., and Spanswick, D. (2003). Orexins induce increased excitability and synchronisation of rat sympathetic preganglionic neurones. *J. Physiol.* **549,** 809–821.

Vanni-Mercier, G., Sakai, K., and Jouvet, M. (1984). 'Waking-state specific' neurons in the caudal hypothalamus of the cat. *C. R. Acad. Sci. III* **298,** 195–200.

Volgin, D. V., Saghir, M., and Kubin, L. (2002). Developmental changes in the orexin 2 receptor mRNA in hypoglossal motoneurons. *Neuroreport* **13,** 433–436.

Williams, R.a.H., Jensen, L. T., Verkhratsky, A., Fugger, L., and Burdakov, D. (2007). Control of hypothalamic orexin neurons by acid and CO_2. *Proc. Natl. Acad. Sci. U.S.A.* **104,** 10685–10690.

Willie, J. T., Chemelli, R. M., Sinton, C. M., Tokita, S., Williams, S. C., Kisanuki, Y. Y., Marcus, J. N., Lee, C., Elmquist, J. K., Kohlmeier, K. A., Leonard, C. S., Richardson, J. A., *et al.* (2003). Distinct narcolepsy syndromes in orexin receptor-2 and orexin null mice: Molecular genetic dissection of non-REM and REM sleep regulatory processes. *Neuron* **38,** 715–730.

Willie, J. T., Chemelli, R. M., Sinton, C. M., and Yanagisawa, M. (2001). To eat or to sleep? Orexin in the regulation of feeding and wakefulness. *Annu. Rev. Neurosci.* **24,** 429–458.

Winsky-Sommerer, R.l., Yamanaka, A., Diano, S., Borok, E., Roberts, A. J., Sakurai, T., Kilduff, T. S., Horvath, T. L., and de Lecea, L. (2004). Interaction between the corticotropin-releasing factor system and hypocretins (orexins): A novel circuit mediating stress response. *J. Neurosci.* **24,** 11439–11448.

Xie, X., Crowder, T. L., Yamanaka, A., Morairty, S. R., LeWinter, R. D., Sakurai, T., and Kilduff, T. S. (2006). $GABA_B$ receptor-mediated modulation of hypocretin/orexin neurones in mouse hypothalamus. *J. Physiol.* **574,** 399–414.

Yamada, H., Okumura, T., Motomura, W., Kobayashi, Y., and Kohgo, Y. (2000). Inhibition of food intake by central injection of anti-orexin antibody in fasted rats. *Biochem. Biophys. Res. Commun.* **267,** 527–531.

Yamanaka, A., Beuckmann, C. T., Willie, J. T., Hara, J., Tsujino, N., Mieda, M., Tominaga, M., Yagami, K.-i., Sugiyama, F., Goto, K., Yanagisawa, M., and Sakurai, T. (2003a). Hypothalamic orexin neurons regulate arousal according to energy balance in mice. *Neuron* **38,** 701–713.

Yamanaka, A., Kunii, K., Nambu, T., Tsujino, N., Sakai, A., Matsuzaki, I., Miwa, Y., Katsutoshi, G., and Sakurai, T. (2000). Orexin-induced food intake involves neuropeptide Y pathway. *Brain Res.* **859,** 404–409.

Yamanaka, A., Muraki, Y., Ichiki, K., Tsujino, N., Kilduff, T. S., Goto, K., and Sakurai, T. (2006). Orexin neurons are directly and indirectly regulated by catecholamines in a complex manner. *J. Neurophysiol.* **96,** 284–298.

Yamanaka, A., Muraki, Y., Tsujino, N., Goto, K., and Sakurai, T. (2003b). Regulation of orexin neurons by the monoaminergic and cholinergic systems. *Biochem. Biophys. Res. Commun.* **303,** 120–129.

Yamanaka, A., Tsujino, N., Funahashi, H., Honda, K., Guan, J.-l., Wang, Q.-P., Tominaga, M., Goto, K., Shioda, S., and Sakurai, T. (2002). Orexins activate histaminergic neurons via the orexin 2 receptor. *Biochem. Biophys. Res. Commun.* **290,** 1237–1245.

Yang, Z.-J., Meguid, M. M., Chai, J.-K., Chen, C., and Oler, A. (1997). Bilateral hypothalamic dopamine infusion in male zucker rat suppresses feeding due to reduced meal size. *Pharmacol. Biochem. Behav.* **58,** 631–635.

Yoshida, K., McCormack, S., España, R. A., Crocker, A., and Scammell, T. E. (2006). Afferents to the orexin neurons of the rat brain. *J. Comp. Neurol.* **494,** 845–861.
Young, J. K., Wu, M., Manaye, K. F., Kc, P., Allard, J. S., Mack, S. O., and Haxhiu, M. A. (2005). Orexin stimulates breathing via medullary and spinal pathways. *J. Appl. Physiol.* **98,** 1387–1395.
Zhang, W., Fukuda, Y., and Kuwaki, T. (2005). Respiratory and cardiovascular actions of orexin-A in mice. *Neurosci. Lett.* **385,** 131–136.

CHAPTER TEN

Hypocretin/Orexin Involvement in Reward and Reinforcement

Rodrigo A. España

Contents

Abstract

Since the discovery of the hypocretins/orexins, a series of observations have indicated that these peptides influence a variety of physiological processes including feeding, sleep/wake function, memory, and stress. More recently, the hypocretins have been implicated in reinforcement and reward-related processes via actions on the mesolimbic dopamine system. Although investigation into the relationship between the hypocretins and reinforcement/reward remains in relatively early stages, accumulating evidence suggests that

Department of Neurobiology and Anatomy, Drexel University College of Medicine, Philadelphia, Pennsylvania, USA

Vitamins and Hormones, Volume 89
ISSN 0083-6729, http://dx.doi.org/10.1016/B978-0-12-394623-2.00010-X

continued research into this area may offer new insights into the addiction process and provide the foundation to generate novel pharmacotherapies for drug abuse. The current chapter will focus on contemporary perspectives of hypocretin regulation of cocaine reward and reinforcement via actions on the mesolimbic dopamine system.

I. Introduction

A. Hypocretin peptide and receptors

The hypocretins (also termed orexins) were discovered in 1998 by two independent research groups (de Lecea *et al.*, 1998; Sakurai *et al.*, 1998) and consist of the hypocretin 1 and hypocretin 2 peptides which are also known as orexin A and B. These peptides are synthesized solely within a restricted portion of the lateral and posterior hypothalamus and perifornical areas (Chemelli *et al.*, 1999; Date *et al.*, 1999; de Lecea *et al.*, 1998; Peyron *et al.*, 1998; Sakurai *et al.*, 1998). While the hypocretin neurons are confined to a relatively circumscribed region, immunohistochemical studies demonstrate widespread projections of these neurons throughout the brain, suggesting varied actions of these peptides (Date *et al.*, 1999; Nambu *et al.*, 1999; Peyron *et al.*, 1998; van Den Pol, 1999).

To date, two G-protein-coupled hypocretin receptor subtypes have been identified. The hypocretin 1 receptor preferentially binds the hypocretin 1 peptide, whereas the hypocretin 2 receptor binds both hypocretin 1 and 2 peptides with equiaffinity (Sakurai *et al.*, 1998). Both the hypocretin 1 and 2 receptors are expressed widely throughout the brain with slight, yet sometimes notable, variations in distribution (Backberg *et al.*, 2002; Bourgin *et al.*, 2000; Cluderay *et al.*, 2002; Greco and Shiromani, 2001; Hervieu *et al.*, 2001; Marcus *et al.*, 2001; Suzuki *et al.*, 2002; Trivedi *et al.*, 1998). For example, hypocretin 1 receptors are observed throughout the cortex, hippocampus, paraventricular thalamic, ventromedial hypothalamic, and arcuate nuclei, as well as the dorsal raphe, locus coeruleus, substantia nigra (SN), and ventral tegmental area (VTA). In contrast, hypocretin 2 receptors are observed in the cortex, septal nuclei, hippocampus, medial thalamic groups, the dorsal and median raphe nuclei, tuberomammillary nucleus, dorsomedial and paraventricular hypothalamic nuclei, SN, and VTA (Backberg *et al.*, 2002; Bourgin *et al.*, 2000; Cluderay *et al.*, 2002; Greco and Shiromani, 2001; Hervieu *et al.*, 2001; Marcus *et al.*, 2001; Suzuki *et al.*, 2002; Trivedi *et al.*, 1998).

Although extensive evidence demonstrates that the lateral hypothalamus receives inputs from much of the central nervous system, only few advances have been made in elucidating the afferent inputs to the hypocretin neurons. Nevertheless, these studies have proven to be valuable at demonstrating that hypocretin neuronal activity is likely influenced by a diverse set of functionally distinct neural structures. For example, studies using classic retrograde and anterograde tracing methods, as well as more novel molecular techniques, demonstrate that hypocretin neurons are innervated by monoaminergic regions such as the dorsal raphe, VTA, and locus coeruleus (Abrahamson *et al.*, 2001; Fadel and Deutch, 2002; Horvath *et al.*, 1999; Sakurai *et al.*, 2005; Yoshida *et al.*, 2006). Although it is generally unclear as to whether these inputs exert excitatory or inhibitory actions, it is evident that hypocretin neurons receive signals from regions that govern motivation, homeostatic drive, behavioral state, and autonomic tone. Thus, the hypocretin neurons are poised to regulate a variety of neural functions.

B. Hypocretin regulates arousal and arousal-related behavioral activity

Despite initial connections between hypocretins and feeding, substantial research now suggests that the hypocretin system plays a critical role in the regulation of arousal, including processes involved in governing sleep and waking. For example, hypocretin neurons are preferentially active during periods of alert waking, novelty, and behavioral arousal and are responsive to wake-promoting drugs (España *et al.*, 2003; Estabrooke *et al.*, 2001; Lee *et al.*, 2005; Mileykovskiy *et al.*, 2005). Further, hypocretin-immunoreactive fibers and hypocretin receptors are located within many arousal-related structures including the noradrenergic, serotonergic, histaminergic, and dopaminergic systems (Brown *et al.*, 2001; Fadel and Deutch, 2002; Hagan *et al.*, 1999; Horvath *et al.*, 1999). Consistent with this, hypocretin levels fluctuate across the day/night cycle with the highest levels observed during the dark-phase when rats are typically awake (Yoshida *et al.*, 2001). Further, intracerebroventricular (i.c.v.) infusions of hypocretin 1 or hypocretin 2 dose-dependently increase waking and suppress sleep and elicit behaviors typical of spontaneous waking and/or high arousal conditions, including those associated with motivated states (España *et al.*, 2001, 2002; Hagan *et al.*, 1999; Ida *et al.*, 1999; Piper *et al.*, 2000). Similar wake-promoting and behavioral-activating effects are also observed when hypocretin 1 is focally delivered to the VTA, locus coeruleus, basal forebrain, and other arousal-related regions (Bourgin *et al.*, 2000; España *et al.*, 2001; Hagan *et al.*, 1999; Vittoz and Berridge, 2006).

Additional evidence for hypocretin involvement in arousal processes comes from clinical and animal studies indicating an important link between dysregulation of hypocretin neurotransmission and the sleep/arousal disorder narcolepsy. Numerous studies using people with narcolepsy have demonstrated that these patients have reduced circulating levels of hypocretin in their cerebrospinal fluid and commonly display a degenerative loss of hypocretin neurons (Blouin *et al.*, 2005; Crocker *et al.*, 2005; Nishino *et al.*, 2000; Peyron *et al.*, 2000; Ripley *et al.*, 2001; Thannickal *et al.*, 2000). Additionally, researchers have detected a genetic defect in the hypocretin 2 receptor gene in a longstanding dog model of narcolepsy (Lin *et al.*, 1999). Like people with narcolepsy, these dogs experience symptoms of excessive daytime sleepiness and cataplexy. Finally, in a mouse model of narcolepsy, hypocretin ligand and hypocretin receptor knockout (KO) mice, as well as transgenic mice with a degenerative loss of hypocretin neurons, also display a phenotype similar to that of human narcolepsy (Chemelli *et al.*, 1999; Hara *et al.*, 2001; Kisanuki *et al.*, 2000). Interestingly, hypocretin ligand KO mice have also been shown to display deficits in reward/reinforcement processes as well as dopamine signaling indicating reduced responsivity to drugs of abuse (see Section II.B and III.B). This is particularly notable given that people with narcolepsy rarely develop addiction, despite treatment with pychostimulant drugs such as amphetamine (Akimoto *et al.*, 1960; Hayduk *et al.*, 1995; Rogers *et al.*, 1997, 2001).

C. Summary

Both basic and clinical research indicate that the hypocretins participate in the regulation of arousal and arousal-related processes via a widespread projection system that acts upon multiple terminal fields. Given that arousal is a critical factor in the accurate expression of all motivated behaviors, these observations have important implications for potential involvement of hypocretin systems on a broad constellation of physiological functions including those associated with drug reward and reinforcement.

II. Hypocretin Regulation of Reward and Reinforcement Processes

An amassing literature indicates that the hypocretin system participates in reward processes and motivated behaviors associated with cocaine. Some of the first evidence to support this emerged from anatomical studies showing prominent hypocretin projections to reward-related brain structures including the VTA and nucleus accumbens (Fadel and Deutch, 2002; Peyron *et al.*, 1998). Additional work also demonstrated that dopamine neurons of the VTA contain both hypocretin 1 and hypocretin 2 receptors and that hypocretins exert excitatory actions on these neurons (Borgland *et al.*, 2006; Korotkova *et al.*, 2003). Given these observations, it is not surprising that multiple reports have focused on the extent to which the hypocretin system influences behavioral and dopamine responses to cocaine and other drugs of abuse.

A. Drugs of abuse recruit the activity of hypocretin neurons

In a series of studies from multiple research groups, it was demonstrated that experience with drugs of abuse results in the activation of hypocretin-producing neurons. For example, acute injections of methamphetamine or nicotine (Ko *et al.*, 2003; Pasumarthi *et al.*, 2006) increased Fos immunoreactivity in hypocretin neurons to over 300% of vehicle-treatment levels. Additionally, chronic nicotine produced an increase of hypocretin mRNA levels, as well as mRNA levels of both hypocretin 1 and 2 receptors (Kane *et al.*, 2000). Discontinuation of chronic drug delivery and subsequent withdrawal can also elicit activation of hypocretin neurons. Indeed, naloxone-induced withdrawal from chronic morphine treatment increases Fos levels of hypocretin peptide mRNA in hypocretin neurons and also increases Fos in the NAc shell (Georgescu *et al.*, 2003; Sharf *et al.*, 2008; Zhou *et al.*, 2006). Interestingly, it appears that hypocretin 1 receptors are important in these actions given that the hypocretin 1 receptor antagonist, SB-334867, reduces the effects of morphine withdrawal on Fos levels in the NAc shell and attenuates symptoms of morphine withdrawal (Sharf *et al.*, 2008). In addition, hypocretin neurons show increased Fos when animals are exposed to cues that once predicted ethanol availability (Dayas *et al.*, 2008).

B. Conditioned place preference

The previous observations suggest that administration of various drugs of abuse appears to engage hypocretin neuronal activity, however, it is possible that the increase in Fos observed with these drugs may be associated with generalized enhancement of arousal, and not with more direct actions on reward mechanisms. Despite this possibility, two studies suggest that this may not be the case for conditioned place preference (CPP) for cocaine or morphine. In those studies, Harris and colleagues demonstrate that the increases in Fos are observed only in animals that developed CPP for morphine or cocaine but not in those that were treated with drug, yet failed to acquire CPP (Harris and Aston-Jones, 2006; Harris *et al.*, 2005). Thus, rats that acquired cocaine or morphine CPP had threefold greater numbers of Fos-positive hypocretin neurons than naïve animals. Animals that were treated with these drugs but did not acquire CPP showed levels of Fos comparable to naïve rats. Interestingly, the degree of Fos activation was also shown to be proportional to the magnitude of CPP induced by chemical activation of hypocretin neurons, further suggesting that the activity of these neurons is associated with the rewarding aspects of these drugs. Consistent with these observations, hypocretin signaling has also been shown to be necessary for reinstatement of CPP. For example, in animals that had been extinguished of morphine CPP behavior, activation of hypocretin neurons or hypocretin 1 injections into the VTA reinstated CPP (Harris *et al.*, 2005).

The importance of hypocretin 1 receptors in reward processes is again highlighted in a series of CPP experiments using SB-334867. Systemic pretreatment with SB-334867 blocks CPP for morphine (Harris *et al.*, 2005) as well as CPP for amphetamine (Hutcheson *et al.*, 2011). Additionally, infusions of SB-334967 into the VTA block morphine CPP (Narita *et al.*, 2006; Sharf *et al.*, 2010), as do unilateral lesions of the lateral hypothalamus combined with contralateral SB-33467 infusions into the VTA (Harris *et al.*, 2007). Surprisingly, while systemic administration of SB-334867 is capable of blocking CPP for morphine (Harris *et al.*, 2005; Sharf *et al.*, 2010) it does not appear to affect CPP for cocaine (Sharf *et et al.*, 2010).

As mentioned above, people with narcolepsy and presumably reduced hypocretin signaling, rarely develop addiction. In this light, it is noteworthy that mice lacking hypocretin peptides show multiple deficits in their responsivity to drugs of abuse. For example, hypocretin KO mice have been shown to be less susceptible than wild types (WT) in developing morphine dependence (Georgescu *et al.*, 2003), they display reduced locomotor and dopamine responses to morphine, and they do not develop CPP for morphine (Narita *et al.*, 2006; Sharf *et al.*, 2010). Recently, we have shown that hypocretin KO mice are also less sensitive to the rewarding properties of cocaine as these mice fail to exhibit CPP for cocaine (España and Jones, 2010). In those studies, and consistent with an extensive literature, WT mice exhibited robust CPP for cocaine, however, hypocretin KO mice showed a nonsignificant trend toward conditioned place aversion. When taken together, these observations suggest that hypocretin signaling is important for CPP behavior associated with cocaine and other drugs and thus normal levels of hypocretins may be a critical participant in regulating the rewarding properties of drugs of abuse.

C. Self-administration

Multiple paradigms are used to examine drug-seeking and drug-taking in rodents. However, intravenous (i.v.) self-administration of drugs is generally accepted as the gold standard for modeling drug abuse. These techniques can be used to model different aspects of drug-taking, including the acquisition and maintenance phases of drug intake as well as the propensity to relapse by measuring reinstatement of operant drug-seeking behavior following a period of forced abstinence. Additionally, researchers often vary the schedules of reinforcement to examine specific aspects of cocaine intake, including drug consumption, diurnal variations in cocaine intake, and the motivation to work for cocaine. The section that follows will provide a summary of recent observations indicating a prominent role for the hypocretin system in self-administration of cocaine and other drugs of abuse.

D. Reinstatement

Reinstatement of drug-seeking behavior is a useful method to assess the persistence of lever pressing when the drug is no longer available. Rats are typically trained to self-administer drugs until stable levels of responding are reached and rats are subsequently exposed to extinction sessions. During extinction, rats quickly learn that drug is no longer available and consequently they cease responding on the lever. Once lever responding is extinguished, rats are presented with a cue associated with cocaine intake, or alternatively, they are exposed to a stressor (e.g., foot shock), which leads to reinstatement of drug-seeking.

Several observations indicate that hypocretin signaling is crucial for normal reinstatement of drug-seeking. For example, i.c.v. infusions of hypocretin 1 are sufficient to reinstate cocaine and nicotine seeking (Boutrel *et al.*, 2005; Plaza-Zabala *et al.*, 2010; Volkow *et al.*, 2009). Consistent with this, SB-334967 reduces cue-induced reinstatement of ethanol and cocaine seeking (Lawrence *et al.*, 2006; Smith *et al.*, 2009) and reinstatement of cocaine-seeking following foot shock and yohimbine-induced stress (Boutrel *et al.*, 2005; Richards *et al.*, 2008). Interestingly, cocaine-primed reinstatement is not attenuated with SB-334867 treatment (Smith *et al.*, 2009), although the mechanisms underlying this difference are not clear. When considered together, these observations indicate that the motivation to seek drug after extinction can be influenced by hypocretin signaling, depending on the parameters used to elicit drug-seeking.

E. Maintenance

The involvement of hypocretins in regulating the reinforcing actions of drugs have been investigated across a battery of self-administration schedules of reinforcement and results have shown varied effects depending on the paradigms used. Initially, observations examining the extent to which the hypocretin system influences ongoing cocaine self-administration suggested that blocking hypocretin signaling had no effect on the maintenance of cocaine intake. In these studies, rats were implanted with a catheter into the right jugular vein and were trained to self-administer cocaine on a fixed ratio 1 (FR1) schedule of reinforcement in which a single lever press resulted in delivery of a relatively large dose of cocaine (Aston-Jones *et al.*, 2009; España *et al.*, 2010). Under these conditions, rats are able to attain preferred blood levels of cocaine with little effort, and thus rats can readily maintain those levels throughout a session. Consequently, responding on an FR1 schedule provides information about an animal's preferred level of cocaine consumption. After reaching stable patterns of cocaine intake, rats were pretreated with either vehicle or SB-334867 and cocaine intake was measured. As previously described (Aston-Jones *et al.*, 2009;

España *et al.*, 2010), treatment with SB-334867 had no effect on cocaine consumption. A similar lack of effect on an FR1 schedule was also observed, when rats were infused with the hypocretin 1 directly into the lateral ventricles (Boutrel *et al.*, 2005; España *et al.*, 2011). Although these data suggested that active cocaine self-administration was not affected by hypocretin signaling, subsequent findings using different schedules of reinforcement with varying availability levels or effort requirements demonstrated significant effects of hypocretin manipulations on self-administration of cocaine and other drugs of abuse.

In a series of studies, we tested the effects of hypocretin manipulations across a battery of self-administration schedules. Using a 24 h access, discrete trials (DT) schedule of reinforcement, rats were kept from maximizing their blood levels of cocaine by restricting cocaine access to three trials per hour. This degree of cocaine access engenders a characteristic pattern of intake in which animals engage in cocaine intake almost exclusively during the dark-phase (Roberts *et al.*, 2002). Although the effort requirement is low in a DT paradigm (one lever response results in cocaine delivery), the complex interaction between dose and availability makes this schedule more susceptible to pharmacological and physiological influences than schedules with less restricted access. As shown in Fig. 10.1, injections of SB-334867 produce a marked reduction of cocaine intake that occurred within 20 min of SB-334867 treatment, particularly in rats treated with the highest dose of SB-334867 (España *et al.*, 2010). In contrast, i.c.v. infusions of hypocretin 1 increased cocaine intake, thereby extending periods of cocaine intake (España *et al.*, 2011). These effects of hypocretin manipulations are similar to other drugs that selectively reduce intake under DT, but not FR1 schedules (Brebner *et al.*, 2000; Smith *et al.*, 2004).

The progressive ratio (PR) schedule of reinforcement is designed to assess an animal's motivation to work for a reinforcer and provides information on changes in the reinforcing efficacy of drugs. During the early portions of a PR session, single cocaine injections are obtained with relatively low effort (few lever responses). However, as the session continues, the lever response requirement increases and thus rats must exert progressively greater effort to obtain a single cocaine injection. Using the PR schedule, we demonstrated that both intraperitoneal (i.p.) and bilateral intra-VTA injections of SB-334867 reduced the motivation for an animal to work for cocaine. Specifically, animals treated with SB-334867 engaged in significantly less lever pressing and reached lower breakpoints (fewer cocaine injections) than animals treated with vehicle (Fig. 10.2A). These effects are similar to recent reports showing that a 10 mg/kg i.p. dose of SB-334867 reduces PR responding for cocaine, as well as for nicotine and heroin (Borgland *et al.*, 2009; Hollander *et al.*, 2008; Smith and Aston-Jones, 2010). Consistent with these findings, enhancement of hypocretin signaling produces the opposite effect. Thus, as shown in Fig. 10.2B, bilateral infusions of the hypocretin 1

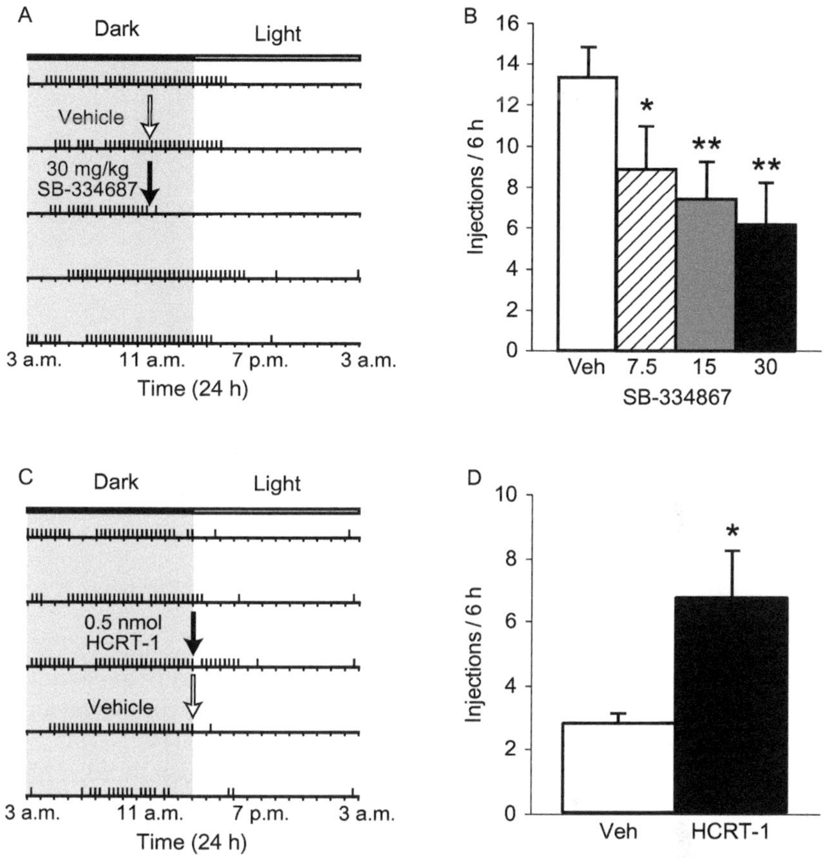

Figure 10.1 Hypocretin signaling regulates cocaine self-administration on a DT schedule of reinforcement. (A) Response pattern from an individual rat that received an i.p. vehicle (white arrow) or 30 mg/kg SB-334867 injection (black arrow). Horizontal rasters represent 24 h periods. Vertical tick marks represent trials in which a 1.5 mg/kg cocaine injection was taken. (B) The mean ± SEM number of cocaine injections taken over the 6-h period following i.p. injections of vehicle ($n=8$) or SB-334867 (7.5, 15, and 30 mg/kg; $n=8$). (C) A response pattern from an individual rat that received vehicle (white arrow) or 0.5 nmol hypocretin-1 (HCRT-1; black arrow) into the lateral ventricle. (D) The mean ± SEM number of cocaine injections taken over the 6-h period following infusion of vehicle ($n=7$) or 0.5 nmol hypocretin-1 ($n=7$). Note that for SB-334867 experiments, rats were treated at 11:00 a.m. when rats are typically awake, whereas for hypocretin-1 experiments, rats were treated at 3:00 p.m. a time when rats typically discontinue taking cocaine. *$P<0.05$, **$P<0.01$ relative to baseline.

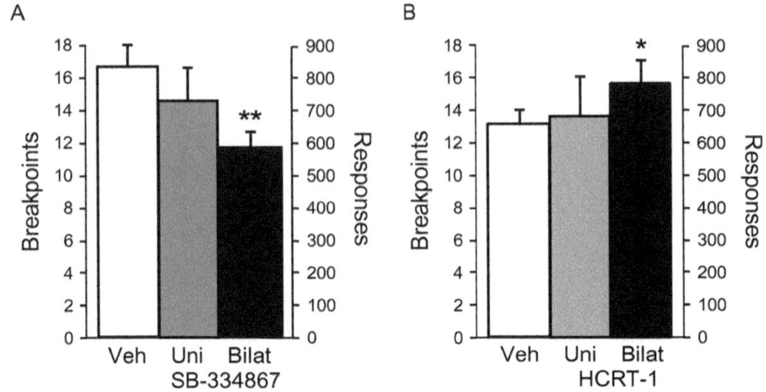

Figure 10.2 Hypocretin signaling within the VTA regulates cocaine self-administration on a PR schedule of reinforcement. (A) The mean ± SEM number of cocaine breakpoints and lever responses following unilateral or bilateral intra-VTA infusions of vehicle (uni, $n=5$; bilat, $n=6$) or 10 nmol SB-334867 (uni, $n=5$; bilat, $n=6$). (B) The mean ± SEM number of cocaine breakpoints and lever responses following unilateral or bilateral intra-VTA infusions of vehicle (uni, $n=5$; bilat, $n=6$) or 0.5 nmol hypocretin-1 (HCRT-1; uni, $n=5$; bilat, $n=6$). $^*P<0.05$, $^{**}P<0.01$ relative to baseline.

directly into the VTA elicit an increase in breakpoints and the number of lever responses, further indicating the importance of hypocretin signaling in cocaine reinforcement (España *et al.*, 2011).

Another self-administration procedure, termed the threshold schedule of reinforcement, has been used to examine both consumption and motivation within a single session (España *et al.*, 2010). In this procedure, lever responses during the early portion of the session result in high doses of cocaine, similar to that observed with an FR1 schedule. During this portion of the session, rats can readily titrate to preferred blood levels of cocaine, and thus it is not surprising that SB-334867 has no effect on cocaine intake under these conditions (Fig. 10.3A). However, as the dose of cocaine per injection is lowered across the session, rats are required to respond more frequently to maintain blood levels of cocaine. This is reminiscent of a PR schedule in which increasingly greater numbers of responses are required to obtain the same amount of drug. At this higher price of cocaine, injections of SB-334867 decrease responding earlier in the session (Fig. 10.3B).

F. Summary

Combined, the described self-administration studies indicate that hypocretin neurotransmission is necessary to support cocaine self-administration under schedules of reinforcement that require high effort or where titrating

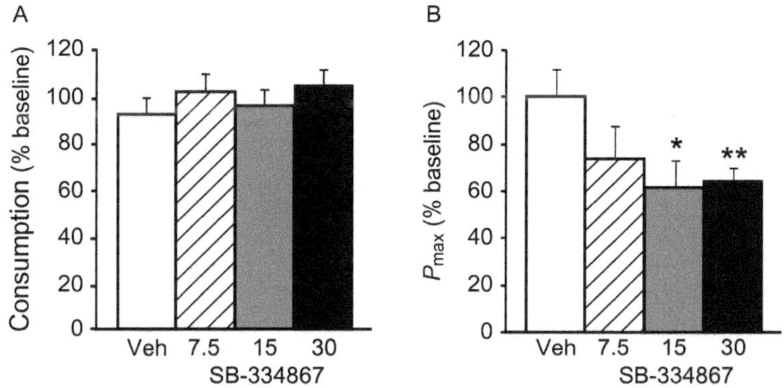

Figure 10.3 SB-334867 reduces responding as the unit price of cocaine is increased. (A) The mean ± SEM percent baseline consumption of cocaine following i.p. injection of vehicle ($n=9$) or SB-334867 (7.5, 15, or 30 mg/kg; $n=9$) on the threshold schedule of reinforcement. (B) The mean ± SEM P_{max} values, expressed as a percentage of baseline, following i.p. injections of vehicle or SB-334867. The maximal unit price, P_{max}, is defined as the point at which maximal responding occurs before an animal discontinues taking cocaine. P_{max} is a measure of the behavioral economic index of price. *$P<0.05$, **$P<0.01$ relative to vehicle.

to preferred blood levels of cocaine is restricted. Furthermore, given that intra-VTA SB-334867 and i.p. SB-334867 reduced cocaine intake to a similar extent, these observations provide strong support for the hypothesis that hypocretin influences cocaine reinforcement, via actions within the VTA.

III. Hypocretin Regulation of Dopamine Signaling

A series of studies using behavioral, genetic, electrophysiological, and neurochemical techniques have expanded our understanding of hypocretin involvement in arousal, particularly as it relates to the regulation of motivated behavior, reward/reinforcement processes, and the neural mechanisms underlying these actions. These studies have shown convincingly that enhancement of hypocretin neurotransmission promotes behavioral and neurochemical responses to drugs of abuse, while manipulations that disrupt hypocretin signaling attenuate these responses. Given that the present review involves a discussion of hypocretin regulation of dopamine function and motivated behaviors reliant on dopamine signaling, it is helpful to briefly review the importance of the mesolimbic dopamine system in the regulation of reward and reinforcement processes associated with cocaine.

A. Dopamine involvement in reward and reinforcement mechanisms

An extensive literature has demonstrated the importance of the mesolimbic projections from the VTA to the ventral striatum in reward and reinforcement processes associated with cocaine and other drugs of abuse (Koob and Le Moal, 1997; Wise, 1996; Woolverton and Johnson, 1992). Cocaine inhibits uptake of dopamine into the presynaptic terminal by blocking the dopamine transporter (DAT) and, through these actions, increases extracellular levels of dopamine and activation of pre- and postsynaptic dopamine receptors in VTA target regions (Fig. 10.4). It is generally believed that this enhancement of dopamine participates in cocaine's rewarding and reinforcing effects.

Pharmacological manipulations were among the first to suggest that enhanced dopamine signaling produced rewarding/reinforcing effects while attenuation of dopamine signaling leads to reduced reinforced behavior. For instance, various dopamine agonists produce CPP (Hoffman and Beninger,

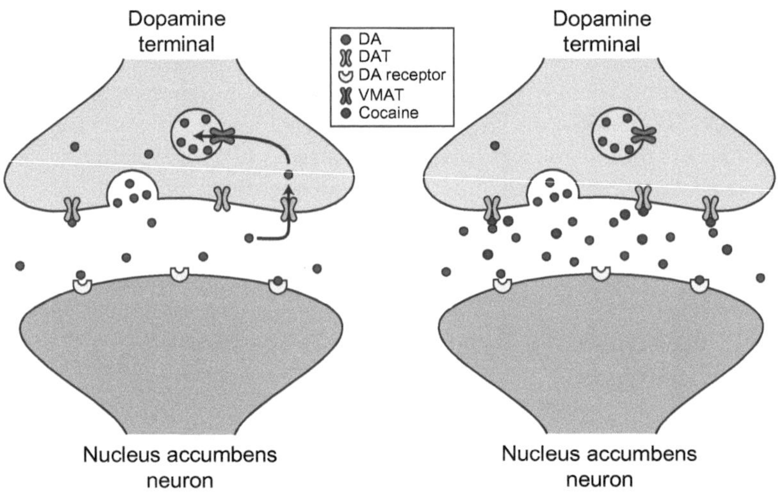

Figure 10.4 Effects of cocaine at the dopamine transporter. (Left) Under normal conditions, dopamine (DA) neuron firing results in dopamine-filled vesicles to fuse with the presynaptic membrane and subsequently release into the synaptic cleft. Once in the synapse, dopamine can bind to postsynaptic dopamine receptors and then is removed from extracellular space by the dopamine transporter (DAT). Once dopamine is back inside the presynaptic terminal, it is repackaged into synaptic vesicles for future release via the vesicular monoamine transporter (VMAT). (Right) Cocaine increases extracellular levels of dopamine by interacting with the DAT and thereby inhibiting dopamine uptake back into the terminal. As dopamine uptake is reduced, levels accumulate in the synapse and dopamine has a greater opportunity to bind to dopamine receptors. (See Color Insert.)

1988, 1989; Hoffman *et al.,* 1988; Papp, 1988; Parker, 1992; White *et al.,* 1991), are readily self-administered (Caine *et al.,* 1999; Self and Stein, 1992; Self *et al.,* 1996; Weed and Woolverton, 1995), and have cocaine-like discriminative stimulus effects (Sinnott and Nader, 2001; Sinnott *et al.,* 1999; Spealman *et al.,* 1991). In contrast, dopamine antagonists can produce conditioned place aversion (Acquas and Di Chiara, 1994; Cervo and Samanin, 1995; Funada and Shippenberg, 1996; Hoffman and Beninger, 1988, 1989; Shippenberg and Herz, 1987; Shippenberg *et al.,* 1991; White *et al.,* 1991), and attenuate cocaine self-administration (Caine and Koob, 1994).

Among the multiple limbic structures involved in dopamine regulation of reward and reinforcement, the NAc stands out as critical participant in psychostimulant self-administration. The vast majority of addictive drugs increase extracellular dopamine in the NAc (Carboni *et al.,* 1989; Di Chiara and Imperato, 1988; Imperato and Di Chiara, 1986) and NAc neurons display discrete discharge activity in response to cocaine-reinforced responding during self-administration (Carelli *et al.,* 1993; Uzwiak *et al.,* 1997). Additionally, lesions and pharmacological suppression of dopamine signaling within the NAc indicate that cocaine self-administration requires an intact NAc (Lyness *et al.,* 1979; McGregor and Roberts, 1995; Roberts *et al.,* 1977). These observations, among many others, support the hypothesis that the mesolimbic dopamine system, including the connection from the VTA to the NAc, is an essential participant in the reinforcing and behavioral effects of cocaine.

B. Hypocretin neurotransmission modulates dopamine responses to cocaine

As mentioned above, hypocretin neurons send relatively strong projections to the VTA where hypocretin fibers make synaptic contacts with dopamine neurons (Fadel and Deutch, 2002; Peyron *et al.,* 1998). Additionally, both hypocretin 1 and 2 induce burst firing of dopamine neurons and potentiate their glutamatergic-mediated excitation (Borgland *et al.,* 2006; Korotkova *et al.,* 2003), indicating that the hypocretin neurons are poised to regulate dopaminergic function. Given these observations and the general involvement of dopamine systems in regulating motivated behaviors associated with drugs of abuse, it is likely that hypocretin influences reinforcement processing via actions on mesolimbic dopamine systems.

Some of the first evidence that hypocretin systems participated in regulating dopamine responses to drugs of abuse came from studies investigating the pharmacological effects of hypocretin agents on dopamine signaling. Under baseline conditions, infusions of hypocretin 1 into the VTA were shown to increase extracellular levels of dopamine in the prefrontal cortex and NAc of rats (Narita *et al.,* 2006; Vittoz and Berridge, 2006; Vittoz *et al.,* 2008). Consistent with this, hypocretin KO mice show reduced dopamine responses to morphine, despite showing normal levels of extracellular dopamine under baseline conditions (Narita *et al.*, 2006). In recent microdialysis and voltammetry studies, we have also shown that hypocretins regulate dopamine signaling, particularly in response to cocaine. In the first set of studies, rats were implanted with microdialysis probes to measure extracellular dopamine levels in the NAc core. On testing days, rats were pretreated with i.p. vehicle or 30 mg/kg SB-334867, 40 min prior to receiving a single 10 mg/kg i.p. injection of cocaine. In rats treated with vehicle, injections of cocaine produced robust increases in extracellular dopamine levels (Fig. 10.5A). In contrast, the effects of cocaine in animals treated with SB-334867 were attenuated to nearly half of what was observed in vehicle

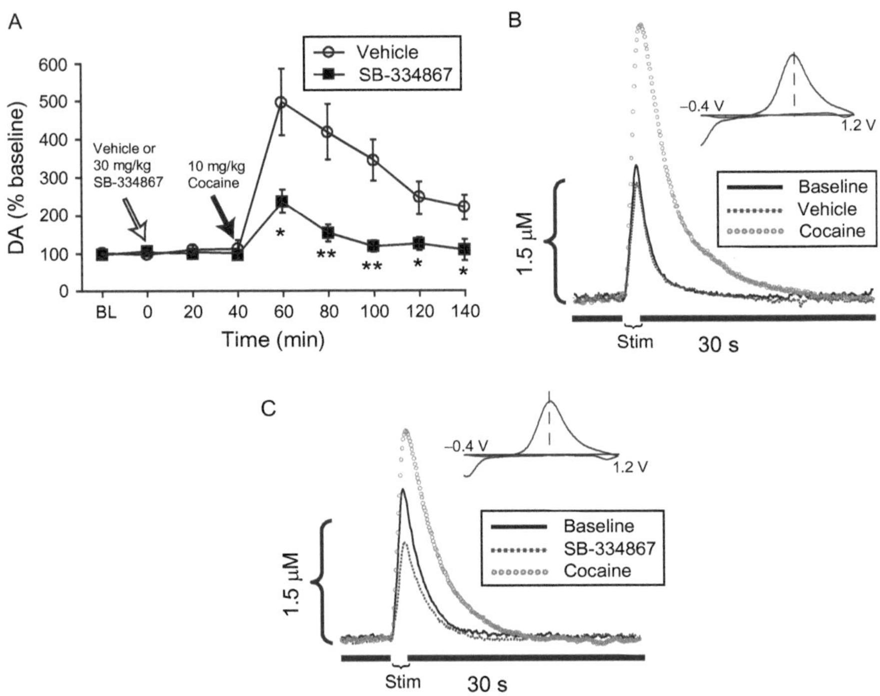

Figure 10.5 SB-334867 attenuates cocaine-induced elevations in dopamine signaling in the NAc core. (A) The mean ± SEM of extracellular levels of dopamine (DA) within the NAc core following i.p. injection of vehicle ($n=6$) or 30 mg/kg SB-334867 ($n=6$). Representative concentration–time plots and cyclic voltammograms (insets) of dopamine responses from rats that received pretreatment infusions of (B) vehicle or (C) 10 nmol SB-334867 into the VTA. Stim represents the time of electrical stimulation (1 s, 60 Hz pulse). (Insets in B and C) Cyclic voltammograms depict two current peaks, one at 600 mV (positive deflection) for dopamine oxidation and another at -200 mV (negative deflection) for reduction of dopamine-*o*-quinone. The position of the peaks identifies the substance as DA. $^{*}P<0.05$, $^{**}P<0.01$ relative to vehicle. (See Color Insert.)

controls (España *et al.,* 2010). In another set of experiments, animals were implanted with probes in the NAc and also with bilateral infusion cannulae in the VTA. Rats were pretreated with vehicle or SB-334867 (10 nmol) directly into the VTA and as before received a single i.p. injection of cocaine. Similar to that observed with i.p. injections, SB-334867 reduced the effects of cocaine on dopamine signaling. Interestingly, unlike that seen with i.p. delivery, SB-334867 into VTA also reduced baseline levels of dopamine prior to cocaine administration.

A similar set of results was also obtained in studies using voltammetry in anesthetized rats. Animals were implanted with an i.v. jugular catheter, a recording electrode in the NAc core, and an infusion cannula/stimulating electrode in the ipsilateral VTA. Following collection of a stable baseline of electrically stimulated dopamine release, rats received an infusion of vehicle or SB-334867 (10 nmol) directly into the VTA. Forty minutes later, rats received a single i.v. injection (1.5 mg/kg) of cocaine and changes in dopamine release and uptake were measured. When compared to vehicle-treated animals, SB-334867 produced a significant reduction in electrically stimulated dopamine release prior to cocaine injection, further indicating that hypocretin signaling regulates dopamine neurotransmission (Fig. 10.5B and C). In addition to these effects, SB-334867 also reduced the effects of cocaine on dopamine signaling. Relative to vehicle treatment, SB-334867 reduced the effects of cocaine on both stimulated dopamine release and dopamine uptake inhibition.

In another set of experiments, we used *in vitro* voltammetry in brain slices from WT and hypocretin KO mice to examine whether a complete loss of hypocretin signaling would also produce deficits in dopamine signaling. Recording and stimulating electrodes were positioned within the NAc core to allow for measurement of locally evoked dopamine release. Following a stable baseline of dopamine release, cocaine was bath-applied to the slice at cumulatively higher concentrations. Under baseline conditions, disruption of hypocretin neurotransmission in KO mice results in disrupted dopamine signaling, with a reduction in both evoked dopamine release and dopamine uptake rate (Fig. 10.6). Furthermore, hypocretin KO mice displayed attenuated dopamine responses to cocaine, showing only half as much dopamine uptake inhibition as WT mice (España *et al.,* 2010).

Given that disruptions in hypocretin signaling reduce dopamine responses to cocaine, we next examined whether enhancement of hypocretin signaling would have the opposite effect. Initial studies used microdialysis to measure extracellular levels of dopamine in the NAc core. Experiments were conducted as described above with the exception that all animals received vehicle or hypocretin 1 (0.5 nmol) directly into the VTA, 20 min prior to receiving a 10 mg/kg cocaine injection. As shown in Fig. 10.7A, infusions of hypocretin 1 had no effect on dopamine levels under baseline conditions (España *et al.,* 2011). Nevertheless, hypocretin 1

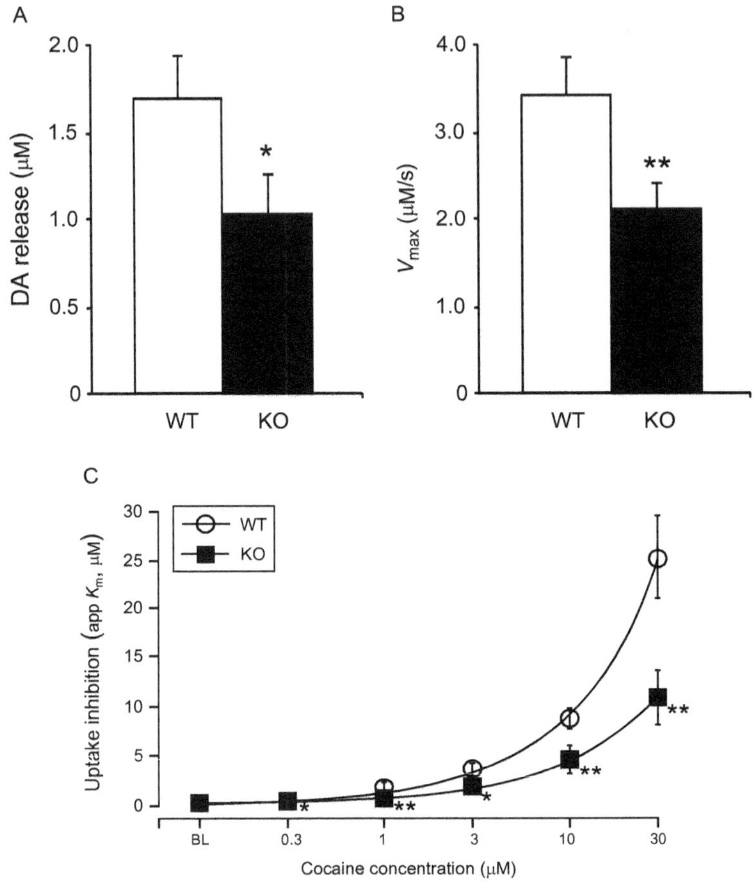

Figure 10.6 Hypocretin knockout mice display disrupted baseline dopamine signaling and attenuated dopamine responses to cocaine. The mean ± SEM of (A) stimulated dopamine (DA) release and (B) maximal dopamine uptake rate (V_{max}) in WT ($n=7$) and hypocretin KO ($n=7$) mouse slices containing the NAc core. (C) The mean ± SEM DA uptake inhibition (apparent K_m) in WT ($n=7$) and hypocretin KO ($n=7$) mouse slices across cumulative doses of cocaine. $^*P<0.05$, $^{**}P<0.01$ relative to vehicle.

significantly augmented the effects of cocaine at increasing dopamine levels. Voltammetry studies in anesthetized rats also showed a hypocretin enhancement of cocaine's effects. In those experiments, rats were pretreated with vehicle or hypocretin 1 (0.5 nmol) into the VTA 20 min prior to receiving an i.v. injection of 1.5 mg/kg cocaine (España *et al.*, 2011). Within 5 min of infusion, hypocretin 1 significantly increased evoked dopamine release prior to cocaine treatment. Further, hypocretin 1 infusions also augmented the effects of cocaine on evoked dopamine release and dopamine uptake inhibition (Fig. 10.7B and C).

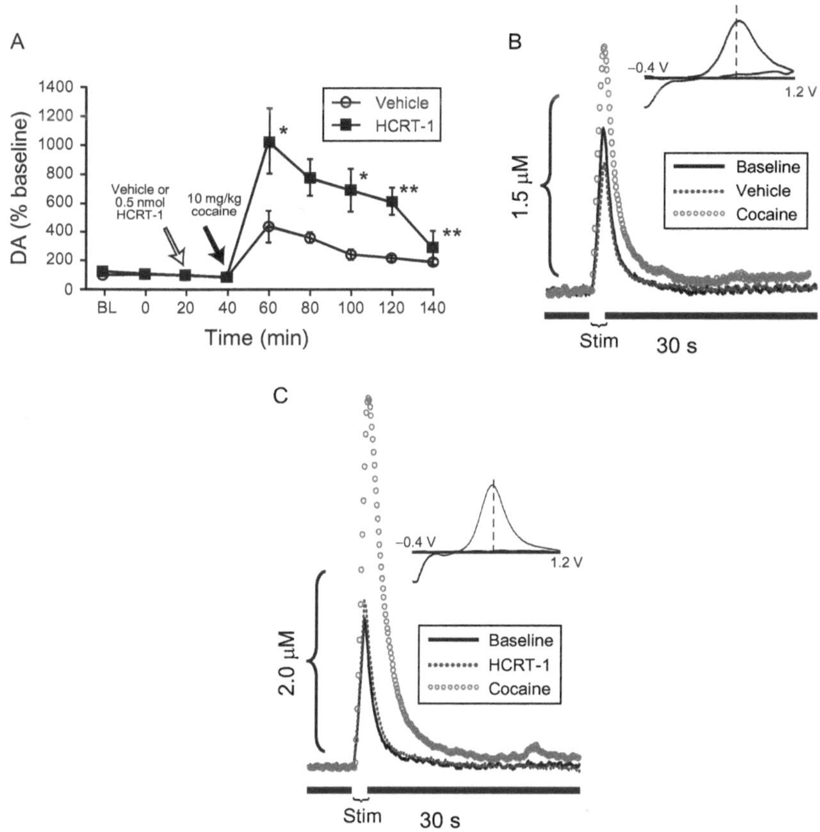

Figure 10.7 Hypocretin-1 augments cocaine-induced elevations in dopamine signaling in the NAc core. (A) The mean ± SEM of extracellular levels of dopamine (DA) within the NAc core following intra-VTA infusion of vehicle ($n=6$) or 0.5 nmol hypocretin-1 (HCRT-1; $n=6$). Representative concentration–time plots and cyclic voltammograms (insets) of dopamine responses from rats that received pretreatment infusions of (B) vehicle or (C) 0.5 nmol hypocretin-1 into the VTA. Stim represents the time of electrical stimulation (1 s, 60 Hz pulse). (Insets in B and C) Cyclic voltammograms depict two current peaks, one at 600 mV (positive deflection) for dopamine oxidation and another at −200 mV (negative deflection) for reduction of dopamine-*o*-quinone. The position of the peaks identifies the substance as DA. $^{*}P<0.05$, $^{**}P<0.01$ relative to vehicle. (See Color Insert.)

C. Summary

The neurochemical studies described above provide compelling evidence for the hypothesis that hypocretin neurotransmission influences dopamine signaling in the NAc core, particularly in response to cocaine. Moreover, given that many of the described experiments used intratissue infusions of agents into the VTA, these studies indicate that the actions of hypocretin on dopamine release and uptake involve signaling within the VTA.

IV. Conclusions

The hypocretin projection to dopamine neurons of the VTA appears to be a critical modulator of reward and reinforcement processing and dopamine signaling in the ventral striatum. As described above, amassing evidence indicates that an intact hypocretin system is necessary for normal behavioral responses to various drugs of abuse, including cocaine. Studies using multiple self-administration schedules of reinforcement demonstrate clearly that disruption of hypocretin signaling reduces the motivation for animals to take cocaine under conditions that require effortful responding or in which access to cocaine is limited. Consistent with these observations, enhancement of hypocretin signaling exerts the opposite influence by increasing the motivation to take cocaine.

The actions of hypocretin on reward and reinforcement behavior are likely to be associated with modulation of dopamine signaling within the striatum. Neurochemical and electrophysiological studies show convincingly that manipulations to hypocretin neurotransmission result in disrupted dopamine signaling that lead to altered dopamine levels within the NAc core both under baseline conditions and in responses to cocaine and other drugs of abuse. When taken together, behavioral, electrophysiological, and neurochemical studies provide significant evidence for the hypothesis that the hypocretin system participates in reward and reinforcement processes, via actions on the mesolimbic system. Further, these observations suggest that continued research in this area of drug addiction may lead to development of rational pharmacotherapies based on hypocretin signaling.

REFERENCES

Abrahamson, E. E., Leak, R. K., and Moore, R. Y. (2001). The suprachiasmatic nucleus projects to posterior hypothalamic arousal systems. *Neuroreport* **12,** 435–440.

Acquas, E., and Di Chiara, G. (1994). D1 receptor blockade stereospecifically impairs the acquisition of drug-conditioned place preference and place aversion. *Behav. Pharmacol.* **5,** 555–569.

Akimoto, H., Honda, Y., and Takahashi, Y. (1960). Pharmacotherapy in narcolepsy. *Dis. Nerv. Syst.* **21,** 704–706.

Aston-Jones, G., Smith, R. J., Moorman, D. E., and Richardson, K. A. (2009). Role of lateral hypothalamic orexin neurons in reward processing and addiction. *Neuropharmacology* **56** (Suppl. 1), 112–121.

Backberg, M., Hervieu, G., Wilson, S., and Meister, B. (2002). Orexin receptor-1 (OX-R1) immunoreactivity in chemically identified neurons of the hypothalamus:

Focus on orexin targets involved in control of food and water intake. *Eur. J. Neurosci.* **15,** 315–328.

Blouin, A. M., Thannickal, T. C., Worley, P. F., Baraban, J. M., Reti, I. M., and Siegel, J. M. (2005). Narp immunostaining of human hypocretin (orexin) neurons: Loss in narcolepsy. *Neurology* **65,** 1189–1192.

Borgland, S. L., Taha, S. A., Sarti, F., Fields, H. L., and Bonci, A. (2006). Orexin A in the VTA is critical for the induction of synaptic plasticity and behavioral sensitization to cocaine. *Neuron* **49,** 589–601.

Borgland, S. L., Chang, S. J., Bowers, M. S., Thompson, J. L., Vittoz, N., Floresco, S. B., Chou, J., Chen, B. T., and Bonci, A. (2009). Orexin A/hypocretin 1 selectively promotes motivation for positive reinforcers. *J. Neurosci.* **29,** 11215–11225.

Bourgin, P., Huitron-Resendiz, S., Spier, A. D., Fabre, V., Morte, B., Criado, J. R., Sutcliffe, J. G., Henriksen, S. J., and de Lecea, L. (2000). Hypocretin-1 modulates rapid eye movement sleep through activation of locus coeruleus neurons. *J. Neurosci.* **20,** 7760–7765.

Boutrel, B., Kenny, P. J., Specio, S. E., Martin-Fardon, R., Markou, A., Koob, G. F., and de Lecea, L. (2005). Role for hypocretin in mediating stress-induced reinstatement of cocaine-seeking behavior. *Proc. Natl. Acad. Sci. U.S.A.* **102,** 19168–19173.

Brebner, K., Phelan, R., and Roberts, D. C. S. (2000). Effect of baclofen on cocaine self-administration in rats reinforced under fixed-ratio 1 and progressive-ratio schedules. *Psychopharmacology (Berl.)* **148,** 314–321.

Brown, R. E., Sergeeva, O., Eriksson, K. S., and Haas, H. L. (2001). Orexin A excites serotonergic neurons in the dorsal raphe nucleus of the rat. *Neuropharmacology* **40,** 457–459.

Caine, S. B., and Koob, G. F. (1994). Effects of dopamine D-1 and D-2 antagonists on cocaine self-administration under different schedules of reinforcement in the rat. *J. Pharmacol. Exp. Ther.* **270,** 209–218.

Caine, S. B., Negus, S. S., Mello, N. K., and Bergman, J. (1999). Effects of dopamine D (1-like) and D(2-like) agonists in rats that self-administer cocaine. *J. Pharmacol. Exp. Ther.* **291,** 353–360.

Carboni, E., Imperato, A., Perezzani, L., and Di Chiara, G. (1989). Amphetamine, cocaine, phencyclidine and nomifensine increase extracellular dopamine concentrations preferentially in the nucleus accumbens of freely moving rats. *Neuroscience* **28,** 653–661.

Carelli, R. M., King, V. C., Hampson, R. E., and Deadwyler, S. A. (1993). Firing patterns of nucleus accumbens neurons during cocaine self-administration in rats. *Brain Res.* **626,** 14–22.

Cervo, L., and Samanin, R. (1995). Effects of dopaminergic and glutamatergic receptor antagonists on the acquisition and expression of cocaine conditioning place preference. *Brain Res.* **673,** 242–250.

Chemelli, R. M., Willie, J. T., Sinton, C. M., Elmquist, J. K., Scammell, T., Lee, C., Richardson, J. A., Williams, S. C., Xiong, Y., Kisanuki, Y., Fitch, T. E., Nakazato, M., *et al.* (1999). Narcolepsy in orexin knockout mice: Molecular genetics of sleep regulation. *Cell* **98,** 437–451.

Cluderay, J. E., Harrison, D. C., and Hervieu, G. J. (2002). Protein distribution of the orexin-2 receptor in the rat central nervous system. *Regul. Pept.* **104,** 131–144.

Crocker, A., Espana, R. A., Papadopoulou, M., Saper, C. B., Faraco, J., Sakurai, T., Honda, M., Mignot, E., and Scammell, T. E. (2005). Concomitant loss of dynorphin, NARP, and orexin in narcolepsy. *Neurology* **65,** 1184–1188.

Date, Y., Ueta, Y., Yamashita, H., Yamaguchi, H., Matsukura, S., Kangawa, K., Sakurai, T., Yanagisawa, M., and Nakazato, M. (1999). Orexins, orexigenic hypothalamic peptides, interact with autonomic, neuroendocrine and neuroregulatory systems. *Proc. Natl. Acad. Sci. U.S.A.* **96,** 748–753.

Dayas, C. V., McGranahan, T. M., Martin-Fardon, R., and Weiss, F. (2008). Stimuli linked to ethanol availability activate hypothalamic CART and orexin neurons in a reinstatement model of relapse. *Biol. Psychiatry* **63,** 152–157.

de Lecea, L., Kilduff, T. S., Peyron, C., Gao, X., Foye, P. E., Danielson, P. E., Fukuhara, C., Battenberg, E. L., Gautvik, V. T., Bartlett, F. S., Frankel, W. N., van Den Pol, A. N., *et al.* (1998). The hypocretins: Hypothalamus-specific peptides with neuroexcitatory activity. *Proc. Natl. Acad. Sci. U.S.A.* **95,** 322–327.

Di Chiara, G., and Imperato, A. (1988). Opposite effects of mu and kappa opiate agonists on dopamine release in the nucleus accumbens and in the dorsal caudate of freely moving rats. *J. Pharmacol. Exp. Ther.* **244,** 1067–1080.

España, R. A., and Jones, S. R. (2010). Hypocretin/Orexin Knockout Mice Display Disrupted Dopamine Responses to Cocaine. Society for Neuroscience, San Diego, CA[668.14].

España, R. A., Baldo, B. A., Kelley, A. E., and Berridge, C. W. (2001). Wake-promoting and sleep-suppressing actions of hypocretin (orexin): Basal forebrain sites of action. *Neuroscience* **106,** 699–715.

España, R. A., Plahn, S., and Berridge, C. W. (2002). Circadian-dependent and circadian-independent behavioral actions of hypocretin/orexin. *Brain Res.* **943,** 224–236.

España, R. A., Valentino, R. J., and Berridge, C. W. (2003). Fos immunoreactivity in hypocretin-synthesizing and hypocretin 1 receptor-expressing neurons: Effects of diurnal and nocturnal spontaneous waking, stress and hypocretin 1 administration. *Neuroscience* **121,** 201–217.

España, R. A., Oleson, E. B., Locke, J. L., Brookshire, B. R., Roberts, D. C. S., and Jones, S. R. (2010). The hypocretin-orexin system regulates cocaine self-administration via actions on the mesolimbic dopamine system. *Eur. J. Neurosci.* **31,** 336–348.

España, R. A., Melchior, J. R., Roberts, D. C. S., and Jones, S. R. (2011). Hypocretin 1/orexin A in the ventral tegmental area enhances dopamine responses to cocaine and promotes cocaine self-administration. *Psychopharmacology* 1–12.

Estabrooke, I. V., McCarthy, M. T., Ko, E., Chou, T. C., Chemelli, R. M., Yanagisawa, M., Saper, C. B., and Scammell, T. E. (2001). Fos expression in orexin neurons varies with behavioral state. *J. Neurosci.* **21,** 1656–1662.

Fadel, J., and Deutch, A. Y. (2002). Anatomical substrates of orexin-dopamine interactions: Lateral hypothalamic projections to the ventral tegmental area. *Neuroscience* **111,** 379–387.

Funada, M., and Shippenberg, T. S. (1996). Differential involvement of D1 and D2 dopamine receptors in the expression of morphine withdrawal signs in rats. *Behav. Pharmacol.* **7,** 448–453.

Georgescu, D., Zachariou, V., Barrot, M., Mieda, M., Willie, J. T., Eisch, A. J., Yanagisawa, M., Nestler, E. J., and DiLeone, R. J. (2003). Involvement of the lateral hypothalamic peptide orexin in morphine dependence and withdrawal. *J. Neurosci.* **23,** 3106–3111.

Greco, M. A., and Shiromani, P. J. (2001). Hypocretin receptor protein and mRNA expression in the dorsolateral pons of rats. *Brain Res. Mol. Brain Res.* **88,** 176–182.

Hagan, J. J., Leslie, R. A., Patel, S., Evans, M. L., Wattam, T. A., Holmes, S., Benham, C. D., Taylor, S. G., Routledge, C., Hemmati, P., Munton, R. P., Ashmeade, T. E., *et al.* (1999). Orexin A activates locus coeruleus cell firing and increases arousal in the rat. *Proc. Natl. Acad. Sci. U.S.A.* **96,** 10911–10916.

Hara, J., Beuckmann, C. T., Nambu, T., Willie, J. T., Chemelli, R. M., Sinton, C. M., Sugiyama, F., Yagami, K., Goto, K., Yanagisawa, M., and Sakurai, T. (2001). Genetic ablation of orexin neurons in mice results in narcolepsy, hypophagia, and obesity. *Neuron* **30,** 345–354.

Harris, G. C., and Aston-Jones, G. (2006). Arousal and reward: A dichotomy in orexin function. *Trends Neurosci.* **29,** 571–577.

Harris, G. C., Wimmer, M., and Aston-Jones, G. (2005). A role for lateral hypothalamic orexin neurons in reward seeking. *Nature* **437,** 556–559.

Harris, G. C., Wimmer, M., Randall-Thompson, J. F., and Aston-Jones, G. (2007). Lateral hypothalamic orexin neurons are critically involved in learning to associate an environment with morphine reward. *Behav. Brain Res.* **183,** 43–51.

Hayduk, R., Erman, M. K., Poceta, J. S., and Mitler, M. M. (1995). Methamphetamine in the treatment of narcolepsy: Serum levels, dosage and MSLT. *Sleep Res.* **24A,** 316.

Hervieu, G. J., Cluderay, J. E., Harrison, D. C., Roberts, J. C., and Leslie, R. A. (2001). Gene expression and protein distribution of the orexin-1 receptor in the rat brain and spinal cord. *Neuroscience* **103,** 777–797.

Hoffman, D. C., and Beninger, R. J. (1988). Selective D1 and D2 dopamine agonists produce opposing effects in place conditioning but not in conditioned taste aversion learning. *Pharmacol. Biochem. Behav.* **31,** 1–8.

Hoffman, D. C., and Beninger, R. J. (1989). The effects of selective dopamine D1 or D2 receptor antagonists on the establishment of agonist-induced place conditioning in rats. *Pharmacol. Biochem. Behav.* **33,** 273–279.

Hoffman, D. C., Dickson, P. R., and Beninger, R. J. (1988). The dopamine D2 receptor agonists, quinpirole and bromocriptine produce conditioned place preferences. *Prog. Neuropsychopharmacol. Biol. Psychiatry* **12,** 315–322.

Hollander, J. A., Lu, Q., Cameron, M. D., Kamenecka, T. M., and Kenny, P. J. (2008). Insular hypocretin transmission regulates nicotine reward. *Proc. Natl. Acad. Sci. U.S.A.* **105,** 19480–19485.

Horvath, T. L., Peyron, C., Diano, S., Ivanov, A., Aston-Jones, G., Kilduff, T. S., and van Den Pol, A. N. (1999). Hypocretin (orexin) activation and synaptic innervation of the locus coeruleus noradrenergic system. *J. Comp. Neurol.* **415,** 145–159.

Hutcheson, D. M., Quarta, D., Halbout, B., Rigal, A., Valerio, E., and Heidbreder, C. (2011). Orexin-1 receptor antagonist SB-334867 reduces the acquisition and expression of cocaine-conditioned reinforcement and the expression of amphetamine-conditioned reward. *Behav. Pharmacol.* **22,** 173–181.

Ida, T., Nakahara, K., Katayama, T., Murakami, N., and Nakazato, M. (1999). Effect of lateral cerebroventricular injection of the appetite-stimulating neuropeptide, orexin and neuropeptide Y, on the various behavioral activities of rats. *Brain Res.* **821,** 526–529.

Imperato, A., and Di Chiara, G. (1986). Preferential stimulation of dopamine release in the nucleus accumbens of freely moving rats by ethanol. *J. Pharmacol. Exp. Ther.* **239,** 219–228.

Kane, J. K., Parker, S. L., Matta, S. G., Fu, Y., Sharp, B. M., and Li, M. D. (2000). Nicotine up-regulates expression of orexin and its receptors in rat brain. *Endocrinology* **141,** 3623–3629.

Kisanuki, Y. Y., Chemelli, R. M., Sinton, C. M., Williams, S. C., and Richardson, J. A. (2000). The role of orexin receptor type-1 (OX1R) in the regulation of sleep. *Sleep* **23,** A91.

Ko, E. M., Estabrooke, I. V., McCarthy, M., and Scammell, T. E. (2003). Wake-related activity of tuberomammillary neurons in rats. *Brain Res.* **992,** 220–226.

Koob, G. F., and Le Moal, M. (1997). Drug abuse: Hedonic homeostatic dysregulation. *Science* **278,** 52–58.

Korotkova, T. M., Sergeeva, O. A., Eriksson, K. S., Haas, H. L., and Brown, R. E. (2003). Excitation of ventral tegmental area dopaminergic and nondopaminergic neurons by orexins/hypocretins. *J. Neurosci.* **23,** 7–11.

Lawrence, A. J., Cowen, M. S., Yang, H. J., Chen, F., and Oldfield, B. (2006). The orexin system regulates alcohol-seeking in rats. *Br. J. Pharmacol.* **148,** 752–759.

Lee, M. G., Hassani, O. K., and Jones, B. E. (2005). Discharge of identified orexin/hypocretin neurons across the sleep-waking cycle. *J. Neurosci.* **25,** 6716–6720.

Lin, L., Faraco, J., Li, R., Kadotani, H., Rogers, W., Lin, X., Qiu, X., de Jong, P. J., Nishino, S., and Mignot, E. (1999). The sleep disorder canine narcolepsy is caused by a mutation in the hypocretin (orexin) receptor 2 gene. *Cell* **98,** 365–376.

Lyness, W. H., Friedle, N. M., and Moore, K. E. (1979). Destruction of dopaminergic nerve terminals in nucleus accumbens: Effect on d-amphetamine self-administration. *Pharmacol. Biochem. Behav.* **11,** 553–556.

Marcus, J. N., Aschkenasi, C. J., Lee, C. E., Chemelli, R. M., Saper, C. B., Yanagisawa, M., and Elmquist, J. K. (2001). Differential expression of orexin receptors 1 and 2 in the rat brain. *J. Comp. Neurol.* **435,** 6–25.

McGregor, A., and Roberts, D. C. S. (1995). Effect of medial prefrontal cortex injections of SCH 23390 on intravenous cocaine self-administration under both a fixed and progressive ratio schedule of reinforcement. *Behav. Brain Res.* **67,** 75–80.

Mileykovskiy, B. Y., Kiyashchenko, L. I., and Siegel, J. M. (2005). Behavioral correlates of activity in identified hypocretin/orexin neurons. *Neuron* **46,** 787–798.

Nambu, T., Sakurai, T., Mizukami, K., Hosoya, Y., Yanagisawa, M., and Goto, K. (1999). Distribution of orexin neurons in the adult rat brain. *Brain Res.* **827,** 243–260.

Narita, M., Nagumo, Y., Hashimoto, S., Narita, M., Khotib, J., Miyatake, M., Sakurai, T., Yanagisawa, M., Nakamachi, T., Shioda, S., and Suzuki, T. (2006). Direct involvement of orexinergic systems in the activation of the mesolimbic dopamine pathway and related behaviors induced by morphine. *J. Neurosci.* **26,** 398–405.

Nishino, S., Ripley, B., Overeem, S., Lammers, G. J., and Mignot, E. (2000). Hypocretin (orexin) deficiency in human narcolepsy. *Lancet* **355,** 39–40.

Papp, M. (1988). Different effects of short- and long-term treatment with imipramine on the apomorphine- and food-induced place preference conditioning in rats. *Pharmacol. Biochem. Behav.* **30,** 889–893.

Parker, L. A. (1992). Place conditioning in a three- or four-choice apparatus: Role of stimulus novelty in drug-induced place conditioning. *Behav. Neurosci.* **106,** 294–306.

Pasumarthi, R. K., Reznikov, L. R., and Fadel, J. (2006). Activation of orexin neurons by acute nicotine. *Eur. J. Pharmacol.* **535,** 172–176.

Peyron, C., Tighe, D. K., van Den Pol, A. N., de Lecea, L., Heller, H. C., Sutcliffe, J. G., and Kilduff, T. S. (1998). Neurons containing hypocretin (orexin) project to multiple neuronal systems. *J. Neurosci.* **18,** 9996–10015.

Peyron, C., Faraco, J., Rogers, W., Ripley, B., Overeem, S., Charnay, Y., Nevsimalova, S., Aldrich, M., Reynolds, D., Albin, R., Li, R., Hungs, M., *et al.* (2000). A mutation in a case of early onset narcolepsy and a generalized absence of hypocretin peptides in human narcoleptic brains. *Nat. Med.* **6,** 991–997.

Piper, D. C., Upton, N., Smith, M. I., and Hunter, A. J. (2000). The novel brain neuropeptide, orexin-A, modulates the sleep–wake cycle of rats. *Eur. J. Neurosci.* **12,** 726–730.

Plaza-Zabala, A., Martin-Garcia, E., de, L. L., Maldonado, R., and Berrendero, F. (2010). Hypocretins regulate the anxiogenic-like effects of nicotine and induce reinstatement of nicotine-seeking behavior. *J. Neurosci.* **30,** 2300–2310.

Richards, J. K., Simms, J. A., Steensland, P., Taha, S. A., Borgland, S. L., Bonci, A., and Bartlett, S. E. (2008). Inhibition of orexin-1/hypocretin 1 receptors inhibits yohimbine-induced reinstatement of ethanol and sucrose seeking in Long-Evans rats. *Psychopharmacology (Berl.)* **199,** 109–117.

Ripley, B., Overeem, S., Fujiki, N., Nevsimalova, S., Uchino, M., Yesavage, J., Di Monte, D., Dohi, K., Melberg, A., Lammers, G. J., Nishida, Y., Roelandse, F. W., *et al.* (2001). CSF hypocretin/orexin levels in narcolepsy and other neurological conditions. *Neurology* **57,** 2253–2258.

Roberts, D. C. S., Corcoran, M. E., and Fibiger, H. C. (1977). On the role of ascending catecholaminergic systems in intravenous self-administration of cocaine. *Pharmacol. Biochem. Behav.* **6,** 615–620.

Roberts, D. C. S., Brebner, K., Vincler, M., and Lynch, W. J. (2002). Patterns of cocaine self-administration in rats produced by various access conditions under a discrete trials procedure. *Drug Alcohol Depend.* **67,** 291–299.

Rogers, A. E., Aldrich, M. S., Berrios, A. M., and Rosenberg, R. S. (1997). Compliance with stimulant medications in patients with narcolepsy. *Sleep* **20,** 28–33.

Rogers, A. E., Aldrich, M. S., and Lin, X. (2001). A comparison of three different sleep schedules for reducing daytime sleepiness in narcolepsy. *Sleep* **24,** 385–391.

Sakurai, T., Amemiya, A., Ishii, M., Matsuzaki, I., Chemelli, R. M., Tanaka, H., Williams, S. C., Richarson, J. A., Kozlowski, G. P., Wilson, S., Arch, J. R., Buckingham, R. E., *et al.* (1998). Orexins and orexin receptors: A family of hypothalamic neuropeptides and G protein-coupled receptors that regulate feeding behavior. *Cell* **92,** 1.

Sakurai, T., Nagata, R., Yamanaka, A., Kawamura, H., Tsujino, N., Muraki, Y., Kageyama, H., Kunita, S., Takahashi, S., Goto, K., Koyama, Y., Shioda, S., *et al.* (2005). Input of orexin/hypocretin neurons revealed by a genetically encoded tracer in mice. *Neuron* **46,** 297–308.

Self, D. W., and Stein, L. (1992). The D1 agonists SKF 82958 and SKF 77434 are self-administered by rats. *Brain Res.* **582,** 349–352.

Self, D. W., Belluzzi, J. D., Kossuth, S., and Stein, L. (1996). Self-administration of the D1 agonist SKF 82958 is mediated by D1, not D2, receptors. *Psychopharmacology (Berl.)* **123,** 303–306.

Sharf, R., Sarhan, M., and DiLeone, R. J. (2008). Orexin mediates the expression of precipitated morphine withdrawal and concurrent activation of the nucleus accumbens shell. *Biol. Psychiatry* **64,** 175–183.

Sharf, R., Guarnieri, D. J., Taylor, J. R., and DiLeone, R. J. (2010). Orexin mediates morphine place preference, but not morphine-induced hyperactivity or sensitization. *Brain Res.* **1317,** 24–32.

Shippenberg, T. S., and Herz, A. (1987). Place preference conditioning reveals the involvement of D1-dopamine receptors in the motivational properties of mu- and kappa-opioid agonists. *Brain Res.* **436,** 169–172.

Shippenberg, T. S., Bals-Kubik, R., Huber, A., and Herz, A. (1991). Neuroanatomical substrates mediating the aversive effects of D-1 dopamine receptor antagonists. *Psychopharmacology (Berl.)* **103,** 209–214.

Sinnott, R. S., and Nader, M. A. (2001). Modulation of cocaine's discriminative stimulus effects by dopamine D(1) agonists in rhesus monkeys. *Pharmacol. Biochem. Behav.* **68,** 301–309.

Sinnott, R. S., Mach, R. H., and Nader, M. A. (1999). Dopamine D2/D3 receptors modulate cocaine's reinforcing and discriminative stimulus effects in rhesus monkeys. *Drug Alcohol Depend.* **54,** 97–110.

Smith, R. J., and Aston-Jones, G. (2010). The Orexin/Hypocretin 1 Receptor Antagonist SB-334867 Reduces Self-Administration and Cue-Induced Reinstatement of Heroin in Rats. Society for Neuroscience, San Diego, CA[67.6].

Smith, M. A., Yancey, D. L., Morgan, D., Liu, Y., Froestl, W., and Roberts, D. C. S. (2004). Effects of positive allosteric modulators of the GABAB receptor on cocaine self-administration in rats. *Psychopharmacology (Berl.)* **173,** 105–111.

Smith, R. J., See, R. E., and Aston-Jones, G. (2009). Orexin/hypocretin signaling at the orexin 1 receptor regulates cue-elicited cocaine-seeking. *Eur. J. Neurosci.* **30,** 493–503.

Spealman, R. D., Bergman, J., Madras, B. K., and Melia, K. F. (1991). Discriminative stimulus effects of cocaine in squirrel monkeys: Involvement of dopamine receptor subtypes. *J. Pharmacol. Exp. Ther.* **258,** 945–953.

Suzuki, R., Shimojima, H., Funahashi, H., Nakajo, S., Yamada, S., Guan, J. L., Tsurugano, S., Uehara, K., Takeyama, Y., Kikuyama, S., and Shioda, S. (2002). Orexin-1 receptor immunoreactivity in chemically identified target neurons in the rat hypothalamus. *Neurosci. Lett.* **324,** 5–8.

Thannickal, T. C., Moore, R. Y., Nienhuis, R., Ramanathan, L., Gulyani, S., Aldrich, M., Cornford, M., and Siegel, J. M. (2000). Reduced number of hypocretin neurons in human narcolepsy. *Neuron* **27,** 469–474.

Trivedi, P., Yu, H., MacNeil, D. J., Van der Ploeg, L. H., and Guan, X. M. (1998). Distribution of orexin receptor mRNA in the rat brain. *FEBS Lett.* **438,** 71–75.

Uzwiak, A. J., Guyette, F. X., West, M. O., and Peoples, L. L. (1997). Neurons in accumbens subterritories of the rat: Phasic firing time-locked within seconds of intravenous cocaine self-infusion. *Brain Res.* **767,** 363–369.

van Den Pol, A. N. (1999). Hypothalamic hypocretin (orexin): Robust innervation of the spinal cord. *J. Neurosci.* **19,** 3171–3182.

Vittoz, N. M., and Berridge, C. W. (2006). Hypocretin/orexin selectively increases dopamine efflux within the prefrontal cortex: Involvement of the ventral tegmental area. *Neuropsychopharmacology* **31,** 384–395.

Vittoz, N. M., Schmeichel, B., and Berridge, C. W. (2008). Hypocretin/orexin preferentially activates caudomedial ventral tegmental area dopamine neurons. *Eur. J. Neurosci.* **28,** 1629–1640.

Volkow, N. D., Fowler, J. S., Logan, J., Alexoff, D., Zhu, W., Telang, F., Wang, G. J., Jayne, M., Hooker, J. M., Wong, C., Hubbard, B., Carter, P., *et al.* (2009). Effects of modafinil on dopamine and dopamine transporters in the male human brain: Clinical implications. *JAMA* **301,** 1148–1154.

Weed, M. R., and Woolverton, W. L. (1995). The reinforcing effects of dopamine D1 receptor agonists in rhesus monkeys. *J. Pharmacol. Exp. Ther.* **275,** 1367–1374.

White, N. M., Packard, M. G., and Hiroi, N. (1991). Place conditioning with dopamine D1 and D2 agonists injected peripherally or into nucleus accumbens. *Psychopharmacology (Berl.)* **103,** 271–276.

Wise, R. A. (1996). Neurobiology of addiction. *Curr. Opin. Neurobiol.* **6,** 243–251.

Woolverton, W. L., and Johnson, K. M. (1992). Neurobiology of cocaine abuse. *Trends Pharmacol. Sci.* **13,** 193–200.

Yoshida, Y., Fujiki, N., Nakajima, T., Ripley, B., Matsumura, H., Yoneda, H., Mignot, E., and Nishino, S. (2001). Fluctuation of extracellular hypocretin 1 (orexin A) levels in the rat in relation to the light-dark cycle and sleep-wake activities. *Eur. J. Neurosci.* **14,** 1075–1081.

Yoshida, K., McCormack, S., España, R. A., Crocker, A., and Scammell, T. E. (2006). Afferents to the orexin neurons of the rat brain. *J. Comp. Neurol.* **494,** 845–861.

Zhou, Y., Bendor, J., Hofmann, L., Randesi, M., Ho, A., and Kreek, M. J. (2006). Mu opioid receptor and orexin/hypocretin mRNA levels in the lateral hypothalamus and striatum are enhanced by morphine withdrawal. *J. Endocrinol.* **191,** 137–145.

CHAPTER ELEVEN

Glutamate and Orexin Neurons

Ozhan Eyigor,* Zehra Minbay,* *and* Ilker M. Kafa†

Contents

Abstract

Orexin neurons are localized in the lateral hypothalamus and regulate many functions including sleep–wake states. Substantial number of neurotransmitters and neuromodulators has been proposed to influence orexinergic system. Glutamate, as the major excitatory amino acid neurotransmitter in the hypothalamus, was shown to mediate orexin neurons in the regulation of wakefulness and feeding. Glutamate is readily present in the lateral hypothalamus, and glutamate receptors are expressed by the neurons of this region. Glutamate agonists initiate excitatory postsynaptic currents in orexin neurons, and this can be blocked by specific antagonists of the glutamate receptors. It is reported that both NMDA and non-NMDA receptors contribute the glutamatergic neurotransmission which affects orexinergic functions. Glutamatergic axon terminals are demonstrated to make contacts with the orexin neurons, as revealed by the presence of vesicular glutamate transporter proteins in the terminals, and these contacts were ultrastructurally confirmed to establish synapses on orexin neurons. This chapter reviews the literature on the glutamatergic regulation of orexin neurons including the data from our laboratory. © 2012 Elsevier Inc.

* Department of Histology and Embryology, Faculty of Medicine, Uludag University, Bursa, Turkey
† Department of Anatomy, Faculty of Medicine, Uludag University, Bursa, Turkey

Vitamins and Hormones, Volume 89
ISSN 0083-6729, http://dx.doi.org/10.1016/B978-0-12-394623-2.00011-1

I. Introduction

Orexin peptides are synthesized and secreted by a group of neurons mostly localized in the lateral hypothalamus including the perifornical area. Small groups of orexin neurons also found in the posterior hypothalamic area and dorsomedial hypothalamic nucleus. Orexin peptides are derived from prepro-orexin, as the common precursor peptide and known as orexin A and orexin B. These peptides are known to play a crucial role in regulating and maintaining the wakefulness. Orexins are also known to participate in the regulation of feeding behavior, control of cardiovascular and neuroendocrine systems as well as the cognitive functions and energy expenditure.

Many neurotransmitter and neuromodulator systems have been identified to regulate the synthesis and secretion of the orexin peptides. These regulatory systems primarily include glutamate, GABA, acetylcholine, noradrenaline, and serotonin. This chapter focuses on the glutamatergic regulation of the orexin neurons, with the data from our laboratory and the review of the literature.

II. Glutamate and Glutamate Receptors in the Lateral Hypothalamus

Glutamate is known to be the major excitatory amino acid neurotransmitter in the hypothalamus (Van den Pol *et al.*, 1990). At the ultrastructural level, electron microscopic immunohistochemistry revealed that glutamate-positive axonal endings make synaptic contacts with dendrites and neuronal cell bodies throughout the lateral hypothalamus (Van den Pol and Trombley, 1993). Receptor binding studies showed that glutamate binds to its receptors to some extend in the lateral hypothalamic area (Maragos *et al.*, 1988; Meeker *et al.*, 1994).

The importance of the localization of glutamate in the lateral hypothalamus and the results of receptor autoradiography studies are further strengthened by the reports analyzing the expression of glutamate receptors in the lateral hypothalamus. Our data on the distribution of ionotropic glutamate receptor subunit mRNAs in the rat hypothalamus showed that almost all subunits are expressed in the lateral hypothalamus including the perifornical area (Eyigor *et al.*, 2001). Although less number of glutamate receptor subunit mRNA-expressing cells was detected in this area when compared to the other regions of the hypothalamus, the intensity of the expression per cell was found to be higher. It is suggested that the localization of these scattered cells with subunit expression overlaps the localization pattern of the orexinergic neurons (de Lecea *et al.*, 1998; Sakurai *et al.*, 1998).

Hybridization signals were detected for relatively higher number of neurons which are expressing kainate receptor subunits of non-NMDA glutamate receptors including KA2 and GluR7 (Eyigor *et al.*, 2001). Similarly, NMDAR1 subunit of the NMDA receptors was found to be expressed in moderate numbers of lateral hypothalamic area neurons. We reported in the aforementioned study that relatively less number of neurons in the lateral hypothalamus expresses GluR1 and GluR2 subunits of AMPA receptors, GluR5 and GluR6 subunits of kainate receptors, and NMDAR2 receptor subunits. Although the localization of glutamate receptor subunit proteins in the hypothalamus has been extensively studied using immunohistochemistry, these reports lack the information about the expression pattern of subunit proteins in the lateral hypothalamus (Eyigor *et al.*, 2005; Gannon and Rea, 1993; Ginsberg *et al.*, 1995; Martin *et al.*, 1993; Pak and Curras-Collazo, 2002; Petralia and Wenthold, 1992, 1996; Petralia *et al.*, 1994a,b). In a previous report, Khan *et al.* (1999) found robust NMDAR1 and moderate levels of NMDAR2A and NMDAR2B expression using Western blot analysis and detected NMDAR2B subunit-immunoreactive neurons in the lateral hypothalamus including the perifornical area. Data from our laboratory showed that KA2- and GLUR6/7-immunoreactive neurons are present in the perifornical area (unpublished data, Eyigor, Minbay, Jennes a representative example is given in Fig. 11.1). The data reviewed above suggest that glutamatergic transmission is an important part of the neurotransmission in the lateral hypothalamus where orexin neurons are localized and that some, if not all,

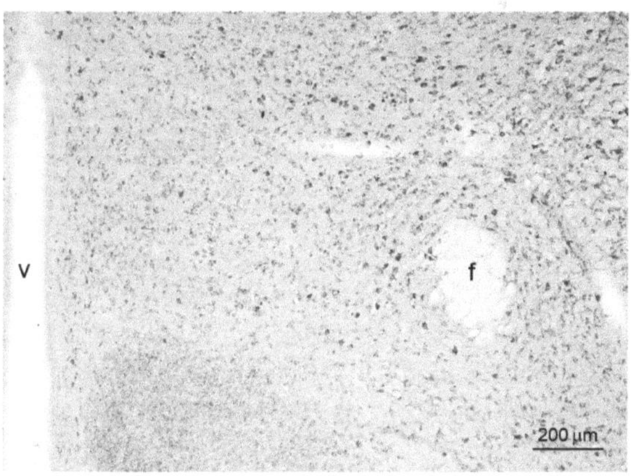

Figure 11.1 Expression of KA2 subunit of kainate receptors in the lateral hypothalamus. Note the abundance of KA2-immunoreactive perikarya in the perifornical area of the lateral hypothalamus (v, third ventricle; f, fornix). KA2 subunit was labeled with a rabbit anti-KA2 polyclonal antibody (1:2000 dilution, R52-4, Eyigor and Jennes, 2000). (See Color Insert.)

of these glutamate receptor subunits may be expressed by orexin neurons, which, in turn, may play an important role in the regulation of sleep–wake states as well as other functions of the orexinergic system.

III. Glutamatergic Afferents of Orexin Neurons

There is substantial evidence that orexin neurons receive glutamatergic afferents in addition to the afferents from other neurotransmitter systems in different nervous system areas. Abundant projections from the lateral septum, basal forebrain, preoptic area, hypothalamus, amygdala, and raphe nuclei using different neurotransmitters such as glutamate, GABA, serotonin, histamine, acetylcholine, and noradrenaline were detected by tracing experiments (Sakurai, 2007; Sakurai and Mieda, 2011; Sakurai *et al.*, 2005; Yamanaka, 2006; Yoshida *et al.*, 2006). In order to differentiate glutamatergic neurons and axon terminals innervating a particular neuron, the expression of the three isoforms of vesicular glutamate transporter (VGluT) proteins has been used as a glutamatergic marker to identify the neurons which use glutamate as the excitatory neurotransmitter (Liguz-Lecznar and Skangiel-Kramska, 2007; Takamori *et al.*, 2000). Studies utilizing VGluT protein immunohistochemistry have revealed that the glutamatergic axonal endings are present in the lateral hypothalamus. Of the three isoforms of VGluTs, VGluT2 protein was found to be the most prominent VGluT in the hypothalamus (Lin *et al.*, 2003; Ziegler *et al.*, 2002). Lin *et al.* (2003) showed that moderate numbers of VGluT2-positive fibers are scattered in the lateral hypothalamus. In addition to VGluT2, VGluT1- and VGluT3-immunoreactive fibers were also demonstrated in the lateral hypothalamic area (Collin *et al.*, 2003; Herzog *et al.*, 2004). VGluT2-immunoreactive (hence glutamatergic) axon terminals were shown in the vicinity of orexin neurons, and most of these terminals were found to be in contact with orexin cell bodies or dendrites (Li *et al.*, 2002). The presence of orexin neuron-contacting VGluT2-immunoreactive fibers was further confirmed by the studies from our (unpublished data, Eyigor, Minbay) and other laboratories (Henny and Jones, 2006; Horvath and Gao, 2005). The contacts of VGluT2-reactive axon terminals on orexin neurons were shown to establish synaptic organization at the ultrastructural level using correlated light and electron microscopy (Horvath and Gao, 2005). We also observed VGluT3-containing appositions on the orexin neurons which points out the possibility of an innervation by a subgroup of glutamate neurons using VGluT3 as the VGluT (unpublished data, Eyigor, Minbay a representative example is given in Fig. 11.2).

Tracing studies suggested that the glutamatergic inputs to the orexin neurons may originate from the neurons located in the basal forebrain (Henny and Jones, 2006) and/or lateral parabrachial nucleus (Hettes *et al.*,

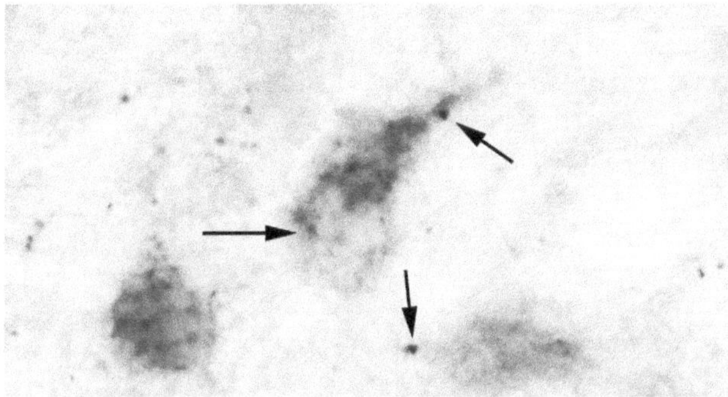

Figure 11.2 Expression of VGluT3 protein on the orexin neurons. Orexin neurons are seen with the cytoplasmic DAB reaction (gray, actual color is brown). The black puncta on the orexin neurons as well as in the vicinity are the Ni-DAB reaction localizing the VGluT3-positive terminals (arrows). Orexin neurons were labeled with a goat anti-orexin A polyclonal antibody (1:1000 dilution, Santa Cruz Biotechnology, USA), while the glutamatergic terminals were labeled with a guinea pig anti-VGluT3 polyclonal antibody (1:5000 dilution, Chemicon International, USA). (See Color Insert.)

2010). Other regions as the source of the glutamatergic innervation to the orexin neurons are yet to be identified, which would include many brain areas known to have projections to the orexinergic neurons (Ohno and Sakurai, 2008; Yoshida *et al.*, 2006). It is challenging, however, to reveal the glutamatergic cell bodies in tract-tracing experiments combined with immunohistochemistry, since the available antibodies for VGluT proteins fail to detect VGluT immunoreactivity without colchicine treatment. Even after this treatment, only a small number of cell bodies can be seen when compared to the results of *in situ* hybridization studies for mRNA expression (Lin *et al.*, 2003).

Glutamatergic interneurons residing in the lateral hypothalamus were also demonstrated to innervate orexinergic neurons (Li *et al.*, 2002). The data of this study suggested that these interneurons may orchestrate the output of the orexin neurons indirectly by conveying a number of signals known to influence the orexin neurons.

In addition to their innervation by glutamatergic endings, it is important to point out that orexin neurons may use glutamate as a neurotransmitter to mediate their own neurotransmission. This idea was suggested by the immunohistochemical findings that the glutamate immunoreactivity is colocalized in the cell bodies (Abrahamson *et al.*, 2001) as well as the axonal terminals of the orexin neurons (Torrealba *et al.*, 2003). Authors of the latter study suggested that glutamate acts in synergy with the orexin peptides to innervate tuberomammillary nucleus neurons (possibly histaminergic) in regulating the wake–sleep states. Additional data confirmed the glutamatergic phenotype of the orexin neurons by demonstrating the expression of VGluT1 and VGlut2 mRNA in orexin neurons (Rosin *et al.*, 2003). The data discussed in this section clearly suggest that the glutamatergic afferents are in the appropriate position within the lateral hypothalamus in order to innervate and activate orexin neurons.

IV. Effects of Glutamate Agonists and Antagonists on the Activation of Orexin Neurons

Transgenic mice with green fluorescent protein (GFP)-expressing orexin neurons have been used in electrophysiological studies to evaluate the effects of glutamate agonists as well as antagonists on orexin neurons. Using brain slices taken from these mice, Li *et al.* (2002) showed that the glutamate agonists AMPA and NMDA induced depolarization and evoked inward currents in the GFP-orexin neurons. In addition, application of AMPA and NMDA antagonists CNQX and AP-5 blocked the depolarization as well as the inward currents. These findings suggest that the functional glutamate receptors are present on the orexin neurons, and it is plausible to assume that the glutamatergic synapses on the orexin neurons regulate these neurons through AMPA and/or NMDA receptor channels. These results were further confirmed in another transgenic mice line in which the orexin neurons express enhanced green fluorescent protein (EGFP) (Yamanaka *et al.*, 2003). When AMPA or NMDA applied on the brain slices of these mice, whole cell current clamping revealed depolarization in the EGFP-expressing orexin neurons. Similar to the previous study, simultaneous application of AP-5 and NBQX as the glutamatergic antagonists almost blocks the excitatory postsynaptic currents (EPSCs) in the orexin neurons. The miniature excitatory postsynaptic currents (mEPSCs) in the orexin neurons were also shown to be sensitive to AMPA receptor antagonists GYKI 52466 and DNQX which abolished the mEPSCs when recorded by whole cell patch clamping (Alberto and Hirasawa, 2010).

The activation of various neurons can also be analyzed by demonstrating the expression of c-Fos mRNA or protein in the nuclei of hypothalamic neurons (Hoffman *et al.*, 1993). In our laboratory, we have used c-Fos immunohistochemistry as a marker of neuronal activation in different neuronal systems (Bora *et al.*, 2004; Eyigor and Jennes, 2000; Eyigor *et al.*, 2012; Minbay *et al.*, 2006). Following the footsteps of the electrophysiological data reviewed above, we, for the first time, reported the histological confirmation of the neuronal activation of the orexinergic system through non-NMDA glutamate receptors (Eyigor *et al.*, 2010). In that study, we observed that the administration of kainic acid (kainate and AMPA receptor agonist) significantly increased the number of c-Fos-positive orexin neurons. Application of non-NMDA glutamate receptor antagonist CNQX significantly diminished the ratio of activated neurons over all orexin-immunoreactive neurons. It is important to point out that kainic acid was not used among the glutamate agonists in the aforementioned electrophysiological experiments, and that the findings of our study added the possibility of kainate receptors to be involved in the regulation of the orexin neurons by glutamatergic innervation. Here, we additionally present previously unpublished data from our laboratory, suggesting similar effects of AMPA and NMDA in the activation of orexin neurons. In these experiments, we observed that the number of activated orexin neurons (c-Fos positive) significantly increased following AMPA administration (5 mg/kg, ip). Statistical analyses revealed that this activation was blocked by CNQX (2 mg/kg, ip) in a significant number of orexin neurons, confirming the electrophysiological findings that the functional AMPA receptors play an important role in conveying the glutamatergic signals to the orexin neurons (Fig. 11.3, left panel). We also analyzed the effects of NMDA on the c-Fos expression in the orexin neurons. NMDA (100 mg/kg, ip) caused statistically significant increase in the number of c-Fos-immunoreactive orexin neuron; however, MK-801 (1.5 mg/kg, ip) failed to block this effect (Fig. 11.3, right panel). Data from these experiments are summarized in Fig. 11.4 and Table 11.1. In contrast to the results obtained in our study about the NMDA effects on orexin neuronal activation, in a recent report, microinjections of 1 or 10 mM NMDA into the perifornical area of the lateral hypothalamus did not significantly affect the percentage of c-Fos-positive orexin neurons (Li *et al.*, 2011). The same study, however, is in agreement with our data that AMPA injections significantly increased the number of activated orexin neurons.

All these studies discussed above strongly suggest that functional ionotropic glutamate receptor channels are present in orexin neurons. It is also plausible to state that the orexin neurons may express all three subgroups of ionotropic glutamate receptors including the subunits of AMPA, kainate, and NMDA receptors.

V. Glutamate Receptor Expression by Orexin Neurons

In order to validate the data discussed in the previous sections, it is important to histologically demonstrate the expression of glutamate receptor subunits in the orexin neurons. Functional glutamate receptors are formed by homomeric or heteromeric combinations of different subunits,

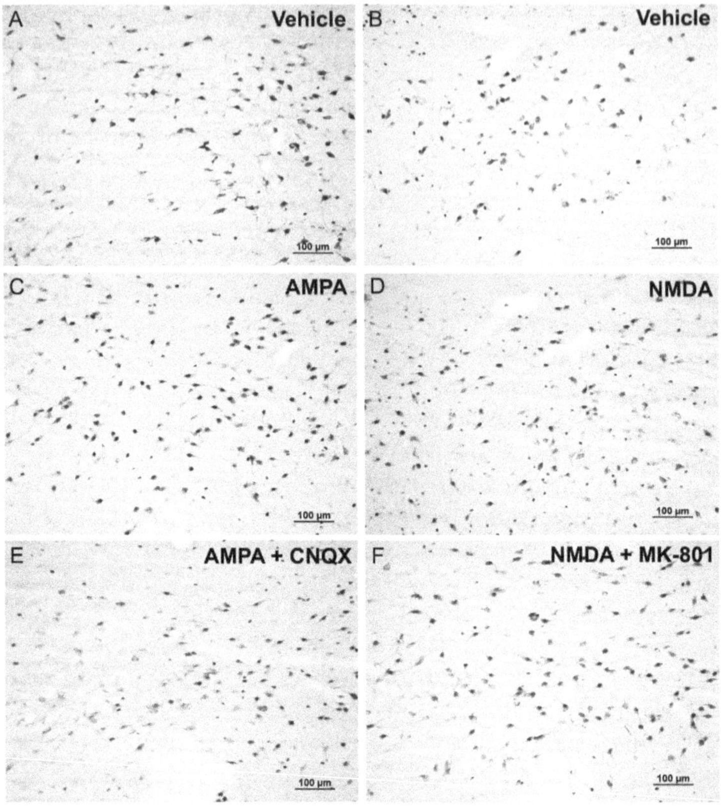

Figure 11.3 Effects of glutamate agonists and antagonists in the activation of orexin neurons. The activated neurons were detected with the black reaction of Ni-DAB in the nuclei localizing the c-Fos immunoreactivity, while orexin neurons possess cytoplasmic staining (gray, actual color is brown). Note that the administration of AMPA (5 mg/kg, ip) or NMDA (100 mg/kg, ip) increased the number of c-Fos-positive orexin neurons (seen in (C) and (D), respectively) when compared to respective vehicle treatments ((A) and (B), respectively). Administration of non-NMDA receptor antagonist CNQX (5 mg/kg, ip) 15 min prior to AMPA diminished the number of activated neurons (seen in (E)). MK-801 administration decreased the number of c-Fos-expressing orexin neurons (seen in (F)), but statistically, this decrease was not significant. Orexin neurons were labeled with a goat anti-orexin A polyclonal antibody (1:1000 dilution, Santa Cruz Biotechnology, USA), while the c-Fos expression was assessed with a rabbit anti-c-Fos polyclonal antibody (1:20,000 dilution, Oncogene, USA). (See Color Insert.)

and the function of the receptor may change accordingly (Howe, 1996). Preliminary data from our laboratory showed that non-NMDA glutamate receptor subunits are expressed in the orexin neurons (Eyigor *et al.*, 2009). Immunoreactivity for kainate receptor subunits was detected in many

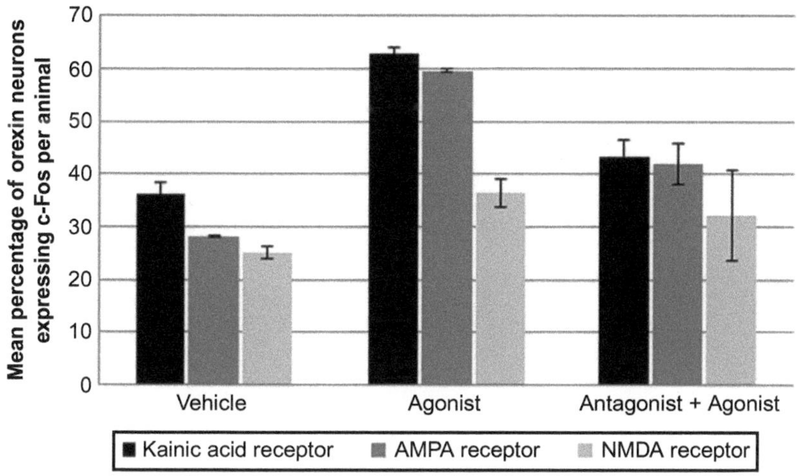

Figure 11.4 Graphical representation of the data seen in Fig. 11.3 and summarized in Table 11.1.

Table 11.1 c-Fos expression in orexin neurons following glutamate receptor agonists and antagonists

Groups	Mean number of orexin neurons counted per animal	Mean number of orexin neurons expressing c-Fos per animal	Mean percentage of orexin neurons expressing c-Fos per animal
Control	534 ± 48.5	196.6 ± 26.2	36.31 ± 2.1*
Kainic acid	473.6 ± 44.6	295.4 ± 25	62.69 ± 1.4
CNQX	683 ± 110.2	309.6 ± 65.8	43.36 ± 3.1*
Control	562 ± 12.1	158.54 ± 10	28.21 ± 0.2*
AMPA	602 ± 35.9	358.73 ± 21.6	59.59 ± 0.3
CNQX	540 ± 61.2	226.3 ± 37.9	41.91 ± 4.0**
Control	367 ± 13.9	92.11 ± 4.9	25.10 ± 1.3**
NMDA	460 ± 30.2	167.85 ± 19.2	36.49 ± 2.7
MK-801	473 ± 23.3	152.35 ± 8.2	32.21 ± 8.7

Data are summarized as the mean ± SEM number or percentage of neurons in the hypothalamus ($n = 5$/each). ANOVA followed by Student–Newman–Keuls test revealed statistical significance for the percentages between agonist and control or antagonist groups ($^{*}p < 0.001$ and $^{**}p < 0.05$ compared to agonist groups).

orexin neurons. Most orexin neurons in the perifornical area were found to be dual labeled with KA2 subunit of the kainate receptors (a representative example is given in Fig. 11.5). Ongoing analyses reveal that orexin neurons also express other subunits of the kainate receptors. In addition to the

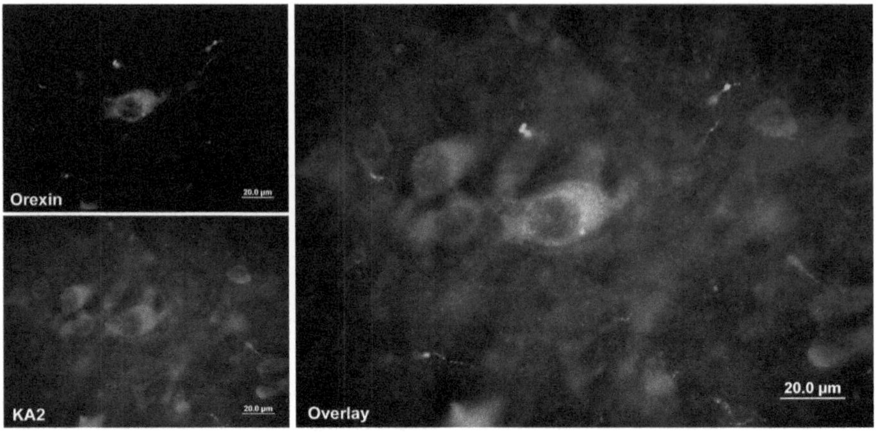

Figure 11.5 Kainate receptor subunit KA2 expression in orexin neurons. Orexin neurons are seen in green (FITC, left top) and KA2-positive neurons are seen in red (Texas red, left bottom). The overlay on the right shows that the KA2 immunoreactivity is colocalized in the orexin-immunoreactive neuron (yellow color). Note that there are other KA2-positive neurons in the vicinity which lack the immunoreaction for orexin A. Orexin neurons were labeled with a goat anti-orexin A polyclonal antibody (1:500 dilution, Santa Cruz Biotechnology), while the KA2 subunit was labeled with a rabbit anti-KA2 polyclonal antibody (1:2000 dilution, Eyigor and Jennes, 2000). (See Color Insert.)

kainate receptor subunits, dual immunofluorescence experiments showed that the orexinergic neurons express GluR1 and GluR2 subunits of the AMPA receptors (unpublished data, Eyigor, Minbay). Although these results need quantification, for the first time, we were able to histologically confirm the existence of glutamate receptors in the orexin neurons.

VI. Conclusion

There is substantial evidence in the literature that glutamate regulates various functions of the orexin neurons. Although it is less studied when compared to the other neurotransmitter systems, glutamate is now known to maintain one of the primary excitatory inputs on the orexinergic system. The studies in the literature suggest that glutamatergic transmission mediates the orexinergic modulation of sleep as well as the feeding behavior. Reports from different laboratories discussed in this chapter, including our own data, revealed that the ionotropic glutamate receptors take part in the regulation of orexin neurons. Both NMDA and non-NMDA receptor activation are crucial for glutamate to affect orexin neurons, and the presence of the glutamatergic synapses on these neurons suggests a possible direct mechanism. Although the findings in the literature support the idea that orexin neurons express functional glutamate receptors and glutamate binds and activates these receptors in a direct fashion, there is also a possibility of an indirect mechanism involving glutamate-receptive interneurons in the vicinity of the orexin neurons. The glutamatergic signals may activate these interneurons which in turn activate orexin neurons using different neurotransmitters. Direct or indirect effects of glutamate on the orexin neurons are clear, and these effects have the potential to initiate the orexinergic modulation in the central nervous system. It is also important to deeper analyze the differential effects of the different glutamate receptors as well as the different subunit combinations in regulating the diverse functions of orexin neurons. Ongoing studies in our laboratory would reveal the differential expression of glutamate receptor subunits in orexin neurons. Future studies are needed to understand the influences of different central nervous system areas, which send glutamatergic axon terminals to the lateral hypothalamus and affect the functions of the orexin neurons.

ACKNOWLEDGMENT

This work was supported by the Scientific and Technological Research Council of Turkey (TUBITAK) through a "Career" Grant (104S286-SBAG-K-74 to O. E.).

REFERENCES

Abrahamson, E. E., Leak, R. K., and Moore, R. Y. (2001). The suprachiasmatic nucleus projects to posterior hypothalamic arousal systems. *Neuroreport* **12,** 435–440.

Alberto, C. O., and Hirasawa, M. (2010). AMPA receptor-mediated miniature EPSCs have heterogeneous time courses in orexin neurons. *Biochem. Biophys. Res. Commun.* **400,** 707–712.

Bora, I., Taskapilioglu, O., Eyigor, O., Kurt, M. A., and Temel, S. (2004). Changing of c-fos levels according to age and time after status epilepticus induced by kainic acid in a rat temporal lobe epilepsy model. *Eur. J. Neurol.* **11,** 88–89.

Collin, M., Backberg, M., Ovesjo, M. L., Fisone, G., Edwards, R. H., Fujiyama, F., and Meister, B. (2003). Plasma membrane and vesicular glutamate transporter mRNAs/ proteins in hypothalamic neurons that regulate body weight. *Eur. J. Neurosci.* **18,** 1265–1278.

de Lecea, L., Kilduff, T. S., Peyron, C., Gao, X., Foye, P. E., Danielson, P. E., Fukuhara, C., Battenberg, E. L., Gautvik, V. T., Bartlett, F. S., Frankel, W. N., Van Den Pol, A. N., *et al.* (1998). The hypocretins: Hypothalamus-specific peptides with neuroexcitatory activity. *Proc. Natl. Acad. Sci. U.S.A.* **95,** 322–327.

Eyigor, O., and Jennes, L. (2000). Kainate receptor subunit-positive gonadotropin-releasing hormone neurons express c-Fos during the steroid-induced luteinizing hormone surge in the female rat. *Endocrinology* **141,** 779–786.

Eyigor, O., Centers, A. P., and Jennes, L. (2001). Distribution of ionotropic glutamate receptor subunit mRNAs in the rat hypothalamus. *J. Comp. Neurol.* **434,** 101–124.

Eyigor, O., Minbay, Z., Cavusoglu, I., and Jennes, L. (2005). Localization of kainate receptor subunit GluR5-immunoreactive cells in the rat hypothalamus. *Brain Res. Mol. Brain Res.* **136,** 38–44.

Eyigor, O., Minbay, F. Z., Cavusoglu, I., and Tosun, F. (2009). Immunohistochemical identification of the presence of glutamatergic innervation on hypothalamic neuroendocrine neurons. *Turkish J. Neurol.* **15**(Suppl. 1), 159–160.

Eyigor, O., Minbay, Z., and Cavusoglu, I. (2010). Activation of orexin neurons through non-NMDA glutamate receptors evidenced by c-Fos immunohistochemistry. *Endocrine* **37,** 167–172.

Eyigor, O., Coskun, C., Cavun, S., and Savci, V. (2012). Intravenous CDP-choline activates neurons in supraoptic and paraventricular nuclei and induces hormone secretion. *Brain Res. Bull.* **87,** 286–294.

Gannon, R. L., and Rea, M. A. (1993). Glutamate receptor immunoreactivity in the rat suprachiasmatic nucleus. *Brain Res.* **622,** 337–342.

Ginsberg, S. D., Price, D. L., Blackstone, C. D., Huganir, R. L., and Martin, L. J. (1995). Non-NMDA glutamate receptors are present throughout the primate hypothalamus. *J. Comp. Neurol.* **353,** 539–552.

Henny, P., and Jones, B. E. (2006). Innervation of orexin/hypocretin neurons by GABAergic, glutamatergic or cholinergic basal forebrain terminals evidenced by immunostaining for presynaptic vesicular transporter and postsynaptic scaffolding proteins. *J. Comp. Neurol.* **499,** 645–661.

Herzog, E., Gilchrist, J., Gras, C., Muzerelle, A., Ravassard, P., Giros, B., Gaspar, P., and El Mestikawy, S. (2004). Localization of VGLUT3, the vesicular glutamate transporter type 3, in the rat brain. *Neuroscience* **123,** 983–1002.

Hettes, S. R., Gonzaga, W. J., Heyming, T. W., Nguyen, J. K., Perez, S., and Stanley, B. G. (2010). Stimulation of lateral hypothalamic AMPA receptors may induce feeding in rats. *Brain Res.* **1346,** 112–120.

Hoffman, G. E., Smith, M. S., and Verbalis, J. G. (1993). c-Fos and related immediate early gene products as markers of activity in neuroendocrine systems. *Front. Neuroendocrinol.* **14,** 173–213.

Horvath, T. L., and Gao, X. B. (2005). Input organization and plasticity of hypocretin neurons: Possible clues to obesity's association with insomnia. *Cell Metab.* **1,** 279–286.

Howe, J. R. (1996). Homomeric and heteromeric ion channels formed from the kainate-type subunits GluR6 and KA2 have very small, but different, unitary conductances. *J. Neurophysiol.* **76,** 510–519.

Khan, A. M., Curras, M. C., Dao, J., Jamal, F. A., Turkowski, C. A., Goel, R. K., Gillard, E. R., Wolfsohn, S. D., and Stanley, B. G. (1999). Lateral hypothalamic NMDA receptor subunits NR2A and/or NR2B mediate eating: Immunochemical/behavioral evidence. *Am. J. Physiol. Regul. Integr. Comp. Physiol.* **276,** R880–R891.

Li, Y., Gao, X. B., Sakurai, T., and Van den Pol, A. N. (2002). Hypocretin/orexin excites hypocretin neurons via a local glutamate neuron—A potential mechanism for orchestrating the hypothalamic arousal system. *Neuron* **36,** 1169–1181.

Li, F. W., Deurveilher, S., and Semba, K. (2011). Behavioural and neuronal activation after microinjections of AMPA and NMDA into the perifornical lateral hypothalamus in rats. *Behav. Brain Res.* **224,** 376–386.

Liguz-Lecznar, M., and Skangiel-Kramska, J. (2007). Vesicular glutamate transporters (VGLUTs): The three musketeers of glutamatergic system. *Acta Neurobiol. Exp. (Wars)* **67,** 207–218.

Lin, W., McKinney, K., Liu, L., Lakhlani, S., and Jennes, L. (2003). Distribution of vesicular glutamate transporter-2 messenger ribonucleic acid and protein in the septum-hypothalamus of the rat. *Endocrinology* **144,** 662–670.

Maragos, W. F., Penney, J. B., and Young, A. B. (1988). Anatomic correlation of Nmda and H-3-Tcp-labeled receptors in rat-brain. *J. Neurosci.* **8,** 493–501.

Martin, L. J., Blackstone, C. D., Levey, A. I., Huganir, R. L., and Price, D. L. (1993). AMPA glutamate receptor subunits are differentially distributed in rat brain. *Neuroscience* **53,** 327–358.

Meeker, R. B., Greenwood, R. S., and Hayward, J. N. (1994). Glutamate receptors in the rat hypothalamus and pituitary. *Endocrinology* **134,** 621–629.

Minbay, F. Z., Eyigor, O., and Cavusoglu, I. (2006). Kainic acid activates oxytocinergic neurons through non-NMDA glutamate receptors. *Int. J. Neurosci.* **116,** 587–600.

Ohno, K., and Sakurai, T. (2008). Orexin neuronal circuitry: Role in the regulation of sleep and wakefulness. *Front. Neuroendocrinol.* **29,** 70–87.

Pak, C. W., and Curras-Collazo, M. C. (2002). Expression and plasticity of glutamate receptors in the supraoptic nucleus of the hypothalamus. *Microsc. Res. Tech.* **56,** 92–100.

Petralia, R. S., and Wenthold, R. J. (1992). Light and electron immunocytochemical localization of AMPA-selective glutamate receptors in the rat brain. *J. Comp. Neurol.* **318,** 329–354.

Petralia, R. S., and Wenthold, R. J. (1996). Types of excitatory amino acid receptors and their localization in nervous system and hypothalamus. *In* "Excitatory Amino Acids: Their Role in Neuroendocrine Function," (D. W. Brann and V. B. Mahesh, Eds.), pp. 55–101. CRC Press, Boca Raton.

Petralia, R. S., Wang, Y. X., and Wenthold, R. J. (1994a). Histological and ultrastructural localization of the kainate receptor subunits, KA2 and GluR6/7, in the rat nervous system using selective antipeptide antibodies. *J. Comp. Neurol.* **349,** 85–110.

Petralia, R. S., Yokotani, N., and Wenthold, R. J. (1994b). Light and electron microscope distribution of the NMDA receptor subunit NMDAR1 in the rat nervous system using a selective anti-peptide antibody. *J. Neurosci.* **14,** 667–696.

Rosin, D. L., Weston, M. C., Sevigny, C. P., Stornetta, R. L., and Guyenet, P. G. (2003). Hypothalamic orexin (hypocretin) neurons express vesicular glutamate transporters VGLUT1 or VGLUT2. *J. Comp. Neurol.* **465,** 593–603.

Sakurai, T. (2007). The neural circuit of orexin (hypocretin): Maintaining sleep and wakefulness. *Nat. Rev. Neurosci.* **8,** 171–181.

Sakurai, T., and Mieda, M. (2011). Connectomics of orexin-producing neurons: Interface of systems of emotion, energy homeostasis and arousal. *Trends Pharmacol. Sci.* **32,** 451–462.

Sakurai, T., Amemiya, A., Ishii, M., Matsuzaki, I., Chemelli, R. M., Tanaka, H., Williams, S. C., Richardson, J. A., Kozlowski, G. P., Wilson, S., Arch, J. R. S., Buckingham, R. E., *et al.* (1998). Orexins and orexin receptors: A family of hypothalamic neuropeptides and G protein-coupled receptors that regulate feeding behavior. *Cell* **92,** 573–585.

Sakurai, T., Nagata, R., Yamanaka, A., Kawamura, H., Tsujino, N., Muraki, Y., Kageyama, H., Kunita, S., Takahashi, S., Goto, K., Koyama, Y., Shioda, S., *et al.* (2005). Input of orexin/hypocretin by a genetically encoded neurons revealed tracer in mice. *Neuron* **46,** 297–308.

Takamori, S., Rhee, J. S., Rosenmund, C., and Jahn, R. (2000). Identification of a vesicular glutamate transporter that defines a glutamatergic phenotype in neurons. *Nature* **407,** 189–194.

Torrealba, F., Yanagisawa, M., and Saper, C. B. (2003). Colocalization of orexin a and glutamate immunoreactivity in axon terminals in the tuberomammillary nucleus in rats. *Neuroscience* **119,** 1033–1044.

Van den Pol, A. N., and Trombley, P. Q. (1993). Glutamate neurons in hypothalamus regulate excitatory transmission. *J. Neurosci.* **13,** 2829–2836.

Van den Pol, A. N., Wuarin, J.-P., and Dudek, F. E. (1990). Glutamate, the dominant excitatory transmitter in neuroendocrine regulation. *Science* **250,** 1276–1278.

Yamanaka, A. (2006). Afferent system of orexin neurons. *In* "The Orexin/Hypocretin System: Physiology and Pathophysiology," (S. Nishino and T. Sakurai, Eds.), pp. 61–70. Humana Press, Totowa.

Yamanaka, A., Muraki, Y., Tsujino, N., Goto, K., and Sakurai, T. (2003). Regulation of orexin neurons by the monoaminergic and cholinergic systems. *Biochem. Biophys. Res. Commun.* **303,** 120–129.

Yoshida, K., McCormack, S., Espana, R. A., Crocker, A., and Scammell, T. E. (2006). Afferents to the orexin neurons of the rat brain. *J. Comp. Neurol.* **494,** 845–861.

Ziegler, D. R., Cullinan, W. E., and Herman, J. P. (2002). Distribution of vesicular glutamate transporter mRNA in rat hypothalamus. *J. Comp. Neurol.* **448,** 217–229.

CHAPTER TWELVE

Serotonin Conflict in Sleep–Feeding

Katsunori Nonogaki

Contents

Abstract

Short sleep duration has been suggested to be a risk factor for weight gain and adiposity. Serotonin (5-HT) substantially contributes to the regulation of sleep and feeding behavior. Although 5-HT predominately promotes waking and satiety, the effects of 5-HT depend on 5-HT receptor function. The 5-HT1A,

Department of Lifestyle Medicine, Translational Research Center, Tohoku University Hospital, Sendai, Miyagi, Japan

Vitamins and Hormones, Volume 89
ISSN 0083-6729, http://dx.doi.org/10.1016/B978-0-12-394623-2.00012-3

5-HT1B, 5-HT2A, 5-HT2C, 5-HT6, and 5-HT7 receptors reportedly contribute to sleep–waking regulation, whereas the 5-HT1B and 5-HT2C receptors contribute to the regulation of satiety. The 5-HT1B and 2C receptors may therefore be involved in the regulation of sleep–feeding.

In genetic studies, 5-HT1B receptor mutant mice display greater amounts of rapid eye movement sleep (REMS) than wild-type mice, while displaying no effects on waking or slow wave sleep (SWS). On the other hand, 5-HT2C receptor mutant mice exhibit increased wakefulness and decreased SWS, without any effect on REMS. Moreover, the 5-HT2C receptor mutants display leptin-independent hyperphagia, leading to a middle-aged onset of obesity, whereas 5-HT1B receptor mutants do not display any effect on food intake. Thus, the genetic deletion of 5-HT2C receptors results in sleep loss-associated hyperphagia, leading to the late onset of obesity. This is a quite different pattern of sleep–feeding behavior than is observed in disturbed leptin signaling, which displays an increase in sleep-associated hyperphagia.

In pharmacologic studies, 5-HT1B and 5-HT2C receptors upregulate wakefulness and downregulate SWS, REMS, and food intake. These findings suggest that 5-HT1B/2C receptor stimulation induces sleep loss-associated anorexia. Thus, the central 5-HT regulation of sleep–feeding can be dissociated. Functional hypothalamic proopiomelanocortin and orexin activities may contribute to the dissociated 5-HT regulation.

I. Introduction

A shortened duration of sleep is suggested to be a risk factor for weight gain in adults and children (Cappuccio *et al.*, 2008; Horne, 2011; Mozaffarian *et al.*, 2011; Patel and Hu, 2008; Spiegel *et al.*, 2009; St-Onge *et al.*, 2011). People with a short sleep duration of <7 h/night have a greater odds of being obese than do those who sleep 7–8 h/night (Patel and Hu, 2008). A sleep period of less than 6 h or more than 8 h is associated with weight gain (Mozaffarian *et al.*, 2011). A reduction in sleep of 4 h/night for five consecutive nights increases energy intake associated with increased fat intake in normal weight individuals, while having no effect on energy expenditure, suggesting that sleep loss-induced increases in energy intake contribute to the development of sleep loss-associated obesity (St-Onge *et al.*, 2011).

Clinical studies of reduced sleep in healthy young men have shown that certain hormones involved in appetite regulation, such as leptin and ghrelin, are altered by changes in sleep duration (Schmid *et al.*, 2008; Spiegel *et al.*, 2004). Sleep curtailment in healthy young men is associated with decreased leptin levels and elevated ghrelin levels that may in turn lead to increased hunger and appetite (Spiegel *et al.*, 2004). Thus, reduced sleep duration may lead to a hormonal state that is conducive to overeating. Many neurochemical systems interact to generate sleep and feeding, so it is important to identify specific factors related to consequent behaviors.

Serotonin (5-HT) activity is highest during wakefulness, decreases during non-rapid eye movement sleep (NREMS), and almost ceases during rapid eye movement sleep (REMS) (Portas *et al.*, 2000). The central 5-HT system has been implicated in the regulation of sleep–feeding behavior via 5-HT receptors. In genetic and pharmacologic studies, 5-HT1A, 5-HT1B, 5-HT2A, 5-HT2C, 5-HT6, and 5-HT7 receptors have been shown to be partially involved in the 5-HT regulation of sleep (Monti, 2010, 2011), whereas the 5-HT1B and 5-HT2C receptors contribute to the regulation of feeding (Nonogaki, 2008; Nonogaki *et al.*, 2006a, 2007b; Tecott, 2007).

In this review, we consider the potential role of 5-HT receptors, especially the 5-HT2C receptors, in the regulation of sleep–feeding behavior based on recent pharmacologic and genetic studies.

II. Brain Areas Involved in the Regulation of Sleep

Electroencephalograms have indicated the existence of three major states of behavior: wakefulness, REMS, and NREMS. NREMS is further divided into stages 1–4. Slow wave sleep (SWS) is the deepest stage of sleep, and this occurs during stages 3 and 4 of NREMS. Wakefulness is promoted by neurons in the pons, midbrain, and posterior hypothalamus. Most of these ascending arousal systems diffusely activate the cortex and other forebrain targets. NREMS is mainly driven by neurons in the preoptic area that inhibit the ascending arousal, while REMS is regulated primarily by neurons in the pons, with additional influence exerted by the hypothalamus. Mutual inhibition between these wake- and sleep-regulating regions likely helps generate both full wakefulness and sleep, along with rapid transitions between these states (Sehgal and Mignot, 2011).

III. The Distribution of the 5-HT Receptors Involved in Regulation of Sleep and Feeding

In studies using microinjections of 5-HT, 5-HT receptor agonists or antagonists into brain sites, the paraventricular nucleus (PVN), the ventromedial (VMN) and dorsomedial nuclei (DMN) have been shown to be involved in 5-HT regulation of satiety (Hutson *et al.*, 1988; Leibowitz *et al.*, 1990; Paez and Leibowitz, 1993; Pasqualetti *et al.*, 1999; Schwartz *et al.*, 1989; Shor-Posner *et al.*, 1986), whereas the dorsal raphe nucleus (DRN), laterodorsal tegmental nucleus, and lateral hypothalamus (LH) are involved in sleep-waking regulation. Subsets of neurons in the arcuate nucleus (ARC) project to the PVN, VMN, LH, and spinal cord sympathetic preganglionic neurons (Cowley *et al.*, 2001; Saper and Loewy, 1980). The neural mechanisms of the central 5-HT influence on sleep and feeding have been highlighted by the discovery of at least 14 functionally diverse subtypes of 5-HT receptors (Hoyer *et al.*, 1994). Studies using gene knockout technology and pharmacological agents with enhanced 5-HT receptor subtype specificity have focused particular attention on the 5-HT2C and 1B receptors as key mediators of 5-HT-induced satiety and wakefulness (Monti, 2010, 2011; Nonogaki, 2008; Nonogaki *et al.*, 2006a,b; Tecott, 2007), although other 5-HT receptor subtypes might also influence sleep–feeding regulation.

The 5-HT2C receptors are widely expressed throughout the neuroaxis and the central nervous system (CNS) (Baxter *et al.*, 1995; Conn *et al.*, 1986; Julius *et al.*, 1988; Wright *et al.*, 1995; Yagaloff and Hartig, 1985). In addition, 5-HT2C receptor expression is found in the white adipose tissue of mice, and leptin downregulates this expression in white adipose tissue but not in the hypothalamus (Nonogaki *et al.*, 2007a). Although 5-HT2C receptor-mediated actions are best characterized in the ARC, 5HT2C receptor transcripts are widely expressed in hypothalamic regions which are especially implicated in appetite and energy balance, including the ARC, PVN, VMN, DMN, and LH (Hoffman and Mezey, 1989; Pasqualetti *et al.*, 1999; Wright *et al.*, 1995). These structures all receive 5-HTergic innervations from the mesencephalic dorsal and/or median raphe nuclei (Petrov *et al.*, 1992; Steinbusch and Nieuwenhuys, 1981).

In addition to 5-HT2C receptors, multiple 5-HT receptor subtypes, including the 5-HT1A receptor, 5-HT1B receptor, 5-HT2A receptor, 5-HT6 receptor, and 5-HT7 receptor, are expressed in the hypothalamic regions implicated in sleep and feeding regulation (Baxter *et al.*, 1995; Bruinvels *et al.*, 1994; Hedlund and Sutcliffe, 2004). Moreover, it should be noted that the 5-HT receptor subtypes, such as the 5-HT1B and 5-HT2C receptors, are coexpressed in certain brainstem locations implicated in ingestion, raising the possibility that their complementary influence on feeding circuits may not be restricted to the hypothalamus (Tecott, 2007).

IV. Role of 5-HT2C Receptors in Sleep–Feeding Behavior

A. Genetic deletion of 5-HT2C receptors

Two- to three-month-old 5-HT2C receptor mutant mice display a significant increase in wakefulness and a reduction of SWS, while exhibiting no effects on REMS (Frank *et al.*, 2002). Despite normal body weight, 5-HT2C receptor mutants display leptin-independent hyperphagia and hyperactivity at

2–3 months of age (Nonogaki *et al.*, 1998, 2003). The changes in feeding behavior are not associated with changes in the plasma leptin, insulin, or corticosterone levels, nor are they associated with glucose or lipid metabolism (Nonogaki *et al.*, 1998). Chronic hyperphagia and hyperactivity lead to a middle age onset of obesity and secondary insulin resistance after 6 months of age. A high-fat diet enhances the development of obesity and insulin resistance, leading to type 2 diabetes in 5-HT2C receptor mutants (Nonogaki *et al.*, 1998). These findings suggest a sleep loss-associated hyperphagia, leading to a late onset of obesity in animals with a genetic ablation of 5-HT2C receptors. This is a quite different behavioral pattern than disturbed leptin signaling, which displays an increase in sleep-associated hyperphagia (Laposky *et al.*, 2006, 2008).

B. Pharmacologic studies

5-HT2C receptors are located on postsynaptic neurons (Barnes and Sharp, 1999). Systemic administration of the 5-HT2C/1B receptor agonist mCPP or the selective 5-HT2C receptor agonist RO 60-0175 increases wakefulness and reduces SWS in rats (Katsuda *et al.*, 1993; Martin *et al.*, 1998). Systemic administration of a selective 5-HT2C receptor antagonist, SB243213, or 5-HT2C receptor blockades, such as cyproheptadine, ritanserin, ketanserin, olanzapine, mirtazapine, and agomelatine, increases SWS and suppresses REMS in rats and humans (Aslan *et al.*, 2002; Sharpley *et al.*, 2000; Smith *et al.*, 2002; Solomon *et al.*, 1989). These pharmacologic findings suggest that 5-HT2C receptors downregulate SWS and upregulate wakefulness.

On the other hand, systemic administration of 5-HT1B/2C receptor agonist, mCPP, or selective 5-HT2C receptor agonists, such as RO 60-0175 and lorcaserin, decreases food intake (Fletcher *et al.*, 2009; Thomsen *et al.*, 2008). The anorexic effects of mCPP are found in both db/db mice with a leptin receptor mutation and A^y mice (Nonogaki *et al.*, 2006a, 2008).

These findings suggest that the pharmacologic stimulation of 5-HT2C receptors-induced anorexia does not result from increased sleep but, rather, is associated with sleep loss. In pharmacologic studies, 5-HT2C receptors may downregulate both food intake and sleep, especially in SWS. Thus, there is a discrepancy between the genetic and pharmacologic study results.

C. The 5-HT2C receptor and the POMC–orexin network

Although the reason for the discrepancy between the pharmacologic and genetic knockout studies is unclear, there is a hypothesis that the greater amount of wakefulness in 5-HT2C receptor-deficient mice could be related to an increase in catecholaminergic neurotransmission, mainly in the noradrenergic and the dopaminergic systems (Frank *et al.*, 2002). 5-HT2C receptors participate in the release of dopamine and noradrenaline, which both promote wakefulness (Fink and Göthert, 2007).

Another hypothesis for this discrepancy may result from a 5-HT2C receptor deletion-induced reduction in proopiomelanocortin (POMC) activity. POMC neurons in the arcuate nuclei of the hypothalamus are suggested to be the downstream target of 5-HT2C receptor signaling (Heisler *et al.*, 2002; Xu *et al.*, 2008). The hypothalamic distribution of 5-HT2C receptors on POMC neurons indicates that 5-HT2C receptors and the melanocortin (MC) pathway might interact in the regulation of feeding. mCPP activates POMC neurons that express 5-HT2C receptors in the ARC *in vitro* (Heisler *et al.*, 2002). Consistent with this hypothesis, 5-HT2C receptor agonists activate α-MSH-containing neurons (Heisler *et al.*, 2002).

Intracerebroventricular (icv) injection of high-dose α-MSH, a POMC-derived peptide, increases wakefulness and reduces REMS and SWS in a dose-dependent manner (Opp *et al.*, 1988). Increased POMC neuronal activity may therefore mediate the stimulation of 5-HT2C receptor-induced increases in wakefulness as well as decreases in SWS and food intake. Icv injection of POMC siRNA oligonucleotide increases daily food consumption, which is attenuated by icv injection of orexin siRNA oligonucleotide. These findings suggest that POMC downregulates central orexin activity (Nonogaki and Kaji, 2010).

Orexin is well known as an orexigenic peptide which promotes wakefulness and decreases SWS and REMS (Ohno and Sakurai, 2008; Tsujino and Sakurai, 2009). Orexin deficiency induces narcolepsy in humans and other mammalian species (Sakurai and Mieda, 2011). Hyperphagia in 5-HT2C receptor mutants is associated with decreased expression of the hypothalamic POMC gene (Nonogaki *et al.*, 2009). Compensatory increased functional orexin activity may therefore contribute to the increases in wakefulness and decreases in SWS in the 5-HT2C receptor mutants.

The anorexic effects of 5-HT2C receptor stimulation require an increase in the hypothalamic POMC activity and functional orexin activity (Nonogaki *et al.*, 2011) that promote wakefulness and decrease SWS. On the other hand, 5-HT2C receptor mutants induce hyperphagia associated with decreases in hypothalamic POMC expression (Nonogaki *et al.*, 2009), which in turn increases hypothalamic orexin activity (Nonogaki and Kaji, 2010). Orexin potentially promotes wakefulness and decreases SWS. Thus, the balance of functional POMC and orexin neuronal activities may play a crucial role in the 5-HT2C receptor-mediated regulation of sleep–feeding.

D. The 5-HT2C receptor and leptin signaling

Although both 5-HT2C and leptin receptors are expressed in the hypothalamic regions that regulate energy balance (Baxter *et al.*, 1995; Conn *et al.*, 1986; Friedman, 2004; Friedman and Halaas, 1998; Hoffman and Mezey, 1989; Julius *et al.*, 1988; Pasqualetti *et al.*, 1999; Wright *et al.*, 1995; Yagaloff and Hartig, 1985), the pattern of physiological changes in the receptor mutants is quite different (Friedman, 2004; Friedman and Halaas, 1998; Nonogaki *et al.*, 1998). 5-HT2CR mutant mice exhibit a primary deficit in the regulation of food consumption rather than in the neural regulation of carbohydrate or fat metabolism (Nonogaki *et al.*, 1998).

Moreover, administration of mCPP suppresses food intake in db/db mice which have leptin receptor deficiency (Nonogaki *et al.*, 2008), whereas the administration of leptin suppressed food intake in young adult 5-HT2C receptor-deficient mice as well as in age-matched wild-type mice (Nonogaki *et al.*, 1998). From such evidence, the leptin receptor and 5-HT2CR signaling downregulate food intake via independent pathways.

In contrast, mice (ob/ob) in which the leptin gene was disrupted, along with mice (db/db) with genetic disturbances of leptin receptor signaling, exhibit hyperphagia, hyperinsulinemia, and decreased sympathetic outflow, leading to obesity early in life (Friedman, 2004; Friedman and Halaas, 1998). In addition, ob/ob mice and db/db mice display an increase in sleep time; increased NREMS (SWS) and decreased REMS (Laposky *et al.*, 2006, 2008). Thus, ob/ob and db/db mice display an increase in sleep-associated hyperphagia that is also quite different than the 5-HT2C receptor mutants, which display sleep loss-associated hyperphagia.

Decreases in hypothalamic orexin expression in addition to the decreases in hypothalamic POMC expression are found in ob/ob and db/db mice (Stricker-Krongrad *et al.*, 2002; Yamamoto *et al.*, 1999). The decreased orexin activity may contribute to the altered sleep–waking cycle in the ob/ob and db/db mice (Fig. 12.1).

E. GLP-1 and 5-HT2C receptors

Glucagon-like peptide 1 (GLP-1) is an incretin hormone released from intestinal L-cells in response to nutrient ingestion (Holst, 2007). GLP-1 potentiates glucose-dependent insulin secretion by activating the GLP-1 receptor (GLP-1R) expressed on pancreatic islet β-cells (Holst, 2007). GLP-1R is also expressed in the CNS, and the extrapancreatic functions of GLP-1 include its effects on the hypothalamus that promote satiety (Holst, 2007; Lovshin and Drucker, 2009).

The 5-HT2C receptor has a major role in the leptin-independent regulation of energy intake (Nonogaki *et al.*, 1998). Systemic administration of GLP-1 suppresses food intake in wild-type mice, whereas the anorexic effects are blunted in 5-HT2C receptor mutant mice and also heterogeneous melanocortin-4 receptor mutants (Asarian, 2009; Nonogaki *et al.*, 2011). These findings suggest that GLP-1 is a stimulator of central 5-HT2C receptors-mediated MC pathways, which can alter sleep–feeding behavior.

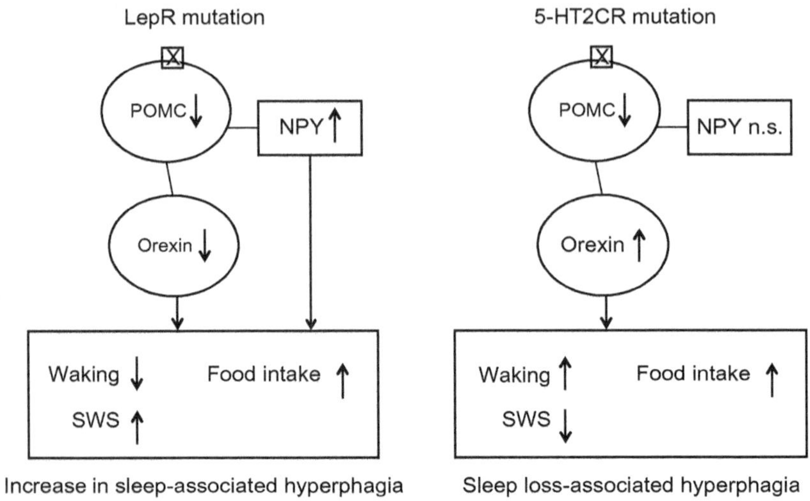

Figure 12.1 Sleep change-associated hyperphagia in db/db mice and 5-HT2C receptor mutants. POMC, proopiomelanocortin; NPY, neuropeptide Y; ↑, increase; ↓, decrease.

V. 5-HT Receptors Other than 5-HT2C Receptors

A. Effects of genetic deletion of 5-HT receptors other than the 5-HT2C receptor on sleep–feeding

5-HT1A and 5-HT1B receptor mutants display increases in REMS, while displaying no effects on wakefulness and SWS (Boutrel *et al.*, 1999, 2002). 5-HT2A receptor mutants as well as 5-HT2C receptor mutants display an increase in wakefulness and a decrease in SWS, while exhibiting no effects on REMS (Popa *et al.*, 2005). 5-HT7 receptor mutants exhibit a reduction in REMS compared with wild-type mice, mainly during the light period (Hedlund *et al.*, 2005), whereas there are no genotypic differences in wakefulness or SWS duration. On the other hand, genetic ablation of the 5-HT1A, 5-HT1B, 5-HT2A, or 5-HT7 receptor has no effect on feeding behavior (Bouwknecht *et al.*, 2001; Tecott, 2007) (Table 12.1).

VI. Pharmacologic Studies of 5-HT Receptors Other than the 5-HT2C Receptor

A. 5-HT1B receptor agonists and antagonists

5-HT1B receptors are located on presynaptic neurons and stimulate 5-HT release, whereas 5-HT2C receptors are located on postsynaptic neurons (Barnes and Sharp, 1999). The 5-HT1B receptor is linked to the inhibition

Table 12.1 Sleep and feeding behavior in 5-HT receptor mutant mice

Mutant mice	Wakefulness	SWS	REMS	Food intake
5-HT1AR	n.s.	n.s.	+	n.s.
5-HT1BR	n.s.	n.s.	+	n.s.
5-HT2CR	+	−	n.s.	+
5-HT2AR	+	−	n.s.	n.s.
5-HT6R	?	?	?	n.s.
5-HT7R	n.s.	n.s.	−	n.s.

+, increase; −, decrease; ?, unknown; n.s., no significant change.
REMS, rapid eye movement sleep; NREMS, non-REM sleep; SWS, slow wave sleep.

of adenylate cyclase and was initially proposed to be located at presynaptic (5-HT axon terminals) and postsynaptic (outside the DRN) sites. The 5-HT1B receptor has also been characterized in the ventromedial DRN, where it is expressed by non-5-HT cells (Heisler *et al.*, 2006).

Systemic administration of the selective 5-HT1B receptor agonists CGS 120668 and CP-94253 significantly increases wakefulness and reduces REMS and SWS in rats (Bjorvatn and Ursin, 1994; Monti *et al.*, 1995). Systemic administration of the 5-HT1B receptor antagonist GR 125939 increases REMS over a period of 4 h (Boutrel *et al.*, 1999). These findings suggest that the 5-HT1B receptor upregulates wakefulness and downregulates SWS and REMS.

mCPP and fenfluramine-induced anorexic effects are attenuated in 5-HT1B receptor-deficient mice (Lee *et al.*, 2004; Lucas *et al.*, 1998). In addition, the administration of a selective 5-HT1B receptor agonist induces appetite-suppressing effects (Halford and Blundell, 1996; Lee and Simansky, 1997). In contrast, 5-HT2C receptor mutant mice are more sensitive to the hypophagia induced by CP 94253, a selective 5-HT1B receptor agonist, than wild-type mice (Nonogaki *et al.*, 2007b). Pharmacological inactivation of 5-HT2C receptors rapidly increases hypothalamic 5-HT1B receptor gene expression, suggesting that 5-HT2C receptors downregulate 5-HT1B receptor gene expression (Nonogaki *et al.*, 2007b) (Fig. 12.2).

These findings suggest that the pharmacologic stimulation of 5-HT1B receptors which induces anorexia does not result from increased sleep but, instead, is associated with sleep loss. Thus, 5-HT1B receptors may downregulate both food intake and sleep, especially in SWS and REMS. These pharmacologic findings, however, are inconsistent with the findings on the genetic ablation of 5-HT1B receptors.

B. The 5-HT1B receptor network

5-HT2C and 5-HT1B receptors display a complementary distribution pattern within the ARC: 5-HT2C receptors are expressed in POMC/cocaine- and amphetamine-related transcript (CART)-expressing neurons,

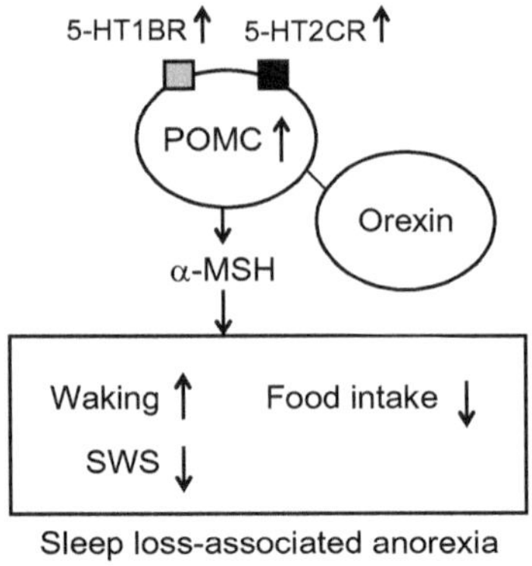

Figure 12.2 Sleep loss-associated anorexia induced by 5-HT2C and 5-HT1B receptor stimulation. POMC, proopiomelanocortin; ↑, increase; ↓, decrease.

whereas 5-HT1B receptors are found in neuropeptide Y (NPY)/Agouti-related peptide (AgRP) neurons (Heisler *et al.*, 2006). Postsynaptic somatodendritic 5-HT1B receptors inhibit NPY/AgRP neuronal activity, while presynaptic 5-HT1B receptors expressed on the axon terminals of these NPY/AgRP neurons suppress the γ-amino butyric acid (GABA)-ergic inhibition of POMC/CART neurons (Heisler *et al.*, 2006).

On the other hand, although it remains to be conclusively proven that 5-HT1B receptors coexist on POMC/CART neurons in the hypothalamus, systemic administration of CP94253, a selective 5-HT1B receptor agonist, rapidly increases hypothalamic POMC and CART gene expression and also decreases hypothalamic orexin gene expression, without altering NPY gene expression (Nonogaki *et al.*, 2007b). The altered expression of hypothalamic neuropeptides is associated with the 5-HT1B receptor agonist-induced feeding suppression (Nonogaki *et al.*, 2007b). This evidence suggests that pharmacologic activation of the 5-HT1B receptor directly activates hypothalamic POMC and CART neurons *in vivo*.

C. The 5-HT1A receptor agonists and antagonists

Systemic injection of flesinoxan, a 5-HT1A receptor agonist, increases wakefulness and reduces SWS and REMS in rats (Monti and Jantos, 2003). Similar effects have been observed following the administration of 8-OH-DPAT, a 5-HT1A receptor agonist, to vehicle-treated and serotonin-depleted animals (Monti *et al.*, 1994). Pretreatment with the mixed β-adrenoceptor and 5-HT1A/1B receptor antagonist (−)-pindolol or *p*-MPPI reversed the effect of 8-OH-DPAT on wakefulness and SWS (Monti *et al.*, 1994; Sørensen *et al.*, 2001).

The findings in these pharmacologic studies suggest that the 5-HT1A receptor upregulates wakefulness and downregulates REMS and SWS.

D. The 5-HT2A receptor antagonists

Systemic administration of selective 5-HT2A receptor antagonists, such as volinanserin and pruvanserin, or the 5-HT2A inverse agonist nelotanserin reduces wakefulness and REMS and increases SWS in rats (Al-Shamma *et al.*, 2010; Morairty *et al.*, 2008). The effects of selective 5-HT2A receptor agonists have not yet been evaluated. These pharmacologic findings suggest that the 5-HT2A receptor upregulates wakefulness and REMS and downregulates SWS. On the other hand, systemic administration of sarpogrelate, a selective 5-HT2A receptor antagonist, suppresses food intake (Nonogaki *et al.*, 2006b).

E. 5-HT6 receptor agonists and antagonists

5-HT6 is a G-protein-coupled receptor, and its primary signal transduction pathway is the stimulation of adenylate cyclase (Ruat *et al.*, 1993). The 5-HT6 receptor is located postsynaptically of 5-HT cells and has been localized in the cerebral cortex, BFB (BNST), limbic system (hippocampus, amygdala), striatum, nucleus accumbens, thalamus, hypothalamus, and mesencephalon of rats and humans (Roberts *et al.*, 2002; Woolley *et al.*, 2004).

The effects of the selective 5-HT6 receptor antagonists on sleep remain uncertain. Systemic administration of selective 5-HT6 receptor antagonists, such as SB-399885 (2.5–10 mg/kg) and RO-4368554 (2.5–10 mg/kg) during the light phase, results in an increase of wakefulness and a reduction of SWS and REMS in rats (Monti and Jantos, 2011). The injection of SB-399885 during the dark period also induced a decrease of REMS (Monti and Jantos, 2011). However, there are reports that systemic administration of RO-4368554 (10 mg/kg) promotes sleep and decreases waking in rats (Morairty *et al.*, 2008). The effects of the genetic ablation of 5-HT6 receptors on sleep have not yet been evaluated, while having no effects on feeding behavior or body weight (Tables 12.2 and 12.3).

VII. Conclusion

5-HT substantially contributes to the regulation of sleep and feeding behavior via 5-HT receptors. Because the results using genetic deletion of 5-HT receptors and those obtained using pharmacologic receptor antagonists and agonists are not consistent, the functions of 5-HT receptors in sleep-waking regulation appear to be highly complex.

Table 12.2 Sleep and feeding behavior in db/db and ob/ob mice, and icv injection of α-MSH

Mutant mice	Wakefulness	NREMS/SWS	REMS	Food intake
db/db (leptin-R)	−	+	−	+
ob/ob (leptin)	−	+	n.s.	+
Icv injection				
α-MSH	+	−	−	−

+, increase; −, decrease; n.s., no significant change.
REMS, rapid eye movement sleep; NREMS, non-REM sleep; SWS, slow wave sleep.

Table 12.3 Effects of systemic administration of selective 5-HT receptor agonists and antagonists on sleep and feeding

5-HTR subtype	Wakefulness	NREMS/SWS	REMS	Food intake
Agonists				
5-HT1AR	+	−	−	n.s.
5-HT1BR	+	−	−	−
5-HT2CR	+	−	−	−
Antagonists				
5-HT2AR	−	+	−	−
5-HT6R	+	−	−	n.s.

+, increase; −, decrease; n.s., no significant change.
REMS, rapid eye movement sleep; NREMS, non-REM sleep; SWS, slow wave sleep.

Pharmacologic studies suggest that 5-HT2C receptors upregulate wakefulness and downregulate SWS. Surprisingly, despite the opposing effects on feeding behavior, 5-HT2C receptor mutants and 5-HT2C receptor agonists display closely similar effects on wakefulness and SWS. The alterations in central neurotransmission induced by 5-HT2C receptor deletion or stimulation may contribute to this discrepancy.

5-HT2C receptor stimulation-induced anorexia requires an increase in the hypothalamic POMC activity and functional orexin activity that promote wakefulness and decrease SWS. On the other hand, genetic deletion of 5-HT2C receptors induces hyperphagia associated with decreases in hypothalamic POMC expression, which in turn increases hypothalamic orexin activity. Orexin potentially promotes wakefulness and decreases SWS. Disturbed leptin signaling observed in db/db mice and ob/ob mice results in an increase in sleep-associated hyperphagia that is associated with decreases in both hypothalamic POMC and orexin activity. Thus, a balancing of functional POMC and orexin neuronal activities may play a crucial role in the 5-HT2C receptor regulation of sleep–feeding behaviors and may be central to an elucidation of the mechanisms by which sleep of short duration is related to obesity.

ACKNOWLEDGMENTS

We thank Ms. Marine Sanuki for her secretary assistance and K. Boru for critical reading of the chapter. This work was supported by a Grant in-Aid for Scientific Research (C2) and Sendai Knowledge Cluster Initiative.

REFERENCES

Al-Shamma, H. A., Anderson, C., Chuang, E., Luthringer, R., Grottick, A. J., Hauser, E., Morgan, M., Shanahan, W., Teegarden, B. R., Thomsen, W. J., and Behan, D. (2010). Nelotanserin, a novel selective human 5-hydroxytryptamine 2A inverse agonist for the treatment of insomnia. *J. Pharmacol. Exp. Ther.* **332,** 281–290.

Asarian, L. (2009). Loss of cholecystokinin and glucagon-like peptide-1-induced satiation in mice lacking serotonin 2C receptors. *Am. J. Physiol. Regul. Integr. Comp. Physiol.* **296,** 51–56.

Aslan, S., Isik, E., and Cosar, B. (2002). The effects of mirtazapine on sleep: A placebo controlled, double-blind study in young healthy volunteers. *Sleep* **25,** 677–679.

Barnes, N. M., and Sharp, T. (1999). A review of central 5-HT receptors and their function. *Neuropharmacology* **38,** 1083–1152.

Baxter, G., Kennett, G., Blaney, F., and Blackburn, T. (1995). 5-HT2 receptor subtypes: A family re-united? *Trends Pharmacol. Sci.* **16,** 105–110.

Bjorvatn, B., and Ursin, R. (1994). Effects of the selective 5-HT1B agonist, CGS 12066B, on sleep/waking stages and EEG power spectrum in rats. *J. Sleep Res.* **3,** 97–105.

Boutrel, B., Franc, B., Hen, R., Hamon, M., and Adrien, J. (1999). Key role of 5-HT1B receptors in the regulation of paradoxical sleep as evidenced in 5-HT1B knock-out mice. *J. Neurosci.* **19,** 3204–3212.

Boutrel, B., Monaca, C., Hen, R., Hamon, M., and Adrien, J. (2002). Involvement of 5-HT1A receptors in homeostatic and stress-induced adaptive regulations of paradoxical sleep: Studies in 5-HT1A knock-out mice. *J. Neurosci.* **22,** 4686–4692.

Bouwknecht, J. A., van der Gugten, J., Hijzen, T. H., Maes, R. A., Hen, R., and Olivier, B. (2001). Male and female 5-HT(1B) receptor knockout mice have higher body weights than wildtypes. *Physiol. Behav.* **74,** 507–516.

Bruinvels, A. T., Landwehrmeyer, B., Gustafson, E. L., Durkin, M. M., Mengod, G., Branchek, T. A., Hoyer, D., and Palacios, J. M. (1994). Localization of 5-HT1B, 5-HT1D alpha, 5-HT1E and 5-HT1F receptor messenger RNA in rodent and primate brain. *Neuropharmacology* **33,** 367–386.

Cappuccio, F. P., Taggart, F. M., Kandala, N. B., Currie, A., Peile, E., Stranges, S., and Miller, M. A. (2008). Meta-analysis of short sleep duration and obesity in children and adults. *Sleep* **31,** 619–626.

Conn, P. J., Sanders-Bush, E., Hoffman, B. J., and Hartig, P. R. (1986). A unique serotonin receptor in choroid plexus is linked to phosphatidylinositol turnover. *Proc. Natl. Acad. Sci. U.S.A.* **83,** 4086–4088.

Cowley, M. A., Smart, J. L., Rubinstein, M., Cerdán, M. G., Diano, S., Horvath, T. L., Cone, R. D., and Low, M. J. (2001). Leptin activates anorexigenic POMC neurons through a neural network in the arcuate nucleus. *Nature* **411,** 480–484.

Fink, K. B., and Göthert, M. (2007). 5-HT receptor regulation of neurotransmitter release. *Pharmacol. Rev.* **59,** 360–417.

Fletcher, P. J., Tampakeras, M., Sinyard, J., Slassi, A., Isaac, M., and Higgins, G. A. (2009). Characterizing the effects of 5-HT(2C) receptor ligands on motor activity and feeding behaviour in 5-HT(2C) receptor knockout mice. *Neuropharmacology* **57,** 259–267.

Frank, M. G., Stryker, M. P., and Tecott, L. H. (2002). Sleep and sleep homeostasis in mice lacking the 5-HT2c receptor. *Neuropsychopharmacology* **27,** 869–873.

Friedman, J. M. (2004). Modern science versus the stigma of obesity. *Nat. Med.* **10,** 563–569.

Friedman, J. M., and Halaas, J. L. (1998). Leptin and the regulation of body weight in mammals. *Nature* **395,** 763–770.

Halford, J. C., and Blundell, J. E. (1996). The 5-HT1B receptor agonist CP-94,253 reduces food intake and preserves the behavioural satiety sequence. *Physiol. Behav.* **60,** 933–939.

Hedlund, P. B., and Sutcliffe, J. G. (2004). Functional, molecular and pharmacological advances in 5-HT7 receptor research. *Trends Pharmacol. Sci.* **25,** 481–486.

Hedlund, P. B., Huitron-Resendiz, S., Henriksen, S. J., and Sutcliffe, J. G. (2005). 5-HT7 receptor inhibition and inactivation induce antidepressantlike behavior and sleep pattern. *Biol. Psychiatry* **58,** 831–837.

Heisler, L. K., Cowley, M. A., Tecott, L. H., Fan, W., Low, M. J., Smart, J. L., Rubinstein, M., Tatro, J. B., Marcus, J. N., Holstege, H., Lee, C. E., Cone, R. D., *et al.* (2002). Activation of central melanocortin pathways by fenfluramine. *Science* **297,** 609–611.

Heisler, L. K., Jobst, E. E., Sutton, G. M., Zhou, L., Borok, E., Thornton-Jones, Z., Liu, H. Y., Zigman, J. M., Balthasar, N., Kishi, T., Lee, C. E., Aschkenasi, C. J., *et al.* (2006). Serotonin reciprocally regulates melanocortin neurons to modulate food intake. *Neuron* **51,** 239–249.

Hoffman, B. J., and Mezey, E. (1989). Distribution of serotonin 5-HT1C receptor mRNA in adult rat brain. *FEBS Lett.* **247,** 453–462.

Holst, J. J. (2007). The physiology of glucagon-like peptide 1. *Physiol. Rev.* **87,** 1409–1439.

Horne, J. (2011). Obesity and short sleep: Unlikely bedfellows? *Obes. Rev.* **12,** 84–94.

Hoyer, D., Clarke, D. E., Fozard, J. R., Hartig, P. R., Martin, G. R., Mylecharane, E. J., Saxena, P. R., and Humphrey, P. P. (1994). International Union of Pharmacology classification of receptors for 5-hydroxytryptamine (Serotonin). *Pharmacol. Rev.* **46,** 157–203.

Hutson, P. H., Donohoe, T. P., and Curzon, G. (1988). Infusion of the 5-hydroxytryptamine agonists RU24969 and TFMPP into the paraventricular nucleus of the hypothalamus causes hypophagia. *Psychopharmacology (Berl.)* **95,** 550–552.

Julius, D., MacDermott, A. B., Axel, R., and Jessell, T. M. (1988). Molecular characterization of a functional cDNA encoding the serotonin 1c receptor. *Science* **241,** 558–564.

Katsuda, Y., Walsh, A. E. S., Ware, C. J., Cowen, P. J., and Sharpley, A. L. (1993). *meta*-Chlorophenylpiperazine decrease slow wave sleep in humans. *Biol. Psychiatry* **33,** 49–51.

Laposky, A. D., Shelton, J., Bass, J., Dugovic, C., Perrino, N., and Turek, F. W. (2006). Altered sleep regulation in leptin-deficient mice. *Am. J. Physiol. Regul. Integr. Comp. Physiol.* **290,** R894–R903.

Laposky, A. D., Bradley, M. A., Williams, D. L., Bass, J., and Turek, F. W. (2008). Sleep-wake regulation is altered in leptin-resistant (db/db) genetically obese and diabetic mice. *Am. J. Physiol. Regul. Integr. Comp. Physiol.* **295,** R2059–R2066.

Lee, M. D., and Simansky, K. J. (1997). CP-94, 253: A selective serotonin1B (5-HT1B) agonist that promotes satiety. *Psychopharmacology* **131,** 264–270.

Lee, M. D., Somerville, E. M., Kennett, G. A., Dourish, C. T., and Clifton, P. G. (2004). Reduced hypophagic effects of D-fenfluramine and the 5-HT2C receptor agonist mCPP in 5-HT1B receptor knockout mice. *Psychopharmacology* **176,** 39–49.

Leibowitz, S. F., Weiss, G. F., and Suh, J. S. (1990). Medial hypothalamic nuclei mediate serotonin's inhibitory effect on feeding behavior. *Pharmacol. Biochem. Behav.* **37,** 735–742.
Lovshin, J. A., and Drucker, D. J. (2009). Incretin-based therapies for type 2 diabetes mellitus. *Nat. Rev. Endocrinol.* **5,** 262–269.
Lucas, J. J., Yamamoto, A., Scearce-Levie, K., Saudou, F., and Hen, R. (1998). Absence of fenfluramine-induced anorexia and reduced c-Fos induction in the hypothalamus and central amygdaloid complex of serotonin 1B receptor knock-out mice. *J. Neurosci.* **18,** 5537–5544.
Martin, J. R., Bös, M., Jenck, F., Moreau, J., Mutel, V., Sleight, A. J., Wichmann, J., Andrews, J. S., Berendsen, H. H., Broekkamp, C. L., Ruigt, G. S., Köhler, C., *et al.* (1998). 5-HT2C receptor agonists: Pharmacological characteristics and therapeutic potential. *J. Pharmacol. Exp. Ther.* **286,** 913–924.
Monti, J. M. (2010). The role of dorsal raphe nucleus serotonergic and non-serotonergic neurons, and of their receptors, in regulating waking and rapid eye movement (REM) sleep. *Sleep Med. Rev.* **14,** 319–327.
Monti, J. M. (2011). Serotonin control of sleep-wake behavior. *Sleep Med. Rev.* **15,** 269–281.
Monti, J. M., and Jantos, H. (2003). Differential effects of the 5-HT1A receptor agonist flesinoxan given locally or systemically on REM sleep in the rat. *Eur. J. Pharmacol.* **478,** 121–130.
Monti, J. M., and Jantos, H. (2011). Effects of the 5-HT1A receptor antagonists SB-399885 and RO-4368554 and of the 5-HT(2A) receptor antagonist EMD 281014 on sleep and wakefulness in the rat during both phases of the light-dark cycle. *Behav. Brain Res.* **216,** 381–388.
Monti, J. M., Jantos, H., Silveira, R., Reyes-Parada, M., Scorza, C., and Prunell, G. (1994). Depletion of brain serotonin by 5,7-DHT: Effects on the 8-OH-DPAT-induced changes of sleep and waking in the rat. *Psychopharmacology* **115,** 273–277.
Monti, J. M., Monti, D., Jantos, H., and Ponzoni, A. (1995). Effects of selective activation of the 5-HT1B receptor with CP-94,253 on sleep and wakefulness in the rat. *Neuropharmacology* **34,** 1647–1651.
Morairty, S. R., Hedley, L., Flores, J., Martin, R., and Kilduff, T. S. (2008). Selective 5HT2A and 5HT6 receptor antagonists promote sleep in rats. *Sleep* **31,** 34–44.
Mozaffarian, D., Hao, T., Rimm, E. B., Willett, W. C., and Hu, F. B. (2011). Changes in diet and lifestyle and long-term weight gain in women and men. *N. Engl. J. Med.* **364,** 2392–2404.
Nonogaki, K. (2008). 5-HT and NA reuptake inhibitors and appetite regulation: The role of the central 5-HT network. *Immun. Endocr. Metab. Agents Med. Chem.* **8,** 303–310.
Nonogaki, K., and Kaji, T. (2010). Hypothalamic orexin and pro-opiomelanocortin activities are essential for the anorexic effects of m-chlorophenylpiperazine in mice. *Int. J. Neuropsychopharmacol.* **13,** 1261–1267.
Nonogaki, K., Strack, A. M., Dallman, M. F., and Tecott, L. H. (1998). Leptin-independent hyperphagia and type 2 diabetes in mice with a mutated serotonin 5-HT2C receptor gene. *Nat. Med.* **4,** 1152–1156.
Nonogaki, K., Abdallah, L., Goulding, E. H., Bonasera, S. J., and Tecott, L. H. (2003). Hyperactivity and reduced energy cost of physical activity in serotonin 5-HT(2C) receptor mutant mice. *Diabetes* **52,** 315–320.
Nonogaki, K., Nozue, K., and Oka, Y. (2006a). Hyperphagia alters expression of hypothalamic 5-HT2C and 5-HT1B receptor genes and plasma des-acyl ghrelin levels in A^y mice. *Endocrinology* **147,** 5893–5900.
Nonogaki, K., Nozue, K., and Oka, Y. (2006b). Increased hypothalamic 5-HT2A receptor gene expression and effects of pharmacologic 5-HT2A receptor inactivation in obese A^y mice. *Biochem. Biophys. Res. Commun.* **351,** 1078–1082.
Nonogaki, K., Nozue, K., and Oka, Y. (2007a). Social isolation affects the development of obesity and type 2 diabetes in mice. *Endocrinology* **148,** 4658–4666.

Nonogaki, K., Nozue, K., Takahashi, Y., Yamashita, N., Hiraoka, S., Kumano, H., Kuboki, T., and Oka, Y. (2007b). Fluvoxamine, a selective serotonin reuptake inhibitor, and 5-HT2C receptor inactivation induce appetite-suppressing effects in mice via 5-HT1B receptors. *Int. J. Neuropsychopharmacol.* **10,** 675–681.

Nonogaki, K., Ohba, Y., Sumii, M., and Oka, Y. (2008). Serotonin systems upregulate the expression of hypothalamic NUCB2 via 5-HT2C receptors and induce anorexia via a leptin-independent pathway in mice. *Biochem. Biophys. Res. Commun.* **372,** 186–190.

Nonogaki, K., Ohba, Y., Wakameda, M., and Tamari, T. (2009). Fluvoxamine exerts anorexic effect in 5-HT2C receptor mutant mice with heterozygous mutation of beta-endorphin gene. *Int. J. Neuropsychopharmacol.* **12,** 547–552.

Nonogaki, K., Suzuki, M., Sanuki, M., Wakameda, M., and Tamari, T. (2011). The contribution of serotonin 5-HT2C and melanocortin-4 receptors to the satiety signaling of glucagon-like peptide 1 and liragultide, a glucagon-like peptide 1 receptor agonist, in mice. *Biochem. Biophys. Res. Commun.* **29**(411), 445–448.

Ohno, K., and Sakurai, T. (2008). Orexin neuronal circuitry: Role in the regulation of sleep and wakefulness. *Front. Neuroendocrinol.* **29,** 70–87.

Opp, M. R., Obál, F., Jr., and Krueger, J. M. (1988). Effects of alpha-MSH on sleep, behavior, and brain temperature: Interactions with IL 1. *Am. J. Physiol.* **255,** R914–R922.

Paez, X., and Leibowitz, S. F. (1993). Changes in extracellular PVN monoamines and macronutrient intake after idazoxan or fluoxetine injection. *Pharmacol. Biochem. Behav.* **46,** 933–941.

Pasqualetti, M., Ori, M., Castagna, M., Marazziti, D., Cassano, G. B., and Nardi, I. (1999). Distribution and cellular localization of the serotonin type 2C receptor messenger RNA in human brain. *Neuroscience* **92,** 601–611.

Patel, S. R., and Hu, F. B. (2008). Short sleep duration and weight gain: A systematic review. *Obesity* **16,** 643–653.

Petrov, T., Krukoff, T. L., and Jhamandas, J. H. (1992). The hypothalamic paraventricular and lateral parabrachial nuclei receive collaterals from raphe nucleus neurons: A combined double retrograde and immunocytochemical study. *J. Comp. Neurol.* **318,** 18–26.

Popa, D., Léna, C., Fabre, V., Prenat, C., Gingrich, J., Escourrou, P., Hamon, M., and Adrien, J. (2005). Contribution of 5-HT2 receptor subtypes to sleep-wakefulness and respiratory control, and functional adaptations in knock-out mice lacking 5-HT2A receptors. *J. Neurosci.* **25,** 11231–11238.

Portas, C. M., Bjorvatn, B., and Ursin, R. (2000). Serotonin and the sleep/wake cycle: Special emphasis on microdialysis studies. *Prog. Neurobiol.* **60,** 13–35.

Roberts, J. C., Reavill, C., East, S. Z., Harrison, P. J., Patel, S., Routledge, C., and Leslie, R. A. (2002). The distribution of 5-HT(6) receptors in rat brain: An autoradiographic binding study using the radiolabelled 5-HT(6) receptor antagonist [(125)I]SB-258585. *Brain Res.* **934,** 49–57.

Ruat, M., Traiffort, E., Arrang, J. M., Tardivel-Lacombe, J., Diaz, J., Leurs, R., and Schwartz, J. C. (1993). A novel rat serotonin (5-HT6) receptor: Molecular cloning, localization and stimulation of cAMP accumulation. *Biochem. Biophys. Res. Commun.* **193,** 268–276.

Sakurai, T., and Mieda, M. (2011). Connectomics of orexin-producing neurons: Interface of systems of emotion, energy homeostasis and arousal. *Trends Pharmacol. Sci.* **32,** 451–462.

Saper, C. B., and Loewy, A. D. (1980). Efferent connections of the parabrachial nucleus in the rat. *Brain Res.* **197,** 291–317.

Schmid, S. M., Hallschmid, M., Jauch-Chara, K., Born, J., and Schultes, B. (2008). A single night of sleep deprivation increases ghrelin levels and feelings of hunger in normal-weight healthy men. *J. Sleep Res.* **17,** 331–334.

Schwartz, D., Hernandez, L., and Hoebel, B. G. (1989). Fenfluramine administered systemically or locally increases extracellular serotonin in the lateral hypothalamus as measured by microdialysis. *Brain Res.* **482,** 261–270.

Sehgal, A., and Mignot, E. (2011). Genetics of sleep and sleep disorders. *Cell* **146,** 194–207.

Sharpley, A. L., Vassallo, C. M., and Cowen, P. J. (2000). Olanzapine increases slow-wave sleep: Evidence for blockade of central 5-HT2C receptors in vivo. *Biol. Psychiatry* **47,** 468–470.

Shor-Posner, G., Grinker, J. A., Marinescu, C., Brown, O., and Leibowitz, S. F. (1986). Hypothalamic serotonin in the control of meal patterns and macronutrient selection. *Brain Res. Bull.* **17,** 663–671.

Smith, M. I., Piper, D. C., Duxon, M. S., and Upton, N. (2002). Effect of SB-243213, a selective 5-HT2C receptor antagonist, on the rat sleep profile: A comparison to paroxetine. *Pharmacol. Biochem. Behav.* **71,** 599–605.

Solomon, R. A., Sharpley, A. L., and Cowen, P. J. (1989). Increased slow wave sleep with 5-HT2 receptor antagonists: Detection by ambulatory EEG recording and automatic sleep stage analysis. *J. Psychopharmacol.* **3,** 125–129.

Sørensen, E., Grønli, J., Bjorvatn, B., and Ursin, R. (2001). The selective 5-HT(1A) receptor antagonist p-MPPI antagonizes sleep–waking and behavioural effects of 8-OH-DPAT in rats. *Behav. Brain Res.* **121,** 181–187.

Spiegel, K., Tasali, E., Penev, P., and Van Cauter, E. (2004). Brief communication: Sleep curtailment in healthy young men is associated with decreased leptin levels, elevated ghrelin levels, and increased hunger and appetite. *Ann. Intern. Med.* **141,** 846–850.

Spiegel, K., Tasali, E., Leproult, R., and Van Cauter, E. (2009). Effects of poor and short sleep on glucose metabolism and obesity risk. *Nat. Rev. Endocrinol.* **5,** 253–261.

Steinbusch, H. W., and Nieuwenhuys, R. (1981). Localization of serotonin-like immunoreactivity in the central nervous system and pituitary of the rat, with special references to the innervation of the hypothalamus. *Adv. Exp. Med. Biol.* **133,** 7–35.

St-Onge, M. P., Roberts, A. L., Chen, J., Kelleman, M., O'Keeffe, M., Roychoudhury, A., and Jones, P. J. (2011). Short sleep duration increases energy intakes but does not change energy expenditure in normal-weight individuals. *Am. J. Clin. Nutr.* **94,** 410–416.

Stricker-Krongrad, A., Richy, S., and Beck, B. (2002). Orexins/hypocretins in the ob/ob mouse: Hypothalamic gene expression, peptide content and metabolic effects. *Regul. Pept.* **104,** 11–20.

Tecott, L. H. (2007). Serotonin and the orchestration of energy balance. *Cell Metab.* **6,** 352–361.

Thomsen, W. J., Grottick, A. J., Menzaghi, F., Reyes-Saldana, H., Espitia, S., Yuskin, D., Whelan, K., Martin, M., Morgan, M., Chen, W., Al-Shamma, H., Smith, B., *et al.* (2008). Lorcaserin, a novel selective human 5-hydroxytryptamine2C agonist: In vitro and in vivo pharmacological characterization. *J. Pharmacol. Exp. Ther.* **325,** 577–587.

Tsujino, N., and Sakurai, T. (2009). Orexin/hypocretin: A neuropeptide at the interface of sleep, energy homeostasis, and reward system. *Pharmacol. Rev.* **61,** 162–176.

Woolley, M. L., Marsden, C. A., and Fone, K. C. (2004). 5-HT6 receptors. *Curr. Drug Targets CNS Neurol. Disord.* **3,** 59–79.

Wright, D. E., Seroogy, K. B., Lundgren, K. H., Davis, B. M., and Jennes, L. (1995). Comparative localization of serotonin1A, 1C, and 2 receptor subtype mRNAs in rat brain. *J. Comp. Neurol.* **351,** 357–373.

Xu, Y., Jones, J. E., Kohno, D., Williams, K. W., Lee, C. E., Choi, M. J., Anderson, J. G., Heisler, L. K., Zigman, J. M., Lowell, B. B., and Elmquist, J. K. (2008). 5-HT2CRs expressed by pro-opiomelanocortin neurons regulate energy homeostasis. *Neuron* **60,** 582–589.

Yagaloff, K. A., and Hartig, P. R. (1985). 125I-lysergic acid diethylamide binds to a novel serotonergic site on rat choroid plexus epithelial cells. *J. Neurosci.* **5,** 3178–3183.

Yamamoto, Y., Ueta, Y., Date, Y., Nakazato, M., Hara, Y., Serino, R., Nomura, M., Shibuya, I., Matsukura, S., and Yamashita, H. (1999). Down regulation of the prepro-orexin gene expression in genetically obese mice. *Brain Res. Mol. Brain Res.* **65,** 14–22.

CHAPTER THIRTEEN

Humoral Sleep Regulation; Interleukin-1 and Tumor Necrosis Factor

Kathryn A. Jewett*,† *and* James M. Krueger*

Contents

Abstract

Two substances, the cytokines interleukin-1 beta (IL1β) and tumor necrosis factor alpha (TNFα), known for their many physiological roles, for example, cognition, synaptic plasticity, and immune function, are also well characterized in their actions of sleep regulation. These substances promote non-rapid eye movement sleep and can induce symptoms associated with sleep loss such as sleepiness, fatigue, and poor cognition. IL1β and TNFα are released from glia in response to extracellular ATP. They bind to their receptors on neurons resulting in neuromodulator and neurotransmitter receptor up/downregulation (e.g., adenosine and glutamate receptors) leading to altered neuronal excitability and function, that is, a state change in the local network. Synchronization of state between local networks leads to emergent whole brain oscillations, such as sleep/wake cycles.

* WWAMI Medical Education Program, Sleep and Performance Research Center, Washington State University, Spokane, Washington, USA
† Department of Veterinary and Comparative Anatomy, Pharmacology and Physiology, Washington State University, Pullman, Washington, USA

Vitamins and Hormones, Volume 89
ISSN 0083-6729, http://dx.doi.org/10.1016/B978-0-12-394623-2.00013-5

I. Introduction

Despite the importance of sleep to our everyday lives, its biochemical regulation continues to confound us. Many studies have provided strong evidence that sleep is regulated, in part, by humoral agents dubbed "sleep-regulatory substances" or SRSs (Borbély and Tobler, 1989; Imeri and Opp, 2009; Inoue, 1989; Jouvet, 1984; Kilduff and Peyron, 2000; Krueger, 2008; Krueger *et al.*, 1990, 2008; Obál *et al.*, 2003; Roky *et al.*, 1995). The first discovery of SRSs that accumulated in cerebrospinal fluid during prolonged waking occurred over a century ago (Ishimori, 1909; Legendre and Piéron, 1913).

To be classified as an SRS, a substance must meet several criteria (Borbély and Tobler, 1980; Imeri and Opp, 2009; Jouvet, 1984; Krueger and Obál, 1994). These include (1) the substance and/or its receptor changes with sleep propensity, (2) administration of the substance increases or decreases sleep, (3) blocking the action or inhibiting the production of the substance changes sleep, (4) levels of the substance change during disease states associated with altered sleep, for example, infection, and finally (5) the substance acts on known sleep-regulatory circuits. While there are many substances meeting some of these criteria, including microRNAs, metabolites, hormones, growth factors, transcription factors, and various proteins and their receptors, only a few meet all the required characteristics.

II. Interleukin-1β and Tumor Necrosis Factor α

Two well-characterized SRSs are the cytokines interleukin-1 beta (IL1β) and tumor necrosis factor alpha (TNFα). While well known for their contribution to signaling in the peripheral immune system, cytokines and their receptors are constitutively expressed in the central nervous system of healthy organisms, supporting the notion that they have functions beyond immune responses (Opp, 2005; Szelényi, 2001).

Electrophysiological, biochemical, and molecular genetic studies of IL1β and TNFα demonstrate specific effects on sleep–wake behavior. They seem to promote sleep via similar mechanisms, for example, both activate nuclear factor kappa-B (NF-κB). Many of their downstream biochemical effectors, for example, adenosine, nitric oxide, nerve growth factor, growth hormone-releasing hormone, and prostaglandins, are also implicated in sleep-regulatory roles in health and disease (reviewed in Churchill *et al.*, 2008; Kapsimalis *et al.*, 2005; Krueger *et al.*, 2008). For instance, injection of IL1β or TNFα into humans (mimicking their endogenous accumulation during wakefulness or sleep loss) induces symptoms associated with sleep loss, such as sensitivity to kindling (Yi *et al.*, 2004) and pain stimuli (Honore *et al.*, 2006; Kawasaki *et al.*,

2008; Kundermann *et al.*, 2008), depression (Anisman and Marali, 2003; Vollmer-Conna *et al.*, 2004), sleepiness (Moldofsky, 1995; Obál *et al.*, 2003; Tringall *et al.*, 2000), fatigue (Anisman and Marali, 2003; Carmichael *et al.*, 2006; Omdal and Gunnarsson, 2005), and impairments in cognition (Baune *et al.*, 2008; Gambino *et al.*, 2007; Trompet *et al.*, 2008), memory (Banks and Dinges, 2007; Dantzer, 2004; Pickering and O'Connor, 2007), and performance (Banks and Dinges, 2007). Some of these symptoms can be blocked with the administration of cytokine inhibitors (Depino *et al.*, 2004; Larsen *et al.*, 2007; Opp and Krueger, 1991). Chronic sleep disruption is also associated with multiple pathologies such as metabolic syndrome (Hristova and Aloe, 2006; Jager *et al.*, 2007; Larsen *et al.*, 2007), chronic inflammation (Frey *et al.*, 2007; Hu *et al.*, 2003), and cardiovascular disease (reviewed in Yndestad *et al.*, 2007), and IL1β and TNFα play a role in the etiology of these diseases.

A. Interleukin-1β

IL1β is a somnogenic cytokine originally described as an endogenous pyrogen that induced fever in rabbits (Atkins and Wood, 1955). Immunologists working independently described lymphocyte-activating factor that subsequently was recognized as endogenous pyrogen, and both were given the new name interleukin-1. IL1β is normally produced in response to infection, injury, or immunologic challenge; at minimal concentrations, it causes fever, hypotension, and production of additional proinflammatory cytokines, such as IL6 (Church *et al.*, 2008; Dinarello, 2000). IL1β is a member of the interleukin 1 family that also includes IL1α and IL1 receptor antagonist (IL1ra) (Gibson *et al.*, 2004). The IL1 family now comprises at least 11 different proteins (IL1F1–11) on the basis of their sequence homology, structure, and receptors (Allan *et al.*, 2005; Barksby *et al.*, 2007). IL1β transcription may be induced by proinflammatory stimuli such as microorganisms or their products (Konsman *et al.*, 2002) and by proinflammatory cytokines, including type I interferons (Brandwein, 1986), TNFα (Williams *et al.*, 2000), and IL1β itself (Churchill *et al.*, 2006; Granowitz *et al.*, 1992).

Almost all nucleated cells produce IL1β (Brough and Rothwell, 2007). IL1β is produced as a large ~36 kDa (Deak *et al.*, 2005) inactive precursor protein (pro-IL1β) that requires cleavage by caspase-1 (also known as IL1β-converting enzyme) to its active form (a 17 kDa protein) (Barksby *et al.*, 2007; Church *et al.*, 2008; Fogal and Hewett, 2008).

IL1β binds to two receptor subtypes, one of which produces downstream signaling and activation and the other of which lacks an intracellular signaling moiety. Both receptors can also bind IL1ra and IL1α. The receptor that produces activation is an 80 kDa membrane-bound receptor named IL1-receptor (IL1-R) type 1 or IL1-R1 which interacts with the cytoplasmic protein IL1-R accessory protein to form a complex that leads to the recruitment of adaptor molecules (Fitzgerald and O'Neill, 2000). This signaling can lead to the activation of NF-κB and mitogen-activated protein (MAP) kinase (Trinchieri and Sher, 2007). IL1β also can bind to the IL1-R2, a receptor that lacks an intracellular signaling domain, and consequently, no signaling is activated, therefore, the IL1-R2 functions as a decoy receptor (Colotta *et al.*, 1993, 1994). In other words, IL1-R2 binds to IL1β and thereby prevents it from associating with IL1-R1 (Allan *et al.*, 2005). Interestingly, IL1-R1 has a higher binding affinity for IL1ra than for IL1β or IL1α allowing IL1ra to act as a strong antagonist, whereas IL1-R2 has a higher affinity for IL1β than for IL1α supporting an important role for the receptor in regulating IL1 activity (Colotta *et al.*, 1993, 1994; Re *et al.*, 1996).

B. Tumor Necrosis Factor α

TNFα was first discovered as a product of lymphocytes and macrophages, capable of lysing certain cell types, especially tumor cells (Carswell *et al.*, 1975). TNFα is now associated with many physiological functions in both the normal and diseased body (Bertazza and Mocellin, 2008; Bradley, 2008; Perry *et al.*, 2002). TNFα is involved in synaptic scaling, neurogenesis, cognition, immune system coordination, systemic inflammation, and induction of apoptosis. However, like many other cytokines, TNFα has emerged as an important cell-signaling molecule with diverse roles in many tissues, including the brain. In the brain, TNFα is expressed in neurons, microglia, and astrocytes (Breder *et al.*, 1993; Inoue *et al.*, 2000).

TNFα is synthesized as a membrane-bound homotrimer (made up of 26 kDa monomers), pro-TNFα, that is cleaved by the TNFα-converting enzyme (Solomon *et al.*, 1999; Tracey *et al.*, 2008). After cleavage, the soluble cytokine is released as the 17 kDa form which can interact with TNFα cell-surface receptors. Additionally, membrane-bound pro-TNFα can function as a receptor for TNFα antagonists and as a ligand, binding to TNFα cell-surface receptors. Both actions can lead to the suppression of cytokine expression and apoptosis (Tracey *et al.*, 2008).

There are two TNFα cell-surface receptors, TNF-R1 and TNF-R2. The receptors are structurally related, forming trimeric complexes. However, they differ in their affinity for ligands, signaling mechanisms, and cellular expression (TNF-R1 is expressed on virtually all cell types, while TNF-R2 is usually inducible and expressed only in endothelial and immune cells) (Palin *et al.*, 2007; Tracey *et al.*, 2008). Both receptors lack intrinsic enzymatic activity in their intracellular domains and therefore signal by recruitment of cytosolic adaptor proteins via protein–protein interaction domains to activate transcription factors such as NF-κB and members of the MAP kinase pathway (Goeddel, 1999; Ledgerwood *et al.*, 1999). The activation of these transcription factors plays an important role in the induction of many other cytokines and immune-regulatory proteins, in many cases mediating an inflammatory response. In some cases, activation of these transcription factors can induce apoptosis or necrosis (Ledgerwood *et al.*, 1999; Liu, 2005).

III. Cytokine Production and Release

IL1β and TNFα mRNAs are detectable in various areas of the brain in several species (reviewed by Vitkovic *et al.*, 2000). Because constitutive expression of IL1β (Medana *et al.*, 1997; Taishi *et al.*, 1997) and TNFα (Bredow *et al.*, 1997) mRNAs is region specific and diurnal, some studies did not find them in normal rodent brains (reviewed by Vitkovic *et al.*, 2000). IL1β protein is present in many areas in both neurons and glia in normal rat and mouse brains (Bandtlow *et al.*, 1990; Hagan *et al.*, 1993; Lechan *et al.*, 1990; Molenaar *et al.*, 1993; Quan *et al.*, 1998). IL1β is detectable in the normal human cortex in glia but not neurons (da Cunha *et al.*, 1993a,b), although, in mice, neurons express IL1β as determined by immunohistochemistry. Neuronal activity stimulated through activation of transfected channelrhodopsin-2 increases IL1β expression in mouse neurons (Jewett *et al.*, 2011). TNFα protein is found in many areas of the rodent brain (Breder *et al.*, 1993; Ignatowski *et al.*, 1997; Saito *et al.*, 1996). TNFα protein has marked diurnal changes, for example, 10-fold changes in the cortex and hypothalamus, and correlates with mRNA rhythms (Bredow *et al.*, 1997; Floyd and Krueger, 1997). TNFα is found in rat neurons as determined by immunohistochemistry, and like IL1β, expression is activity dependent. Whisker stimulation increases TNFα expression in the correspondingly activated somatosensory cortical columns (Churchill *et al.*, 2008).

Glia synthesize and exocytose a variety of molecules, including IL1β and TNFα, that when injected either systemically or into the brain can increase sleep time or intensity (Halassa *et al.*, 2009; Pascual *et al.*, 2005). For example, IL1β derived from cultured mouse astrocytes increases non-rapid eye movement sleep (NREMS) in rats when administered into the ventricles (Tobler *et al.*, 1984). Astrocytes release IL1β and TNFα in response to neuronal signals, including extracellular ATP acting at purine type 2 (P2) receptors (Bianco *et al.*, 2005; Krueger *et al.*, 2010; Solle *et al.*, 2001; Suzuki *et al.*, 2004; Verderio and Matteoli, 2011). Microglia also synthesize and release cytokines such as IL1β and TNFα in response to extracellular ATP, for example, during ischemia or inflammation (Ferrari *et al.*, 1997; Hide *et al.*, 2000; Inoue, 2002).

IV. Cytokines and Sleep

Cytokines have important roles in multiple physiological functions, including sleep regulation (Krueger *et al.*, 2001), memory (Yirmiya and Goshen, 2011), appetite (Andréasson *et al.*, 2007), cerebral circulation (Faraci and Heistad, 1998), temperature regulation (Leon, 2002), and insulin production (Fu *et al.*, 2006). Several cytokines, including the proinflammatory cytokines IL1α, IL1β, IL6, IFNα, IFNγ, TNFα, and TNFβ, have the capacity to enhance NREMS (reviewed by Krueger and Majde, 2003; Krueger *et al.*, 2001). Two cytokines studied extensively for their relationship with sleep are IL1β and TNFα (Opp, 2005). Endogenous production of IL1β and TNFα and conditions that enhance their production, for example, excessive food intake (Hansen *et al.*, 1998) or infectious disease (Toth and Krueger, 1988), promote NREMS (Krueger *et al.*, 2007; Obál and Krueger, 2003). IL1β and TNFα are constitutively expressed in the brain. In rats, IL1β and TNFα mRNA and protein levels exhibit a diurnal variation in certain areas of the brain, with higher concentrations correlating with higher sleep propensity (Bredow *et al.*, 1997; Taishi *et al.*, 1997). Furthermore, after sleep deprivation, increases in NREMS as well as increases in IL1β and TNFα expression in the brain occur (Krueger *et al.*, 2001; Taishi *et al.*, 1998; Takahashi *et al.*, 1997).

The sleep-promoting actions of IL1β were initially demonstrated in rabbits. Central administration of IL1β enhances NREMS in this species (Krueger *et al.*, 1983, 1984). Further, intracerebroventricular (ICV) injection with an IL1-R1 fragment, an IL1β inhibitor, reduces sleep (Takahashi *et al.*, 1999). In rats, enhanced NREMS occurs after ICV injection of low doses of IL1β (Opp *et al.*, 1991). In contrast, anti-IL1 antibodies or IL1ra reduce spontaneous sleep and inhibit sleep rebound after sleep deprivation (Obál, *et al.*, 1990). Mice display a robust increase in NREMS and suppressed rapid eye movement sleep (REMS) after intraperitoneal injection with IL1β. These effects are abolished IL1-R1 knockout mice; the knockout mice also have less spontaneous sleep than corresponding controls (Fang *et al.*, 1998). Exogenous administration of IL1β also increases NREMS in other species such as cats (Susić and Totić, 1989), monkeys (Friedman *et al.*, 1995), and humans (Dinarello, 1991). In humans, plasma IL1β peaks at slow-wave sleep onset (Moldofsky *et al.*, 1986). The firing rate of hypothalamic sleep-active neurons is enhanced by IL1β; it inhibits wake-active neurons (Alam *et al.*, 2004). IL1β injected into the locus coeruleus (De Sarro *et al.*, 1997) or the dorsal raphe nuclei (Manfridi *et al.*, 2003) promotes NREMS. These results suggest a role for IL1β in the regulation of physiological sleep (Krueger, 2008).

The somnogenic effects of TNFα were first described after ICV injection of recombinant TNFα into rabbits (Shoham *et al.*, 1987). Intravenous or ICV administration of exogenous TNFα enhances the duration and intensity of NREMS and decreases REMS in this species (Kapás and Krueger, 1992; Shoham *et al.*, 1987). The use of anti-TNFα antibodies or the TNF-soluble receptor attenuates spontaneous sleep and reduces sleep rebound after sleep deprivation (Krueger *et al.*, 2001; Takahashi *et al.*, 1995, 1996). In rats, peripheral administration of TNFα increases NREMS (Kubota *et al.*, 2001). Unilateral microinjection of TNFα into the preoptic area of the anterior hypothalamus or the locus coeruleus increases NREMS in a dose-dependent manner (De Sarro *et al.*, 1997; Kubota *et al.*, 2002; Terao *et al.*, 1998). After intraperitoneal injection of TNFα, mice show a dose-dependent increase in NREMS. This effect is not observed in TNF-R1 knockout mice; they also have significantly less baseline NREMS and REMS than controls (Fang *et al.*, 1997). Finally, in sheep, ICV injection of TNFα results in an increase in NREMS (Dickstein *et al.*, 1999). These results suggest that TNFα also has a role in the regulation of physiological sleep (Krueger and Majde, 2003).

The sleep-regulatory roles of IL1β and TNFα are closely related to each other (Baracchi and Opp, 2008). For example, IL1-R1/TNF-R1 double knockout mice have a reduced NREMS rebound (compared with wild type) and do not exhibit an REMS rebound in response to sleep deprivation (Baracchi and Opp, 2008). Furthermore, in TNF-R1 knockout mice that are nonresponsive to TNFα, whereas an injection of IL1β increases NREMS in these mice (Fang *et al.*, 1997). Similarly, the IL1-R1 knockout mice show increased NREMS and decreased REMS after administration of TNFα (Fang *et al.*, 1998).

In addition to increasing time spent sleeping, central injection of IL1β and TNFα can enhance electroencephalographic (EEG) delta (0.5–4 Hz) power (a measure of sleep intensity), also known as slow-wave activity (SWA), during NREMS but not during REMS or waking. Enhanced SWA is also seen after sleep deprivation (Borbély and Tobler, 1989; Pappenheimer *et al.*, 1975), suggesting that IL1β and TNFα injections mimic the effects of sleep loss.

V. Cytokines in Sleep Regulation

The dominant paradigm in sleep research posits that sleep is initiated and regulated by subcortical neuronal networks (reviewed in Szymusiak and McGinty, 2008).

The arousal systems, for example, the noradrenergic locus coeruleus, serotonergic dorsal raphe nucleus, cholinergic neurons in the basal forebrain, and histaminergic neurons in the tuberomammillary nucleus, provide activating inputs to the diencephalon, limbic system, and neocortex (Saper, 1987). The hypocretin (orexin) neurons in the perifornical region of the lateral hypothalamus constitute another functionally important arousal regulatory cell group (Peyron *et al.*, 1998). GABAergic neurons with enhanced activity during and just prior to sleep are found in the ventrolateral preoptic area of anterior hypothalamus (Sherin *et al.*, 1996, 1998; Szymusiak *et al.*, 1998). These neurons are posited to impose sleep on the rest of the brain by their inhibition of the various arousal/activating systems (reviewed by Saper *et al.*, 2005).

There are many well-known phenomena that cannot be explained by the top-down sleep-regulatory center-imposed sleep paradigm. The most substantial evidence against a necessary top-down sleep-regulatory mechanism comes from lesion studies; if an animal or human survives a brain lesion (e.g., stroke) in any location, it will sleep. There are no reported cases of a complete loss of sleep, including in patients with fatal familial insomnia (Montagna, 2005). The top-down paradigm has little explanatory value for sleep homeostatic mechanisms or how performance is restored during sleep. The existence of parasomnias, such as sleepwalking, indicates that areas of the brain can be awake while other areas are asleep (Mahowald and Schenck, 2005). Many species of birds and marine mammals exhibit unihemispheric sleep (Lyamin *et al.*, 2002, 2008; Rattenborg *et al.*, 2001). Finally, isolated cortical islands retaining their blood flow but no afferent projections show periods of high-amplitude delta waves measured from the cortical surface (Kristiansen and Courtois, 1949).

Such considerations led to the theory that sleep is a local use-dependent phenomenon. The functional states (i.e., asleep or awake) of different parts of the brain can vary. For example, dolphins do not exhibit high-amplitude EEG slow waves simultaneously in both cerebral hemispheres (Mukhametov *et al.*, 1977). During a visual discrimination task, when a monkey becomes drowsy, but is still behaving, some neurons in the cortical visual receptive fields exhibit the burst-pause sleep-like pattern before others as the animal enters sleep (Pigarev *et al.*, 1997). Which neurons switch to the burst-pause pattern depends on their topographic location within their receptive field, indicating that the transition from wake to sleep is a local network phenomenon. Similarly, using surface-evoked response potentials to characterize cortical column state, Rector *et al.* (2005) demonstrated that individual columns semiautonomously oscillate between sleep- and wake-like states. The duration of the localized sleep-like state of a cortical column is dependent on its prior wake-like state duration, suggesting that the local functional state of the column is use-dependent and homeostatic (Rector *et al.*, 2009).

Other studies also suggest the use-dependent regulation of local sleep. For example, during the first NREMS episode after a hand is stimulated prior to sleep by vibration, the EEG SWA is enhanced in the somatosensory cortex contralateral to the stimulated hand as compared to the ipsilateral side (Kattler *et al.*, 1994). Cerebral blood flow during sleep is increased in areas which are disproportionately stimulated during prior waking (Maquet, 2001). The neuronal electrical firing in the cortex and hippocampus during sleep replays the activation pattern learned during a waking task (Ji and Wilson, 2007). After a special motor-learning task just prior to sleep, the cortical area activated by this learning task has enhanced subsequent EEG SWA as compared to the unstimulated regions (Huber *et al.*, 2004).

The use-dependent regulation of sleep is, at least in part, mediated by the SRSs that are produced and released locally in response to the neuronal and glial activity during wakefulness. For instance, in rats, stimulation of whiskers leads to increased expression of TNFα in the corresponding cortical columns (Churchill *et al.*, 2008). When TNFα is applied directly to the cortex unilaterally, EEG SWA is enhanced on the side of injection (Yoshida *et al.*, 2004), and the sleep-like state of the underlying cortical column is increased (Churchill *et al.*, 2008). In addition, unilateral application of a TNFα small-interfering RNA to the cortex inhibits local EEG SWA and neuronal TNFα expression (Taishi *et al.*, 2007). Collectively, these experiments suggest that the production of SRSs depends on the prior activity of the cortical columns, and the functional states of cortical columns are affected by the SRSs. These studies support the theory that sleep is initiated at a local network level in the circuits most active during prior waking. Whole organism sleep is posited to emerge with the synchronization of local network state changes orchestrated in part by the known sleep-regulatory circuits (Krueger *et al.*, 2008; Roy *et al.*, 2008).

A mechanism linking cellular activity to sleep is based on extracellular adenosine triphosphate (ATP) and cytokines. ATP is released into the extracellular space during neuro and gliotransmission (reviewed in Burnstock, 2006, 2007; Halassa *et al.*, 2009). Extracellular ATP induces the release of SRSs like IL1β and TNFα from glia via P2 receptors (reviewed by Bianco *et al.*, 2005; Hide *et al.*, 2000; Krueger *et al.*, 2010; Solle *et al.*, 2001; Suzuki *et al.*, 2004; Verderio and Matteoli, 2011). Thus local levels of SRSs reflect prior local network activity. These substances can then bind to receptors of nearby neurons, directly altering electrical activity (fast process) and altering gene transcription and translation (slow process), leading to changes in receptor populations such as AMPA and adenosine receptors (reviewed by Obál and Krueger, 2003). Extracellular ATP can also be hydrolyzed by ectonucleotidases releasing extracellular adenosine that in turn acts on adenosine receptors (Fields and Stevens, 2000). All these processes can alter the responsiveness of neurons and their input–output relationships, leading to state changes and ultimately sleep.

ACKNOWLEDGMENT

This work was supported by grants from the National Institutes of Health, NS025378, NS031453, and HD36520.

REFERENCES

Alam, M. N., McGinty, D., Bashir, T., Kumar, S., Imeri, L., Opp, M. R., and Szymusiak, R. (2004). Interleukin-1beta modulates state-dependent discharge activity of preoptic area and basal forebrain neurons: Role in sleep regulation. *Eur. J. Neurosci.* **20**(1), 207–216.

Allan, S., Tyrrell, P., and Rothwell, N. (2005). Interleukin-1 and neuronal injury. *Nat. Rev. Immunol.* **5,** 629–640.

Andréasson, A., Arborelius, L., Erlanson-Albertsson, C., and Lekander, M. (2007). A putative role for cytokines in the impaired appetite in depression. *Brain Behav. Immun.* **21**(2), 147–152.

Anisman, H., and Marali, Z. (2003). Cytokines, stress and depressive illness: Brain-immune interactions. *Ann. Med.* **35,** 2–11.

Atkins, E., and Wood, W. (1955). Studies on the pathogenesis of fever. I. The presence of transferable pyrogen in the blood stream following the injection of typhoid vaccine. *J. Exp. Med.* **101,** 519–528.

Bandtlow, C., Meyer, M., Lindholm, D., Spranger, M., Heumann, R., and Thoenen, H. (1990). Regional and cellular codistribution of interleukin-1β and nerve growth factor mRNA in the adult rat brain: Possible relationship to the regulation of nerve growth factor synthesis. *J. Cell Biol.* **111,** 1701–1711.

Banks, S., and Dinges, D. F. (2007). Behavioral and physiological consequences of sleep restriction. *J. Clin. Sleep Med.* **3,** 519–528.

Baracchi, F., and Opp, M. R. (2008). Sleep-wake behavior and responses to sleep deprivation of mice lacking both interleukin-1beta receptor 1 and tumor necrosis factor-alpha receptor 1. *Brain Behav. Immun.* **22**(6), 982–993.

Barksby, H., Lea, S., Preshaw, P., and Taylor, J. (2007). The expanding family of interleukin-1 cytokines and their role in destructive inflammatory disorders. *Clin. Exp. Immunol.* **49,** 217–225.

Baune, B. T., Ponath, G., Rothermundt, M., Riess, O., Funke, H., and Berger, K. (2008). Association between genetic variants of IL-1beta, IL-6 and TNF-alpha cytokines and cognitive performance in the elderly general population of the MEMO-study. *Psychoneuroendocrinology* **33,** 68–76.

Bertazza, L., and Mocellin, S. (2008). Tumor necrosis factor (TNF) biology and cell death. *Front. Biosci.* **13,** 2736–2743.

Bianco, F., Pravettoni, E., Colombo, A., Schenk, U., Möller, T., Matteoli, M., and Verderio, C. (2005). Astrocyte-derived ATP induces vesicle shedding and IL-1β release from microglia. *J. Immunol.* **174**(11), 7269–7277.

Borbély, A. A., and Tobler, I. (1980). The search for an endogenous sleep substances. *TIPS* **1,** 356–358.

Borbély, A. A., and Tobler, I. (1989). Endogenous sleep-promoting substances and sleep regulation. *Physiol. Rev.* **69,** 605–670.

Bradley, J. (2008). TNF-mediated inflammatory disease. *J. Pathol.* **214,** 149–160.

Brandwein, S. (1986). Regulation of interleukin 1 production by mouse peritoneal macrophages. Effects of arachidonic acid metabolites, cyclic nucleotides, and interferons. *J. Biol. Chem.* **261,** 8624–8632.

Breder, C., Tsujimoto, M., Terano, Y., Scott, D., and Saper, C. (1993). Distribution and characterization of tumor necrosis factor-alpha-like immunoreactivity in the murine central nervous system. *J. Comp. Neurol.* **337,** 543–567.

Bredow, S., Guha-Thakurta, N., Taishi, P., Obál, F., Jr., and Krueger, J. M. (1997). Diurnal variations of tumor necrosis factor alpha mRNA and alpha-tubulin mRNA in rat brain. *Neuroimmunomodulation* **4,** 84–90.

Brough, D., and Rothwell, N. (2007). Caspase-1-dependent processing of pro-interleukin-1 beta is cytosolic and precedes cell death. *J. Cell Sci.* **120**(Pt 5), 772–781.

Burnstock, G. (2006). Purinergic signaling—An overview. *Novartis Found. Symp.* **276,** 26–48.

Burnstock, G. (2007). Physiology and pathophysiology of purinergic neurotransmission. *Physiol. Rev.* **87,** 659–797.

Carmichael, M. D., Davis, J. M., Murphy, E. A., Brown, A. S., Carson, J. A., Mayer, E. P., and Ghaffar, A. (2006). Role of brain IL-1β on fatigue after exercise induced muscle damage. *Am. J. Physiol. Regul. Integr. Comp. Physiol.* **291**(5), R1344–R1348.

Carswell, E., Old, L., Kassel, R., Green, S., Fiore, N., and Williamson, B. (1975). An endotoxin-induced serum factor that causes necrosis of tumors. *Proc. Natl. Acad. Sci. U.S.A.* **72,** 3666–3670.

Church, L., Cook, G., and McDermott, M. (2008). Primer: Inflammasomes and interleukin 1beta in inflammatory disorders. *Nat. Clin. Pract. Rheumatol.* **4,** 34–42.

Churchill, L., Taishi, P., Wang, M., Brandt, J., Cearley, C., Rehman, A., and Krueger, J. M. (2006). Brain distribution of cytokine mRNA induced by systemic administration of interleukin-1β or tumor necrosis factor α. *Brain Res.* **1120,** 64–73.

Churchill, L., Rector, D. M., Yasuda, K., Fix, C., Rojas, M. J., Yasuda, T., and Krueger, J. M. (2008). Tumor necrosis factor alpha: Activity dependent expression and promotion of cortical column sleep in rats. *Neuroscience* **156,** 71–80.

Colotta, F., Re, F., Muzio, M., Bertini, R., Polentarutti, N., Sironi, M., Giri, J., Dower, S., Sims, J., and Mantovani, A. (1993). Interleukin-1 type II receptor: A decoy target for IL-1 that is regulated by IL-4. *Science* **261,** 472–475.

Colotta, F., Dower, S. K., Sims, J. E., and Mantovani, A. (1994). The type II "decoy" receptor: A novel regulatory pathway for interleukin 1. *Immunol. Today* **15**(12), 562–566.

Da Cunha, A., Jefferson, J. A., Jackson, R. W., and Vitkovic, L. (1993a). Glial cell-specific mechanisms of TGF-beta 1 induction by IL-1 in cerebral cortex. *J. Neuroimmunol.* **42,** 71–85.

Da Cunha, A., Jefferson, J. J., Tyor, W. R., Glass, J. D., Jannotta, F. S., and Vitkovic, L. (1993b). Control of astrocytosis by interleukin-1 and transforming growth factor-beta 1 in human brain. *Brain Res.* **631,** 39–45.

Dantzer, R. (2004). Cytokin-induced sickness behavior: A neuroimmune response to activation of innate immunity. *Eur. J. Pharmacol.* **500,** 399–411.

De Sarro, G., Gareri, P., Sinopoli, V. A., David, E., and Rotiroti, D. (1997). Comparative, behavioural and electrocortical effects of tumor necrosis factor-alpha and interleukin-1 microinjected into the locus coeruleus of rat. *Life Sci.* **60,** 555–564.

Deak, T., Bordner, K., McElderry, N., Barnum, C., Blandino, P., Deak, M., and Tammariello, S. (2005). Stress-induced increases in hypothalamic IL-1: A systematic analysis of multiple stressor paradigms. *Brain Res. Bull.* **64,** 541–556.

Depino, A. M., Alonso, M., Ferrari, C., del Rey, A., Anthony, D., Besedovsky, H., Medina, J. H., and Pitossi, F. (2004). Learning modulation by endogenous hippocampal IL-1: Blockade of endogenous IL-1 facilitates memory formation. *Hippocampus* **14,** 526–535.

Dickstein, J., Moldofsky, H., Lue, F., and Hay, J. (1999). Intracerebroventricular injection of TNF-alpha promotes sleep and is recovered in cervical lymph. *Am. J. Physiol.* **276,** R1018–R1022.

Dinarello, C. A. (1991). Interleukin-1 and interleukin-1 antagonism. *Blood* **77,** 1627–1652.

Dinarello, C. (2000). Proinflammatory cytokines. *Chest* **118,** 503–508.

Fang, J., Wang, Y., and Krueger, J. M. (1997). Mice lacking the TNF 55 kDa receptor fail to sleep more after TNFalpha treatment. *J. Neurosci.* **17,** 5949–5955.

Fang, J., Wang, Y., and Krueger, J. M. (1998). Effects of interleukin-1 beta on sleep are mediated by the type I receptor. *Am. J. Physiol.* **274,** R655–R660.

Faraci, F. M., and Heistad, D. D. (1998). Regulation of the cerebral circulation: Role of endothelium and potassium channels. *Physiol. Rev.* **78**(1), 53–97.

Ferrari, D., Chiozzi, P., Falzoni, S., Hanau, S., and Di Virgilio, F. (1997). Purinergic modulation of interleukin-1 beta release from microglial cells stimulated with bacterial endotoxin. *J. Exp. Med.* **185**(3), 579–582.

Fields, R. D., and Stevens, B. (2000). ATP: An extracellular signaling molecule between neurons and glia. *Trends Neurosci.* **23**(12), 625–633.

Fitzgerald, K., and O'Neill, L. (2000). The role of the interleukin-1/Toll-like receptor superfamily in inflammation and host defence. *Microbes Infect.* **2,** 933–943.

Floyd, R., and Krueger, J. M. (1997). Diurnal variation of TNF alpha in the rat brain. *Neuroreport* **8,** 915–918.

Fogal, B., and Hewett, S. (2008). Interleukin-1beta: A bridge between inflammation and excitotoxicity? *J. Neurochem.* **106**(1), 1–23.

Frey, D. J., Fleshner, M., and Wright, K. P., Jr. (2007). The effects of 40 hours of total sleep deprivation on inflammatory markers in healthy young adults. *Brain Behav. Immun.* **21,** 1050–1057.

Friedman, E., Boinski, S., and Coe, C. (1995). Interleukin-1 induces sleep-like behaviour and alters call structure in juvenile rhesus macaques. *Am. J. Primatol.* **35,** 145–153.

Fu, Y., Luo, L., Luo, N., and Garvey, W. T. (2006). Proinflammatory cytokine production and insulin sensitivity regulated by overexpression of resistin in 3T3-L1 adipocytes. *Nutr. Metab. (Lond)* **3,** 28.

Gambino, F., Pavlowsky, A., Béglé, A., Dupont, J. L., Bahi, N., Courjaret, R., Gardette, R., Hadjkacem, J., Skala, H., Poulain, B., Chelly, J., Vitale, N., *et al.* (2007). IL1-receptor accessory protein-like 1 (IL1RAPL1), a protein involved in cognitive functions, regulates N-type Ca2+ channel and neurite elongation. *Proc. Natl. Acad. Sci. U.S.A.* **104,** 9063–9068.

Gibson, R., Rothwell, N., and Le Feuvre, R. (2004). CNS injury: The role of the cytokine IL-1. *Vet. J.* **168,** 230–237.

Goeddel, D. V. (1999). Signal transduction by tumor necrosis factor. *Chest* **116,** 69S–73S.

Granowitz, E., Clark, B., Vannier, E., Callahan, M., and Dinarello, C. A. (1992). Effect of interleukin-1 (IL-1) blockade on cytokine synthesis: I. IL-1 receptor antagonist inhibits IL-1-induced cytokine synthesis and blocks the binding of IL-1 to its type II receptor on human monocytes. *Blood* **79,** 2356–2363.

Hagan, P., Poole, S., and Bristow, A. F. (1993). Endotoxin-stimulated production of rat hypothalamic interleukin-1 beta in vivo and in vitro, measured by specific immunoradiometric assay. *J. Mol. Endocrinol.* **11,** 31–36.

Halassa, M. M., Fellin, T., and Haydon, P. G. (2009). Tripartite synapses: Roles for astrocyte purines in the control of synaptic physiology and behavior. *Neuropharmacology* **57,** 343–346.

Hansen, M. K., Taishi, P., Chen, Z., and Krueger, J. M. (1998). Cafeteria feeding induces interleukin-1beta mRNA expression in rat liver and brain. *Am. J. Physiol.* **274**(6 Pt 2), R1734–R1739.

Hide, I., Tanaka, M., Inoue, A., Nakajima, K., Kohsaka, S., Inoue, K., and Nakata, Y. (2000). Extracellular ATP triggers tumor necrosis factor-alpha release from rat microglia. *J. Neurochem.* **75,** 965–972.

Honore, P., Donnelly-Roberts, D., Namovic, M. T., Hsieh, G., Zhu, C. Z., Mikusa, J. P., Hernandez, G., Zhong, C., Gauvin, D. M., Chandran, P., Harris, R., Perez Medrano, A., *et al.* (2006). A-740003 [N-(1-{[(cyanoimino)(5-quinolinylamino) methyl]amin}-2,2-dimethylpropyl)-2-(3,4-dimethoxyphenyl)acetamide], a novel and selective P2X7 receptor antagonist, dose-dependently reduces neuropathic pain in the rat. *J. Pharmacol. Exp. Ther.* **319,** 1376–1385.

Hristova, M., and Aloe, L. (2006). Metabolic syndrome-neurotrophic hypothesis. *Med. Hypotheses* **66,** 545–549.

Hu, J., Chen, Z., Gorczynski, C. P., Gorczynski, L. Y., Kai, Y., Lee, L., Manuel, J., and Gorczynski, R. M. (2003). Sleep-deprived mice show altered cytokine production manifest by perturbations in serum IL-1ra, TNFa, and IL-6 levels. *Brain Behav. Immun.* **17,** 498–504.

Huber, R., Ghilardi, M. F., Massimini, M., and Tononi, G. (2004). Local sleep and learning. *Nature* **430,** 27–28.

Ignatowski, T., Noble, B., Wright, J., Gorfien, J., Heffner, R., and Spengler, R. (1997). Neuronal-associated tumor necrosis factor (TNF alpha): Its role in noradrenergic functioning and modification of its expression following antidepressant drug administration. *J. Neuroimmunol.* **79,** 84–90.

Imeri, L., and Opp, M. R. (2009). How (and why) the immune system makes us sleep. *Nat. Rev. Neurosci.* **10,** 199–210.

Inoue, S. (1989). Biology of Sleep Substances. CRC Press, Inc., Boca Raton, FL.

Inoue, K. (2002). Microglial activation by purines and pyrimidines. *Glia* **40**(2), 156–163.

Inoue, J., Ishida, T., Tsukamoto, N., Kobayashi, N., Naito, A., Azuma, S., and Yamamoto, T. (2000). Tumor necrosis factor receptor-associated factor (TRAF) family: Adapter protein that mediate cytokine signaling. *Exp. Cell Res.* **254,** 14–24.

Ishimori, K. (1909). True cause of sleep—A hynogenic substance as evidenced in the brain sleep-deprived animals. *Tokyo Igakkai Zasshi* **23,** 429–459.

Jager, J., Grémeaux, T., Cormont, M., LeMarchand-Brustel, Y., and Tanti, J. F. (2007). Interleukin-1beta-induced insulin resistance in adipocytes through down-regulation of insulin receptor substrate-1 expression. *Endocrinology* **148,** 241–251.

Jewett, K., Sengupta, P., Kirkpatrick, R., Clinton, J. M., and Krueger, J. M. (2011). Optogenetic stimulation enhances c-fos and interleukin-1 beta levels in cultured neurons. *Sleep* **34,** A14.

Ji, D., and Wilson, M. A. (2007). Coordinated memory replay in the visual cortex and hippocampus during sleep. *Nat. Neurosci.* **10**(1), 100–107.

Jouvet, M. (1984). Neuromediateurs et facteurs hypnogenes. *Rev. Neurol. (Paris)* **140,** 389–400.

Kapás, L., and Krueger, J. M. (1992). Tumor necrosis factor-beta induces sleep, fever, and anorexia. *Am. J. Physiol.* **263**(3 Pt. 2), R703–R707.

Kapsimalis, F., Richardson, G., Opp, M. R., and Kryger, M. (2005). Cytokines and normal sleep. *Curr. Opin. Pulm. Med.* **11**(6), 481–484.

Kattler, H., Dijk, D. J., and Borbély, A. A. (1994). Effect of unilateral somatosensory stimulation prior to sleep on the sleep EEG in humans. *J. Sleep Res.* **3,** 159–164.

Kawasaki, Y., Zhang, L., Cheng, J.-K., and Ji, R.-R. (2008). Cytokine mechanisms of central sensitization: Distinct and overlapping role of interleukin-1β, interleukin-6 and tumor necrosis factor-α in regulating synaptic and neuronal activity in the superficial spinal cord. *J. Neurosci.* **28,** 5189–5194.

Kilduff, T. S., and Peyron, C. (2000). The hypocretin/orexin ligand-receptor system: Implications for sleep and sleep disorders. *Trends Neurosci.* **23,** 359–365.

Konsman, J., Parnet, P., and Dantzer, R. (2002). Cytokine-induced sickness behavior: Mechanisms and implications. *Trends Neurosci.* **25,** 154–159.

Kristiansen, K., and Courtois, G. (1949). Rhythmic electrical activity from isolated cerebral cortex. *Electroencephalogr. Clin. Neurophysiol.* **1**(1–4), 265–272.

Krueger, J. M. (2008). The role of cytokines in sleep regulation. *Curr. Pharm. Des.* **14**(32), 3408–3416.

Krueger, J. M., and Majde, J. (2003). Humoral links between sleep and the immune system. *Ann. N. Y. Acad. Sci.* **992,** 9–20.

Krueger, J. M., and Obál, F., Jr. (1994). Sleep factors. *In* "Sleep and Breathing," (N. A. Saunders and C. E. Sullivan, Eds.), pp. 79–112. Marcel Dekker, Inc., New York.

Krueger, J. M., Dinarello, C. A., and Chedid, L. (1983). Promotion of slow-wave sleep (SWS) by a purified interleukin-1 (IL-1) preparation. *Fed. Proc.* **42,** 356.

Krueger, J. M., Walter, J., Dinarello, C. A., Wolff, S. M., and Chedid, L. (1984). Sleep-promoting effects of endogenous pyrogen (interleukin-1). *Am. J. Physiol.* **246**(6 Pt. 2), R994–R999.

Krueger, J. M., Obál, F., Jr., Opp, M. R., Toth, L., Johannsen, L., and Cady, A. B. (1990). Somnogenic cytokines and models concerning their effects on sleep. *Yale J. Biol. Med.* **63,** 157–172.

Krueger, J. M., Obál, F., Jr., Fang, J., Kubota, P., and Taishi, P. (2001). The role of cytokines in physiological sleep regulation. *Ann. N. Y. Acad. Sci.* **933,** 211–221.

Krueger, J. M., Rector, D. M., and Churchill, L. (2007). Sleep and cytokines. *Sleep Med. Clinics* **2,** 161–169.

Krueger, J. M., Rector, D. M., Roy, S., Van Dongen, H. P. A., Belenky, G., and Panksepp, J. (2008). Sleep as a fundamental property of neuronal assemblies. *Nat. Rev. Neurosci.* **9,** 910–919.

Krueger, J. M., Taishi, P., De, A., Davis, C., Winters, B. D., Clinton, J., Szentirmai, E., and Zielinski, M. R. (2010). ATP and the purine type 2 X7 receptor affect sleep. *J. Appl. Physiol.* **109,** 1318–1327.

Kubota, T., Fang, J., Guan, Z., Brown, R., and Krueger, J. M. (2001). Vagotomy attenuates tumor necrosis factor-alpha-induced sleep and EEG delta-activity in rats. *Am. J. Physiol. Regul. Integr. Comp. Physiol.* **280,** R1213–R1220.

Kubota, T., Li, N., Guan, Z., Brown, R., and Krueger, J. M. (2002). Intrapreoptic microinjection of TNF-alpha enhances non-REM sleep in rats. *Brain Res.* **932,** 37–44.

Kundermann, B., Hemmeter-Spernal, J., Huber, M. T., Krieg, J. C., and Lautenbacher, S. (2008). Effects of total sleep deprivation in major depression: Overnight improvement of mood is accompanied by increased pain sensitivity and augmented pain complaints. *Psychosom. Med.* **70,** 92–101.

Larsen, C. M., Faulenbach, M., Vaag, A., Vølund, A., Ehses, J. A., Seifert, B., Mandrup-Poulsen, T., and Donath, M. Y. (2007). Interleukin-1-receptor antagonist in type 2 diabetes mellitus. *N. Engl. J. Med.* **356,** 1517–1526.

Lechan, R., Toni, R., Clark, B., Cannon, J., Shaw, A., Dinarello, C. A., and Reichlin, S. (1990). Immunoreactive interleukin-1β localization in the rat forebrain. *Brain Res.* **514,** 135–140.

Ledgerwood, E. C., Pober, J. S., and Bradley, J. R. (1999). Recent advances in the molecular basis of TNF signal transduction. *Lab. Invest.* **79,** 1041–1050.

Legendre, R., and Piéron, H. (1913). Recherches sur le besoin de sommeil consécutif à une vielle prolongée. *Z. Allg. Physiol.* **14,** 235–262.

Leon, L. R. (2002). Invited review: Cytokine regulation of fever: Studies using gene knockout mice. *J. Appl. Physiol.* **92**(6), 2648–2655.

Liu, Z. G. (2005). Molecular mechanism of TNF signaling and beyond. *Cell Res.* **15**(1), 24–27.

Lyamin, O. I., Mukhametov, L. M., Siegel, J. M., Nazarenko, E. A., Polyakova, I. G., and Shpak, O. V. (2002). Unihemispheric slow wave sleep and the state of the eyes in a white whale. *Behav. Brain Res.* **129,** 125–129.

Lyamin, O. I., Lapierre, J. L., Kosenko, P. O., Mukhametov, L. M., and Siegel, J. M. (2008). Electroencephalogram asymmetry and spectral power during sleep in the northern fur seal. *J. Sleep Res.* **17,** 154–165.

Mahowald, M. W., and Schenck, C. H. (2005). Insights from studying human sleep disorders. *Nature* **437,** 1279–1285.

Manfridi, A., Brambilla, D., Bianchi, S., Mariotti, M., Opp, M. R., and Imeri, L. (2003). Interleukin-1beta enhances non-rapid eye movement sleep when microinjected into the dorsal raphe nucleus and inhibits serotonergic neurons in vitro. *Eur. J. Neurosci.* **18**(5), 1041–1049.

Maquet, P. (2001). The role of sleep in learning and memory. *Science* **294,** 1048–1052.

Medana, I., Hunt, N., and Chaudhri, G. (1997). Tumor necrosis factor alpha expression in the brain during fatal murine cerebral malaria. *Am. J. Pathol.* **150,** 1473–1486.

Moldofsky, H. (1995). Sleep, neuroimmune and neuroendocrine functions in fibromyalgia and chronic fatigue syndrome. *Adv. Neuroimmunol.* **5,** 39–56.

Moldofsky, H., Lue, F. A., Eisen, J., Keystone, E., and Gorczynski, R. M. (1986). The relationship of interleukin-1 and immune functions to sleep in humans. *Psychosom. Med.* **48**(5), 309–318.

Molenaar, G. J., Berkenbosch, F., Van Dam, A. M., and Lugard, C. M. (1993). Distribution of interleukin 1 beta immunoreactivity within the porcine hypothalamus. *Brain Res.* **608,** 169–174.

Montagna, P. (2005). Fatal familial insomnia: A model disease in sleep physiopathology. *Sleep Med. Rev.* **9,** 339–353.

Mukhametov, L. M., Supin, A. Y., and Polyakova, I. G. (1977). Interhemispheric asymmetry of the electroencephalographic sleep patterns in dolphins. *Brain Res.* **134**(3), 581–584.

Obál, F., Jr., and Krueger, J. M. (2003). Biochemical regulation of non-rapid-eye-movement sleep. *Front. Biosci.* **8,** d520–d550.

Obál, F., Jr., Opp, M. R., Cady, A., Johannsen, L., Postlethwaite, A., Poppleton, H., Seyer, J., and Krueger, J. M. (1990). Interleukin 1 alpha and an interleukin 1 beta fragment are somnogenic. *Am. J. Physiol.* **259,** R439–R446.

Obál, F., Jr., Alt, J., Taishi, P., Gardi, J., and Krueger, J. M. (2003). Sleep in mice with nonfunctional growth hormone-releasing hormone receptors. *Am. J. Physiol.* **284,** R131–R139.

Omdal, R., and Gunnarsson, R. (2005). The effect of interleukin-1 blockade on fatigue in rheumatoid arthritis—A pilot study. *Rheumatol. Int.* **25,** 481–484.

Opp, M. R. (2005). Cytokines and sleep. *Sleep Med. Rev.* **9,** 355–364.

Opp, M. R., and Krueger, J. M. (1991). Interleukin 1 receptor antagonist blocks interleukin 1-induced sleep and fever. *Am. J. Physiol.* **260,** R453–R457.

Opp, M. R., Obál, F., Jr., and Krueger, J. M. (1991). Interleukin 1 alters rat sleep: Temporal and dose-related effects. *Am. J. Physiol.* **260,** R52–R58.

Palin, K., Bluthé, R., McCusker, R., Moos, F., Dantzer, R., and Kelley, K. (2007). TNF alpha-induced sickness behavior in mice with functional 55 kD TNF receptors is blocked by central IGF-I. *J. Neuroimmunol.* **187,** 55–60.

Pappenheimer, J. R., Koski, G., Fencl, V., Karnovsky, M. L., and Krueger, J. (1975). Extraction of sleep-promoting factor S from cerebrospinal fluid and from brains of sleep-deprived animals. *J. Neurophysiol.* **38**(6), 1299–1311.

Pascual, O., Casper, K. B., Kubera, C., Zhang, J., Revilla-Sanchez, R., Sul, J. Y., Takano, H., Moss, S. J., McCarthy, K., and Haydon, P. G. (2005). Astrocytic purinergic signaling coordinates synaptic networks. *Science* **310,** 113–116.

Perry, S., Dewhurst, S., Bellizzi, M., and Gelbard, H. (2002). Tumor necrosis factor-alpha in normal and diseased brain: Conflicting effects via intraneuronal receptor crosstalk? *J. Neurovirol.* **8,** 611–624.

Peyron, C., Tighe, D. K., van den Pol, A. N., de Lecea, L., Heller, H. C., Sutcliffe, J. G., and Kilduff, T. S. (1998). Neurons containing hypocretin (orexin) project to multiple neuronal systems. *J. Neurosci.* **18**(23), 9996–10015.

Pickering, M., and O'Connor, J. J. (2007). Pro-inflammatory cytokines and their effects in the dentate gyrus. *Prog. Brain Res.* **163,** 339–354.

Pigarev, I. N., Nothdurft, H. C., and Kastner, S. (1997). Evidence for asynchronous development of sleep in cortical areas. *Neuroreport* **8**(11), 2557–2560.

Quan, N., Whiteside, M., and Herkenham, M. (1998). Time course and localization patterns of interleukin-1 beta mRNA expression in brain and pituitary after peripheral administration of lipopolysaccharide. *Neuroscience* **83,** 281–293.

Rattenborg, N. C., Amlaner, C. J., and Lima, S. L. (2001). Unilateral eye closure and interhemispheric EEG asymmetry during sleep in the pigion (Columba livia). *Brain Behav. Evol.* **58,** 323–332.

Re, F., Sironi, M., Muzio, M., Matteucci, C., Introna, M., Orlando, S., Penton-Rol, G., Dower, S. K., Sims, J. E., Colotta, F., and Mantovani, A. (1996). Inhibition of interleukin-1 responsiveness by type II receptor gene transfer: A surface "receptor" with anti-interleukin-1 function. *J. Exp. Med.* **183**(4), 1841–1850.

Rector, D. M., Topchiy, I. A., Carter, K. M., and Rojas, M. J. (2005). Local functional state differences between rat cortical columns. *Brain Res.* **1047,** 45–55.

Rector, D. M., Schei, J. L., and Rojas, M. J. (2009). Mechanisms underlying state dependent surface-evoked response patterns. *Neuroscience* **159**(1), 115–126.

Roky, R., Obál, F., Jr., Valatx, J. L., Bredow, S., Fang, J., Pagano, L. P., and Krueger, J. M. (1995). Prolactin and rapid eye movement. *Sleep* **18,** 536–542.

Roy, S., Krueger, J. M., Rector, D. M., and Wan, Y. (2008). Network models for activity-dependent sleep regulation. *J. Theor. Biol.* **253,** 462–468.

Saito, K., Suyama, K., Nishida, K., Sei, Y., and Basile, A. (1996). Early increases in TNF-α, IL-6 and IL-1β levels following transient cerebral ischemia in gerbil brain. *Neurosci. Lett.* **206,** 149–152.

Saper, C. B. (1987). Diffuse cortical projection systems: Anatomical organization and role in cortical function. *In* "Handbook of Physiology. The Nervous System V," (F. Plum, Ed.), pp. 169–210. American Physiological Society, Bethesda, MD.

Saper, C. B., Scammell, T. E., and Lu, J. (2005). Hypothalamic regulation of sleep and circadian rhythms. *Nature* **437**(7063), 1257–1263.

Sherin, J. E., Shiromani, P. J., McCarley, R. W., and Saper, C. B. (1996). Activation of ventrolateral preoptic neurons during sleep. *Science* **271**(5246), 216–219.

Sherin, J. E., Elmquist, J. K., Torrealba, F., and Saper, C. B. (1998). Innervation of histaminergic tuberomammillary neurons by GABAergic and galaninergic neurons in the ventrolateral preoptic nucleus of the rat. *J. Neurosci.* **18**(12), 4705–4721.

Shoham, S., Davenne, D., Cady, A., Dinarello, C. A., and Krueger, J. M. (1987). Recombinant tumor necrosis factor and interleukin 1 enhance slow-wave sleep. *Am. J. Physiol.* **253,** R142–R149.

Solle, M., Labasi, J., Perregaux, D. G., Stam, E., Petrushova, N., Koller, B. H., Griffiths, R. J., and Gabel, C. A. (2001). Altered cytokine production in mice lacking P2X7 receptors. *J. Biol. Chem.* **276,** 125–132.

Solomon, K., Pesti, N., Wu, G., and Newton, R. (1999). Cutting edge: A dominant negative form of TNF-alpha converting enzyme inhibits proTNF and TNFRII secretion. *J. Immunol.* **163,** 4105–4108.

Susić, V., and Totić, S. (1989). "Recovery" function of sleep: Effects of purified human interleukin-1 on the sleep and febrile response of cats. *Metab. Brain Dis.* **4,** 73–80.

Suzuki, T., Hide, I., Ido, K., Kohsaka, S., Inoue, K., and Nakata, Y. (2004). Production and release of neuroprotective tumor necrosis factor by P2X7 receptor-activated microglia. *J. Neurosci.* **7,** 1–7.

Szelényi, J. (2001). Cytokines and the central nervous system. *Brain Res. Bull.* **54**(4), 329–338.

Szymusiak, R., and McGinty, D. (2008). Hypothalamic regulation of sleep and arousal. *Ann. N. Y. Acad. Sci.* **1129,** 275–286.

Szymusiak, R., Alam, N., Steininger, T. L., and McGinty, D. (1998). Sleep-waking discharge patterns of ventrolateral preoptic/anterior hypothalamic neurons in rats. *Brain Res.* **803**(1–2), 178–188.

Taishi, P., Bredow, S., Guha-Thakurta, N., Obal, F., Jr., and Krueger, J. M. (1997). Diurnal variations of interleukin-1 beta mRNA and beta-actin mRNA in rat brain. *J. Neuroimmunol.* **75,** 69–74.

Taishi, P., Chen, Z., Obál, F., Jr., Hansen, M., Zhang, J., Fang, J., and Krueger, J. M. (1998). Sleep-associated changes in interleukin-1beta mRNA in the brain. *J. Interferon Cytokine Res.* **18,** 793–798.

Taishi, P., Churchill, L., Wang, M., Kay, D., Davis, C. J., Guan, X., De, A., Yasuda, T., Liao, F., and Krueger, J. M. (2007). TNFα siRNA reduces brain TNF and EEG delta wave activity in rats. *Brain Res.* **1156,** 125–132.

Takahashi, S., Kapás, L., Fang, J., and Krueger, J. M. (1995). An anti-tumor necrosis factor antibody suppresses sleep in rats and rabbits. *Brain Res.* **690,** 241–244.

Takahashi, S., Kapás, L., and Krueger, J. M. (1996). A tumor necrosis factor (TNF) receptor fragment attenuates TNF-alpha- and muramyl dipeptide-induced sleep and fever in rabbits. *J. Sleep Res.* **5,** 106–114.

Takahashi, S., Fang, J., Kapás, L., Wang, Y., and Krueger, J. M. (1997). Inhibition of brain interleukin-1 attenuates sleep rebound after sleep deprivation in rabbits. *Am. J. Physiol.* **273,** R677–R682.

Takahashi, S., Kapás, L., Fang, J., and Krueger, J. M. (1999). Somnogenic relationships between tumor necrosis factor and interleukin-1. *Am. J. Physiol.* **276,** R1132–R1140.

Terao, A., Matsumura, H., Yoneda, H., and Saito, M. (1998). Enhancement of slow-wave sleep by tumor necrosis factor-alpha is mediated by cyclooxygenase-2 in rats. *Neuroreport* **9,** 3791–3796.

Tobler, I., Borbély, A. A., Schwyzer, M., and Fontana, A. (1984). Interleukin-1 derived from astrocytes enhances slow wave activity in sleep EEG of the rat. *Eur. J. Pharmacol.* **104,** 191–192.

Toth, L. A., and Krueger, J. M. (1988). Alteration of sleep in rabbits by Staphylococcus aureus infection. *Infect. Immun.* **56**(7), 1785–1791.

Tracey, D., Klareskog, L., Sasso, E., Salfeld, J., and Tak, P. (2008). Tumor necrosis factor antagonist mechanisms of action: A comprehensive review. *Pharmacol. Ther.* **117,** 244–279.

Trinchieri, G., and Sher, A. (2007). Cooperation of Toll-like receptor signals in innate immune defence. *Nat. Rev. Immunol.* **7,** 179–190.

Tringall, G., Dello Russo, C., Preziosi, P., and Navarra, P. (2000). Interleukin-1 in the central nervous system: From physiology to pathology. *Therapie* **55,** 171–175.

Trompet, S., de Craen, A. J., Slagboom, P., Shepherd, J., Blauw, G. J., Murphy, M. B., Bollen, E. L., Buckley, B. M., Ford, I., Gaw, A., Macfarlane, P. W., Packard, C. J., *et al.* (2008). Genetic variation in the interleukin-1 beta-converting enzyme associates with cognitive function. The PROSPER study. *Brain* **131,** 1069–1077.

Verderio, C., and Matteoli, M. (2011). ATP in neuron-glia bidirectional signaling. *Brain Res. Rev.* **66,** 106–114.

Vitkovic, L., Bockaert, J., and Jacque, C. (2000). "Inflammatory" cytokines: Neuromodulators in normal brain? *J. Neurochem.* **74**(2), 457–471.

Vollmer-Conna, U., Fazou, C., Cameron, B., Li, H., Brennan, C., Luck, L., Davenport, T., Wakefield, D., Hickie, I., and Lloyd, A. (2004). Production of pro-inflammatory cytokines correlates with the symptoms of acute sickness behavior in humans. *Psychol. Med.* **34,** 128–1297.

Williams, R., Marinova-Mutafchieva, L., Feldmann, M., and Maini, R. (2000). Evaluation of TNF-alpha and IL-1 blockade in collagen-induced arthritis and comparison with combined anti-TNF-alpha/anti-CD4 therapy. *J. Immunol.* **165,** 7240–7245.

Yi, P. L., Tsai, C. H., Lin, J. G., Lee, C. C., and Chang, F. C. (2004). Kindling stimuli delivered at different times in the sleep-wake cycle. *Sleep* **27,** 203–212.

Yirmiya, R., and Goshen, I. (2011). Immune modulation of learning, memory, neural plasticity and neurogenesis. *Brain Behav. Immun.* **25,** 181–213.

Yndestad, A., Damås, J. K., Øie, E., Ueland, T., Gullestad, L., and Aukrust, P. (2007). Role of inflammation in the progression of heart failure. *Curr. Cardiol. Rep.* **9,** 236–241.

Yoshida, H., Peterfi, Z., Garcia-Garcia, F., Kirkpatrick, R., Yasuda, T., and Krueger, J. M. (2004). State-specific asymmetries in EEG slow wave activity induced by local application of TNF alpha. *Brain Res.* **1009,** 129–136.

CHAPTER FOURTEEN

Action of Modafinil Through Histaminergic and Orexinergic Neurons

Tomoko Ishizuka,[1] Tomotaka Murotani,[2] *and* Atsushi Yamatodani

Contents

Abstract

Modafinil is a wake-promoting drug used for the treatment of excessive daytime sleepiness due to narcolepsy as well as excessive sleepiness associated with obstructive sleep apnea and shift work disorder. Although the wake-promoting effect of modafinil is expressed through the dopaminergic and the norepinephrinergic systems similar to that of classical psychostimulants, the mechanism of action is distinct from those compounds in terms of the involvement of the histaminergic and the orexinergic systems. Modafinil activates the histaminergic system in an indirect manner, presumably via attenuation of the inhibitory GABAergic input to the histaminergic neurons. The orexinergic system controls arousal through the histaminergic system, and the modafinil-induced increment of histamine release is abolished in orexin neuron-ablated mice, suggesting

Department of Medical Science and Technology, Graduate School of Allied Health Sciences, Faculty of Medicine, Osaka University, Osaka, Japan

[1] Present address: Department of Pharmacology, Osaka Dental University, 8-1 Kuzuhahanazono-cho, Hirakata, Osaka 573-1121, Japan.

[2] Present address: Kobe University School of Medicine, 7-5-1 Kusunoki-cho, Chuo-ku, Kobe, Hyogo 650-0017, Japan.

Vitamins and Hormones, Volume 89
ISSN 0083-6729, http://dx.doi.org/10.1016/B978-0-12-394623-2.00014-7

that modafinil increases histaminergic tone via orexinergic neurons. Clinical and experimental investigations have suggested less importance of the orexinergic system in the wake-promoting effect of modafinil, but the orexinergic system is considered to be involved in modafinil-induced alertness or synaptic plasticity.

I. Introduction

Narcolepsy is a chronic, neurologic sleep disorder affecting 0.03–0.18% of the general population (Nishino *et al.*, 2000a). It is characterized by symptoms of excessive daytime sleepiness and abnormal rapid eye movement (REM) sleep including cataplexy (a sudden loss of bilateral skeletal muscle tone due to strong emotions), sleep paralysis, and hypnagogic hallucinations. In most narcoleptic patients, excessive daytime sleepiness and cataplexy are more troublesome symptoms.

Excessive daytime sleepiness and cataplexy can be pharmacologically treated, but not cured. Excessive daytime sleepiness has typically been treated with traditional psychostimulants, such as methylphenidate or dextroamphetamine, while cataplexy has been treated using antidepressant compounds, such as venlafaxine or atomoxetine. Among the existing pharmacological treatments for excessive daytime sleepiness, modafinil is now the most generally prescribed drug because it has fewer sympathomimetic actions and side effects and listed in Schedule IV of the controlled substances act in the United States. Although traditional psychostimulants are not always effective due to their significant adverse side effects, modafinil promotes wakefulness in daytime without tolerance and drug dependence and does not disturb nocturnal sleep (Bastuji and Jouvet, 1988; Touret *et al.*, 1995).

II. Neuronal Targets of Modafinil

A. Catecholamine

Based on the characteristics of modafinil, it has been postulated that the pharmacological profile of modafinil differs from those of other psychostimulants. Psychostimulants exert their robust wake-promoting actions via the dopaminergic system (Kanbayashi *et al.*, 2000; Nishino *et al.*, 1998). Dopaminergic neurons are dense in the striatum and cortex, the brain area excited by psychostimulants. However, the brain areas stimulated by modafinil have been proven to be, in part, distinct from those of psychostimulants. Lin *et al.* (1996) studied the neuronal targets for modafinil by c-Fos expression in cats. The proto-oncogene c-Fos is expressed in the activated brain areas in response to stimuli, thus serving as a marker of neuronal excitation (Sagar *et al.*, 1988). They found that the c-Fos positive cells induced by modafinil localized in the anterior hypothalamus and adjacent areas, while either amphetamine or methylphenidate evoked a robust induction of c-Fos expression in the striatum and whole cortex. Subsequent study using rats (Engber *et al.*, 1998) also showed that modafinil-induced c-Fos expression in the anterior hypothalamus and suprachiasmatic nuclei but not in the frontal cortex or striatum, supporting the idea that the potential pharmacological targets of modafinil differ from those of amphetamine and methylphenidate.

Based on these findings, earlier studies focused on the actions of modafinil that are dissociated from the dopaminergic system. Modafinil did not increase synaptic dopamine levels in the caudate nucleus (De Sereville *et al.*, 1994) and [^{3}H]dopamine release from the mouse synaptosomes preloaded with [^{3}H]dopamine (Simon *et al.*, 1995) and did not modify the firing pattern of dopaminergic neurons in the ventral tegmental area (Akaoka *et al.*, 1991). Moreover, α-methyl-DL-*p*-tyrosine methyl ester, an inhibitor of catecholamine synthesis, only slightly reduced the waking effect of modafinil (Lin *et al.*, 1992) and did not suppress locomotor activity induced by modafinil (Simon *et al.*, 1995). D_1- and D_2-antagonist did not block modafinil-induced wakefulness in mice (Simon *et al.*, 1995) and cats (Lin *et al.*, 1992).

However, as research progressed, a substantial amount of data indicating that the dopaminergic system is likely to be one of the important targets of modafinil has been accumulated. Modafinil has a weak affinity for the dopamine transporter (Madras *et al.*, 2006; Mignot *et al.*, 1994) and has an agonistic action on dopamine D_2-like receptors (Korotkova *et al.*, 2007). Several microdialysis studies also demonstrated the potency of modafinil in facilitating extracellular dopamine release in the rat prefrontal cortex (de Saint Hilaire *et al.*, 2001), the rat nucleus accumbens (Murillo-Rodríguez *et al.*, 2007), and the narcoleptic canine caudate (Wisor *et al.*, 2001). The wake-promoting effect of modafinil is attenuated in dopamine transporter knockout (KO) mice (Wisor *et al.*, 2001), while amplified in dopamine β-hydroxylase KO mice which are hypersensitive to dopaminergic signaling (Mitchell *et al.*, 2008). Since modafinil also has an affinity for the norepinephrine transporter (Madras *et al.*, 2006), the involvement of norepinephrine in the arousal effect of modafinil has been investigated. Modafinil can increase norepinephrine levels both in rat prefrontal cortex and in the medial hypothalamus area (de Saint Hilaire *et al.*, 2001). Pretreatments with selective α1-antagonists significantly attenuated the arousal effect of modafinil in cats (Lin *et al.*, 1992) and mice (Stone *et al.*, 2002). In α1B-receptors-ablated mice, there was also a significant attenuation of gross movement in response to modafinil (Stone *et al.*, 2002). These findings indicate that catecholamines are a major target of modafinil.

B. Newly discovered targets of modafinil

Meanwhile, the possible involvement of the hypothalamus in the action of modafinil is expected by the pattern of c-Fos immunoreactivity. Although the mode of action of modafinil resembles those of psychostimulants in terms of the participation of catecholaminergic systems, modafinil is characterized by its powerful action on the hypothalamus and the microinjection of modafinil into the anterior hypothalamus enhanced wakefulness (Arias-Carrión *et al.*, 2011).

The hypothalamus is the important area for natural sleep–wake regulation; thus, it seems reasonable that neurotransmitters, which control arousal function in the hypothalamus, should be involved in the action of modafinil. Another immunohistochemical investigation by Scammell *et al.* (2000) showed that modafinil increased c-Fos expression in the tuberomammillary nucleus (TMN) and in the perifornical area, two regions implicated in the regulation of wakefulness. Since the TMN is the sole source of histaminergic neurons and the perifornical area is that of orexinergic neurons, both the histaminergic and the orexinergic systems are thought to be candidates for the pharmacological targets of modafinil.

1. The histaminergic system

The overall picture of the central histaminergic system was demonstrated in 1984 (Panula *et al.*, 1984; Watanabe *et al.*, 1984). The cell bodies of histamine neurons are located exclusively in the TMN in the posterior hypothalamus, and their fibers project to almost all brain regions. In the brain, there are three types of histamine receptors, postsynaptic H_1, H_2, and presynaptic H_3 receptor.

It is well known that the classical antihistamines penetrating the central nervous system cause drowsiness; thus, histamine is known as an important neurotransmitter controlling the arousal state in the hypothalamus. Histamine release from the rat hypothalamus has a clear circadian rhythm, being high during the active phase and low during the resting phase (Mochizuki *et al.*, 1992). Histaminergic tuberomammillary neurons are active only during wakefulness, and they show delayed response in firing during transitions from sleep to wakefulness (Takahashi *et al.*, 2006), indicating that the histaminergic system takes part in the maintenance of wakefulness. Both depletion of neuronal histamine (Kiyono *et al.*, 1985; Lin *et al.*, 1988, 1994) and injection of classical H_1-antagonists (Lin *et al.*, 1988, 1994) increase slow-wave sleep and REM sleep during the resting phase and decrease arousal during the active phase.

When endogenous histamine levels were increased by H_3-receptor-inverse agonist (Lin *et al.*, 1990; Parmentier *et al.*, 2002) or an inhibitor of histamine catabolic enzyme (Lin *et al.*, 1988), prolonged wakefulness was observed. Similarly, injection of histamine itself also increased wakefulness and reduced slow-wave sleep and REM sleep (Lin *et al.*, 1994). The effects of the H_3-inverse agonist on wakefulness are attenuated in H_1 receptor KO mice, but not in H_2 receptor KO mice (Parmentier *et al.*, 2007). These reports support the idea that histamine maintains wakefulness via histamine H_1 receptors.

2. The orexinergic system

The neuropeptides orexin-A and -B (also called hypocretin-1 and -2) were discovered by two independent groups of researchers around the same time (de Lecea *et al.*, 1998; Sakurai *et al.*, 1998). Orexins are located exclusively in neurons of the lateral hypothalamus, and their projections are widely distributed throughout the brain (Peyron *et al.*, 1998). There are two kinds of orexin receptors, orexin-1 receptor and orexin-2 receptor (also called hypocretin 1 receptor and hypocretin 2 receptor). Orexin-1 receptor is selective for orexin-A, while orexin-2 receptor has an affinity for both orexin-A and -B (Sakurai *et al.*, 1998). Initially, the physiological role of orexin was focused on feeding regulation and energy homeostasis because orexin-A and -B stimulated food consumption when administered centrally (Sakurai *et al.*, 1998). However, morphological feature of the orexinergic system which densely innervates brain regions important for the control of vigilance, such as the locus coeruleus and the raphe nuclei (Peyron *et al.*, 1998), predicted sleep–wake regulation by orexins. Extracellular orexin levels in the lateral hypothalamus of cats (Kiyashchenko *et al.*, 2002) and rats (Yoshida *et al.*, 2001) exhibited a robust diurnal fluctuation, being higher during the active phase than during the resting phase. The microinjection of orexin (Hagan *et al.*, 1999; Piper *et al.*, 2000) and optogenetic stimulation of the orexinergic neurons (Adamantidis *et al.*, 2007) strongly promote wakefulness. Forced wake causes an increase in orexin-A levels in the hypothalamus (Yoshida *et al.*, 2001) or cerebrospinal fluid (CSF) (Deboer *et al.*, 2004). These reports clarified that the orexinergic system was the key wake-promoting system.

Despite earlier discovery of symptoms of narcolepsy, its etiology remained uncertain until recently: during the late 1990s, it was demonstrated that orexin and its receptor in the brain play crucial roles in narcolepsy. Emerging evidence that linked narcolepsy with the orexinergic system was based on the finding that familial narcoleptic canines had a mutation in the *orexin-2 receptor* gene (Lin *et al.*, 1999). Another group also showed that mice lacking orexin ligands due to *prepro-orexin* gene KO showed abnormalities in sleep control resembling aspects of narcolepsy (Chemelli *et al.*, 1999). Either genetic ablation (Hara *et al.*, 2001) or pharmacological lesion of orexin-containing neurons (Gerashchenko *et al.*, 2001) also induced a phenotype similar to human narcolepsy. Based on these findings, orexin-related genes (orexin and its receptor) are considered "narcolepsy genes," and it has been speculated that dysfunction of the orexinergic system occurs in human narcolepsy. After mutation screening research in human narcolepsy, mutation in the orexin precursor gene or orexin receptor gene was shown to be extremely rare (Peyron *et al.*, 2000), but 85–95% of orexinergic neurons have been lost in narcoleptic patients (Thannickal *et al.*, 2000), and the level of orexin in the CSF of narcolepsy patients is significantly lower than that of healthy controls (Kanbayashi *et al.*, 2002; Nishino *et al.*, 2000b, 2001b). Interestingly, since low orexin levels in the CSF are very specific to narcolepsy–cataplexy compared with those of other sleep disorders (Mignot *et al.*, 2002; Ripley *et al.*, 2001), measurement of CSF orexin level was newly included in the revised international diagnostic criteria of narcolepsy–cataplexy in 2005.

III. The Interplay Between the Histaminergic and the Orexinergic Systems

Several lines of evidence indicated a functional relationship between the histaminergic and the orexinergic systems in the control of arousal. Orexinergic neurons densely send fibers to the TMN (Peyron *et al.*, 1998). Furthermore, orexin-2 receptors are enriched in the area (Marcus *et al.*, 2001), and both orexin-A and -B activate histamine neurons in the TMN (Bayer *et al.*, 2001; Eriksson *et al.*, 2001; Yamanaka *et al.*, 2002). Moreover, in orexin-2 receptor KO mice, orexin-A-evoked intracellular calcium transients in the TMN were not detectable, demonstrating the importance of orexin-2 receptor in orexin-mediated excitation of the TMN neurons (Willie *et al.*, 2003).

Figure 14.1 shows microdialysis data which studied the effects of orexins on hypothalamic histamine release in rats. The intracerebroventricular injections of both orexin peptides significantly increase histamine release in the rat anterior hypothalamus, although a fivefold dose of orexin-B (5 nmol) is required to achieve an effect equivalent to that of orexin-A (1 nmol) on histamine release (Fig. 14.1; Ishizuka *et al.*, 2002). Huang *et al.* (2001) also reported that direct perfusion of orexin-A into the TMN enhanced waking time concomitant with a reduction of slow-wave sleep and REM sleep and increased histamine release in the medial preoptic area and the frontal cortex. Orexin-A-induced wakefulness cannot be observed in histamine H_1 receptor KO mice (Huang *et al.*, 2001), in rats with pharmacological depletion of neuronal histamine (Yasuko *et al.*, 2010), and in rats pretreated with H_1-antagonist (Yamanaka *et al.*, 2002). Taken together, orexin exerts its arousal effect through the histaminergic system mediated by histamine H_1 receptors.

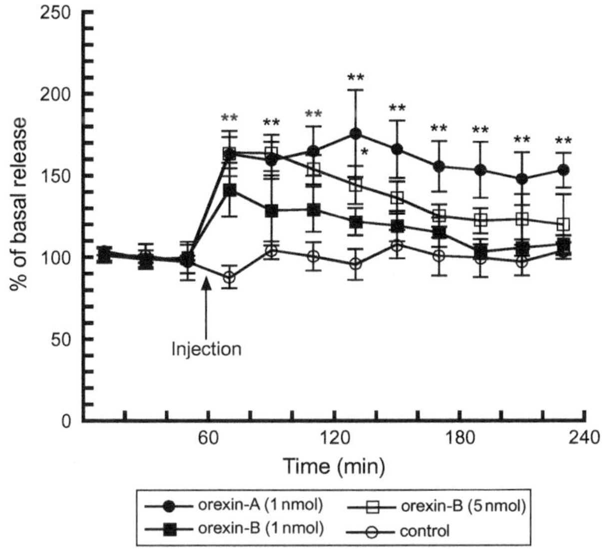

Figure 14.1 The effects of orexin-A (1 nmol, i.c.v., $n = 4$) and orexin-B (1 and 5 nmol, i.c.v., $n = 4$ of each) on the release of histamine from the rat anterior hypothalamus (Ishizuka *et al.*, 2002). The average mean value in the first three samples was taken as 100%. Values are presented as percentages of the mean basal release and SEM. $^{**}p < 0.01$ compared with the basal release in each group.

These findings suggest that reduced orexin signaling in narcoleptic animals invokes low histaminergic transmission. Nishino *et al.* (2001a) found a significant decrease in histamine content in the cortex and thalamus in orexin-2 receptor-mutated narcoleptic Dobermans and in hypocretin ligand-deficient sporadic narcoleptic dogs. In this context, recent research reported that CSF histamine levels are reduced in narcoleptic patients (Kanbayashi *et al.*, 2009; Nishino *et al.*, 2009). In addition, histamine H_3-inverse agonist can increase wakefulness in *prepro-orexin* gene KO mice (Guo *et al.*, 2009; Lin *et al.*, 2008) and narcoleptic patients (Lin *et al.*, 2008). H_3-inverse agonist also significantly reduced cataplexy in familial narcoleptic Dobermans using the standard food elicited cataplexy test (Bonaventure *et al.*, 2007) and also decreased direct transitions from wakefulness to REM sleep corresponding to murine cataplectic episodes in *prepro-orexin* gene KO mice (Lin *et al.*, 2008). Thus, some symptoms of narcolepsy, excessive daytime sleepiness, and cataplexy may be circumvented by direct activation of the histaminergic system. However, the involvement of histamine itself in the pathology of narcolepsy seems negative because histidine decarboxylase KO mice, which cannot synthesize histamine from histidine, do not demonstrate narcoleptic symptoms in contrast with that in orexin KO mice (Parmentier *et al.*, 2002).

IV. The Effects of Modafinil on the Histaminergic and the Orexinergic Systems

As indicated above, immunohistochemical investigation demonstrated that modafinil (150 mg/kg, i.p.), at a dose that promotes vigilance, induced c-Fos-positive cells in the TMN (Scammell *et al.*, 2000), suggesting that the histaminergic system is one of the targets for the action of modafinil. Hypothalamic histamine release was significantly increased by modafinil over the basal release when it was intraperitoneally (150 mg/kg) or intracerebroventricularly (1 nmol) injected to urethane-anesthetized rats (Fig. 14.2; Ishizuka *et al.*, 2003). In this study, relatively delayed response of histamine release was observed: modafinil increased histamine release about 2 h and an hour after intraperitoneal administration and intracerebroventricular injection, respectively. A similar microdialysis study using freely moving rats also displayed an increment of hypothalamic histamine release following intraperitoneal injection of modafinil (75 and 150 mg/kg) concomitant with enhanced locomotor activity, which is proportional to waking time thus available as a surrogate measure of wakefulness (Edgar and Seidel, 1997) (Fig. 14.3; Ishizuka *et al.*, 2008). Compared with the results obtained from anesthetized rats, the dynamic responses of histamine release in freely moving rats were promptly observed. This could be partly due to the urethane anesthesia we used for anesthetized rats because urethane

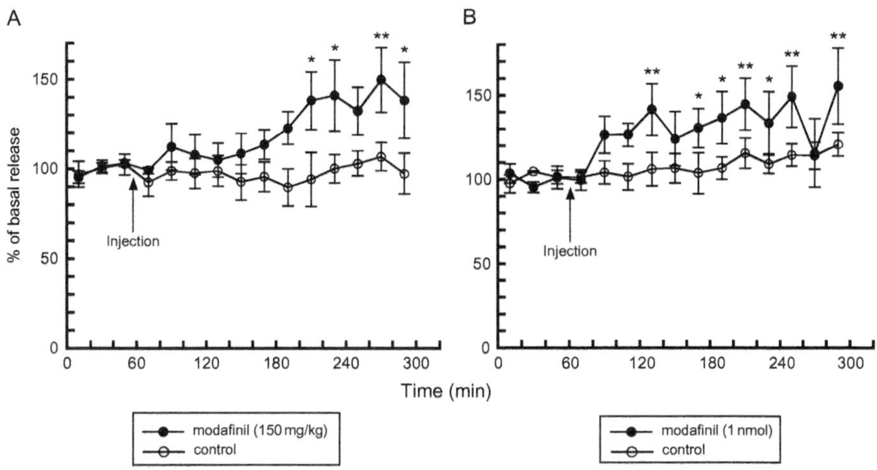

Figure 14.2 The effects of modafinil (A) 150 mg/kg, i.p. ($n=7$) and (B) 1 nmol, i.c.v. ($n=6$) on the release of histamine from the rat anterior hypothalamus (Ishizuka *et al.*, 2008). The average mean value in the first three samples was taken as 100%. Values are presented as percentages of the mean basal release and SEM. $^{*}p<0.05$, $^{**}p<0.01$ compared with the basal release of each group.

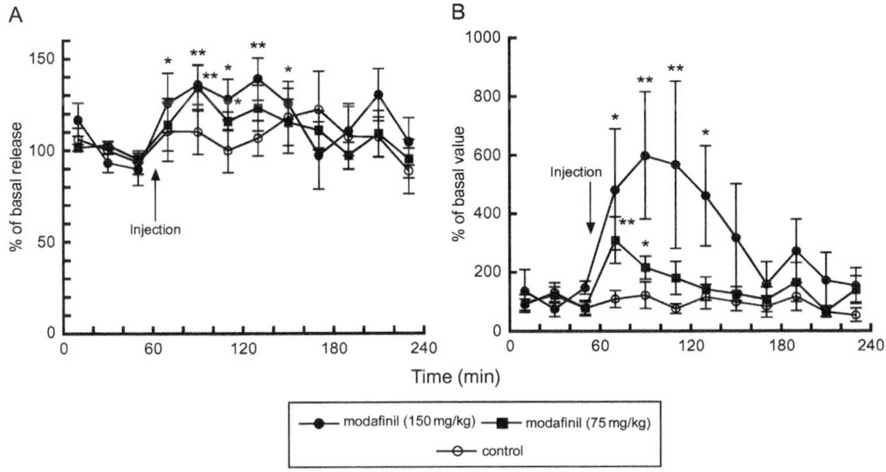

Figure 14.3 The effects of modafinil (75 and 150 mg/kg, i.p., $n=6$ and 5, respectively) on (A) hypothalamic histamine release and (B) locomotor activity in freely moving rats (Ishizuka *et al.*, 2008). The average mean values in the first three samples (A) and bins (B) were taken as 100%. Values are presented as percentages of the mean basal release and SEM. $^{*}p<0.05$, $^{**}p<0.01$ compared with the basal release of each group.

anesthesia might inhibit the TMN via $GABA_A$ receptors (Ishizuka *et al.*, 2008). Other researchers (Lin *et al.*, 2008) also showed that orally injected modafinil increased the level of *tele*-methylhistamine, a histamine metabolite, in the mouse cerebral cortex, further supporting the theory that modafinil activates the central histaminergic system.

In contrast, when methylphenidate (3 mg/kg), the drug widely used for daytime somnolence of narcolepsy, is injected to freely moving rats, histamine release was not enhanced but rather showed a significant decline by methylphenidate although this compound enhanced locomotor activity at the same extent of modafinil (Fig. 14.4; Ishizuka *et al.*, 2008). Together with the above finding (Fig. 14.3), selective activation of the histaminergic system by modafinil is clarified. Furthermore, the depletion of neuronal histamine by pretreatment of α-fluoromethylhistidine, an irreversible inhibitor of histamine forming enzyme, blocked modafinil-induced locomotor activity, but not methylphenidate-induced locomotor activity (Fig. 14.5; Ishizuka *et al.*, 2008). These findings clearly demonstrated that the effects of modafinil and methylphenidate are different in terms of the involvement of the histaminergic system.

However, when modafinil (1 nmol) was injected directly into the TMN, histamine release was not altered (Fig. 14.6; Ishizuka *et al.*, 2003). According to this observation, the histaminergic system does not seem to be a direct pharmacological target of modafinil, and it is postulated that the histaminergic system is the indirect and/or secondary target of modafinil. Modafinil reduces c-Fos expression in the ventrolateral preoptic area

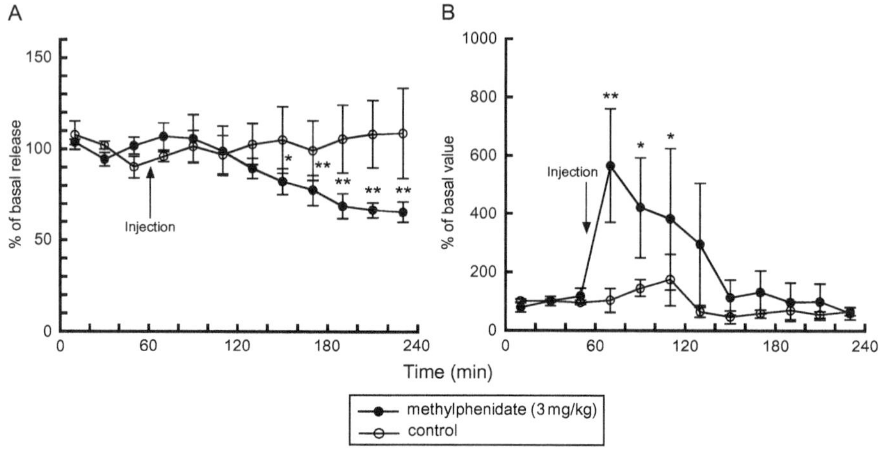

Figure 14.4 The effects of methylphenidate (3 mg/kg, i.p., $n = 5$) on (A) hypothalamic histamine release and (B) locomotor activity in freely moving rats (Ishizuka *et al.*, 2008). Saline is a vehicle for methylphenidate. The average mean values in the first three samples (A) and bins (B) were taken as 100%. Values are presented as percentages of the mean basal release and SEM. $^{*}p < 0.05$, $^{**}p < 0.01$ compared with the basal release of each group.

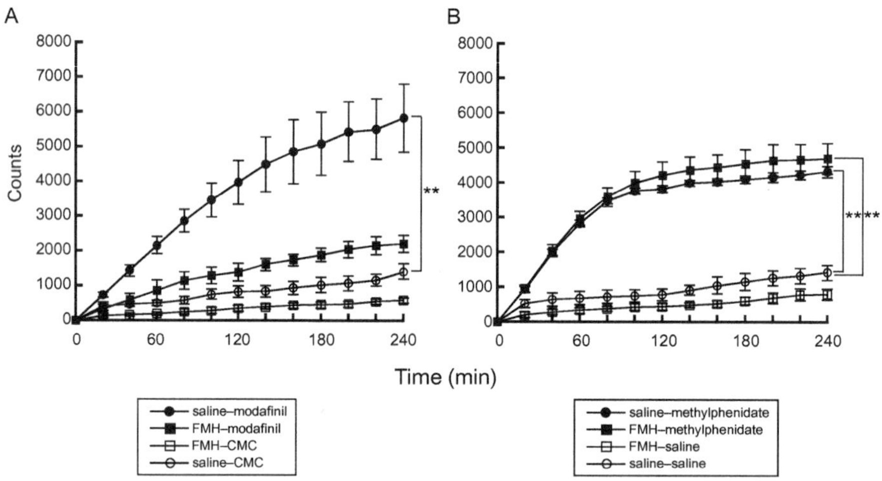

Figure 14.5 The effects of α-fluoromethylhistidine (FMH), an irreversible inhibitor of histamine forming enzyme, on (A) modafinil (150 mg/kg, i.p.)-induced and (B) methylphenidate (20 mg/kg, i.p.)-induced hyperactivity in mice (Ishizuka *et al.*, 2008). CMC is a vehicle for modafinil, and saline is a vehicle for FMH and methylphenidate. FMH (100 mg/kg, i.p.) was injected 2 h before modafinil treatment to achieve complete depletion of neuronal histamine. Each value represents the means and SEM. $^{**}p < 0.01$ between groups.

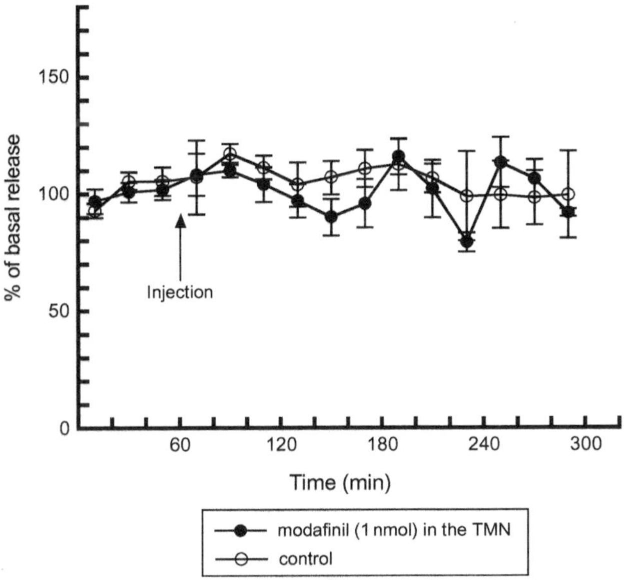

Figure 14.6 The effects of intra-TMN modafinil (1 nmol, $n=5$) on the release of histamine from the rat anterior hypothalamus (Ishizuka *et al.*, 2002). The average mean value in the first three samples was taken as 100%. Values are presented as percentages of the mean basal release and SEM.

(Scammell *et al.*, 2000), a necessary part of the brain to induce sleep (Lu *et al.*, 2000); thus, modafinil promotes wakefulness by inhibition of sleep-active neurons in the ventrolateral preoptic nucleus. These neurons provide the inhibitory GABAergic input to the TMN (Sherin *et al.*, 1998), and modafinil reduces outflow of GABA in the posterior hypothalamus (Ferraro *et al.*, 1996). Additionally, Beck *et al.* (2008) demonstrated that modafinil induces arousal by opening gap junctions between neurons, indicating that modafinil increases electrical coupling which is thought to decrease input resistance of GABAergic neurons and thereby decrease their output. Thus, modafinil is likely to disinhibit the histaminergic TMN neurons by decreasing the GABAergic activity from the ventrolateral preoptic area neurons.

Another possibility is that modafinil secondarily activates the histaminergic system via the orexinergic system because modafinil induces c-Fos expression in orexin neurons (Chemelli *et al.*, 1999; Scammell *et al.*, 2000), and histamine functionally exists downstream of orexin. Neurochemical and immunohistochemical studies have clearly demonstrated differences in the effects of modafinil on wild-type mice and transgenic mice in which orexin-containing neurons were completely ablated (Hara *et al.*, 2001). Modafinil (150 mg/kg, i.p.) significantly increased hypothalamic histamine

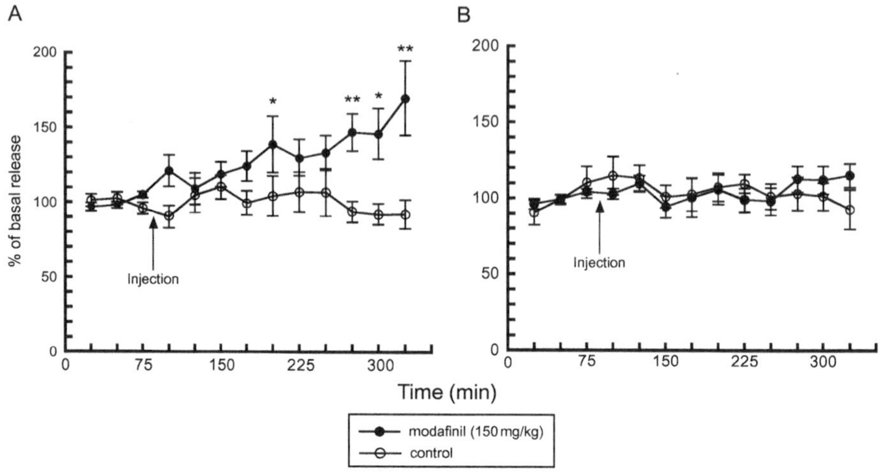

Figure 14.7 The effects of modafinil (150 mg/kg, i.p.) on hypothalamic histamine release in (A) wild-type ($n = 5$) and (B) orexin neuron-deficient mice ($n = 5$) (Ishizuka *et al.*, 2010). The average mean values in the first three samples were taken as 100%. Values are presented as percentages of the mean basal release and SEM. $^{*}p < 0.05$, $^{**}p < 0.01$ compared with the basal release of each group.

release in wild-type mice (Fig. 14.7A; Ishizuka *et al.*, 2010), being consistent with the previous finding using urethane-anesthetized rats (Fig. 14.2A; Ishizuka *et al.*, 2003). In contrast, modafinil did not influence histamine release in orexin neuron-deficient mice (Fig. 14.7B; Ishizuka *et al.*, 2010). Moreover, wild-type mice treated with the same dose of modafinil showed a substantial increase in c-Fos expression in the TMN, while orexin neuron-deficient mice did not (Fig. 14.8; Ishizuka *et al.*, 2010). These findings demonstrated that modafinil activates the histaminergic system via orexinergic neurons. Previous studies revealed that the dopaminergic and the norepinephrinergic systems are prime targets for the action of modafinil, but these findings indicate that the histaminergic and orexinergic systems are in part responsible for the pharmacological effects of modafinil.

V. Modafinil and Orexin—What Is the Physiological Role?

The involvement of orexin in the actions of modafinil was implicated by studies using c-Fos immunohistochemistry; modafinil treatment strongly enhanced c-Fos expression in the orexin neurons (Chemelli *et al.*, 1999; Scammell *et al.*, 2000), and the orexinergic system is thought to be associated

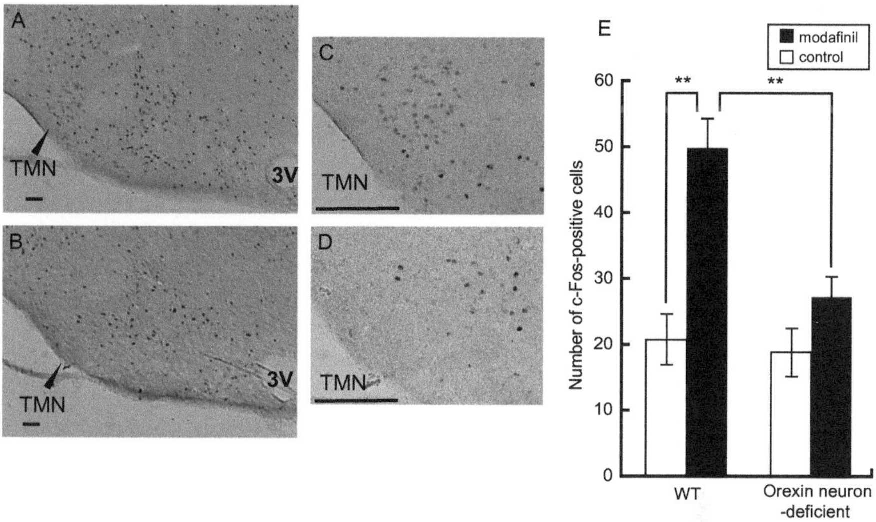

Figure 14.8 Representative photomicrographs of c-Fos expression induced by modafinil (150 mg/kg, i.p.) in (A) wild-type and (B) orexin neuron-deficient mice of the TMN (Ishizuka *et al.*, 2010). The magnification of the TMN of (C) wild-type (WT) and (D) orexin neuron-deficient mice. Scale bars, 100 μm; 3V, third ventricle; TMN, the tuberomammillary nucleus. (E) Cell counts of c-Fos-positive cells in the TMN. Each column represents the mean and SEM ($n = 4$–5). $^{**}p < 0.01$. (See Color Insert.)

with the effect of modafinil. However, since modafinil does not have an affinity to the orexin receptor expressed on SK-N-MC cells or the recombinant orexin-1 receptor (Wieland *et al.*, 2002), modafinil does not appear to have a direct agonistic effect on orexin receptors.

As opposed to these immunohistochemical studies, some researchers demonstrated that modafinil is still effective in promoting wakefulness in orexin KO mice (Lin *et al.*, 2008; Willie *et al.*, 2005), and they concluded that the presence of orexin is not required for the wake-promoting action of modafinil. These findings appear reasonable because most human narcoleptic patients have a deficiency in orexinergic transmission. Therefore, the presence of orexin does not seem to be essential for the arousal effect of modafinil in narcoleptic patients.

However, possible roles of orexin in modafinil-induced physiological effect other than wake promotion are supposed. On detailed analysis of electroencephalograms, orexin KO mice exhibited reduced power in the θ band (8–9 Hz) during the active waking period compared with that in wild-type mice under baseline conditions (Diniz Behn *et al.*, 2010; Willie *et al.*, 2005). Electroencephalogram oscillation in the θ range is derived from the hippocampus and is regarded as an index of alertness or attention during wakefulness in rodents (Huerta and Lisman, 1993). Modafinil (100 mg/kg) had less effect on the θ power of orexin KO mice, while modafinil increased the θ power in wild-type mice (Willie *et al.*, 2005), suggesting that orexin appears to participate in the modafinil-induced improvement of alertness or attention during wakefulness.

In addition, θ-burst stimulation is known to effectively induce long-term potentiation in the rat hippocampus, which is one of the major mechanisms involved in learning and memory (Nguyen and Kandel, 1997). Considering that modafinil facilitates water maze performance with the enhancement of postsynaptic potentials correlated selectively with θ rhythm augmentation in normal rats (Tsanov *et al.*, 2010) and that orexin-A induces synaptic plasticity in the mouse CA1 region of the hippocampus via stimulation of sharp wave and θ-concurrent activity (Selbach *et al.*, 2004), it is plausible that modafinil enhances learning and memory via orexin-induced θ rhythm augmentation. Thus, orexin may play a role in modafinil-induced synaptic plasticity as well.

As described above, narcolepsy–cataplexy is characterized by a loss of approximately 90% of orexin neurons and a very low CSF orexin level. This orexin deficiency is tightly associated with cataplexy (Kanbayashi *et al.*, 2002), but in narcoleptic patients, more than a quarter of narcoleptic patients with a normal CSF orexin level do not exhibit cataplexy (Longstreth *et al.*, 2007). From postmortem study, it is reported that orexin neurons partially remained in the brains of patients with narcolepsy but without cataplexy (Thannickal *et al.*, 2009). At present, there are no epidemiological data that compare the efficacy of modafinil between patients with low CSF and those with normal CSF orexin level. However, orexinergic activation followed by histaminergic activation could occur in patients with orexin neurons, resulting in more effective promotion of wakefulness (as well as alertness and synaptic plasticity) by modafinil.

VI. Conclusion and Perspectives

Figure 14.9 shows putative pathways of action of modafinil discussed in this chapter. Modafinil expresses its wake-promoting effect primarily though the dopaminergic and the norepinephrinergic systems. Although the histaminergic system also seems to be one of the targets of modafinil, it may not be a direct target of modafinil. The histaminergic system is activated by diminishing the inhibitory input of the GABAergic system from the ventrolateral preoptic area and by activation of the orexinergic system. Several studies show that modafinil affects not only the state of vigilance but also other physiological functions, such as alertness or synaptic plasticity, and it is possible that the orexinergic system enhanced by modafinil is involved in such functions in a histamine-dependent and/or -independent manner.

Modafinil is a very useful and effective compound to improve excessive daytime sleepiness while having no effect on the other major symptom of

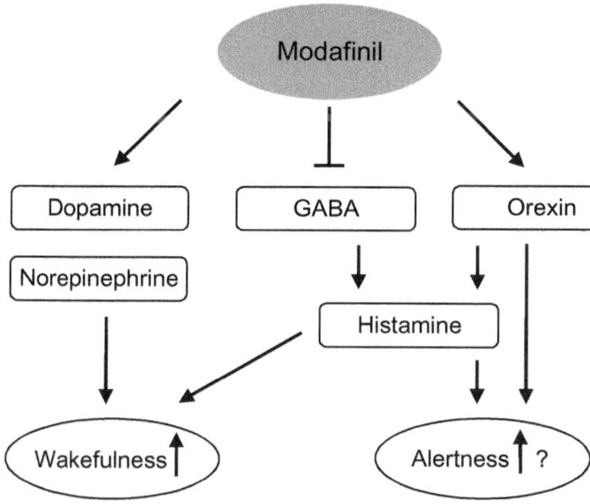

Figure 14.9 Possible pathways of neurotransmitters through which the action of modafinil on various physiological functions is induced.

narcolepsy, cataplexy (Billiard *et al.*, 2006). In fact, modafinil did not affect the direct transitions from wakefulness to REM sleep in narcoleptic orexin KO mice (Lin *et al.*, 2008), suggesting that a combination of medications is needed to manage these two symptoms of narcolepsy. To date, some antidepressant compounds are being used to manage cataplexy and certain histamine H_3-inverse agonists are thought to be a promising drug for the treatment of cataplexy (Lin *et al.*, 2008), but perhaps the most effective approach is to directly facilitate orexinergic signals in the brain using orexin analogs or agonists, because a deficit in the orexin level has been observed in patients of narcolepsy with cataplexy (Kanbayashi *et al.*, 2002). Such compounds are not yet available because of the chemical properties of orexin peptides, which cannot effectively penetrate the brain when applied peripherally. Development of orexin analogs and agonists that can reach the central nervous system seems a very important issue to resolve, and the combination of modafinil and orexin-related compounds is expected to provide a new treatment option for narcolepsy–cataplexy in the near future.

REFERENCES

Adamantidis, A. R., Zhang, F., Aravanis, A. M., Deisseroth, K., and de Lecea, L. (2007). Neural substrates of awakening probed with optogenetic control of hypocretin neurons. *Nature* **450,** 420–424.

Akaoka, H., Roussel, B., Lin, J. S., Chouvet, G., and Jouvet, M. (1991). Effect of modafinil and amphetamine on the rat catecholaminergic neuron activity. *Neurosci. Lett.* **123,** 20–22.

Arias-Carrión, O., Palomero-Rivero, M., Millán-Aldaco, D., Haro, R., Drucker-Colín, R., and Murillo-Rodríguez, E. (2011). Infusion of modafinil into anterior hypothalamus or pedunculopontine tegmental nucleus at different time-points enhances waking and blocks the expression of recovery sleep in rats after sleep deprivation. *Exp. Neurol.* **229,** 358–363.

Bastuji, H., and Jouvet, M. (1988). Successful treatment of idiopathic hypersomnia and narcolepsy with modafinil. *Prog. Neuropsychopharmacol. Biol. Psychiatry* **12,** 695–700.

Bayer, L., Eggermann, E., Serafin, M., Saint-Mleux, B., Machard, D., Jones, B., and Mühlethaler, M. (2001). Orexins (hypocretins) directly excite tuberomammillary neurons. *Eur. J. Neurosci.* **14,** 1571–1575.

Beck, P., Odle, A., Wallace-Huitt, T., Skinner, R. D., and Garcia-Rill, E. (2008). Modafinil increases arousal determined by P13 potential amplitude: An effect blocked by gap junction antagonists. *Sleep* **31,** 1647–1654.

Billiard, M., Bassetti, C., Dauvilliers, Y., Dolenc-Groselj, L., Lammers, G. J., Mayer, G., Pollmächer, T., Reading, P., and Sonka, K. (2006). EFNS guidelines on management of narcolepsy. *Eur. J. Neurol.* **13,** 1035–1048.

Bonaventure, P., Letavic, M., Dugovic, C., Wilson, S., Aluisio, L., Pudiak, C., Lord, B., Mazur, C., Kamme, F., Nishino, S., Carruthers, N., and Lovenberg, T. (2007). Histamine H_3 receptor antagonists: From target identification to drug leads. *Biochem. Pharmacol.* **73,** 1084–1096.

Chemelli, R. M., Willie, J. T., Sinton, C. M., Elmquist, J. K., Scammell, T., Lee, C., Richardson, J. A., Williams, S. C., Xiong, Y., Kisanuki, Y., Fitch, T. E., Nakazato, M., *et al.* (1999). Narcolepsy in orexin knockout mice: Molecular genetics of sleep regulation. *Cell* **98,** 437–451.

de Lecea, L., Kilduff, T. S., Peyron, C., Gao, X., Foye, P. E., Danielson, P. E., Fukuhara, C., Battenberg, E. L., Gautvik, V. T., Bartlett, F. S., Frankel, W. N., van den Pol, A. N., *et al.* (1998). The hypocretins: Hypothalamus-specific peptides with neuroexcitatory activity. *Proc. Natl. Acad. Sci. U.S.A.* **95,** 322–327.

de Saint Hilaire, Z., Orosco, M., Rouch, C., Blanc, G., and Nicolaidis, S. (2001). Variations in extracellular monoamines in the prefrontal cortex and medial hypothalamus after modafinil administration: A microdialysis study in rats. *Neuroreport* **12,** 3533–3537.

De Sereville, J. E., Boer, C., Rambert, F. A., and Duteil, J. (1994). Lack of pre-synaptic dopaminergic involvement in modafinil activity in anaesthetized mice: In vivo voltammetry studies. *Neuropharmacology* **33,** 755–761.

Deboer, T., Overeem, S., Visser, N. A., Duindam, H., Frölich, M., Lammers, G. J., and Meijer, J. H. (2004). Convergence of circadian and sleep regulatory mechanisms on hypocretin-1. *Neuroscience* **129,** 727–732.

Diniz Behn, C. G., Klerman, E. B., Mochizuki, T., Lin, S. C., and Scammell, T. E. (2010). Abnormal sleep/wake dynamics in orexin knockout mice. *Sleep* **33,** 297–306.

Edgar, D. M., and Seidel, W. F. (1997). Modafinil induces wakefulness without intensifying motor activity or subsequent rebound hypersomnolence in the rat. *J. Pharmacol. Exp. Ther.* **283,** 757–769.

Engber, T. M., Koury, E. J., Dennis, S. A., Miller, M. S., Contreras, P. C., and Bhat, R. V. (1998). Differential patterns of regional c-Fos induction in the rat brain by amphetamine and the novel wakefulness-promoting agent modafinil. *Neurosci. Lett.* **241,** 95–98.

Eriksson, K. S., Sergeeva, O., Brown, R. E., and Haas, H. L. (2001). Orexin/hypocretin excites the histaminergic neurons of the tuberomammillary nucleus. *J. Neurosci.* **21,** 9273–9279.

Ferraro, L., Tanganelli, S., O'Connor, W. T., Antonelli, T., Rambert, F., and Fuxe, K. (1996). The vigilance promoting drug modafinil decreases GABA release in the medial preoptic area and in the posterior hypothalamus of the awake rat: Possible involvement of the serotonergic 5-HT_3 receptor. *Neurosci. Lett.* **220,** 5–8.

Gerashchenko, D., Kohls, M. D., Greco, M., Waleh, N. S., Salin-Pascual, R., Kilduff, T. S., Lappi, D. A., and Shiromani, P. J. (2001). Hypocretin-2-saporin lesions of the lateral hypothalamus produce narcoleptic-like sleep behavior in the rat. *J. Neurosci.* **21,** 7273–7283.

Guo, R. X., Anaclet, C., Roberts, J. C., Parmentier, R., Zhang, M., Guidon, G., Buda, C., Sastre, J. P., Feng, J. Q., Franco, P., Brown, S. H., Upton, N., *et al.* (2009). Differential effects of acute and repeat dosing with the H_3 antagonist GSK189254 on the sleep-wake cycle and narcoleptic episodes in Ox−/− mice. *Br. J. Pharmacol.* **157,** 104–117.

Hagan, J. J., Leslie, R. A., Patel, S., Evans, M. L., Wattam, T. A., Holmes, S., Benham, C. D., Taylor, S. G., Routledge, C., Hemmati, P., Munton, R. P., Ashmeade, T. E., *et al.* (1999). Orexin A activates locus coeruleus cell firing and increases arousal in the rat. *Proc. Natl. Acad. Sci. U.S.A.* **96,** 10911–10916.

Hara, J., Beuckmann, C. T., Nambu, T., Willie, J. T., Chemelli, R. M., Sinton, C. M., Sugiyama, F., Yagami, K., Goto, K., Yanagisawa, M., and Sakurai, T. (2001). Genetic ablation of orexin neurons in mice results in narcolepsy, hypophagia, and obesity. *Neuron* **30,** 345–354.

Huang, Z. L., Qu, W. M., Li, W. D., Mochizuki, T., Eguchi, N., Watanabe, T., Urade, Y., and Hayaishi, O. (2001). Arousal effect of orexin A depends on activation of the histaminergic system. *Proc. Natl. Acad. Sci. U.S.A.* **98,** 9965–9970.

Huerta, P. T., and Lisman, J. E. (1993). Heightened synaptic plasticity of hippocampal CA1 neurons during a cholinergically induced rhythmic state. *Nature* **364,** 723–725.

Ishizuka, T., Yamamoto, Y., and Yamatodani, A. (2002). The effect of orexin-A and -B on the histamine release in the anterior hypothalamus in rats. *Neurosci. Lett.* **323,** 93–96.

Ishizuka, T., Sakamoto, Y., Sakurai, T., and Yamatodani, A. (2003). Modafinil increases histamine release in the anterior hypothalamus of rats. *Neurosci. Lett.* **339,** 143–146.

Ishizuka, T., Murakami, M., and Yamatodani, A. (2008). Involvement of central histaminergic systems in modafinil-induced but not methylphenidate-induced increases in locomotor activity in rats. *Eur. J. Pharmacol.* **578,** 209–215.

Ishizuka, T., Murotani, T., and Yamatodani, A. (2010). Modanifil activates the histaminergic system through the orexinergic neurons. *Neurosci. Lett.* **483,** 193–196.

Kanbayashi, T., Honda, K., Kodama, T., Mignot, E., and Nishino, S. (2000). Implication of dopaminergic mechanisms in the wake-promoting effects of amphetamine: A study of D- and L-derivatives in canine narcolepsy. *Neuroscience* **99,** 651–659.

Kanbayashi, T., Inoue, Y., Chiba, S., Aizawa, R., Saito, Y., Tsukamoto, H., Fujii, Y., Nishino, S., and Shimizu, T. (2002). CSF hypocretin-1 (orexin-A) concentrations in narcolepsy with and without cataplexy and idiopathic hypersomnia. *J. Sleep Res.* **11,** 91–93.

Kanbayashi, T., Kodama, T., Kondo, H., Satoh, S., Inoue, Y., Chiba, S., Shimizu, T., and Nishino, S. (2009). CSF histamine contents in narcolepsy, idiopathic hypersomnia and obstructive sleep apnea syndrome. *Sleep* **32,** 181–187.

Kiyashchenko, L. I., Mileykovskiy, B. Y., Maidment, N., Lam, H. A., Wu, M. F., John, J., Peever, J., and Siegel, J. M. (2002). Release of hypocretin (orexin) during waking and sleep states. *J. Neurosci.* **22,** 5282–5286.

Kiyono, S., Seo, M. L., Shibagaki, M., Watanabe, T., Maeyama, K., and Wada, H. (1985). Effects of α-fluoromethylhistidine on sleep-waking parameters in rats. *Physiol. Behav.* **34,** 615–617.

Korotkova, T. M., Klyuch, B. P., Ponomarenko, A. A., Lin, J. S., Haas, H. L., and Sergeeva, O. A. (2007). Modafinil inhibits rat midbrain dopaminergic neurons through D_2-like receptors. *Neuropharmacology* **52,** 626–633.

Lin, J. S., Sakai, K., and Jouvet, M. (1988). Evidence for histaminergic arousal mechanisms in the hypothalamus of cat. *Neuropharmacology* **27,** 111–122.

Lin, J. S., Sakai, K., Vanni-Mercier, G., Arrang, J. M., Garbarg, M., Schwartz, J. C., and Jouvet, M. (1990). Involvement of histaminergic neurons in arousal mechanisms demonstrated with H_3-receptor ligands in the cat. *Brain Res.* **523,** 325–330.
Lin, J. S., Roussel, B., Akaoka, H., Fort, P., Debilly, G., and Jouvet, M. (1992). Role of catecholamines in the modafinil and amphetamine induced wakefulness, a comparative pharmacological study in the cat. *Brain Res.* **88,** 319–326.
Lin, J. S., Sakai, K., and Jouvet, M. (1994). Hypothalamo-preoptic histaminergic projections in sleep-wake control in the cat. *Eur. J. Neurosci.* **6,** 618–625.
Lin, J. S., Hou, Y., and Jouvet, M. (1996). Potential brain neuronal targets for amphetamine-, methylphenidate-, and modafinil-induced wakefulness, evidenced by c-fos immunocytochemistry in the cat. *Proc. Natl. Acad. Sci. U.S.A.* **93,** 14128–14133.
Lin, L., Faraco, J., Li, R., Kadotani, H., Rogers, W., Lin, X., Qiu, X., de Jong, P. J., Nishino, S., and Mignot, E. (1999). The sleep disorder canine narcolepsy is caused by a mutation in the hypocretin (orexin) receptor 2 gene. *Cell* **98,** 365–376.
Lin, J. S., Dauvilliers, Y., Arnulf, I., Bastuji, H., Anaclet, C., Parmentier, R., Kocher, L., Yanagisawa, M., Lehert, P., Ligneau, X., Perrin, D., Robert, P., *et al.* (2008). An inverse agonist of the histamine H_3 receptor improves wakefulness in narcolepsy: Studies in orexin −/− mice and patients. *Neurobiol. Dis.* **30,** 74–83.
Longstreth, W. T., Koepsell, T. D., Ton, T. G., Hendrickson, A. F., and van Belle, G. (2007). The epidemiology of narcolepsy. *Sleep* **30,** 13–26.
Lu, J., Greco, M. A., Shiromani, P., and Saper, C. B. (2000). Effect of lesions of the ventrolateral preoptic nucleus on NREM and REM sleep. *J. Neurosci.* **20,** 3830–3842.
Madras, B. K., Xie, Z., Lin, Z., Jassen, A., Panas, H., Lynch, L., Johnson, R., Livni, E., Spencer, T. J., Bonab, A. A., Miller, G. M., and Fischman, A. J. (2006). Modafinil occupies dopamine and norepinephrine transporters in vivo and modulates the transporters and trace amine activity in vitro. *J. Pharmacol. Exp. Ther.* **319,** 561–569.
Marcus, J. N., Aschkenasi, C. J., Lee, C. E., Chemelli, R. M., Saper, C. B., Yanagisawa, M., and Elmquist, J. K. (2001). Differential expression of orexin receptors 1 and 2 in the rat brain. *J. Comp. Neurol.* **435,** 6–25.
Mignot, E., Nishino, S., Guilleminault, C., and Dement, W. C. (1994). Modafinil binds to the dopamine uptake carrier site with low affinity. *Sleep* **17,** 436–437.
Mignot, E., Lammers, G. J., Ripley, B., Okun, M., Nevsimalova, S., Overeem, S., Vankova, J., Black, J., Harsh, J., Bassetti, C., Schrader, H., and Nishino, S. (2002). The role of cerebrospinal fluid hypocretin measurement in the diagnosis of narcolepsy and other hypersomnias. *Arch. Neurol.* **59,** 1553–1562.
Mitchell, H. A., Bogenpohl, J. W., Liles, L. C., Epstein, M. P., Bozyczko-Coyne, D., Williams, M., and Weinshenker, D. (2008). Behavioral responses of dopamine beta-hydroxylase knockout mice to modafinil suggest a dual noradrenergic-dopaminergic mechanism of action. *Pharmacol. Biochem. Behav.* **91,** 217–222.
Mochizuki, T., Yamatodani, A., Okakura, K., Horii, A., Inagaki, N., and Wada, H. (1992). Circadian rhythm of histamine release from the hypothalamus of freely moving rats. *Physiol. Behav.* **51,** 391–394.
Murillo-Rodríguez, E., Haro, R., Palomero-Rivero, M., Millán-Aldaco, D., and Drucker-Colín, R. (2007). Modafinil enhances extracellular levels of dopamine in the nucleus accumbens and increases wakefulness in rats. *Behav. Brain Res.* **176,** 353–357.
Nguyen, P. V., and Kandel, E. R. (1997). Brief theta-burst stimulation induces a transcription-dependent late phase of LTP requiring cAMP in area CA1 of the mouse hippocampus. *Learn. Mem.* **4,** 230–243.
Nishino, S., Mao, J., Sampathkumaran, R., and Shelton, J. (1998). Increased dopaminergic transmission mediates the wake-promoting effects of CNS stimulants. *Sleep Res. Online* **1,** 49–61.

Nishino, S., Okura, M., and Mignot, E. (2000a). Narcolepsy: Genetic predisposition and neuropharmacological mechanisms. REVIEW ARTICLE. *Sleep Med. Rev.* **4,** 57–99.

Nishino, S., Ripley, B., Overeem, S., Lammers, G. J., and Mignot, E. (2000b). Hypocretin (orexin) deficiency in human narcolepsy. *Lancet* **355,** 39–40.

Nishino, S., Fujiki, N., Ripley, B., Sakurai, E., Kato, M., Watanabe, T., Mignot, E., and Yanai, K. (2001a). Decreased brain histamine content in hypocretin/orexin receptor-2 mutated narcoleptic dogs. *Neurosci. Lett.* **313,** 125–128.

Nishino, S., Ripley, B., Overeem, S., Nevsimalova, S., Lammers, G. J., Vankova, J., Okun, M., Rogers, W., Brooks, S., and Mignot, E. (2001b). Low cerebrospinal fluid hypocretin (Orexin) and altered energy homeostasis in human narcolepsy. *Ann. Neurol.* **50,** 381–388.

Nishino, S., Sakurai, E., Nevsimalova, S., Yoshida, Y., Watanabe, T., Yanai, K., and Mignot, E. (2009). Decreased CSF histamine in narcolepsy with and without low CSF hypocretin-1 in comparison to healthy controls. *Sleep* **32,** 175–180.

Panula, P., Yang, H. Y., and Costa, E. (1984). Histamine-containing neurons in the rat hypothalamus. *Proc. Natl. Acad. Sci. U.S.A.* **81,** 2572–2576.

Parmentier, R., Ohtsu, H., Djebbara-Hannas, Z., Valatx, J. L., Watanabe, T., and Lin, J. S. (2002). Anatomical, physiological, and pharmacological characteristics of histidine decarboxylase knock-out mice: Evidence for the role of brain histamine in behavioral and sleep-wake control. *J. Neurosci.* **22,** 7695–7711.

Parmentier, R., Anaclet, C., Guhennec, C., Brousseau, E., Bricout, D., Giboulot, T., Bozyczko-Coyne, D., Spiegel, K., Ohtsu, H., Williams, M., and Lin, J. S. (2007). The brain H_3-receptor as a novel therapeutic target for vigilance and sleep-wake disorders. *Biochem. Pharmacol.* **73,** 1157–1171.

Peyron, C., Tighe, D. K., van den Pol, A. N., de Lecea, L., Heller, H. C., Sutcliffe, J. G., and Kilduff, T. S. (1998). Neurons containing hypocretin (orexin) project to multiple neuronal systems. *J. Neurosci.* **18,** 9996–10015.

Peyron, C., Faraco, J., Rogers, W., Ripley, B., Overeem, S., Charnay, Y., Nevsimalova, S., Aldrich, M., Reynolds, D., Albin, R., Li, R., Hungs, M., *et al.* (2000). A mutation in a case of early onset narcolepsy and a generalized absence of hypocretin peptides in human narcoleptic brains. *Nat. Med.* **6,** 991–997.

Piper, D. C., Upton, N., Smith, M. I., and Hunter, A. J. (2000). The novel brain neuropeptide, orexin-A, modulates the sleep-wake cycle of rats. *Eur. J. Neurosci.* **12,** 726–730.

Ripley, B., Overeem, S., Fujiki, N., Nevsimalova, S., Uchino, M., Yesavage, J., Di Monte, D., Dohi, K., Melberg, A., Lammers, G. J., Nishida, Y., Roelandse, F. W., *et al.* (2001). CSF hypocretin/orexin levels in narcolepsy and other neurological conditions. *Neurology* **57,** 2253–2258.

Sagar, S. M., Sharp, F. R., and Curran, T. (1988). Expression of c-fos protein in brain: Metabolic mapping at the cellular level. *Science* **240,** 1328–1331.

Sakurai, T., Amemiya, A., Ishii, M., Matsuzaki, I., Chemelli, R. M., Tanaka, H., Williams, S. C., Richardson, J. A., Kozlowski, G. P., Wilson, S., Arch, J. R., Buckingham, R. E., *et al.* (1998). Orexins and orexin receptors: A family of hypothalamic neuropeptides and G protein-coupled receptors that regulate feeding behavior. *Cell* **92,** 573–585.

Scammell, T. E., Estabrooke, I. V., McCarthy, M. T., Chemelli, R. M., Yanagisawa, M., Miller, M. S., and Saper, C. B. (2000). Hypothalamic arousal regions are activated during modafinil-induced wakefulness. *J. Neurosci.* **20,** 8620–8628.

Selbach, O., Doreulee, N., Bohla, C., Eriksson, K. S., Sergeeva, O. A., Poelchen, W., Brown, R. E., and Haas, H. L. (2004). Orexins/hypocretins cause sharp wave- and theta-related synaptic plasticity in the hippocampus via glutamatergic, gabaergic, noradrenergic, and cholinergic signaling. *Neuroscience* **127,** 519–528.

Sherin, J. E., Elmquist, J. K., Torrealba, F., and Saper, C. B. (1998). Innervation of histaminergic tuberomammillary neurons by GABAergic and galaninergic neurons in the ventrolateral preoptic nucleus of the rat. *J. Neurosci.* **18,** 4705–4721.

Simon, P., Hemet, C., Ramassamy, C., and Costentin, J. (1995). Non-amphetaminic mechanism of stimulant locomotor effect of modafinil in mice. *Eur. Neuropsychopharmacol.* **5,** 509–514.

Stone, E. A., Cotecchia, S., Lin, Y., and Quartermain, D. (2002). Role of brain alpha 1B-adrenoceptors in modafinil-induced behavioral activity. *Synapse* **46,** 269–270.

Takahashi, K., Lin, J. S., and Sakai, K. (2006). Neuronal activity of histaminergic tuberomammillary neurons during wake-sleep states in the mouse. *J. Neurosci.* **26,** 10292–10298.

Thannickal, T. C., Moore, R. Y., Nienhuis, R., Ramanathan, L., Gulyani, S., Aldrich, M., Cornford, M., and Siegel, J. M. (2000). Reduced number of hypocretin neurons in human narcolepsy. *Neuron* **27,** 469–474.

Thannickal, T. C., Nienhuis, R., and Siegel, J. M. (2009). Localized loss of hypocretin (orexin) cells in narcolepsy without cataplexy. *Sleep* **32,** 993–998.

Touret, M., Sallanon-Moulin, M., and Jouvet, M. (1995). Awakening properties of modafinil without paradoxical sleep rebound: Comparative study with amphetamine in the rat. *Neurosci. Lett.* **189,** 43–46.

Tsanov, M., Lyons, D. G., Barlow, S., González Reyes, R. E., and O'Mara, S. M. (2010). The psychostimulant modafinil facilitates water maze performance and augments synaptic potentiation in dentate gyrus. *Neuropharmacology* **59,** 9–19.

Watanabe, T., Taguchi, Y., Shiosaka, S., Tanaka, J., Kubota, H., Terano, Y., Tohyama, M., and Wada, H. (1984). Distribution of the histaminergic neuron system in the central nervous system of rats; a fluorescent immunohistochemical analysis with histidine decarboxylase as a marker. *Brain Res.* **295,** 13–25.

Wieland, H. A., Soll, R. M., Doods, H. N., Stenkamp, D., Hurnaus, R., Lammle, B., and Beck-Sickinger, A. G. (2002). The SK-N-MC cell line expresses an orexin binding site different from recombinant orexin 1-type receptor. *Eur. J. Biochem.* **269,** 1128–1135.

Willie, J. T., Chemelli, R. M., Sinton, C. M., Tokita, S., Williams, S. C., Kisanuki, Y. Y., Marcus, J. N., Lee, C., Elmquist, J. K., Kohlmeier, K. A., Leonard, C. S., Richardson, J. A., *et al.* (2003). Distinct narcolepsy syndromes in Orexin receptor-2 and Orexin null mice: Molecular genetic dissection of Non-REM and REM sleep regulatory processes. *Neuron* **38,** 715–730.

Willie, J. T., Renthal, W., Chemelli, R. M., Miller, M. S., Scammell, T. E., Yanagisawa, M., and Sinton, C. M. (2005). Modafinil more effectively induces wakefulness in orexin-null mice than in wild-type littermates. *Neuroscience* **130,** 983–995.

Wisor, J. P., Nishino, S., Sora, I., Uhl, G. H., Mignot, E., and Edgar, D. M. (2001). Dopaminergic role in stimulant-induced wakefulness. *J. Neurosci.* **21,** 1787–1794.

Yamanaka, A., Tsujino, N., Funahashi, H., Honda, K., Guan, J. L., Wang, Q. P., Tominaga, M., Goto, K., Shioda, S., and Sakurai, T. (2002). Orexins activate histaminergic neurons via the orexin 2 receptor. *Biochem. Biophys. Res. Commun.* **290,** 1237–1245.

Yasuko, S., Atanda, A. M., Masato, M., Kazuhiko, Y., and Kazuki, H. (2010). Alpha-fluoromethylhistidine, a histamine synthesis inhibitor, inhibits orexin-induced wakefulness in rats. *Behav. Brain Res.* **207,** 151–154.

Yoshida, Y., Fujiki, N., Nakajima, T., Ripley, B., Matsumura, H., Yoneda, H., Mignot, E., and Nishino, S. (2001). Fluctuation of extracellular hypocretin-1 (orexin A) levels in the rat in relation to the light-dark cycle and sleep-wake activities. *Eur. J. Neurosci.* **14,** 1075–1081.

CHAPTER FIFTEEN

Anti-Parkinson Drugs and Orexin Neurons

Hiroshi Katsuki* *and* Shotaro Michinaga†

Contents

Abstract

Non-ergot-type dopamine receptor agonists such as ropinirole are used for treatment of Parkinson disease, but they frequently produce adverse actions characterized by sleepiness and sleep attacks. Because these symptoms are similar to those observed in patients with narcolepsy, a sleep disorder caused by degeneration of hypothalamic orexin neurons, involvement of orexinergic system in the adverse drug actions is suspected. We found that ropinirole and other non-ergot dopamine D_2 receptor agonists cause selective loss of orexin-immunoreactive neurons in organotypic slice culture of rat hypothalamus. The mechanism of this action is considered to involve D_2 receptor-mediated presynaptic suppression of glutamatergic excitatory inputs to orexin neurons because continuous silencing of excitatory activity of orexin neurons can deplete orexin from cell bodies.

* Department of Chemico-Pharmacological Sciences, Graduate School of Pharmaceutical Sciences, Kumamoto University, Kumamoto, Japan
† Laboratory of Pharmacology, Faculty of Pharmacy, Osaka Ohtani University, Osaka, Japan

Vitamins and Hormones, Volume 89
ISSN 0083-6729, http://dx.doi.org/10.1016/B978-0-12-394623-2.00015-9

In addition, Parkinson disease itself may accompany loss of orexin neurons. Disturbance of orexinergic system may play an important role in sleep/arousal dysfunctions under these and other clinical conditions.

I. Introduction

Neural mechanisms involved in regulation of sleep and arousal are still incompletely understood but are being revealed by recent intensive efforts in basic and clinical researches. One of the most important advances in the last decade in this field is identification and characterization of neuropeptides in the hypothalamus, named orexins or hypocretins. Substantial lines of evidence indicate that orexins play a pivotal role in maintaining arousal state (Sakurai and Mieda, 2011), and neural pathways involving orexinergic system that maintains consolidated sleep and wakefulness have been proposed (Tsujino and Sakurai, 2009).

With these advances in our hands, now we may be able to address or reevaluate the mechanisms of therapeutic actions and/or adverse actions of centrally acting drugs that affect sleep and wakefulness. Here, we pick up and discuss the adverse action of ropinirole (Ravikumar and Sridhar, 2006), a dopamine receptor agonist used for treatment of Parkinson disease (PD), in the context of manipulation of orexinergic neural system.

II. Parkinson Disease and Adverse Actions of Anti-Parkinson Drugs

PD is a major neurodegenerative disorder affecting about 2% of populations at ages over 70. A hallmark of neuropathology of this disorder is progressive decline in the number of dopaminergic neurons in the substantia nigra pars compacta in the midbrain (Lees *et al.*, 2009). Because these neurons normally send axonal projections to the striatum, loss of these neurons results in shortage of dopamine supply to the striatum, leading to imbalance between the direct and the indirect pathways of the extrapyramidal system and manifestation of the symptoms associated with the disease such as akinesia, rigidity, and tremor. On the therapeutic basis, neuroprotective strategies are unavailable at present, and current pharmaceutical treatments are mainly aimed to counterbalance the shortage of dopamine in the striatum. A straightforward approach is administration of levodopa as a dopamine precursor. Levodopa is indeed one of the most effective drugs in PD treatment, but long-term usage of this drug is usually associated with many problems including fluctuations of the efficacy (on–off and delayed-on phenomena) and adverse actions such as dyskinesia. Therefore, drugs other than levodopa are preferred for the treatment of PD patients at early stage of the disease.

In this regard, dopamine receptor agonists are useful drugs for the therapy of PD (Foley *et al.*, 2004; Katzenschlager and Lees, 2002). Activation of dopamine D_2 receptors in the striatum by these drugs nullifies shortage of dopamine signaling, normalizes the balance of activities of neural connections involved in motor control, and alleviates the symptoms associated with the disease. Among various dopamine receptor agonists, ergot-type compounds such as bromocriptine and pergolide have been used for a long time, either alone or in combination with levodopa. However, these drugs have mixed agonist activity on D_1 and D_2 receptors and exhibit adverse actions that frequently appear as gastrointestinal damages and cardiac valvular disease (Horvath *et al.*, 2004).

Non-ergot-type compounds such as ropinirole, pramipexole, and talipexole (Hobson *et al.*, 1999) are another class of dopamine agonists used for the treatment of PD. Non-ergot-type compounds are considered to stimulate D_2 family of dopamine receptors selectively and have little adverse actions compared to ergot-type drugs (Steiger *et al.*, 2009). However, these compounds also are not free from several undesirable effects. The most characteristic one of the adverse actions is increased daytime sleepiness and occurrence of sudden sleep attacks (Frucht *et al.*, 1999; Paus *et al.*, 2003). The cellular mechanisms of the disturbance of sleep and wakefulness by non-ergot type D_2 receptor agonists remain unknown, but the symptoms observed are reminiscent of narcolepsy, a representative sleep disorder.

III. Properties of Orexin Neurons

A. Orexin neurons as sleep/arousal regulators relevant to narcolepsy

Narcolepsy is a neurological disorder associated with disturbance of sleep and wakefulness such as excessive daytime sleepiness, sleep attacks, sleep paralysis, and intrusions of rapid-eye-movement sleep into wakefulness (Zeitzer *et al.*, 2006). Extensive studies on the patients as well as on experimental animals have established that deficiency of orexins is responsible for this neurological disorder. Orexin-A and orexin-B, also called as hypocretin-1 and hypocretin-2, are neuropeptides produced from a common precursor peptide prepro-orexin. Orexin-containing neurons constitute a small subset of neurons located in the lateral hypothalamic area and the perifornical area of the hypothalamus (Sakurai, 2007). Notably, the number of orexin neurons is substantially decreased in the postmortem brain of narcoleptic patients (Peyron *et al.*, 2000; Thannickal *et al.*, 2000). The decrease is specific to orexin neurons because melanin-concentrating hormone

(MCH)-containing neurons that are distributed in similar regions to orexin neurons show no change. Moreover, orexin-deficient mice exhibit a phenotype including disturbed sleep/arousal regulation that closely resembles the symptoms observed in narcoleptic patients (Chemelli *et al.*, 1999).

In contrast to the confined localization of cell bodies in the hypothalamus, axonal projections of orexin neurons as well as expression of orexin receptors are widely distributed throughout the central nervous system. This widespread distribution forms a basis of divergent functions of orexins including regulation of sleep/arousal, feeding and energy homeostasis, reward and drug dependence, and neuroendocrine functions (Tsujino and Sakurai, 2009). In playing these multiple roles in the central nervous system, orexin neurons interact with various kinds of neurotransmitter systems, which has been reviewed elsewhere (Sakurai and Mieda, 2011). Because the topic of this chapter is on the actions of dopamine receptor agonists, below we briefly summarize the role of dopaminergic system in the regulation of activity of orexin neurons.

B. Regulation of activities of orexin neurons by dopamine

Dopaminergic regulation of electrophysiological activities of orexin neurons has been addressed in several studies using acute hypothalamic slices (Alberto *et al.*, 2006; Li and van den Pol, 2005; Yamanaka *et al.*, 2006) and has been shown to involve multiple modes of actions. Dopamine at 20–50 μM decreases action potential firing and hyperpolarizes membrane potential of mouse orexin neurons, and the effect is blocked by eticlopride, a D_2 receptor antagonist (Li and van den Pol, 2005). Another study has proposed that direct hyperpolarizing effect of dopamine on orexin neurons may not be mediated by dopamine receptors but by α_2 adrenergic receptors: hyperpolarization of mouse orexin neurons induced by 300 μM dopamine was inhibited by idazoxan, an α_2 receptor antagonist (Yamanaka *et al.*, 2006). On the other hand, bidirectional actions of dopamine on excitatory inputs to orexin neurons have been reported in a study on rat hypothalamic slices by Alberto *et al.* (2006). That is, dopamine at a low concentration (1 μM) increased frequency of miniature excitatory postsynaptic currents (mEPSCs) in a D_1 receptor-dependent manner, whereas dopamine at higher concentrations (10–100 μM) decreased mEPSC frequency via activation of D_2 receptors.

Assessment of the activity of orexin neurons *in vivo* by c-Fos immunoreactivity reveals a different aspect of dopaminergic regulation. Administration of a D1-like agonist A-77636 or a D_2-like agonist quinpirole, as well as a mixed dopamine agonist apomorphine, induced c-Fos expression in orexin neurons in rats (Bubser *et al.*, 2005). These authors have also demonstrated that the lateral hypothalamic area and the perifornical area, where orexin neurons are concentrated, did not exhibit appreciable expression of mRNAs encoding dopamine receptors. Accordingly, they concluded that the effect of apomorphine may be mediated *trans*-synaptically, rather than via direct actions onto orexin neurons.

Overall, these findings are consistent with the idea that dopamine receptor stimulation can modify neuronal activity of orexin neurons. However, depending on conditions where orexin neurons are situated, the direction of the actions can be either excitatory or inhibitory.

C. Neural activity-dependent depletion of orexin

We have developed experimental setup of hypothalamic slice cultures and have been investigating the properties of orexin neurons to give insight into the mechanisms of loss of orexin neurons in narcolepsy. One of the reasons for employing organotypic slice cultures is that the absolute number of orexin neurons is very small, which has been estimated to be only about 4000 in adult rat brain (Kilduff and Peyron, 2000). In addition, according to a study on developmental changes of orexin expression (Yamamoto *et al.*, 2000), orexin-immunoreactive neurons in rat brain were not detectable until postnatal day 15, then their number markedly increased between postnatal days 15 and 20, reaching adult level. These characteristics hamper preparation of dissociated primary cell culture of orexin neurons. Organotypic slice cultures are advantageous in that they can be prepared from postnatal animals and are expected to maintain cell viability with preserved tissue architecture. Indeed, we could successfully maintain rat hypothalamic slices in culture for weeks, and by immunohistochemical methods, we observed that both orexin neurons and MCH neurons were present in areas that corresponded to the region reported to contain these neuronal populations *in vivo* (Katsuki and Akaike, 2004).

Using this preparation, we found several lines of evidence suggesting that the properties of turnover of orexin as a peptide neurotransmitter differ from those of other hypothalamic neuropeptides such as MCH. For example, application of a sodium channel blocker tetrodotoxin (TTX) to hypothalamic slice cultures for 3–72 h resulted in a substantial decrease in the number of orexin-immunoreactive neurons, but not of MCH-immunoreactive neurons (Michinaga *et al.*, 2010b). Elevation of extracellular Mg^{2+}, a treatment leading to suppression of neuronal firing, caused a similar effect. These effects may result from depletion of orexin stored within neurons rather than occurrence of cell death because the number of orexin-immunoreactive neurons recovered 72 h after washout of TTX or added Mg^{2+}. Absence of cell death under these conditions was also verified by assessment with propidium iodide fluorescence. We also found that treatment with TTX and Mg^{2+} decreased expression level of mRNA encoding prepro-orexin. Taken together, the effect of TTX and Mg^{2+} on orexin neurons suggests that spontaneous neuronal activity is required to maintain orexin expression.

In line with this idea, when we applied ω-conotoxin MVIIC, a blocker of N- and P/Q-type Ca^{2+} channels that mediate presynaptic Ca^{2+} entry, we again observed selective decrease in the number of orexin-immunoreactive neurons. Moreover, antagonists at *N*-methyl-D-aspartate (NMDA) subtype of glutamate receptors also caused loss of orexin-immunoreactive neurons, which is consistent with the fact that glutamatergic excitatory synaptic inputs regulate the electrical activity of orexin neurons (Acuna-Goycolea *et al.*, 2004; Li *et al.*, 2002). Finally, the effect of TTX on orexin neurons was abrogated by concurrent application of a moderate concentration of NMDA (Michinaga *et al.*, 2010b). Overall, these findings indicate that Ca^{2+} entry associated with nontoxic levels of spontaneous activity of glutamatergic inputs plays an important role in the maintenance of orexin neurons.

On the other hand, selective loss of orexin neurons in slice culture can also be induced by continuous, mild depolarizing conditions (Katsuki *et al.*, 2010). That is, elevation of extracellular K^+ concentration (10–30 mM) or application of veratridine, a Na^+ channel activator, for 24–72 h resulted in a decrease in the number of orexin-immunoreactive neurons but not of MCH-immunoreactive neurons. In these cases, the loss of orexin neurons was again attributable to depletion of orexin stored within neurons because there was no sign of cell death and also because prepro-orexin mRNA level did not decline. However, in contrast to the cases with neuronal activity inhibition, depolarization-induced loss of orexin-immunoreactive neurons appeared to be irreversible at least to some extent. The precise mechanisms of orexin depletion by mild depolarizing conditions are unclear at present because the amount of orexin released extracellularly was paradoxically decreased by treatment with elevated K^+ and veratridine. Notably, disappearance of orexin immunoreactivity in cell bodies induced by elevated K^+ and veratridine was frequently associated with an apparent increase in orexin immunoreactivity in axon-like processes. In addition, concomitant application of colchicine, a drug that inhibits tubulin polymerization and axonal transport, completely prevented the decrease in the number of orexin-immunoreactive cell bodies by elevated K^+ and veratridine. Therefore, redistribution of orexin within neurons may be one mechanism that contributes to the disappearance of orexin in the cell body.

IV. Possible Dysfunctions of Orexin Neurons Associated with Parkinson Disease

A. Depletion of orexin in slice culture by anti-Parkinson drugs

The findings in slice cultures mentioned above altogether suggest that orexin neurons are particularly sensitive to alterations of neural activities. Both suppression and enhancement of neuronal excitatory activities may eventually lead to dysfunction of orexin neurons that is manifested as depletion of stored orexin peptide. Obtaining these findings, we postulated that adverse actions of centrally acting drugs related to sleep/arousal disturbance might result from dysfunction of orexin neurons. Then we set out for the experiments to examine the effect of ropinirole, a non-ergot-type D_2 dopamine receptor agonist, on the integrity of orexin neurons (Michinaga *et al.*, 2010a). As discussed earlier, ropinirole has been used for treatment of PD, and promotion of sleepiness is well recognized as a characteristic adverse action of this drug (Frucht *et al.*, 1999). Reportedly, about 10% of patients treated with combination of ropinirole and levodopa experience sleep attacks (Paus *et al.*, 2003).

Ropinirole at various concentrations (50 μM to 1 mM) was applied for 72 h to hypothalamic slice cultures. We found that ropinirole caused a concentration-dependent decrease in the number of orexin-immunoreactive neurons (Fig. 15.1). In contrast, the number of MCH-immunoreactive neurons within the same slice cultures showed no change after treatment with ropinirole. With 1 mM ropinirole, a significant decrease in the number of orexin-immunoreactive neurons was evident already at 6 h after initiation of treatment, and the number of orexin-immunoreactive neurons gradually decreased in a time-dependent manner to reach a plateau level at 24 h. Similar effects on orexin neurons were observed with talipexole and pramipexole, other non-ergot drugs used for the treatment of PD, although the degree of the decrease was smaller than that induced by ropinirole.

Disappearance of orexin immunoreactivity induced by ropinirole was considered to result from depletion of the orexin peptide because (1) the decrease of orexin-immunoreactive neurons was reversible after washout of ropinirole, and (2) treatment of slice cultures with ropinirole for 24–72 h did not increase propidium iodide uptake within tissues, a hallmark of cell death induction. As with the case with TTX, ropinirole-induced decrease in the number of orexin-immunoreactive neurons was prevented by concomitant application of a low concentration (20 μM) of NMDA. Moreover, the effect of ropinirole and that of MK-801, an NMDA receptor antagonist, in reducing the number of orexin-immunoreactive neurons were not additive. The effect of ropinirole was significantly attenuated by an antagonist at dopamine D_2 receptors (sulpiride).

These results with ropinirole can be interpreted as follows: ropinirole may inhibit excitatory activity of orexin neurons, thereby causing reversible depletion of orexin peptide, as is the case with TTX and Mg^{2+}. Orexin neurons themselves do not appear to possess dopamine D_2 receptors (Sakurai, 2007) because D_2 receptor mRNAs are rarely expressed in the lateral hypothalamus and the perifornical area where orexin neurons are located (Bubser *et al.*, 2005) as already discussed. However, stimulation of dopamine D_2 receptors has been shown to reduce the frequency of mEPSCs recorded from orexin neurons in acute hypothalamic slices (Alberto *et al.*, 2006). Therefore, depletion of orexin

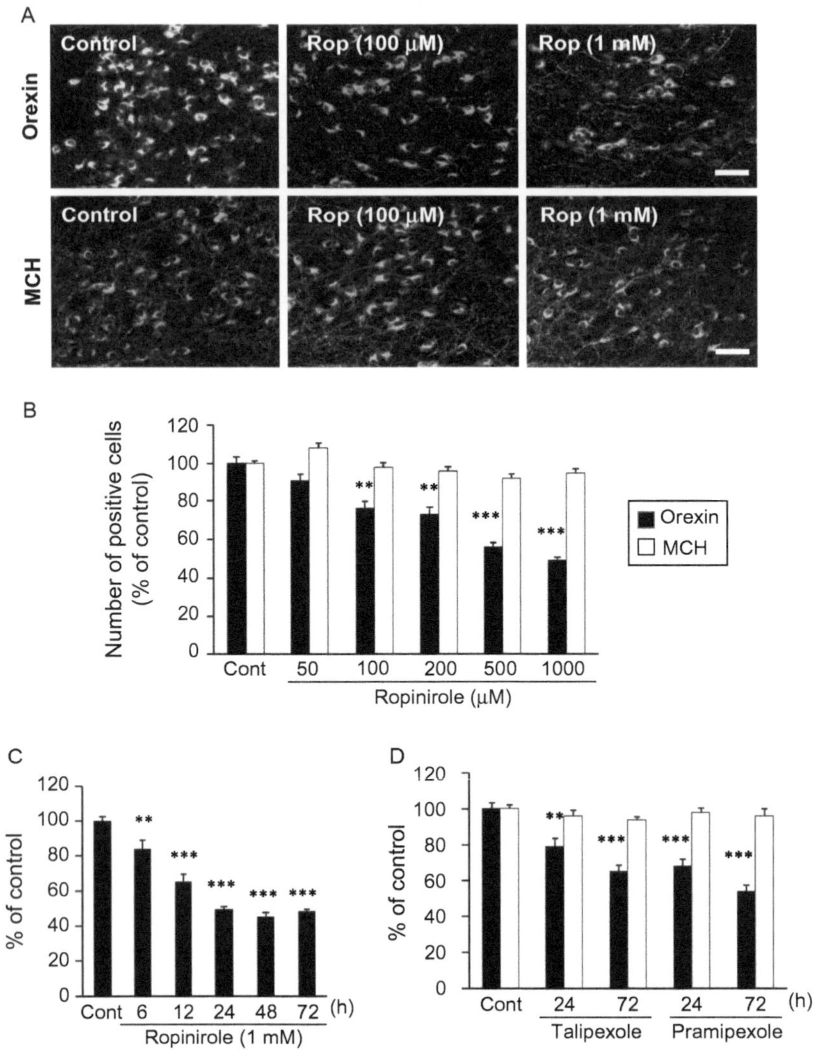

Figure 15.1 Non-ergot dopamine receptor agonists induce a selective decrease of orexin neurons in hypothalamic slice culture. (A) Representative photographs of orexin- and MCH-immunoreactive neurons in hypothalamus slice culture. Ropinirole at indicated concentrations was applied for 72 h. Scale bars = 50 μm. (B) Concentration dependency of the effect of ropinirole applied for 72 h on the number of orexin- and MCH-immunoreactive neurons. (C) Time course of the effect of 1 mM ropinirole on the number of orexin-immunoreactive neurons. (D) Selective decrease of orexin neurons by 1-mM talipexole and pramipexole. Drugs were applied for indicated periods. $n = 12–18$ for each condition in panels B–D. $^{**}p < 0.01$, $^{***}p < 0.001$ versus control. Reproduced with permission from Michinaga *et al.* (2010a).

by ropinirole may be caused by D_2 receptor-mediated presynaptic suppression of glutamatergic excitatory inputs to orexin neurons.

Unfortunately, we cannot simply relate these findings obtained from *in vitro* experiments to clinical conditions because ropinirole at or over 100 μM, concentrations that were beyond the therapeutic range, was required to affect the number of orexin-immunoreactive neurons. However, the observed effect of ropinirole on orexin neurons was mediated by the principal action of this drug as anti-Parkinson drug, that is, stimulation of dopamine D_2 receptors. Moreover, provided that suppression of presynaptic glutamate release was responsible for the effect of ropinirole, the effect might have been diminished in slice cultures that have lost several neural connections present *in vivo*. Furthermore, the effect of ropinirole was determined within a short period (up to 72 h), whereas long-term treatment for months or years is common in the case of treatment of PD. Finally, several reports have shown that the hypothalamus of PD patients exhibits a reduced number of orexin neurons, as discussed below.

B. Orexin neurons in Parkinson disease and other neurological disorders

An important point that should be taken into consideration is that PD *per se* is associated with dysfunctions of orexinergic system. That is, loss of orexin neurons may occur in the brain of PD patients. An early study demonstrated that orexin-A levels measured in 19 PD patients were lower than those in neurologic controls (Drouot *et al.*, 2003). Subsequently, two groups independently reported that the hypothalamus of the postmortem brain of PD patients contains lower number of orexin neurons than that of age-matched controls (Fronczek *et al.*, 2007; Thannickal *et al.*, 2007). The percentage loss of orexin neurons was greater in advanced stage of patients than in stage I patients (Thannickal *et al.*, 2007). Orexin-A concentration in the prefrontal cortex of PD patients was also lower than that of controls (Fronczek *et al.*, 2007).

In a recent study on 25 patients with PD, lower orexin levels in the cerebrospinal fluid were associated with longer disease duration, which has been linked to higher incidence of sleep attacks (Asai *et al.*, 2009). Interestingly, switching drug treatment from pramipexole or high dose of levodopa to pergolide resulted in a significant recovery of orexin levels in the cerebrospinal fluid of the patients. Authors proposed a possibility that D_3 dopamine receptor stimulation is responsible for suppression of orexinergic system and for sleep attacks promoted by anti-Parkinson drugs (Asai *et al.*, 2009). Overall, it is postulated that the decrease in the absolute number of orexin neurons in the brain of PD patients contributes to dysregulation of sleep/arousal, in conjunction with adverse actions of anti-Parkinson drugs such as decreased levels of orexin expression induced by long-term treatment with non-ergot D_2 receptor agonists.

Additional point to be considered is that narcolepsy-like syndromes in PD patients may not be solely and simply attributable to dysfunctions of orexin neurotransmission. Several lines of evidence have suggested that sleepiness exists already before the onset of Parkinsonian symptoms and before initiation of drug treatment (Arnulf and Leu-Semenescu, 2009). Neurotransmitter systems other than orexinergic system may also be affected by the disease. They include noradrenergic system originating from the locus coeruleus, cholinergic system from the pontine nucleus and the basal forebrain, and serotonergic system from the raphe nuclei (Arnulf and Leu-Semenescu, 2009). Therefore, symptoms related to sleep/arousal dysfunctions in PD patients may well involve divergent sets of disorganized regulation by these nondopaminergic projections.

Disruption of sleep and wakefulness is frequently observed in patients with other psychiatric and neurodegenerative disorders, including major depression, schizophrenia, Alzheimer disease, and Huntington disease (Wulff *et al.*, 2010). With regard to orexin, Huntington disease is reportedly associated with a decrease in the number of orexin neurons in the patients (Aziz *et al.*, 2008; Petersén *et al.*, 2005). In addition, aging, which is a major risk factor of various neurodegenerative disorders, might be a contributing factor to the dysfunctions of orexin neurons: age-related loss of orexin neurons is observed in aged rats (Kessler *et al.*, 2011). Regardless of whether orexinergic system is involved or not, elucidation of the mechanisms of sleep dysregulation associated with divergent neurological disorders is an important issue to develop new kinds of therapeutics to improve patients' quality of life.

V. Conclusions and Perspectives

Here, we discussed potential mechanisms of adverse actions of anti-Parkinson drugs, with reference to dysregulation of sleep/arousal. According to the similarities of symptoms between drug-induced and narcolepsy-associated sleep/arousal disturbance, we postulated that orexinergic system is related to manifestation of adverse actions of ropinirole and other non-ergot dopamine receptor agonists. Experiments on organotypic slice cultures indeed demonstrated that ropinirole could induce selective loss of functions of orexin neurons (i.e., depletion of orexin). However, *in vivo* and/or clinical relevance of this adverse action *in vitro* remains to be clarified. Notably, PD as well as other neurodegenerative disorders is associated with a decline in the number of orexin neurons, which may also contribute to problems of sleep/arousal disturbance experienced by the patients. Further investigations are required to clarify contribution of orexinergic system to disturbed regulation of sleep and wakefulness associated with various pathological and clinical conditions.

ACKNOWLEDGMENTS

Our work cited and discussed in this chapter was supported by Grants-in-Aid for Scientific Research from The Ministry of Education, Culture, Sports, Science and Technology, Japan.

REFERENCES

Acuna-Goycolea, C., Li, Y., and van den Pol, A. N. (2004). Group III metabotropic glutamate receptors maintain tonic inhibition of excitatory synaptic input to hypocretin/orexin neurons. *J. Neurosci.* **24,** 3013–3022.

Alberto, C. O., Trask, R. B., Quinlan, M. E., and Hirasawa, M. (2006). Bidirectional dopaminergic modulation of excitatory synaptic transmission in orexin neurons. *J. Neurosci.* **26,** 10043–10050.

Arnulf, I., and Leu-Semenescu, S. (2009). Sleepiness in Parkinson's disease. *Parkinsonism Relat. Disord.* **15,** S101–S104.

Asai, H., Hirano, M., Furiya, Y., Udaka, F., Morikawa, M., Kanbayashi, T., Shimizu, T., and Ueno, S. (2009). Cerebrospinal fluid-orexin levels and sleep attacks in four patients with Parkinson's disease. *Clin. Neurol. Neurosurg.* **111,** 341–344.

Aziz, A., Fronczek, R., Maat-Schieman, M., Unmehopa, U., Roelandse, F., Overeem, S., van Duinen, S., Lammers, G. J., Swaab, D., and Roos, R. (2008). Hypocretin and melanin-concentrating hormone in patients with Huntington disease. *Brain Pathol.* **18,** 474–483.

Bubser, M., Fadel, J. R., Jackson, L. L., Meador-Woodruff, J. H., Jing, D., and Deutch, A. Y. (2005). Dopaminergic regulation of orexin neurons. *Eur. J. Neurosci.* **21,** 2993–3001.

Chemelli, R. M., Willie, J. T., Sinton, C. M., Elmquist, J. K., Scammell, T., Lee, C., Richardson, J. A., Williams, S. C., Xiong, Y., Kisanuki, Y., Fitch, T. E., Nakazato, M., *et al.* (1999). Narcolepsy in orexin knockout mice: Molecular genetics of sleep regulation. *Cell* **98,** 437–451.

Drouot, X., Moutereau, S., Nguyen, J. P., Lefaucheur, J. P., Créange, A., Remy, P., Goldenberg, F., and d'Ortho, M. P. (2003). Low levels of ventricular CSF orexin/hypocretin in advanced PD. *Neurology* **61,** 540–543.

Foley, P., Gerlach, M., Double, K. L., and Riederer, P. (2004). Dopamine receptor agonists in the therapy of Parkinson's disease. *J. Neural Transm.* **111,** 1375–1446.

Fronczek, R., Overeem, S., Lee, S. Y., Hegeman, I. M., van Pelt, J., van Duinen, S. G., Lammers, G. J., and Swaab, D. F. (2007). Hypocretin (orexin) loss in Parkinson's disease. *Brain* **130,** 1577–1585.

Frucht, S., Rogers, J. D., Greene, P. E., Gordon, M. F., and Fahn, S. (1999). Falling asleep at the wheel: Motor vehicle mishaps in persons taking pramipexole and ropinirole. *Neurology* **52,** 1908–1910.

Hobson, D. E., Pourcher, E., and Martin, W. R. (1999). Ropinirole and pramipexole, the new agonists. *Can. J. Neurol. Sci.* **26,** S27–S33.

Horvath, J., Fross, R. D., Kleiner-Fisman, G., Lerch, R., Stalder, H., Liaudat, S., Raskoff, W. J., Flachsbart, K. D., Rakowski, H., Pache, J. C., Burkhard, P. R., and Lang, A. E. (2004). Severe multivalvular heart disease: A new complication of the ergot derivative dopamine agonists. *Mov. Disord.* **19,** 611–613.

Katsuki, H., and Akaike, A. (2004). Excitotoxic degeneration of hypothalamic orexin neurons in slice culture. *Neurobiol. Dis.* **15,** 61–69.

Katsuki, H., Kurosu, S., Michinaga, S., Hisatsune, A., Isohama, Y., Izumi, Y., Kume, T., and Akaike, A. (2010). Depolarizing stimuli cause persistent and selective loss of orexin in rat hypothalamic slice culture. *Peptides* **31,** 1131–1138.

Katzenschlager, R., and Lees, A. J. (2002). Treatment of Parkinson's disease: Levodopa as the first choice. *J. Neurol.* **249,** II19–II24.
Kessler, B. A., Stanley, E. M., Frederick-Duus, D., and Fadel, J. (2011). Age-related loss of orexin/hypocretin neurons. *Neuroscience* **178,** 82–88.
Kilduff, T. S., and Peyron, C. (2000). The hypocretin/orexin ligand-receptor system: Implications for sleep and sleep disorders. *Trends Neurosci.* **23,** 359–365.
Lees, A. J., Hardy, J., and Revesz, T. (2009). Parkinson's disease. *Lancet* **373,** 2055–2066.
Li, Y., and van den Pol, A. N. (2005). Direct and indirect inhibition by catecholamines of hypocretin/orexin neurons. *J. Neurosci.* **25,** 173–183.
Li, Y., Gao, X. B., Sakurai, T., and van den Pol, A. N. (2002). Hypocretin/orexin excites hypocretin neurons via a local glutamate neuron—A potential mechanism for orchestrating the hypothalamic arousal system. *Neuron* **36,** 1169–1181.
Michinaga, S., Hisatsune, A., Isohama, Y., and Katsuki, H. (2010a). An anti-Parkinson drug ropinirole depletes orexin from rat hypothalamic slice culture. *Neurosci. Res.* **68,** 315–321.
Michinaga, S., Hisatsune, A., Isohama, Y., and Katsuki, H. (2010b). Inhibition of neural activity depletes orexin from rat hypothalamic slice culture. *J. Neurosci. Res.* **88,** 214–221.
Paus, S., Brecht, H. M., Köster, J., Seeger, G., Klockgether, T., and Wüllner, U. (2003). Sleep attacks, daytime sleepiness, and dopamine agonists in Parkinson's disease. *Mov. Disord.* **18,** 659–667.
Petersén, A., Gil, J., Maat-Schieman, M. L., Björkqvist, M., Tanila, H., Araújo, I. M., Smith, R., Popovic, N., Wierup, N., Norlén, P., Li, J. Y., Roos, R. A., *et al.* (2005). Orexin loss in Huntington's disease. *Hum. Mol. Genet.* **14,** 39–47.
Peyron, C., Faraco, J., Rogers, W., Ripley, B., Overeem, S., Charnay, Y., Nevsimalova, S., Aldrich, M., Reynolds, D., Albin, R., Li, R., Hungs, M., *et al.* (2000). A mutation in a case of early onset narcolepsy and a generalized absence of hypocretin peptides in human narcoleptic brains. *Nat. Med.* **6,** 991–997.
Ravikumar, K., and Sridhar, B. (2006). Ropinirole hydrochloride, a dopamine agonist. *Acta Crystallogr. C* **62,** o265–o267.
Sakurai, T. (2007). The neural circuit of orexin (hypocretin): Maintaining sleep and wakefulness. *Nat. Rev. Neurosci.* **8,** 171–181.
Sakurai, T., and Mieda, M. (2011). Connectomics of orexin-producing neurons: Interface of systems of emotion, energy homeostasis and arousal. *Trends Pharmacol. Sci.* **32,** 451–462.
Steiger, M., Jost, W., Grandas, F., and Van Camp, G. (2009). Risk of valvular heart disease associated with the use of dopamine agonists in Parkinson's disease: A systematic review. *J. Neural Transm.* **116,** 179–191.
Thannickal, T. C., Moore, R. Y., Nienhuis, R., Ramanathan, L., Gulyani, S., Aldrich, M., Cornford, M., and Siegel, J. M. (2000). Reduced number of hypocretin neurons in human narcolepsy. *Neuron* **27,** 469–474.
Thannickal, T. C., Lai, Y. Y., and Siegel, J. M. (2007). Hypocretin (orexin) cell loss in Parkinson's disease. *Brain* **130,** 1586–1595.
Tsujino, N., and Sakurai, T. (2009). Orexin/hypocretin: A neuropeptide at the interface of sleep, energy homeostasis, and reward system. *Pharmacol. Rev.* **61,** 162–176.
Wulff, K., Gatti, S., Wettstein, J. G., and Foster, R. G. (2010). Sleep and circadian rhythm disruption in psychiatric and neurodegenerative disease. *Nat. Rev. Neurosci.* **11,** 589–599.
Yamamoto, Y., Ueta, Y., Hara, Y., Serino, R., Nomura, M., Shibuya, I., Shirahata, A., and Yamashita, H. (2000). Postnatal development of orexin/hypocretin in rats. *Mol. Brain Res.* **78,** 108–119.
Yamanaka, A., Muraki, Y., Ichiki, K., Tsujino, N., Kilduff, T. S., Goto, K., and Sakurai, T. (2006). Orexin neurons are directly and indirectly regulated by catecholamines in a complex manner. *J. Neurophysiol.* **96,** 284–298.
Zeitzer, J. M., Nishino, S., and Mignot, E. (2006). The neurobiology of hypocretins (orexins), narcolepsy and related therapeutic interventions. *Trends Pharmacol. Sci.* **27,** 368–374.

CHAPTER SIXTEEN

Cocaine and Nicotine Research Illustrates a Range of Hypocretin Mechanisms in Addiction

Corey Baimel,* Stephanie L. Borgland,* *and* William Corrigall†

Contents

Abstract

Hypocretins (also known as orexins) are neuropeptides synthesized in the lateral hypothalamus and perifornical region and projecting widely throughout the brain. They play an important modulatory role in plasticity related to addictive behavior. Hypocretin signaling to the ventral tegmental area (VTA) promotes synaptic plasticity by potentiating glutamatergic inputs to dopamine neurons and is required for the plasticity induced by stimulant drugs like cocaine. Plasticity in the VTA leads to increased output of dopamine neurons and increased release of dopamine in projection areas, which is associated with the development of addiction-related behaviors. Antagonists of hypocretin receptors inhibit some of these behaviors, particularly those with high effort

* Department of Anesthesiology, Pharmacology & Therapeutics, University of British Columbia, Vancouver, British Columbia, Canada
† Department of Psychiatry, University of Minnesota, Minneapolis, Minnesota, USA

Vitamins and Hormones, Volume 89
ISSN 0083-6729, http://dx.doi.org/10.1016/B978-0-12-394623-2.00016-0

requirements, suggesting a significant role of hypocretin in the motivation to obtain drugs. Furthermore, hypocretin neurons are also targeted by drugs of abuse, such as nicotine. Projections of hypocretin neurons to regions beyond the VTA may also play a significant role in motivation and addiction. Taken together, the hypocretin system may be a prime drug target for treatment of addiction and related disorders.

I. Addiction and the Mesolimbic Dopamine System

The mesolimbic dopamine system consists of the dopamine neurons originating in the ventral tegmental area (VTA) and their projections including the nucleus accumbens (NAc), the prefrontal cortex (PFC), the hippocampus, bed nucleus of the stria terminalis (BNST), and the amygdala. Plasticity in this system has been implicated in a variety of addictive behaviors (Jones and Bonci, 2005; Kalivas, 2007; Luscher and Malenka, 2011; Thomas *et al.*, 2008; Wolf and Ferrario, 2010). Specifically, initial *in vivo* drug exposure resulted in long-lasting changes at excitatory synapses in the VTA and the NAc (Borgland *et al.*, 2004; Fitzgerald *et al.*, 1996; Mameli *et al.*, 2009; Martin *et al.*, 2006; Saal *et al.*, 2003; Thomas *et al.*, 2001; Ungless *et al.*, 2001; Wolf *et al.*, 2004), which are proposed to underlie some of the long-term effects of chronic drug use (Borgland *et al.*, 2004; Chen *et al.*, 2008; Kauer, 2004; Nogueira *et al.*, 2006; Wolf *et al.*, 2004). The current proposed hypothesis is that drugs of abuse induce a strengthening of glutamatergic synapses in the VTA causing a change in the firing patterns of dopamine neurons from tonic to burst firing and leading to increased dopamine release in projection areas (Jones and Bonci, 2005). Increased release of dopamine in regions like the NAc is important for the association of environmental cues and context with the drug-taking experience (Aston-Jones *et al.*, 2009).

II. Hypocretin Involvement with the Mesolimbic Dopamine System

Recently, substantial evidence has linked the lateral hypothalamic (LH) hypocretin (hcrt) system with the mesolimbic dopamine system and reward and reinforcement (Aston-Jones *et al.*, 2009). There is a substantial projection of hcrt neurons from the LH to VTA (Baldo *et al.*, 2003; Fadel and Deutch, 2002), and although only 5% of these projections form direct synapses (Balcita-Pedicino and Sesack, 2007), the presence of intra-VTA hypocretin-containing dense-cored vesicles (Balcita-Pedicino and Sesack, 2007) indicates that the hcrt peptides are likely released extrasynaptically from en-passant fibers. Hypocretin-1 (hcrt-1) and hypocretin-2 (hcrt-2) activate Gq-coupled hypocretin-1 receptors (hcrt-R1), whereas hcrt-2 preferentially activates hypocretin-2 receptors (hcrt-R2). Both hcrt receptor subtypes are expressed on dopamine and GABA neurons within the VTA (Korotkova *et al.*, 2003; Narita *et al.*, 2006), and hcrt-1 or hcrt-2 application to the VTA increases dopamine and GABA neuron firing rates (Korotkova *et al.*, 2003; Muschamp *et al.*, 2007). Taken together, this suggests that the hcrt projections to the VTA may be implicated in the cellular and behavioral responses to drug exposure.

III. Hypocretin-1 Effects on NMDAR Currents in Dopamine Neurons

Using whole-cell patch clamp electrophysiology, Borgland *et al.* (2006) demonstrated that hcrt-1, acting primarily through hcrt-R1, caused a dose-dependent potentiation of *N*-methyl-D-aspartate receptor (NMDAR) excitatory postsynaptic current (EPSC) amplitudes measured in VTA dopamine neurons. This potentiation was due to activation of a protein kinase C/phospholipase C (PKC/PLC) intracellular signaling pathway and resulted in increased trafficking of NMDARs to the membrane (Borgland *et al.*, 2006). Additionally, NMDAR miniature EPSC (mEPSC) amplitude was increased 15 min after hcrt-1 application but not 3–4 h later, further indicating that hcrt-1 induces short-term plastic effects of NMDARs in VTA dopamine neurons (Borgland *et al.*, 2006). One of the major roles of NMDARs in dopamine neurons is the promotion of burst firing (Overton and Clark, 1992; Suaud-Chagny *et al.*, 1992; Tong *et al.*, 1996), a phenomenon associated with more efficient dopamine release in projecting areas, and although not normally observed *in vitro*, it can be mimicked with bath NMDA application (Johnson *et al.*, 1992). Therefore, hcrt-1-induced potentiation of NMDAR input to the VTA may result in increased dopamine neuron activity and increased dopamine release in projecting regions. Hcrt-1 application to the VTA increased the firing rate of dopamine neurons and in some cases was found to induce burst firing (Korotkova *et al.*, 2003; Muschamp *et al.*, 2007), although it is still unknown if this increase in the firing rate is dependent on glutamatergic potentiation. Furthermore, intra-VTA injections of hcrt-1 was associated with increased dopamine release in the NAc and the development of a conditioned place preference (CPP), both of which were blocked by administration of PKC and PLC inhibitors (Narita *et al.*, 2006, 2007). Hcrt-1 also induces increased dopamine release in the PFC (Vittoz and Berridge, 2006; Vittoz *et al.*, 2008).

IV. Hypocretin-1 Effects on AMPAR EPSCs in Dopamine Neurons

Another major role of NMDARs in dopamine neurons is the induction of long-term potentiation (LTP), a form of long-term plasticity often measured as a change in the ratio of AMPAR-mediated to NMDAR-mediated currents in dopamine neurons (Borgland *et al.*, 2004; Saal *et al.*, 2003; Ungless *et al.*, 2001). It is therefore possible that hcrt-1-induced potentiation of NMDAR EPSCs facilitates the induction of synaptic plasticity (Borgland *et al.*, 2006). Unlike NMDAR EPSCs, AMPAR current amplitudes are unchanged when measured 15 min following hcrt-1 administration (Borgland *et al.*, 2006). However, hcrt-1 induced an increase in the AMPAR/NMDAR ratio when measured 3–4 h postapplication and was associated with an increase in both the frequency and the amplitude of AMPAR mEPSCs (Borgland *et al.*, 2006). The increase in mEPSC amplitude, but not the frequency, was inhibited by application of the NMDAR antagonist APV (Borgland *et al.*, 2006). This suggested that AMPAR EPSCs were potentiated through a NMDAR-dependent postsynaptic mechanism as well as a NMDAR-independent increase in glutamate release (Borgland *et al.*, 2006). Future experiments will determine whether AMPAR potentiation is due to functional changes in existing AMPARs or by trafficking of new AMPARs to the membrane.

V. Hypocretin-2 and Plasticity of Dopamine Neurons

Although less studied in the context of addiction, hcrt-2 is presumably coreleased with hcrt-1 into the VTA (Borgland *et al.*, 2008) and can also increase the firing rate of dopamine neurons (Korotkova *et al.*, 2003). Hcrt-2 caused a dose-dependent increase in both NMDAR and AMPAR EPSCs (Borgland *et al.*, 2008). Hcrt-2 in the VTA signals primarily through hcrt-R2 (Borgland *et al.*, 2008) and induces a postsynaptic potentiation of NMDAR EPSCs via a PKC-dependent mechanism. Additionally, hcrt-2 caused a presynaptic increase in glutamate release affecting both NMDARs and AMPARs (Borgland *et al.*, 2008). This was reflected by a decrease in paired-pulse ratio and an increase in the frequency, but not the amplitude, of AMPAR mEPSCs (Borgland *et al.*, 2008). Surprisingly, the effect of hcrt-2 on AMPAR mEPSC frequency was not blocked by antagonists for either hcrt-R1 or hcrt-R2 suggesting that the enhanced presynaptic glutamate release may be due to hcrt-2 or one of its metabolites acting at an unidentified PKC-coupled receptor (Borgland *et al.*, 2008).

Hcrt-2 injected directly into the VTA induced a place preference and increased dopamine release in the NAc, both of which required intact PKC signaling (Narita *et al.*, 2007). While hcrt-2 primarily signals through hcrt-R2, other studies have demonstrated that these receptors do not play a primary role in addiction-related behaviors (Smith *et al.*, 2009; Wang *et al.*, 2009). Therefore, it has been proposed that signaling through hcrt-R1 in the VTA mediates behaviors associated with addiction, whereas signaling through hcrt-R2 mediates arousal-related functions (Aston-Jones *et al.*, 2010).

VI. Hypocretin and Drug-Induced Synaptic Plasticity

It has been well characterized that *in vivo* exposure to drugs of abuse induces an LTP-like potentiation of AMPAR-mediated responses in VTA dopamine neurons (Borgland *et al.*, 2004; Saal *et al.*, 2003; Ungless *et al.*, 2001). Induction of AMPAR potentiation is an NMDAR-dependent process (Kauer and Malenka, 2007) and promotes an increase in phasic firing of dopamine neurons and downstream increases in dopamine release in projection regions (Johnson *et al.*, 1992; Murase *et al.*, 1993; Suaud-Chagny *et al.*, 1992). Furthermore, NMDARs in the VTA are potentiated by acute cocaine treatment (Argilli *et al.*, 2008). Because hcrt-1 potentiated NMDARs of VTA dopamine neurons, hcrt-R1 signaling may underlie cocaine-induced plasticity. Following 5 days of cocaine treatment with or without the hcrt-R1 antagonist, SB-334867, Borgland *et al.* (2006) measured the relative contribution of AMPAR and NMDARs at glutamatergic synapses of dopamine neurons. Systemic pretreatment with SB-334867 blocked cocaine-induced potentiation of the AMPAR/NMDAR ratio (Borgland *et al.*, 2006). These results suggest that hcrt signaling in the VTA plays a critical role in drug-induced synaptic plasticity. Furthermore, España *et al.* (2010) demonstrated that both systemic and intra-VTA administration of SB-334867 attenuates cocaine-induced increases in dopamine concentrations in the NAc core. Conversely, intra-VTA infusion of hcrt-1 increases dopamine concentrations in the NAc and increases the efficacy of cocaine-mediated dopamine reuptake inhibition (España *et al.*, 2011). Taken together, blockade of hcrt-1 signaling in the VTA can inhibit cocaine-mediated strengthening of synapses and output of VTA dopamine neurons (España *et al.*, 2010).

Long-term drug exposure can also alter hcrt signaling in the VTA. In rats trained to self-administer cocaine, regular- or high-fat food, hcrt-1-induced potentiation of NMDARs in VTA dopamine neurons was significantly enhanced only in cocaine or high-fat self-administering rats (Borgland *et al.*, 2009). This was accompanied by an increase in the frequency of AMPAR mEPSCs, suggesting that cocaine or high-fat self-administration increased the probability of presynaptic glutamate release (Borgland *et al.*, 2009). Furthermore, application of an ineffective concentration of hcrt-1 in naïve animals induced potentiation of NMDARs only in cocaine or high-fat self-administering rats, suggesting the drug treatment increased the sensitivity to hcrt possibly by increasing the availability of receptors or signal transduction machinery (Borgland *et al.*, 2009). Taken together, both pre- and postsynaptic modulation of glutamatergic transmission by hcrt can occur after drug treatment. The VTA receives several glutamatergic inputs to the VTA that can potentially be modulated by hcrt-1. The medial PFC sends direct glutamatergic inputs to the VTA (Sesack and Pickel, 1992; Sesack *et al.*, 1989), and stimulation of these inputs can activate dopamine neurons *in vivo* (Murase *et al.*, 1993). Electrical stimulation of mPFC inputs in anesthetized rats evoked a burst of action potentials in the VTA (Moorman and Aston-Jones, 2010). Application of hcrt-1 into the VTA enhanced basal firing in addition to mPFC-evoked bursts (Moorman and Aston-Jones, 2010), suggesting that hcrt-1 can modulate mPFC glutamatergic inputs to the VTA.

VII. Hypocretin and Behavioral Plasticity

Drug-induced synaptic plasticity in the VTA underlies some of the behavioral features of addiction. Behavioral sensitization involves increased locomotor activity and dopamine neurotransmission with repeated administration of a drug and persists long after drug exposure is discontinued (Robinson and Berridge, 1993). Sensitization is dependent on activation of NMDARs in the VTA (Kalivas and Alesdatter, 1993). Preadministration of SB-334867 both systemically and intra-VTA prior to drug exposure significantly inhibited the acquisition of sensitization to cocaine (Borgland *et al.*, 2006), amphetamine (Quarta *et al.*, 2009), but not morphine (Sharf *et al.*, 2010) and was ineffective at blocking the expression of this behavior in previously cocaine sensitized animals (Borgland *et al.*, 2006). Sensitization is representative of drug-induced neural adaptations associated with drug craving (Boileau *et al.*, 2006). Thus, inhibiting hcrt transmission in the VTA likely reduces the motivational significance of stimulant drugs and a subsequent reduction in the animal's drive to obtain the drug.

In CPP paradigms, whereby preferences for drug-paired contexts are measured, hcrt neurons from rats conditioned with food, morphine, or cocaine displayed greater cFos expression with the drug-paired environment (Harris *et al.*, 2005). SB-334867 blocked the development and the expression of morphine preference (Harris *et al.*, 2005; Narita *et al.*, 2006; Sharf *et al.*, 2010), but not the expression of cocaine preference (Sharf *et al.*, 2010) or the development of ethanol preference (Voorhees and Cunningham, 2011).

Moreover, microinjections of hcrt-1 into the VTA robustly reinstated extinguished morphine preference behavior (Harris *et al.*, 2005). Furthermore, in a bilateral disconnection study, a unilateral LH lesion blocked the acquisition of morphine CPP when SB-334867 was injected into the contralateral VTA (Harris *et al.*, 2007). Taken together, this demonstrates that hcrt projections to the VTA play an important role in the acquisition and the expression of drug preference, although this may be dependent on the drug used.

VIII. Hypocretin and the Motivation for Drugs

There are several lines of evidence that point to a role for hcrt signaling in the motivation to obtain drugs of abuse. In self-administration studies, animals are placed in operant chambers and are required to lever press in order to obtain reward. Responding for ethanol is reduced by SB-334867 (Lawrence *et al.*, 2006) and increased by intracranial hcrt-1 (Schneider *et al.*, 2007) on fixed-ratio (FR) schedules of reinforcement. Interestingly, cocaine self-administration is not affected by SB-334867 administration under these conditions (Boutrel *et al.*, 2005; España *et al.*, 2010; Smith *et al.*, 2009). However, on a progressive ratio (PR) schedule of reinforcement, where increased effort is required to obtain each subsequent reinforcer, SB-334867 reduced the breakpoint and the total lever pressing for cocaine (Borgland *et al.*, 2009; España *et al.*, 2010) or nicotine (Hollander *et al.*, 2008) injections. SB-334867 had little effect on cocaine self-administration when the response requirement was low; however, as the effort required to obtain the drug was increased, inhibition mediated by SB-334867 was greater (Borgland *et al.*, 2009; España *et al.*, 2010). This effect is replicated with intra-VTA bilateral injections of SB-334867 (España *et al.*, 2010), suggesting that hcrt signaling in the VTA is necessary for effort-based tasks. Consistent with this, hcrt-1 in the VTA increased breakpoints and total lever responding for cocaine (España *et al.*, 2010). Finally, in a threshold experiment in which the dose of cocaine is progressively decreased within a given testing session making it increasingly difficult to titrate blood levels, SB-334867 had no effect on the beginning of the session when titration of blood levels is easily achieved but did significantly inhibit responding later in sessions when animals were required to work harder to receive the same quantity of drug (España *et al.*, 2010).

Relapse to drug seeking is a common characteristic of addiction which can be modeled in rats. Stress, cues, as well as small doses of the drug (drug prime) can all induce reinstatement to drug seeking. Interestingly, SB-334867 can block cue-induced reinstatement of cocaine self-administration, but not drug-primed reinstatement (Smith *et al.*, 2009).

Based on these findings, it is clear that hcrt signaling to the VTA plays an important role in both the cellular and the behavioral plasticity induced by stimulant drugs like cocaine. Because this plasticity is not unique to stimulants, it would be beneficial for future research to characterize the role of hcrt in the plasticity induced by other classes of abused drugs. Doing so would enable the development of a more complete understanding of the role of hcrt in addiction and motivated behaviors.

In addition to hcrt modulating plasticity of dopamine neurons induced by drugs of abuse, certain drugs have direct effects on hcrt neurons themselves. Furthermore, the projections of hcrt neurons from the LH to brain regions associated with addiction are not limited to the VTA. Thus, hcrt likely has a role modulating brain regions outside the mesolimbic dopamine system in the context of drug-seeking behaviors. This concept will be further discussed below in relation to nicotine.

IX. Existing Studies of Hypocretin Mechanisms in the Effects of Nicotine

Compared to studies of the interactions of the hcrt system with cocaine and other drugs, research exploring hcrt mechanisms in the effects of nicotine has been much more limited. Nonetheless, a few studies do provide evidence that experimenter-administered or self-administered nicotine delivered either acutely or chronically has effects on hcrt neurons. Chronic administration of nicotine by repetitive injection over a period of 10–14 days was found to alter the expression of mRNA for prepro-hypocretin itself and its receptors and peptide ligands (Kane *et al.*, 2000, 2001). It has also been shown that nicotine, administered acutely at behaviorally relevant doses equivalent to those which produce locomotor activation, dose-dependently increases the proportion of hcrt-containing neurons in the LH and perifornical area (PFA) that express Fos (Pasumarthi *et al.*, 2006). LeSage *et al.* (2010) examined gene expression for the hcrt system (mRNA for hcrt, hcrt-R1, and hcrt-R2) in animals following a 19-day period of nicotine self-administration on a simple fixed-ratio 1 (FR1) schedule (each lever press results in the delivery of a drug infusion, as long as the response is temporally after a time-out period that follows the previous drug delivery). A selection of brain regions was examined; however, statistically significant changes were confined to the hypothalamic region. In tissue collected immediately following the last self-administration session, there was a decrease in mRNA for hcrt-R1 in the rostral LH; in tissue collected 5 h after the last self-administration session (to allow nicotine levels to decrease), there was an increase in hcrt-R1 mRNA in the arcuate nucleus. The difference between these groups suggests either that the amount of nicotine present at the time of tissue collection is a factor, or that change in the hcrt system is very labile. If, as suggested by studies of hcrt mechanisms in the behavioral pharmacology of cocaine, workload or motivational effects play a role in the manifestation of hcrt effects (e.g., Borgland *et al.*, 2009; España *et al.*, 2010), then the absence of involvement of other brain regions may be related to the use of a FR1 schedule for the self-administration of nicotine. Recently, Huang *et al.* (2011) reported electrophysiological evidence that nicotine could excite hcrt-containing neurons in the LH/PFA; nicotine depolarized hcrt neurons and increased spike frequency, although to a lesser extent than it affected proopiomelanocortin or neuropeptide Y cells of the hypothalamic arcuate nucleus. Collectively, these studies provide a small but convincing dataset showing that nicotine can alter hcrt-containing neurons in the LH/PFA.

Nicotine–hcrt interactions have also been observed in several behavioral measures of the rewarding, reinforcing, and motivational effects of nicotine in addition to the LeSage *et al.* study noted above, and in indirect measures that likely relate to motivational effects such as arousal and attention. With respect to the latter, Fos protein expressed in hcrt-containing neurons of the LH/PFA subsequent to nicotine treatment has been found to be located predominantly in those hcrt neurons that project to the basal forebrain and the paraventricular nucleus of the dorsal thalamus (Pasumarthi and Fadel, 2008), providing candidate mechanisms through which nicotine could produce arousal (via nicotine activation of a LH-to-PVT hcrt pathway which in turn activates neurons projecting to the PFC) and attentional effects (via hcrt activation of the basal forebrain cholinergic system). A potential attentional mechanism in common for nicotine and hcrt is also suggested by the finding that nicotine and hcrt, the latter through hcrt-R2 receptors, both excite the same thalamocortical synapses and improve performance in a behavioral task requiring attention (Lambe *et al.*, 2005).

Hollander *et al.* (2008) reported the first studies of hcrt manipulations on the rewarding and reinforcing effects of nicotine. In their research, presession administration of the hcrt-R1 antagonist SB-334867 attenuated nicotine self-administration maintained on both a FR5 and a PR schedule, in which the response requirement to obtain each successive drug infusion increases according to a given algorithm throughout the session. FR schedules measure drug reinforcement, whereas PR schedules are believed to measure the motivation of the animal to obtain the drug. In addition, microinfusion of SB-334867 into the insular cortex also reduced self-administration on the FR schedule. It has previously been shown that tobacco smokers with damage to the insula are more likely than normals to quit smoking without relapse and the recurrence of urges to smoke (Naqvi *et al.*, 2007). Speculation regarding possible mechanisms for hcrt effects in the insula on nicotine reinforcement includes a direct effect the drug on hcrt projections to the insula or effects on dopaminergic and/or other inputs to it from the VTA or other reward-related regions of the brain.

Another aspect of the LeSage *et al.* study noted earlier was comparison of the effects of the hcrt-R1 antagonist SB-334867 and the dual hcrt-R1/2 antagonist almorexant on nicotine self-administration maintained on a FR5 schedule. Although both antagonists reduced nicotine self-administration to a similar extent, the observation is insufficient evidence to rule out a role for the hcrt-R2 receptor in the effects of nicotine, which will require use of a selective antagonist for the hcrt-R2 receptor.

The attenuation of responding for nicotine in these two self-administration studies appears to be selective based on the parallel observations that responding for food pellets in similarly designed operant experiments was not affected. Although this may at first glance appear to be curious, given the orexigenic action of hcrt in feeding, control experiments with food-maintained responding are possible, at least for the SB-334867 compound, because its effect is to advance satiety, with apparently no effect on the microstructure of feeding behavior prior to reaching satiety (Rodgers *et al.*, 2001). In consequence, studies that utilize animals maintained on a regimen of limited access to food with responding delivering only small amounts of food do not observe effects with SB-334867 treatment. In contrast, when animals can obtain greater amounts of food and/or the food is high fat/high carbohydrate in content, effects of SB-334867 are clearly evident (Nair *et al.*, 2008). It is less obvious that the effect of the hcrt-R1/2 antagonist almorexant on nicotine self-administration is specific because there were effects on food-maintained responding at antagonist doses that are comparable to those which attenuate self-administration (LeSage *et al.*, 2010). Whether this effect is due to the hcrt-R2 component of the antagonist, dual antagonism, or some other property remains unknown.

The potential influence of hcrt has been examined in several other tasks that measure motivation-related effects, both positive and negative. Plaza-Zabala *et al.* (2010) reported that hcrt-1 could reinstate extinguished drug-seeking behavior in mice in which the operant was nose-poke behavior. This effect was reversed by SB-334867 but not by the CRF1 antagonist antalarmin, suggesting a dissociation from stress-related mechanisms. Indeed, reinstatement induced by footshock was reversed by the CRF1 antagonist but not by the hcrt antagonist, supporting this conclusion. However, nicotine-induced anxiogenesis in the plus-maze task was reduced by treatment with SB-334867 and diminished in prepro-hcrt KO mice, leaving open the possibility that hcrt effects related to stress and anxiogenesis might depend on the behavioral test that is employed. In a second recent report, Plaza-Zabala *et al.* (2011) implicated hcrt-R1 mechanisms in the paraventricular nucleus of the hypothalamus (PVN) in nicotine withdrawal. They found that somatic withdrawal signs in chronically treated mice were attenuated by SB-334867 administered systemically and following microinfusion into the PVN, and in prepro-hcrt KO animals. However, withdrawal signs were not attenuated by systemic administration of a hcrt-R2 antagonist.

Another indication of nicotine's enhancement of brain reward systems is its ability to lower the threshold for intracranial self-stimulation; Hollander *et al.* (2008) found that systemic administration of SB-334867 reversed the threshold-lowering effect of nicotine in this behavioral measure.

To date, there has been only one report of a possible role for hcrt mechanisms in human subjects who are tobacco users (von der Goltz *et al.*, 2010). In this study, hcrt levels were measured in blood samples obtained from smokers 3 h postsmoking a cigarette and compared to levels in nonsmokers. There were no differences between the groups, but there was a negative correlation between plasma nicotine level and nicotine craving as assessed by the Questionnaire of Smoking Urges. Although one cannot exclude that the hcrt differences observed might be due to changes outside the brain, this study does provide intriguing human subjects data that should be confirmed and extended. Superficially at least, the negative correlation of hcrt with craving scores in human subjects and the reduction in nicotine self-administration produced by an hcrt antagonist in animals could be construed to be similar directions of effect. On the other hand, it is difficult to reconcile the effects in this human subjects study with those of Plaza-Zabala *et al.* in mice in which hcrt-1 provoked relapse to drug-taking behavior.

In view of the limited number of studies to date, it is not possible to draw wide-ranging conclusions about hcrt influences in the effects of nicotine. However, it does appear conclusive that the hcrt system plays a role in some of the behavioral effects of nicotine related to addiction.

Even in those effects of nicotine, which appear to involve hcrt system, the nature of the hcrt involvement remains largely unknown. For example, although there is some convergent evidence that nicotine interacts with hcrt-containing neurons in the LH/PFA, we must guess that this likely occurs through the alpha4beta2-containing nicotinic cholinergic receptor (nAChR) which is the predominant subtype in this brain region (Gotti *et al.*, 2006). Recently, Pasumarthi and Fadel (2010) showed that the effects of acutely administered nicotine in the LH/PFA appear to be mediated by acetylcholine from the basal forebrain and glutamate from the PFC, so it may be that these presumptive alpha4beta2 nAChRs, or other nicotinic receptor subtypes, such as alpha7 which is often associated with glutamate terminals, are located on these extrinsic inputs to the LH/PFA where they might facilitate transmitter release as they do in dopamine terminal fields in the striatum (Exley *et al.*, 2008; Grady *et al.*, 2007; Livingstone and Wonnacott, 2009). However, this too is conjecture. In addition, there has been no exploration of whether the magnitude of the rewarding/reinforcing effects of nicotine correlates with the extent of change produced by nicotine in the LH/PFA hcrt system. With opioids, for example, the extent of the preference conditioned for an environment paired with morphine is correlated with the amount of Fos expression in hcrt cells of the LH/PFA (Harris *et al.*, 2005). Similar data with nicotine would help confirm that the observed effects are causal and that they register characteristics of the reinforced behavior. More generally, further investigation of the situational and motivational factors that modify nicotine–hcrt interactions are needed. For example, as commented earlier, hcrt-R1 antagonist effects in cocaine self-administration are apparent with more complex schedules of reinforcement than with simpler ones (España *et al.*, 2010), which may relate to whether animals can achieve "satiation" levels of cocaine intake or to workload and task demand, and hcrt-R1 antagonism can influence motivation to obtain a preferred reward such as high-fat chocolate versus regular food (Borgland *et al.*, 2009) which again may also depend on the extent of effort required to attain the reward.

X. Rationale for Further Study of Hcrt Mechanisms in the Preclinical Effects of Nicotine

Although they have been little studied, hcrt mechanisms are compelling candidates as potential substrates in nicotine addiction (Corrigall, 2009). Beyond the obvious benefit that would derive from an increased understanding of the function of the brain, a better understanding of the nature of hcrt mechanisms in nicotine addiction might be exploited to advantage in drug discovery for tobacco dependence where medications that yield better treatment outcomes are required. At present, medications to treat tobacco dependence consist of a variety of nicotine replacement therapies, the antidepressant bupropion (Zyban®), the nicotinic ligand varenicline (Chantix®; Champix®), and several second-line pharmacotherapies, medications which are effective but for which that effectiveness is limited (Polosa and Benowitz, 2011). Compounding this issue, the use of bupropion and varenicline is likely to be reduced by the fact that the FDA has required "black-box" warnings for both medications due to psychiatric side effects. Although the "pipeline" from preclinical to Phase 3 has been populated by a diverse slate of candidates based on a range of CNS targets, altering nicotine metabolism and preventing nicotine access to the brain, they have consistently failed at various stages of development. The most recent victim is the nicotine vaccine NicVAX which recently failed in Phase 3.[1] Hcrt mechanisms may be useful to explore as a platform for drug discovery for tobacco dependence for several reasons. First, hcrts affect alertness and arousal; attendant to withdrawal from smoking is a deficit in attention and concentration; hence, hcrt ligands might be useful after tobacco cessation to sustain treatment gains and prevent relapse. Second, the nature of hcrt mechanisms in nicotine craving and relapse and the direction of

[1] See Nabi Biopharmaceuticals, www.nabi.com/pipeline/.

the effect need to be confirmed, not only because it might provide another avenue for drug discovery but also because pro-relapse effects of hcrt agonists would potentially trump efforts to use such compounds for attention/arousal-enhancing effects. Of course, in such a case, hcrt antagonists may be useful. Third, hcrt mechanisms play a role in nicotine reinforcement in animals, with evidence to date implicating targets (insular cortex, LH/PFA) outside the mesolimbic dopamine system, which has been the frequent focus of drug reinforcement research. Hence, research into the function of the hcrt system in reinforcement would broaden the mechanism discovery horizon and may show the way to new mechanisms by which drug-taking behavior may be altered selectively.

These possibilities notwithstanding, it is clear that drug development based on the hcrt system carries risk, as evidenced by the recent failure of the mixed hcrt-R1/2 antagonist almorexant in Phase 3 clinical trial for sleep disorders.[2] At this time, one can only speculate as to the cause (REM sleep imbalances, narcoleptic side effects, etc.), but it is reasonable to expect that hcrt mechanisms will play a different role in nicotine addiction than in sleep, and that lessons from the adverse effects in the almorexant trials may benefit other developmental work with the hcrt system. Certainly, there appears to be sustained pharmaceutical interest in the hcrt target for sleep disorders (Scammell and Winrow, 2011), and at least at the preclinical level for other substance use disorders (Shoblock *et al.*, 2011) as well as medicinal chemistry activity in ligand development (Di Fabio *et al.*, 2011; Roecker and Coleman, 2008). Finally, it is also to be expected that hcrt effects in nicotine addiction will be through markedly different mechanisms that those for psychomotor stimulants and opioids. Thus, it seems timely for preclinical research to elaborate the mechanisms of hcrt in addiction-related effects of nicotine.

XI. Questions for a Preclinical Discovery Research Agenda

As an example of how one might proceed to develop a broader understanding of the role of hcrt mechanisms in nicotine reinforcement, consider the mesocorticolimbic dopamine system (MDS). A substantial amount of research has focused on the MDS, particularly on the projection from the A10 dopamine neurons in the VTA to the NAc. The interaction of nicotine with this neuronal pathway has been studied extensively at the behavioral and nAChR levels (Balfour, 2004, 2009; Wonnacott *et al.*, 2005).

[2] See www.gsk.com/media/pressreleases/2011/2011_pressrelease_10019.htm.

There is no question that hcrt mechanisms influence neurons in the VTA. Projections of hcrt-containing neurons are present in the VTA (Balcita-Pedicino and Sesack, 2007; Fadel and Deutch, 2002; Nakamura *et al.*, 2000) as are both hcrt receptors (Marcus *et al.*, 2001), and hcrt mechanisms alter Ca^{2+} flux in dopaminergic cells, the firing of both dopaminergic and nondopaminergic cells in the VTA, as well as NMDA-mediated synaptic transmission in the region (Borgland *et al.*, 2006; Korotkova *et al.*, 2003, 2006; Nakamura *et al.*, 2000; Uramura *et al.*, 2001).

Nicotine acts through nAChRs which exist as subtypes composed of five protein subunits, alpha 1–10, and beta 2–4, typically combined to form heteromeric receptors consisting of both alpha and beta subunits, although there are also some homomeric receptors composed of five identical alpha subunits, such as the alpha7 receptor. In the VTA, the two most important subtypes are the alpha4beta2- and alpha6beta2-containing receptors.

The alpha4beta2 nAChR, widely distributed in the brain, was long believed to be the key site for the interaction of smoke-delivered nicotine with the CNS; indeed, it was the target for the development of the smoking cessation medication varenicline (Chantix®; Champix®) by Pfizer. Recently, it has become clear that the stoichiometry of this receptor is more complex than previously thought, at least *in vitro*, the receptor can exist as a high-sensitivity form composed of three alpha4 subunits in combination with two beta2 subunits, and in a low-sensitivity stoichiometry composed of three alpha4 and two beta2 subunits (Nelson *et al.*, 2003) which also appears to have an additional binding site at which ligands may act as allosteric modulators (Harpsøe *et al.*, 2011). The alpha6beta2-containing nAChR has a more restricted distribution than the alpha4beta2 subtype, being localized prominently to the A9 and A10 midbrain dopamine neurons of the VTA and substantia nigra pars compacta (SNc), their synaptic fields in the dorsal and ventral striatum, and in the locus coeruleus (Gotti *et al.*, 2006).

Nicotine self-administration depends on both alpha4- and alpha6-containing receptors in the VTA where there is evidence they may regulate dopamine neurons differentially (Exley *et al.*, 2011; Gotti *et al.*, 2010; Pons *et al.*, 2008; Zhao-Shea *et al.*, 2011). These nAChR populations in the VTA coexist with moderate levels of mRNA for both hcrt receptors (Marcus *et al.*, 2001). Thus, research to elucidate the effects of hcrt manipulations on nicotine action in the VTA could be insightful.

The role of dopamine in addictive behavior has been studied extensively, yielding clearly useful findings. However, it is less clear that the dopamine itself will be a "drug-able" target for medication development in nicotine addiction. The last viable option appears to be the dopamine D3 receptor which has shown some specificity in addiction-related behaviors and which has a relatively restricted CNS distribution which may be of benefit in limiting off-target effects (Heidbreder and Newman, 2010). In the interim, it would be prudent to broaden the preclinical knowledge base.

Beyond the VTA, the wide distribution of the alpha4beta2 nAChR overlaps in many CNS regions with hcrt projections and receptors. High levels of hcrt-R1 and hcrt-R2 mRNA are present in the thalamus, hypothalamus, and hippocampus, and the amygdala contains high levels of message for hcrt-R1 (Marcus *et al.*, 2001). Moderate levels of message for hcrt-R1/2 are present in alpha4beta2-containing regions, including throughout the cortex, the substantia nigra and VTA, and raphe nuclei, with hcrt-R1 expressed at moderate levels in the pedunculopontine tegmental (PPTg) and laterodorsal tegmental (LDTg) nuclei. These are all areas in which alpha4beta2 nAChRs are expressed. This is depicted schematically in Fig. 16.1. A similar although more restricted overlap occurs for alpha6beta2. As noted above, mRNA for

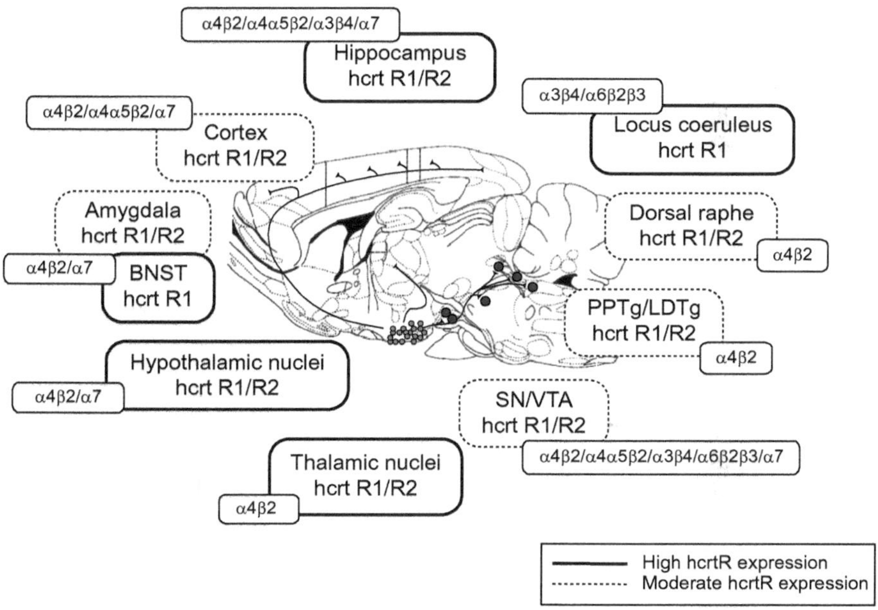

Figure 16.1 Schematic representation of a selection of brain regions according to whether they have been found to have high or moderate expression of mRNA for the hypocretin 1 receptor (hcrt-R1) or the hypocretin 2 receptor (hcrt-R2), based on the data in Marcus *et al.* (2001). The nAChR subtypes that have been found within each region are indicated in the associated boxes (Changeux, 2010; Gotti *et al.*, 2006). For the hypothalamic nuclei, there is both high and moderate expression of mRNA for both hcrt receptors, depending on the particular nucleus in question. Similarly for the thalamic and amygdalar regions, there is a range of expression of hcrt receptor mRNA. In the thalamus, both the paraventricular and rhomboid nuclei exhibit high levels for hcrt-R1 and -R2, respectively; in the amygdala, the levels are moderate, with high expression of message for hcrt-R1 in the bed nucleus of the stria terminalis. The six large gray circles indicate hcrt projection sites in the substantia nigra, ventral tegmental area, pedunculopontine and laterodorsal tegmental nuclei, locus coeruleus, and dorsal raphe nucleus.

both hcrt-R1 and hcrt-R2 exists in SN/VTA, and there is high expression of hcrt-R2 in the locus coeruleus, again affording the opportunity for interactions between hcrt and this distinct population of nAChR subtypes (Fig. 16.1). Thus based on coexistence of receptor populations alone, there is ample opportunity for hcrt to interact with nicotine. For example, the tuberomammillary nucleus (TMN) has a high density of mRNA for hcrt-R2 (Marcus *et al.*, 2001), and the histaminergic neurons in TMN express alpha7 receptors and respond to alpha7-directed ligands (Uteshev *et al.*, 1996, 2002). The intersection of these effects has not been investigated with respect to nicotine addiction, but it well might be: some of the multifunction aspects of the TMN (Wada *et al.*, 1991), particularly arousal, wakefulness, and sleep, might be linked to addictive processes for nicotine, as might alpha7 mechanisms linked to cognitive function (Graef *et al.*, 2011; Haydar and Dunlop, 2010). Given the overlap between nAChRs and hcrt-Rs, there are a number of brain regions where such theoretically relevant interactions might occur.

It would also be valuable to have more information regarding hcrt in some CNS regions. For example, recent gene-wide association studies in humans have implicated several SNPs in CHRNA5/A3/B4 in tobacco smoking, specifically in early onset of smoking and heaviness of use (see overview in Saccone *et al.*, 2010), suggesting that alpha3beta4 and alpha5-containing nAChRs might be important elements in nicotine addiction. These nAChRs are found in several areas of the brain, again ones with presumptive hcrt receptors (Fig. 16.1). In animal studies, nicotine self-administration appears to be under a negative influence of the $\alpha5^{\star}$ receptor in that mice in which the receptor has been knocked-out shown an increase in nicotine self-administration (Fowler *et al.*, 2011). Notably $\alpha5^{\star}$ nAChRs are also found in the medial habenula where lentiviral replacement of the knocked-out receptor in the mouse leads to a recovery of wild-type behavior in nicotine self-administration, implicating a medial habenula–interpeduncular nucleus pathway in the effect. To date, it appears that there have been no studies of the possible expression of hcrt in either of these brain regions, or proximal influence on them, and this would be useful to know.

Continuing in the vein of broadening the research agenda, it is noteworthy that hcrt projections modulate a number of brain stem sites. Hcrt excites wake-active monoaminergic neurons of the locus coeruleus, dorsal raphe, and TMN as well as cholinergic wake-on–REM-on cells in the PPTg and LDTg nuclei (Kilduff and Peyron, 2000). Functionally, most of the hcrt-containing fibers in VTA appear to make very few synapses, projecting directly to caudal brainstem structures (Balcita-Pedicino and Sesack, 2007). The existence of apparent hcrt storage/release vesicles in hcrt fibers in VTA raises the possibility of volume transmission within VTA, and the en passant nature of the projection raises the possible synchronous activation of these more caudally located brainstem regions by hcrt (Fig. 16.1). Nicotine acting at the LH/PFA could stimulate this synchrony, while acting on nAChRs in the target brainstem areas. Relevant to this point, nicotine increases Fos expression in the PPTg (Jose Lança *et al.*, 2000), and lesions of the PPTg attenuate both the acquisition and maintenance of nicotine self-administration (Alderson *et al.*, 2006; Lança *et al.*, 2000) and reverse the preference for an environment associated with experimenter-administered nicotine (Laviolette *et al.*, 2002). It is interesting to note that those hcrt neurons which project to the VTA have maximal activity during exploratory behavior (Mileykovskiy *et al.*, 2005). Do these brainstem sites represent loci at which hcrt and nicotine influence arousal, and at which some of the "value" of nicotine to the tobacco user derives from this effect? If so, this could be a mechanism to explore in drug discovery for tobacco dependence.

The fact that a small research effort has been expended to understand the potential effects of hcrt in nicotine addiction is perhaps understood in light of the relative newness of the hcrt field and the historically greater emphasis in drug addiction research on psychomotor stimulants and opioids. However, the paucity of studies is surprising given the theoretical opportunity to understand how this neuropeptide might contribute to drug use that is mediated by a distinct and widely distributed set of receptors and via circuitry that may well recruit very different populations of neurons than do other drugs. A ramped-up research effort into the role of hcrt mechanisms in nicotine addiction may show the way to further broadening of the research agenda in nicotine addiction, an outcome which is sorely needed.

REFERENCES

Alderson, H. L., Latimer, M. P., and Winn, P. (2006). Intravenous self-administration of nicotine is altered by lesions of the posterior, but not anterior, pedunculopontine tegmental nucleus. *Eur. J. Neurosci.* **23,** 2169–2175.

Argilli, E., Sibley, D. R., Malenka, R. C., England, P. M., and Bonci, A. (2008). Mechanism and time course of cocaine-induced long-term potentiation in the ventral tegmental area. *J. Neurosci.* **28,** 9092–9100.

Aston-Jones, G., Smith, R. J., Moorman, D. E., and Richardson, K. A. (2009). Role of lateral hypothalamic orexin neurons in reward processing and addiction. *Neuropharmacology* **56**(Suppl. 1), 112–121.

Aston-Jones, G., Smith, R. J., Sartor, G. C., Moorman, D. E., Massi, L., Tahsili-Fahadan, P., and Richardson, K. A. (2010). Lateral hypothalamic orexin/hypocretin neurons: A role in reward-seeking and addiction. *Brain Res.* **1314,** 74–90.

Balcita-Pedicino, J. J., and Sesack, S. R. (2007). Orexin axons in the rat ventral tegmental area synapse infrequently onto dopamine and gamma-aminobutyric acid neurons. *J. Comp. Neurol.* **503,** 668–684.

Baldo, B. A., Daniel, R. A., Berridge, C. W., and Kelley, A. E. (2003). Overlapping distributions of orexin/hypocretin- and dopamine-beta-hydroxylase immunoreactive fibers in rat brain regions mediating arousal, motivation, and stress. *J. Comp. Neurol.* **464,** 220–237.

Balfour, D. J. (2004). The neurobiology of tobacco dependence: A preclinical perspective on the role of the dopamine projections to the nucleus accumbens. *Nicotine Tob. Res.* **6,** 899–912.

Balfour, D. J. (2009). The neuronal pathways mediating the behavioral and addictive properties of nicotine. *Handb. Exp. Pharmacol.* **192,** 209–233.

Boileau, I., Dagher, A., Leyton, M., Gunn, R. N., Baker, G. B., Diksic, M., and Benkelfat, C. (2006). Modeling sensitization to stimulants in humans: An [11C]raclopride/positron emission tomography study in healthy men. *Arch. Gen. Psychiatry* **63,** 1386–1395.

Borgland, S. L., Malenka, R. C., and Bonci, A. (2004). Acute and chronic cocaine-induced potentiation of synaptic strength in the ventral tegmental area: Electrophysiological and behavioral correlates in individual rats. *J. Neurosci.* **24,** 7482–7490.

Borgland, S. L., Taha, S. A., Sarti, F., Fields, H. L., and Bonci, A. (2006). Orexin A in the VTA is critical for the induction of synaptic plasticity and behavioral sensitization to cocaine. *Neuron* **49,** 589–601.

Borgland, S. L., Storm, E., and Bonci, A. (2008). Orexin B/hypocretin 2 increases glutamatergic transmission to ventral tegmental area neurons. *Eur. J. Neurosci.* **28,** 1545–1556.

Borgland, S. L., Chang, S. J., Bowers, M. S., Thompson, J. L., Vittoz, N., Floresco, S. B., Chou, J., Chen, B. T., and Bonci, A. (2009). Orexin A/hypocretin-a selectively promotes motivation for positive reinforcers. *J. Neurosci.* **29,** 11215–11225.

Boutrel, B., Kenny, P. J., Specio, S. E., Martin-Fardon, R., Markou, A., Koob, G. F., and de Lecea, L. (2005). Role for hypocretin in mediating stress-induced reinstatement of cocaine-seeking behavior. *Proc. Natl. Acad. Sci. U.S.A.* **102,** 19168–19173.

Changeux, J. P. (2010). Nicotine addiction and nicotine receptors: Lessons learned from genetically modified mice. *Nat. Rev. Neurosci.* **11,** 389–401.

Chen, B. T., Bowers, M. S., Martin, M., Hopf, F. W., Guillory, A. M., Carelli, R. M., Chou, J. K., and Bonci, A. (2008). Cocaine but not natural reward self-administration nor passive cocaine infusion produces persistent LTP in the VTA. *Neuron* **59,** 288–297.

Corrigall, W. A. (2009). Hypocretin mechanisms in nicotine addiction: Evidence and speculation. *Psychopharmacology (Berl.)* **206,** 23–37.

Di Fabio, R., Pellacani, A., Faedo, S., Roth, A., Piccoli, L., Gerrard, P., Porter, R. A., Johnson, C. N., Thewlis, K., Donati, D., Stasi, L., Spada, S., *et al.* (2011). Discovery process and pharmacological characterization of a novel dual orexin 1 and orexin 2 receptor antagonist useful for treatment of sleep disorders. *Bioorg. Med. Chem. Lett.* **21,** 5562–5567.

España, R. A., Oleson, E. B., Locke, J. L., Brookshire, B. R., Roberts, D. C., and Jones, S. R. (2010). The hypocretin-orexin system regulates cocaine self-administration via actions on the mesolimbic dopamine system. *Eur. J. Neurosci.* **31,** 336–348.

España, R. A., Melchior, J. R., Roberts, D. C., and Jones, S. R. (2011). Hypocretin 1/orexin A in the ventral tegmental area enhances dopamine responses to cocaine and promotes cocaine self-administration. *Psychopharmacology (Berl.)* **214,** 415–426.

Exley, R., Clements, M. A., Hartung, H., McIntosh, J. M., and Cragg, S. J. (2008). Alpha6-containing nicotinic acetylcholine receptors dominate the nicotine control of dopamine neurotransmission in nucleus accumbens. *Neuropsychopharmacology* **33,** 2158–2166.

Exley, R., Maubourguet, N., David, V., Eddine, R., Evrard, A., Pons, S., Marti, F., Threlfell, S., Cazala, P., McIntosh, J. M., Changeux, J. P., Maskos, U., *et al.* (2011). Distinct contributions of nicotinic acetylcholine receptor subunit alpha4 and subunit alpha6 to the reinforcing effects of nicotine. *Proc. Natl. Acad. Sci. U.S.A.* **108,** 7577–7582.

Fadel, J., and Deutch, A. Y. (2002). Anatomical substrates of orexin-dopamine interactions: Lateral hypothalamic projections to the ventral tegmental area. *Neuroscience* **111,** 379–387.

Fitzgerald, L. W., Ortiz, J., Hamedani, A. G., and Nestler, E. J. (1996). Drugs of abuse and stress increase the expression of GluR1 and NMDAR1 glutamate receptor subunits in the rat ventral tegmental area: Common adaptations among cross-sensitizing agents. *J. Neurosci.* **16,** 274–282.

Fowler, C. D., Lu, Q., Johnson, P. M., Marks, M. J., and Kenny, P. J. (2011). Habenular α5 nicotinic receptor subunit signalling controls nicotine intake. *Nature* **471,** 597–601.

Gotti, C., Zoli, M., and Clementi, F. (2006). Brain nicotinic acetylcholine receptors: Native subtypes and their relevance. *Trends Pharmacol. Sci.* **27,** 482–491.

Gotti, C., Guiducci, S., Tedesco, V., Corbioli, S., Zanetti, L., Moretti, M., Zanardi, A., Rimondini, R., Mugnaini, M., Clementi, F., Chiamulera, C., and Zoli, M. (2010). Nicotinic acetylcholine receptors in the mesolimbic pathway: Primary role of ventral tegmental area alpha6beta2* receptors in mediating systemic nicotine effects on dopamine release, locomotion, and reinforcement. *J. Neurosci.* **30,** 5311–5325.

Grady, S. R., Salminen, O., Laverty, D. C., Whiteaker, P., McIntosh, J. M., Collins, A. C., and Marks, M. J. (2007). The subtypes of nicotinic acetylcholine receptors on dopaminergic terminals of mouse striatum. *Biochem. Pharmacol.* **74,** 1235–11246.

Graef, S., Schönknecht, P., Sabri, O., and Hegerl, U. (2011). Cholinergic receptor subtypes and their role in cognition, emotion, and vigilance control: An overview of preclinical and clinical findings. *Psychopharmacology (Berl.)* **215,** 205–229.

Harpsøe, K., Ahring, P. K., Christensen, J. K., Jensen, M. L., Peters, D., and Balle, T. (2011). Unraveling the high- and low-sensitivity agonist responses of nicotinic acetylcholine receptors. *J. Neurosci.* **31,** 10759–10766.

Harris, G. C., Wimmer, M., and Aston-Jones, G. (2005). A role for lateral hypothalamic orexin neurons in reward seeking. *Nature* **437,** 556–559.

Harris, G. C., Wimmer, M., Randall-Thompson, J. F., and Aston-Jones, G. (2007). Lateral hypothalamic orexin neurons are critically involved in learning to associate an environment with morphine reward. *Behav. Brain Res.* **183,** 43–51.

Haydar, S. N., and Dunlop, J. (2010). Neuronal nicotinic acetylcholine receptors—Targets for the development of drugs to treat cognitive impairment associated with schizophrenia and Alzheimer's disease. *Curr. Top. Med. Chem.* **10,** 144–152.

Heidbreder, C. A., and Newman, A. H. (2010). Current perspectives on selective dopamine D(3) receptor antagonists as pharmacotherapeutics for addictions and related disorders. *Ann. N. Y. Acad. Sci.* **1187,** 4–34.

Hollander, J. A., Lu, Q., Cameron, M. D., Kamenecka, T. M., and Kenny, P. J. (2008). Insular hypocretin transmission regulates nicotine reward. *Proc. Natl. Acad. Sci. U.S.A.* **105,** 19480–19485.

Huang, H., Xu, Y., and van den Pol, A. (2011). Nicotine excites hypothalamic arcuate anorexigenic proopiomelanocortin neurons and orexigenic neuropeptide Y neurons: Similarities and differences. *J. Neurophysiol.* **106,** 1191–1202.

Johnson, S. W., Seutin, V., and North, R. A. (1992). Burst firing in dopamine neurons induced by N-methyl-D-aspartate: Role of electrogenic sodium pump. *Science* **258,** 665–667.

Jones, S., and Bonci, A. (2005). Synaptic plasticity and drug addiction. *Curr. Opin. Pharmacol.* **5,** 20–25.

Jose Lança, A., Sanelli, T. R., and Corrigall, W. A. (2000). Nicotine-induced fos expression in the pedunculopontine mesencephalic tegmentum in the rat. *Neuropharmacology* **39,** 2808–2817.

Kalivas, P. W. (2007). Cocaine and amphetamine-like psychostimulants: Neurocircuitry and glutamate neuroplasticity. *Dialogues Clin. Neurosci.* **9,** 389–397.

Kalivas, P. W., and Alesdatter, J. E. (1993). Involvement of N-methyl-D-aspartate receptor stimulation in the ventral tegmental area and amygdala in behavioral sensitization to cocaine. *J. Pharmacol. Exp. Ther.* **267,** 486–495.

Kane, J. K., Parker, S. L., Matta, S. G., Fu, Y., Sharp, B. M., and Li, M. D. (2000). Nicotine up-regulates expression of orexin and its receptors in rat brain. *Endocrinology* **141,** 3623–3629.

Kane, J. K., Parker, S. L., and Li, M. D. (2001). Hypothalamic orexin-A binding sites are downregulated by chronic nicotine treatment in the rat. *Neurosci. Lett.* **298,** 1–4.

Kauer, J. A. (2004). Learning mechanisms in addiction: Synaptic plasticity in the ventral tegmental area as a result of exposure to drugs of abuse. *Annu. Rev. Physiol.* **66,** 447–475.

Kauer, J. A., and Malenka, R. C. (2007). Synaptic plasticity and addiction. *Nat. Rev. Neurosci.* **8,** 844–858.

Kilduff, T. S., and Peyron, C. (2000). The hypocretin/orexin ligand-receptor system: Implications for sleep and sleep disorders. *Trends Neurosci.* **23,** 359–365.

Korotkova, T. M., Sergeeva, O. A., Eriksson, K. S., Haas, H. L., and Brown, R. E. (2003). Excitation of ventral tegmental area dopaminergic and nondopaminergic neurons by orexins/hypocretins. *J. Neurosci.* **23,** 7–11.

Korotkova, T. M., Brown, R. E., Sergeeva, O. A., Ponomarenko, A. A., and Haas, H. L. (2006). Effects of arousal- and feeding-related neuropeptides on dopaminergic and GABAergic neurons in the ventral tegmental area of the rat. *Eur. J. Neurosci.* **23,** 2677–2685.

Lambe, E. K., Olausson, P., Horst, N. K., Taylor, J. R., and Aghajanian, G. K. (2005). Hypocretin and nicotine excite the same thalamocortical synapses in prefrontal cortex: Correlation with improved attention in rat. *J. Neurosci.* **25,** 5225–5229.

Lança, A. J., Adamson, K. L., Coen, K. M., Chow, B. L., and Corrigall, W. A. (2000). The pedunculopontine tegmental nucleus and the role of cholinergic neurons in nicotine self-administration in the rat: A correlative neuroanatomical and behavioral study. *Neuroscience* **96,** 735–742.

Laviolette, S. R., Alexson, T. O., and van der Kooy, D. (2002). Lesions of the tegmental pedunculopontine nucleus block the rewarding effects and reveal the aversive effects of nicotine in the ventral tegmental area. *J. Neurosci.* **22,** 8653–8660.

Lawrence, A. J., Cowen, M. S., Yang, H. J., Chen, F., and Oldfield, B. (2006). The orexin system regulates alcohol-seeking in rats. *Br. J. Pharmacol.* **148,** 752–759.

LeSage, M. G., Perry, J. L., Kotz, C. M., Shelley, D., and Corrigall, W. A. (2010). Nicotine self-administration in the rat: Effects of hypocretin antagonists and changes in hypocretin mRNA. *Psychopharmacology (Berl.)* **209,** 203–212.

Livingstone, P. D., and Wonnacott, S. (2009). Nicotinic acetylcholine receptors and the ascending dopamine pathways. *Biochem. Pharmacol.* **78,** 744–755.

Luscher, C., and Malenka, R. C. (2011). Drug-evoked synaptic plasticity in addiction: From molecular changes to circuit remodeling. *Neuron* **69,** 650–663.

Mameli, M., Halbout, B., Creton, C., Engblom, D., Parkitna, J. R., Spanagel, R., and Luscher, C. (2009). Cocaine-evoked synaptic plasticity: Persistence in the VTA triggers adaptations in the NAc. *Nat. Neurosci.* **12,** 1036–1041.

Marcus, J. N., Aschkenasi, C. J., Lee, C. E., Chemelli, R. M., Saper, C. B., Yanagisawa, M., and Elmquist, J. K. (2001). Differential expression of orexin receptors 1 and 2 in the rat brain. *J. Comp. Neurol.* **435,** 6–25.

Martin, M., Chen, B. T., Hopf, F. W., Bowers, M. S., and Bonci, A. (2006). Cocaine self-administration selectively abolishes LTD in the core of the nucleus accumbens. *Nat. Neurosci.* **9,** 868–869.

Mileykovskiy, B. Y., Kiyashchenko, L. I., and Siegel, J. M. (2005). Behavioral correlates of activity in identified hypocretin/orexin neurons. *Neuron* **46,** 787–798.

Moorman, D. E., and Aston-Jones, G. (2010). Orexin/hypocretin modulates response of ventral tegmental dopamine neurons to prefrontal activation: Diurnal influences. *J. Neurosci.* **30,** 15585–15599.

Murase, S., Grenhoff, J., Chouvet, G., Gonon, F. G., and Svensson, T. H. (1993). Prefrontal cortex regulates burst firing and transmitter release in rat mesolimbic dopamine neurons studied in vivo. *Neurosci. Lett.* **157,** 53–56.

Muschamp, J. W., Dominguez, J. M., Sato, S. M., Shen, R. Y., and Hull, E. M. (2007). A role for hypocretin (orexin) in male sexual behavior. *J. Neurosci.* **27,** 2837–2845.

Nair, S. G., Golden, S. A., and Shaham, Y. (2008). Differential effects of the hypocretin 1 receptor antagonist SB 334867 on high-fat food self-administration and reinstatement of food seeking in rats. *Br. J. Pharmacol.* **154,** 406–416.

Nakamura, T., Uramura, K., Nambu, T., Yada, T., Goto, K., Yanagisawa, M., and Sakurai, T. (2000). Orexin-induced hyperlocomotion and stereotypy are mediated by the dopaminergic system. *Brain Res.* **873,** 181–187.

Naqvi, N. H., Rudrauf, D., Damasio, H., and Bechara, A. (2007). Damage to the insula disrupts addiction to cigarette smoking. *Science* **315,** 531–534.

Narita, M., Nagumo, Y., Hashimoto, S., Khotib, J., Miyatake, M., Sakurai, T., Yanagisawa, M., Nakamachi, T., Shioda, S., and Suzuki, T. (2006). Direct involvement of orexinergic systems in the activation of the mesolimbic dopamine pathway and related behaviors induced by morphine. *J. Neurosci.* **26,** 398–405.

Narita, M., Nagumo, Y., Miyatake, M., Ikegami, D., Kurahashi, K., and Suzuki, T. (2007). Implication of protein kinase C in the orexin-induced elevation of extracellular dopamine levels and its rewarding effect. *Eur. J. Neurosci.* **25,** 1537–1545.

Nelson, M. E., Kuryatov, A., Choi, C. H., Zhou, Y., and Lindstrom, J. (2003). Alternate stoichiometries of alpha4beta2 nicotinic acetylcholine receptors. *Mol. Pharmacol.* **63,** 332–341.

Nogueira, L., Kalivas, P. W., and Lavin, A. (2006). Long-term neuroadaptations produced by withdrawal from repeated cocaine treatment: Role of dopaminergic receptors in modulating cortical excitability. *J. Neurosci.* **26,** 12308–12313.

Overton, P., and Clark, D. (1992). Iontophoretically administered drugs acting at the N-methyl-D-aspartate receptor modulate burst firing in A9 dopamine neurons in the rat. *Synapse* **10,** 131–140.

Pasumarthi, R. K., and Fadel, J. (2008). Activation of orexin/hypocretin projections to basal forebrain and paraventricular thalamus by acute nicotine. *Brain Res. Bull.* **77,** 367–373.

Pasumarthi, R. K., and Fadel, J. (2010). Stimulation of lateral hypothalamic glutamate and acetylcholine efflux by nicotine: Implications for mechanisms of nicotine-induced activation of orexin neurons. *J. Neurochem.* **113,** 1023–1035.

Pasumarthi, R. K., Reznikov, L. R., and Fadel, J. (2006). Activation of orexin neurons by acute nicotine. *Eur. J. Pharmacol.* **535,** 172–176.

Plaza-Zabala, A., Martín-García, E., de Lecea, L., Maldonado, R., and Berrendero, F. (2010). Hypocretins regulate the anxiogenic-like effects of nicotine and induce reinstatement of nicotine-seeking behavior. *J. Neurosci.* **30,** 2300–2310.

Plaza-Zabala, A., Flores, A., Maldonado, R., and Berrendero, F. (2011). Hypocretin/orexin signaling in the hypothalamic paraventricular nucleus is essential for the expression of nicotine withdrawal. *Biol. Psychiatry* **71,** 214–223.

Polosa, R., and Benowitz, N. L. (2011). Treatment of nicotine addiction: Present therapeutic options and pipeline developments. *Trends Pharmacol. Sci.* **32,** 281–289.

Pons, S., Fattore, L., Cossu, G., Tolu, S., Porcu, E., McIntosh, J. M., Changeux, J. P., Maskos, U., and Fratta, W. (2008). Crucial role of alpha4 and alpha6 nicotinic acetylcholine receptor subunits from ventral tegmental area in systemic nicotine self-administration. *J. Neurosci.* **28,** 12318–12327.

Quarta, D., Valerio, E., Hutcheson, D. M., Hedou, G., and Heidbreder, C. (2009). The orexin-1 receptor antagonist SB-334867 reduces amphetamine-evoked dopamine outflow in the shell of the nucleus accumbens and decreases the expression of amphetamine sensitization. *Neurochem. Int.* **56,** 11–15.

Robinson, T. E., and Berridge, K. C. (1993). The neural basis of drug craving: An incentive-sensitization theory of addiction. *Brain Res. Brain Res. Rev.* **18,** 247–291.

Rodgers, R. J., Halford, J. C., Nunes de Souza, R. L., Canto de Souze, A. L., Piper, D. C., Arch, J. R., Upton, N., Porter, R. A., Johns, A., and Blundell, J. E. (2001). SB-334867, a selective orexin-1 receptor antagonist, enhances behavioural satiety and blocks the hyperphagic effect of orexin-A in rats. *Eur. J. Neurosci.* **13,** 1444–1452.

Roecker, A. J., and Coleman, P. J. (2008). Orexin receptor antagonists: Medicinal chemistry and therapeutic potential. *Curr. Top. Med. Chem.* **8,** 977–987.

Saal, D., Dong, Y., Bonci, A., and Malenka, R. C. (2003). Drugs of abuse and stress trigger a common synaptic adaptation in dopamine neurons. *Neuron* **37,** 577–582.

Saccone, N. L., Culverhouse, R. C., Schwantes-An, T. H., Cannon, D. S., Chen, X., Cichon, S., Giegling, I., Han, S., Han, Y., Keskitalo-Vuokko, K., Kong, X., Landi, M. T., *et al.* (2010). Multiple independent loci at chromosome 15q25.1 affect smoking quantity: A meta-analysis and comparison with lung cancer and COPD. *PLoS Genet.* **6**pii: e1001053.

Scammell, T. E., and Winrow, C. J. (2011). Orexin receptors: Pharmacology and therapeutic opportunities. *Annu. Rev. Pharmacol. Toxicol.* **51,** 243–266.

Schneider, E. R., Rada, P., Darby, R. D., Leibowitz, S. F., and Hoebel, B. G. (2007). Orexigenic peptides and alcohol intake: Differential effects of orexin, galanin, and ghrelin. *Alcohol. Clin. Exp. Res.* **31,** 1858–1865.

Sesack, S. R., and Pickel, V. M. (1992). Prefrontal cortical efferents in the rat synapse on unlabeled neuronal targets of catecholamine terminals in the nucleus accumbens septi and on dopamine neurons in the ventral tegmental area. *J. Comp. Neurol.* **320,** 145–160.

Sesack, S. R., Deutch, A. Y., Roth, R. H., and Bunney, B. S. (1989). Topographical organization of the efferent projections of the medial prefrontal cortex in the rat: An anterograde tract-tracing study with *Phaseolus vulgaris* leucoagglutinin. *J. Comp. Neurol.* **290,** 213–242.

Sharf, R., Guarnieri, D. J., Taylor, J. R., and DiLeone, R. J. (2010). Orexin mediates morphine place preference, but not morphine-induced hyperactivity or sensitization. *Brain Res.* **1317,** 24–32.

Shoblock, J. R., Welty, N., Aluisio, L., Fraser, I., Motley, S. T., Morton, K., Palmer, J., Bonaventure, P., Carruthers, N. I., Lovenberg, T. W., Boggs, J., and Galici, R. (2011). Selective blockade of the orexin-2 receptor attenuates ethanol self-administration, place preference, and reinstatement. *Psychopharmacology (Berl.)* **215,** 191–203.

Smith, R. J., See, R. E., and Aston-Jones, G. (2009). Orexin/hypocretin signaling at the orexin 1 receptor regulates cue-elicited cocaine-seeking. *Eur. J. Neurosci.* **30,** 493–503.

Suaud-Chagny, M. F., Chergui, K., Chouvet, G., and Gonon, F. (1992). Relationship between dopamine release in the rat nucleus accumbens and the discharge activity of dopaminergic neurons during local in vivo application of amino acids in the ventral tegmental area. *Neuroscience* **49,** 63–72.

Thomas, M. J., Beurrier, C., Bonci, A., and Malenka, R. C. (2001). Long-term depression in the nucleus accumbens: A neural correlate of behavioral sensitization to cocaine. *Nat. Neurosci.* **4,** 1217–12123.

Thomas, M. J., Kalivas, P. W., and Shaham, Y. (2008). Neuroplasticity in the mesolimbic dopamine system and cocaine addiction. *Br. J. Pharmacol.* **154,** 327–342.

Tong, Z. Y., Overton, P. G., and Clark, D. (1996). Antagonism of NMDA receptors but not AMPA/kainate receptors blocks bursting in dopaminergic neurons induced by electrical stimulation of the prefrontal cortex. *J. Neural Transm.* **103,** 889–904.

Ungless, M. A., Whistler, J. L., Malenka, R. C., and Bonci, A. (2001). Single cocaine exposure in vivo induces long-term potentiation in dopamine neurons. *Nature* **411,** 583–587.

Uramura, K., Funahashi, H., Muroya, S., Shioda, S., Takigawa, M., and Yada, T. (2001). Orexin-a activates phospholipase C- and protein kinase C-mediated Ca^{2+} signaling in dopamine neurons of the ventral tegmental area. *Neuroreport* **12,** 1885–1889.

Uteshev, V. V., Stevens, D. R., and Haas, H. L. (1996). Alpha-bungarotoxin-sensitive nicotinic responses in rat tuberomammillary neurons. *Pflugers Arch.* **432,** 607–613.

Uteshev, V. V., Meyer, E. M., and Papke, R. L. (2002). Activation and inhibition of native neuronal alpha-bungarotoxin-sensitive nicotinic ACh receptors. *Brain Res.* **948,** 33–46.

Vittoz, N. M., and Berridge, C. W. (2006). Hypocretin/orexin selectively increases dopamine efflux within the prefrontal cortex: Involvement of the ventral tegmental area. *Neuropsychopharmacology* **31,** 384–395.

Vittoz, N. M., Schmeichel, B., and Berridge, C. W. (2008). Hypocretin/orexin preferentially activates caudomedial ventral tegmental area dopamine neurons. *Eur. J. Neurosci.* **28,** 1629–1640.

von der Goltz, C., Koopmann, A., Dinter, C., Richter, A., Rockenbach, C., Grosshans, M., Nakovics, H., Wiedemann, K., Mann, K., Winterer, G., and Kiefer, F. (2010). Orexin and leptin are associated with nicotine craving: A link between smoking, appetite and reward. *Psychoneuroendocrinology* **35,** 570–577.

Voorhees, C. M., and Cunningham, C. L. (2011). Involvement of the orexin/hypocretin system in ethanol conditioned place preference. *Psychopharmacology (Berl.)* **214,** 805–818.

Wada, H., Inagaki, N., Yamatodani, A., and Watanabe, T. (1991). Is the histaminergic neuron system a regulatory center for whole-brain activity? *Trends Neurosci.* **14,** 415–418.

Wang, B., You, Z. B., and Wise, R. A. (2009). Reinstatement of cocaine seeking by hypocretin (orexin) in the ventral tegmental area: Independence from the local corticotropin-releasing factor network. *Biol. Psychiatry* **65,** 857–862.

Wolf, M. E., and Ferrario, C. R. (2010). AMPA receptor plasticity in the nucleus accumbens after repeated exposure to cocaine. *Neurosci. Biobehav. Rev.* **35,** 185–211.

Wolf, M. E., Sun, X., Mangiavacchi, S., and Chao, S. Z. (2004). Psychomotor stimulants and neuronal plasticity. *Neuropharmacology* **47**(Suppl. 1), 61–79.

Wonnacott, S., Sidhpura, N., and Balfour, D. J. (2005). Nicotine: From molecular mechanisms to behaviour. *Curr. Opin. Pharmacol.* **5,** 53–59.

Zhao-Shea, R., Liu, L., Soll, L. G., Improgo, M. R., Meyers, E. E., McIntosh, J. M., Grady, S. R., Marks, M. J., Gardner, P. D., and Tapper, A. R. (2011). Nicotine-mediated activation of dopaminergic neurons in distinct regions of the ventral tegmental area. *Neuropsychopharmacology* **36,** 1021–1032.

CHAPTER SEVENTEEN

Sleep and Orexins in Nonmammalian Vertebrates

Hélène Volkoff*,†

Contents

Abstract

Although a precise definition of "sleep" has yet to be established, sleep-like behaviors have been observed in all animals studied to date including mammals and nonmammalian vertebrates. Orexins are hypothalamic neuropeptides that are involved in the regulation of many physiological functions, including feeding, thermoregulation, cardiovascular control, as well as the control of the sleep–wakefulness cycle.

To date, the knowledge on the functions of orexins in nonmammalian vertebrates is still limited, but the similarity of the structures of orexins and their receptors among vertebrates suggest that they have similar conserved physiological functions. This review describes our current knowledge on sleep in nonmammalian vertebrates (birds, reptiles, amphibians, and fish) and the possible role of orexins in the regulation of their energy homeostasis and arousal states.

* Department of Biology, Memorial University of Newfoundland, St John's, Newfoundland, Canada
† Department of Biochemistry, Memorial University of Newfoundland, St John's, Newfoundland, Canada

Vitamins and Hormones, Volume 89
ISSN 0083-6729, http://dx.doi.org/10.1016/B978-0-12-394623-2.00017-2

I. Introduction

Although a clear definition of sleep has yet to be established, sleep could be described as a behavioral state of rapidly reversible immobility characterized in part by (1) a species-specific sleeping posture and site, (2) an increased response threshold to external stimulation, and (3) a change in the neurophysiology of the brain (Hartse, 2011; Rattenborg and Amlaner, 2002; Roth *et al.*, 2010; Tobler, 1995). Most, if not all, animals examined to date appear to display some kind of sleep-like behavior (Campbell and Tobler, 1984; Cirelli and Tononi, 2008, 2011). Most often, sleep follows 24-h rhythms, with inactivity periods occurring at night (diurnal animals) or during the day (nocturnal animals) (Huang *et al.*, 2011). The actual functions of sleep are still unclear (Cirelli *et al.*, 2004; Rechtschaffen, 1998), but evidence in mammals suggests that sleep is associated with learning, neurogenesis, immune system regulation, and reversal of oxidative stress in mammals (Siegel, 2009). At least in mammals, sleep is essential to survival and has important restorative functions, as long-term sleep-deprivation studies suggest that severe lack of sleep has negative effects on health and might even induce death (Grandner *et al.*, 2010).

In mammals and birds, sleep is characterized by two main states based on electroencephalograph (EEG) patterns: rapid eye movement (REM) sleep and slow-wave sleep (SWS or non-REM sleep) (Lesku *et al.*, 2009b; Rattenborg *et al.*, 2009). During REM sleep, the EEG resembles the low-amplitude, high-frequency pattern that occurs during wakefulness, whereas during SWS, the EEG shows high-amplitude, low-frequency activity. In contrast to wakefulness, however, REM sleep is characterized by decreased responsiveness to the environment and a reduction in electromyogram (EMG, i.e., muscle tone). In fish, reptiles, and amphibians, sleep-like states have been reported in which activity and responsiveness are diminished. However, in these ectothermic animals, sleep is most often defined by behavioral parameters, as studies measuring the brain activity have produced inconsistent results, making it difficult to establish definitive sleep patterns (Hartse, 1994; Lesku *et al.*, 2009b; Rattenborg *et al.*, 2007; Roth *et al.*, 2010). Therefore, the term "rest" is usually used rather than "sleep" (Cirelli and Tononi, 2008).

Sleep/rest and metabolism are closely related both at the physiological and behavioral levels, and the brain plays a major role in their regulation and interactions (Huang *et al.*, 2011; Rolls *et al.*, 2010). In addition to the hormone melatonin secreted by the pineal gland, several neurotransmitters and neuromodulators such as acetylcholine, noradrenaline, dopamine, serotonin (5-HT), and histamine have been shown to be involved in the regulation of sleep/wake cycles (Espana and Scammell, 2011; McCarley, 2007; Richey and Krystal, 2011). There is also increasing evidence that hypothalamic hormones are involved in the maintenance of wakefulness in addition to regulating other hypothalamic functions, such as the regulation of food intake and metabolism. Among these hormones are melanin concentrating hormone (Peyron *et al.*, 2011; Torterolo *et al.*, 2011) and orexins (OXs) (Nishino, 2011).

II. Orexins

OXs A and B (or hypocretin 1 and 2), two hormones derived from a single gene precursor, prepro-OX, were first identified in rats by two distinct groups in 1998 (de Lecea *et al.*, 1998; Sakurai *et al.*, 1998). In mammals, these neuropeptides have been implicated in the regulation of many physiological functions, including feeding, reproduction, cardiovascular function, and thermoregulation, as well as the control of the sleep–wake cycles (Sakurai and Mieda, 2011; Teske *et al.*, 2010). Some of these actions might be due to interactions between the OX and monoamine (noradrenergic, serotonergic, dopaminergic, histaminergic, and cholinergic) systems as anatomical connections between OX and monoamine neurons have been demonstrated in the posterior hypothalamus (Eriksson *et al.*, 2010). Early studies in mammals have shown that central injections of OXs increase feeding behavior (Sakurai *et al.*, 1998). In mammals, OX treatments also induce arousal and locomotor activity and decrease both non-REM and REM sleep (Hagan *et al.*, 1999), and loss of OX neurons or mutations in the OX gene are associated with excessive daytime sleepiness (narcolepsy) (Chemelli *et al.*, 1999; Nishino, 2011). In rats, OX-immunoreactive (ir) fibers and OX receptors are present in the pineal gland, and orexin A treatment partially inhibits NA-mediated melatonin release, suggesting that OXs may regulate sleep by modulating pineal function (Mikkelsen *et al.*, 2001). Similarly, in ewes, OX treatments affect melatonin secretion by pineal explants *in vitro* (Zieba *et al.*, 2011).

The structures of the OX genes and peptides and that of their receptors appear somewhat conserved among vertebrates (Fig. 17.1), suggesting that their physiological functions might also be conserved (Wong *et al.*, 2011). In lower vertebrates, OXs have been cloned in birds [chicken *Gallus gallus* (Ohkubo *et al.*, 2002), turkey *Meleagris gallopavo* (Genbank accession number XM_003213134), and zebra finch *Taeniopygia guttata* (Genbank accession number XM_002197738)], amphibians [*Xenopus laevis* (Shibahara *et al.*, 1999)], and a number of fish species [zebrafish (*Danio rerio*) and pufferfish (*Fugu* sp.) (Alvarez and Sutcliffe, 2002), tilapia *Oreochromis niloticus* (Genbank accession number FJ871159), stickleback *Gasterosteus aculeatus* and medaka *Oryzias latipes* (Yokogawa *et al.*, 2007), orange spotted grouper *Epinephelus coioides* (Yan *et al.*, 2011), goldfish *Carassius auratus* (Hoskins *et al.*, 2008), Lake trout *Salvelinus namaycush* (Volkoff, H., unpublished results), cavefish *Astyanax mexicanus* (Volkoff, H., unpublished results), Atlantic cod *Gadus morhua* (Xu and Volkoff, 2007), winter flounder *Pleuronectes americanus* (Buckley *et al.*, 2011), winter skate *Raja ocellata* (MacDonald and Volkoff, 2010), and Nile tilapia *O. niloticus* (Chen *et al.*, 2011)].

In mammals, OXs act via two G-protein-coupled receptors, the orexin-1 receptor (OXR1), which has a higher affinity for orexin A than orexin B, and the orexin-2 receptor (OXR2), which binds equally to the two peptides (Mieda and Sakurai, 2009; Steward *et al.*, 2003). In mammals, both receptors have been implicated in the regulation of sleep, although they seem to play differential roles through distinct neuronal pathways (Mieda *et al.*, 2011). Within lower vertebrates, cDNAs encoding OX receptors have been cloned in birds [chicken (Ohkubo *et al.*, 2003)], amphibians [*X. laevis* (Tam *et al.*, 2011)], and fish [zebrafish, pufferfish, medaka,

A

```
Rat          -QPLP-DCC-RQKTCSCRLYELL--H---G-------------AG-NHAAGILTL 33
Chicken      -QSLP-ECC-RQKTCSCRIYDLL--H---G-------------MG-NHAAGILTL 33
Turkey       -QSLP-ECC-RQKTCSCRIYDLL--H---G-------------MG-NHAAGILTL 33
Finch        -HSLP-HCC-RQKTCPCRVYDLL--H---G-------------MG-NHAAGILTL 33
Xenopus      SHGAP-DCC-REKTCSCRIYDIL--R---G-------------TG-NHAAGILTL 34
Danio        -EGVA-SCCARAP-GSCKLYEML-CR--AGRRNDSSVARHLVHLNNDAAVGILTL 49
Goldfish     -EGVA-TCCSSAS-RSCKLYEIL-CR--AGRRNDTSIARHIGRFNNDAAVGILTL 49
Astyanax     -EGVS-ACCVRRP-RACGLYGVR-CN--S---TDSKPVR----VSSGAAVGILTL 42
Trout        -QGVA-NCC-RQKSHSCRLYVLL-CR--SGDGTGTRGPL----TD-DAAAGILTL 44
Medaka       -HSVA-ECC-RKPSRSCPLYALF-CG--SGN-KSFGGAR----AG-DAAAGILTL 43
Stickleback  -HSLS-QCC-RQPARSCRLAVIL-CR--SGS-KNFGGE-----PG-DDAAGILTL 42
Puffer       -HSMS-ECC-RQPSRSCRLYVLL-CR--SGS-KPLGRPL----TG-DAAAGILTL 43
Tilapia      -HSVS-ECC-REPSRPCRLYVLL-CR--SGN-KGPGGVL----TD-DAAAGILTL 43
Grouper      -HSVS-ECC-RQPPRNCRLHVLL-CR--SGS-KNLGGTL----TG-DAAAGILTL 43
Flounder     -HSMS-DCC-RQPSRSCRLYALL-CR--TGS-KTMGGTL----SG-DAAAGILTL 43
Cod          -HSVSASCCSREPPRACRLYVLLLCGPVGGAGRALGGMH----LGEDASAGILTL 50
Skate        SPRVP-KCC-CQQTCSCKVIDLL--R---G-------------TG-NHAAGILTL 34
                  .  **       * :  :                  . . :.*****
```

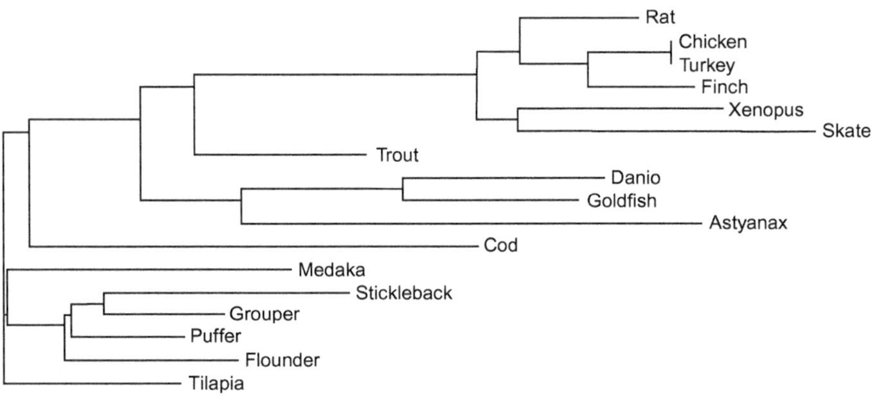

Figure 17.1

B

```
Rat               RPGPPGLQGRLQRLLQA-NGNHAAGILTM 28
Chicken           KSIPPAFQSRLYRLLHG-SGNHAAGILTI 28
Turkey            KSVPPAFQSRLYRLLHG-SGNHAAGILTM 28
Finch             KSVPLTFQSRLYRLLHG-SGNHAAGILTM 28
Xenopus           RSDFQTMQSRLQRLLQG-SGNHAAGILTM 28
Danio             KVGESRVHDRLQQLLHN-SRNQAAGILTM 28
Goldfish          KVGERRVQDRLQQLLHG-SRNQAAGILTV 28
Astyanax          RTAGNRYQDRLQHLLHG-TRNQAAGILTM 28
Trout             ETDERRFQSRLNQLLHG-SRNQAAGILTM 28
Medaka            NEEEHRLESRLQQLLHS-SRNQAAGILTM 28
Stickleback       NEEEHNLQSRLNQLLQG-SRSQAAGILTM 28
Tilapia           KEDEYRFQSRLQQLLQG-SRNQAAGILTM 28
Puffer            VEDEERFQSRLHQLLHG-SRNQAAGILTM 28
Grouper           REDD-RLQSRLHQLLQG-SRNQAAGILTM 27
Flounder          KEEEHRLHSRLHHLLHV-SRNQAAGILTM 28
Cod               EAEEQHFHSRLHQLLRGGARNQAAGILTM 29
Skate             KTNAQPLQNRLHHLLHG-LENQATGILTM 28
                         ..** :**:    .:*:****:
```

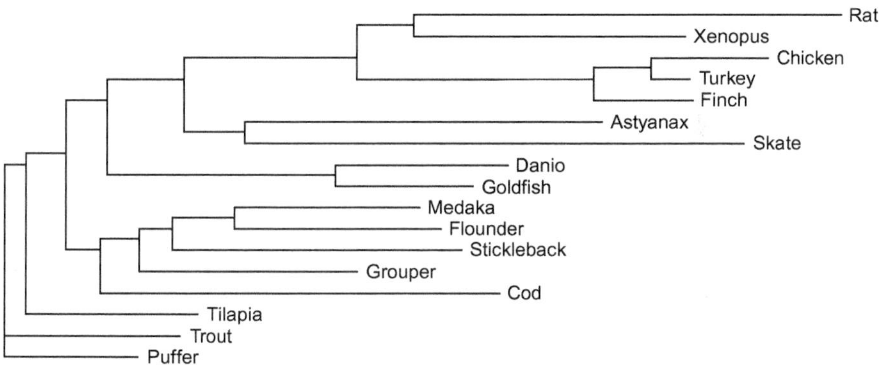

Figure 17.1—cont'd Protein sequence alignments and phylogenetic trees for orexin A (A) and orexin B (B) in lower vertebrates. Multiple alignments of amino acid sequences and N–J trees were performed using ClustalW software (http://align.genome.jp). Refer to text for references and Genbank accession numbers. Symbols on the bottom row of the alignment indicate the degree of sequence similarity between sequences: "*": identical; ":": strong similarity; ".": weak similarity.

stickleback (Panula, 2010; Yokogawa *et al.*, 2007), goldfish (Abbott and Volkoff, 2011), and ornate wrasse *Thalassoma pavo* (Facciolo *et al.*, 2009)]. Unlike mammals, birds and fish appear to have only one OX receptor gene. Birds and most fish appear to have type 2-like receptors, although a type 1-like receptor has been reported in ornate wrasse (Facciolo *et al.*, 2009).

III. Sleep and OXs in Birds

Behavioral sleep has been observed in a number of bird species. Most terrestrial birds sleep sitting or standing with their head drawn in toward the body or resting on the back or wing (Rattenborg and Amlaner, 2002). Some aquatic birds, such as the lesser black-backed Gull *Larus fuscus*, sit on the sea surface drifting passively with the current, resting at sea rather than on land (Shamoun-Baranes *et al.*, 2011). During sleep, the eyes are usually closed. Birds have developed mechanisms to reduce their vulnerability to predation while sleeping: some species [e.g., blackbird *Turdus merula* (Szymczak *et al.*, 1996), mallard *Anas platyrhynchos* (Javůrková *et al.*, 2011), and chicken (Bobbo *et al.*, 2006)] use "vigilant sleep," a state in which sleep is interrupted by short periods where one or both eyes are open as a result of unihemispheric slow-wave sleep (USWS). The latter is a unique state during which one cerebral hemisphere sleeps while the other remains awake, allowing birds to monitor their environment while they sleep (Lima *et al.*, 2005; Rattenborg *et al.*, 2000). In species that live in groups, such as the loafing gulls (*Larus* spp.) (Beauchamp, 2011) or southern lapwing (*Vanellus chilensis*) (Maruyama *et al.*, 2010), birds sleep in "waves," that is, not all individuals sleep at the same time thus allowing vigilant individuals to detect potential threats.

Birds show dramatic changes in sleep duration across seasons, related to day length and migratory status and seem to sleep considerably less during the migratory season (Jones *et al.*, 2010). In captive white-crowned sparrows (*Zonotrichia leucophrys gambelii*), migratory sparrows spend 60% less time sleeping than nonmigratory birds (Rattenborg *et al.*, 2004). Avian sleep is also influenced by environmental temperature and lighting (Dewasmes *et al.*, 2001; Szymczak, 1989) and by geographical latitude (Amlaner and Ball, 1983). In particular, it has been suggested that 5-HT and its receptors play an important role in wakefulness during light periods, as activation of 5-HT_{1A} receptors increases activity and reduces sleep in ring dove, *Columba palumbus* (Tejada *et al.*, 2011).

Although some birds can spend long periods of time in constant flight, there is no true evidence that they sleep during flight (Lesku *et al.*, 2009b). Two studies on pigeons (*Columba livia*) suggest that this species is capable of surviving prolonged sleep deprivation, as animals sleep deprived for several days show no or low increases in sleep time and do not exhibit the typical mammalian symptoms of sleep deprivation such as hyperphagia, weight loss, and debilitation (Berger and Phillips, 1994; Newman *et al.*, 2008, 2009). However, despite being more resistant than mammals to the effects of sleep loss, pigeons nevertheless do show recovery sleep patterns similar to those seen in mammals (Newman *et al.*, 2008, 2009).

As in mammals, sleep in birds is composed of REM sleep (low-amplitude brain activity similar to wakefulness) and non-REM sleep (or SWS, with high-amplitude, low-frequency waves) (Jones *et al.*, 2008; Lesku *et al.*, 2009a; Rattenborg *et al.*, 2004). The SWS is characterized by a decrease in EMG (reduced motor tone as seen in dropping of the head), as well as in respiratory and heart rates, brain temperatures, and metabolic rates (Rattenborg, 2006). However, it is unclear whether the similarities in sleep patterns between mammals and birds necessarily reflect similarities in function (Lesku *et al.*, 2011; Roth *et al.*, 2006).

The brain distribution of OXs in birds is widespread and appears to be conserved among species, suggesting that these peptides play similar roles among birds, and that they might be involved in the regulation of several behavioral and physiological functions (Singletary *et al.*, 2006). In chicken (Ohkubo *et al.*, 2002), house finch, *Carpodacus mexicanus* (Singletary *et al.*, 2006) and Japanese quail, *Coturnix japonica* (Phillips-Singh *et al.*, 2003), OX-ir neurons are located in the paraventricular nucleus of the hypothalamus and the lateral hypothalamic area, whereas OX-ir fibers are seen throughout the brain, with the highest density within the preoptic area, hypothalamus, and thalamus. In chicken, OXR mRNA is widely distributed throughout the brain and is present in peripheral tissues such as adrenal gland and testis (Ohkubo *et al.*, 2003).

It appears that, in birds, OXs may be primarily involved in the control of physiological functions other than energy homeostasis. In both chicken (Ohkubo *et al.*, 2002) and Japanese quail (Phillips-Singh *et al.*, 2003), a 24-h fast does not induce changes in prepro-OX brain expression. Central injections of OXs do not affect food intake in chicks (Furuse *et al.*, 1999; Ohkubo *et al.*, 2002) or feeding and drinking behaviors in pigeons (da Silva *et al.*, 2008). Interestingly, continuous infusion of recombinant chicken leptin results in a significant reduction in food intake in 3-week-old broiler chickens and decreases OX brain expression (Dridi *et al.*, 2005), and central administration of beta-melanocyte-stimulating-hormone in chicks significantly suppresses food intake (Berger and Phillips, 1994) and increases OX mRNA levels and plasma glucose concentrations (Kamisoyama *et al.*, 2009), suggesting that the OX system might play a role in mediating the effects of other appetite-related hormones.

OXs appear to play a role in the regulation of arousal in birds, although inconsistencies have been reported. Intracerebroventricular treatment with orexin A increases arousal and metabolic turnover in neonatal layer chicks but not in broiler chicks, whereas orexin B does not affect arousal in either layer or broiler chicks (Katayama *et al.*, 2010a). In chicks, the orexin A-induced arousal appears to occur via the stimulation of monoaminergic pathways by monoamine oxidase-A (Katayama *et al.*, 2011) but does not involve the hypothalamic–pituitary–adrenal axis (Katayama *et al.*, 2010b). In pigeons, orexin A, but not orexin B, treatments induce a dose-related increase in exploratory behaviors and a reduction in time spent in immobility and sleep-like postures, suggesting a role of OX in vigilance control in that species (da Silva *et al.*, 2008).

IV. Sleep and OXs in Reptiles

Behavioral signs of sleep have been observed in reptiles, including chelonia (turtles), crocodilia (alligators and crocodiles), and squamata (lizards and snakes). "Sleeping" reptiles display periods of immobility, eyelid closure, maximum relaxation of body musculature (usually with their legs drawn up along their bodies), lowered respiratory and cardiac activities, and low behavioral responsiveness to stimulation (elevated arousal thresholds) (Ayala-Guerrero and Mexicano, 2008; Rattenborg and Amlaner, 2002). Some reptiles, such as the Desert Iguanas (*Dipsosaurus dorsalis*), exhibit behavioral sleep plasticity in response to predation risk as they will not sleep and remain vigilant when a predator (a rattle snake) is in close proximity (Revell and Hayes, 2009). Similar to birds, unilateral eye closure has been observed in reptiles, but, to date, there is no true evidence of reptilian USWS (Rattenborg *et al.*, 2000).

Although the relationship between behavioral sleep and electrophysiological parameters is still not clear in reptiles, changes in EEG have been reported during behavioral sleep/inactivity in several species. For example, in caimans, *Caiman sclerops*, behavioral sleep, as seen by decreased respiratory rates and EMG activity and elevated arousal thresholds, is accompanied by high-voltage, slow EEG (Meglasson and Huggins, 1979). In turtles (*Pseudemys* sp.) and geckos (*Gekko* sp.), large sharp waves similar to mammalian hippocampal sharp waves—patterns of irregular slow waves in hippocampal EEG that occur during sleep or resting states—are correlated to decreased arousal (Gaztelu *et al.*, 1991). In the tortoise *Testudo denticulata*, EEG spiking is seen during behaviorally inactive periods but not upon arousal (Walker and Berger, 1973), and in the lizard *Ctenosaura pectinata*, sleep, in contrast with wakefulness, is characterized by a decrease of electrical activity in the forebrain and midbrain (Tauber *et al.*, 1968). The cerebral activity of reptiles during sleep, thus, differs from that of mammals and birds, possibly due to a less developed brain (Ayala-Guerrero and Mexicano, 2008; Lesku *et al.*, 2009a). It has recently been suggested that, behaviorally, reptiles might present two sleep phases, quiet sleep (similar to SWS, but without the EEG slow-wave activity observed in mammals and birds) and active sleep (similar to REM). In addition, in ectothermic reptiles, sleep and the amplitude of EEGs are greatly affected by ambient temperature, with warmer temperatures increasing both activity levels and EEG amplitudes (Rial *et al.*, 2010).

Although the sequences for OXs have not yet been established in reptiles, a few studies have examined the distribution of OXs within the reptilian brain using microscopy techniques. In the green anole lizard *Anolis carolinensis* (Farrell *et al.*, 2003), the lizard *Gekko gecko*, and the turtle *Pseudemys scripta elegans* (Dominguez *et al.*, 2010), most OX-ir neurons are found in the periventricular and the infundibular hypothalamus, whereas OX-ir fibers have a widespread distribution and are found in several brain regions including forebrain and hindbrain. In *Gecko* and *Pseudemis*, orexinergic innervation is seen in dopaminergic, noradrenergic, and serotonergic cell groups, such as the substantia nigra and ventral tegmental area in the midbrain tegmentum, the locus coeruleus, the nucleus of the solitary tract, and the raphe nuclei (Dominguez *et al.*, 2010), all regions of the brain that have been shown to regulate sleep/wake cycles in mammals (Monti and Jantos, 2008). Despite the lack of direct evidence for a role physiological of OXs in reptiles, the presence and distribution of OX fibers within the reptilian brain might suggest a role for these peptides in energy homeostasis and arousal in this vertebrate group.

V. Sleep and OXs in Amphibians

Early observations report that amphibians display sleep-like behavior. Following several experiments on frogs in 1909, W. J. Sibis wrote "I could not help coming to the conclusion that there are such states as sleep in frogs and that those states can be induced under conditions very similar to those we had found in human beings. Still I greatly hesitated to term the states induced in frogs 'sleep;' I termed them 'rest states'" (Sidis, 1909). In most frogs and toads studied to date, periods of elevated arousal thresholds have been observed, with animals sitting motionless with their eyelids closed (Rattenborg and Amlaner, 2002). However, an early study on American bullfrogs (*Rana catesbeiana*) reports a lack of apparent sign of behavioral sleep in this species, as noxious cutaneous stimuli induce change in respiratory responses, even during the resting phase (Hobson, 1967a). Another study reports no obvious behavioral sleep in blind cave salamanders *Proteus anguinus* (Roth and Schlegel, 1988). Sleep-like states in amphibians appear to be associated with decreases in both EEG activity and respiratory rates, as seen in bullfrog (Hobson, 1967b) and ranid frogs (*Hyla* sp.) (Hobson *et al.*, 1968). There is no true evidence of unilateral eye closure in amphibians, and although this phenomena has been reported in bullfrog, it was not associated with behavioral sleep (Hobson, 1967a).

In amphibian brain, most OX-ir neurons seem to be located in the diencephalic nuclei, in particular the preoptic area/hypothalamus, whereas OX-ir fibers are abundant throughout the brain and spinal cord (Lopez *et al.*, 2009a), suggesting that, in amphibians, OXs act as neuropeptides and/or neuromodulators. This distribution pattern has been shown in anurans [*Rana ridibunda* (Galas *et al.*, 2001), *Hyla cinerea* (Singletary *et al.*, 2005), *Rana perezi*, *X. laevis*, *Bufo calamita*, and *Bombina orientalis* (Lopez *et al.*, 2009a)], urodeles [ribbed newt *Pleurodeles waltl*, tiger salamander *Ambystoma tigrinum* (Lopez *et al.*, 2009a), and axolotl *Ambystoma mexicanum* (Suzuki *et al.*, 2008)], and gymnophionans [Mexican burrowing caecilian, *Dermophis mexicanus* (Lopez *et al.*, 2009a)], although species-specific differences in localization exist.

Similar to mammals, orexinergic innervation is present in monoaminergic cell bodies in the amphibian midbrain, including in catecholaminergic (Lopez *et al.*, 2009a) and serotonergic (Suzuki *et al.*, 2008) cells, suggesting that the OX system might regulate arousal in amphibians as these compounds have been involved in the regulation of sleep/wake cycle in vertebrates including mammals (Richey and Krystal, 2011) and amphibians (Kulikov *et al.*, 1994).

Although several studies have failed to detect OX-ir in the amphibian pituitary (Galas *et al.*, 2001; Lopez *et al.*, 2009a; Singletary *et al.*, 2005), OX-ir cells have been reported in Xenopus and bullfrog (*R. catesbeiana*) pituitary glands, where they colocalize with thyroid-stimulating hormone (TSH)- and prolactin (PRL)-containing cells. These results suggest that some hypophyseal cells might store and secrete both an orexin-A-like substance and PRL or TSH (Suzuki *et al.*, 2007b; Yamamoto *et al.*, 2004). In mammals, interactions between the OX system and both the hypothalamic–pituitary–thyroid and the lactotroph axes have been demonstrated (Lopez *et al.*, 2010). As OXs and these axes are closely associated with sleep and arousal, these hormones might interact to regulate sleep–wake cycles. The presence of similar interactions in amphibians suggests that OXs might be linked to TSH and PRL to regulate arousal in this vertebrate group. It is also noteworthy that both the hypothalamic–pituitary–thyroid and the lactotroph axes play an important role in amphibian metamorphosis (Tata, 2006), suggesting that OXs might also be a mediator of metamorphic events in amphibians.

Volatile (such as isoflurane and halothane; Smith and Stump, 2000) and intravenous anesthetics (i.e., pentobarbital; Cakir and Strauch, 2005) have an anesthetizing effect in amphibians, and their hypnotic effects are mediated by the inhibition of chloride currents (Minami *et al.*, 2007; Takizuka *et al.*, 2007). In Xenopus oocytes expressing OX1Rs, orexin A treatment induces chloride currents (Minami *et al.*, 2007; Takizuka *et al.*, 2007), and these anesthetics act via the inhibition of OX1R function (Minami *et al.*, 2007), which indirectly suggests that OXs might have a stimulatory role in arousal in amphibians.

VI. Sleep and OXs in Fish

Most fish studied to date show behavioral signs of sleep such as lying motionless on the bottom or burying under the sand, as well as "physiological quietness," including reduced cardiovascular and respiratory rates (Rattenborg and Amlaner, 2002; Zhdanova, 2009). For example, diurnal fish such as *Mozambique tilapia, Tilapia mossambica* (Shapiro and Hepburn, 1976), cunner *Tautogolabrus adspersus* (Dew, 1976), convict cichlid (*Cichlasoma nigrofasciatum*) and goldfish (Tobler and Borbely, 1985), Princess Parrotfish (*Scarus taeniopterus*) (Dubin and Baker, 1982), some crevice-dwelling coral fishes [e.g., *Dascyllus* sp. (Goldshmid *et al.*, 2004), and cleaner wrasse *Labroides dimidiatus* (Lenke, 1988)] display rest-activity rhythms: they display periods of activity with high respiratory rates during the day- and nighttime "resting" states in which the fish are quiet and display no eye movement and higher stimulus–response thresholds (Shapiro and Hepburn, 1976). Similarly, in zebrafish (Norton and Bally-Cuif, 2010; Prober *et al.*, 2006; Zhdanova, 2011) and cave fish *A. mexicanus* (Duboue *et al.*, 2011), periods of inactivity in which the fish float, making small pectoral fin movements and reduced mouth and operculum movements have been observed. Some fish that spend the night in corals exhibit a unique behavior, termed "sleep swimming," in which energetic, high-frequency fin motions occur—possibly to avoid hypoxia—while the fish hold a fixed position (Goldshmid *et al.*, 2004). Some fish such as parrotfishes (Dubin and Baker, 1982; Grutter *et al.*, 2011) and wrasses (*Labroides* sp.) (Lenke, 1991) sleep in mucous cocoons possibly to protect themselves from predation and parasites. Some Mediterranean blennies leave the water and have excursions on the land at night to "sleep" (Gibson, 1993; Louisy, 1987). In electric fish, several studies show that the electric discharge frequency is lower in resting fish than in active fish (Kramer, 1990), although similar frequencies during sleeping and active fish have been reported in the electric fish *Gymnotus carapo*, perhaps as a mean to detect predators during sleep (Stopa and Hoshino, 1999).

It is noteworthy that fish do not have eyelids and consequently sleep with their eyes open. Although a few fish may have a thin membrane capable of covering the eyeball partially or totally ["adipose eyelid" in teleost fish such as clupeiformes (sardines), salmonids, and gonorynchiformes (milk fish *Chanos chanos*) or a nictitating membrane in some shark species (Chang *et al.*, 2009; Harman, 1899; Nelson, 2006)], these structures appear to have strictly a protective function against physical and UV light damages and are not directly correlated to "resting" behavior (Chang *et al.*, 2009). Although true eye closure and thus unilateral eye closure is not present in fish, unihemispherical sleep could theoretically be present in fish but has never been reported (Rattenborg *et al.*, 2000).

Fish that are thought to swim continuously, such as some sharks or tuna, may survive prolonged periods of sleep deprivation or sleep while swimming (Esteban *et al.*, 2005). Although there is no direct evidence for such a behavior, studies in the spiny dogfish shark (*Squalus acanthias*) show that swimming movements are coordinated through a "central pattern generator" in the spinal cord, and that they exhibit spontaneous locomotion even after a spinal transection (Grillner *et al.*, 1977), suggesting that these animals could swim even while unconscious/asleep. Continuous swimming without rest is seen in migrating fish. For example, wrasse submitted to environmental conditions mimicking time of migration will switch from a diurnal rhythm to continuous activity patterns (Olla and Studholme, 1978).

It seems that light is a powerful arousing stimulus that affects sleep–wake cycles in fish. Continuous light exposure has been shown to drastically reduce sleep in both zebrafish (Prober *et al.*, 2006; Yokogawa *et al.*, 2007;

Zhdanova *et al.*, 2001) and *M. tilapia* (Shapiro and Hepburn, 1976), and larval zebrafish "turn off" their visual system at night when they are not active (Emran *et al.*, 2010). Interestingly, in contrast to surface eyed fish, blind—eyeless—cave fish display reduced sleep and do not appear to consolidate sleep during either daytime or nighttime (Duboue *et al.*, 2011; Parzefall, 1993).

In fish, there is no clear evidence of a correlation between brain activity and "sleep." However, it has been reported that, in cod and goldfish, electrical brain patterns in the midbrain show a dominant rhythm of 8–13 Hz—which resembles the alpha rhythm of mammals—in fish resting in the dark, but a dominant rhythm of 18–32 Hz in fish aroused by light (Marshall, 1972).

Among molecules that regulate arousal states in fish are melatonin, serotonin, and OXs. Melatonin, produced by the pineal gland, decreases locomotor activity in goldfish (Azpeleta *et al.*, 2010) and promotes sleep-like states in zebrafish (Maximino and Herculano, 2010; Zhdanova *et al.*, 2001). Injections of serotonin, serotonin reuptake inhibitors, or serotonin agonists have tranquilizing effects in zebrafish (Bencan *et al.*, 2009), goldfish (Satake, 1979), and cleaner wrasse (Lenke, 1988); decrease aggressive behavior in several species [e.g., Gulf toadfish, *Opsanus beta* (McDonald *et al.*, 2011), and fighting fish, *Betta splendens* (Clotfelter *et al.*, 2010)]; and decrease the time spent searching for a sleeping place (or sleep-appetitive behavior) in the cleaner wrasse (Lenke, 1988), suggesting that as in mammals (Monti and Jantos, 2008) this monoamine neurotransmitter regulates arousal states in fish.

The OX system has been studied in a variety of fish. Whereas in tetrapods, most of the OX-producing cells are localized in the hypothalamus, it appears that, in fish, they have wider distributions within the brain. OX cells have been detected not only in the hypothalamus but also in the preoptic area of zebrafish (Appelbaum *et al.*, 2009; Faraco *et al.*, 2006; Kaslin *et al.*, 2004), goldfish (Huesa *et al.*, 2005; Kojima *et al.*, 2009), medaka (Amiya *et al.*, 2007), and lungfish (Lopez *et al.*, 2009b) and in the telencephalon of lungfish (Lopez *et al.*, 2009b). Similarly, OX mRNA has been detected not only in hypothalamus but also in a number of extra hypothalamic areas in goldfish (Abbott and Volkoff, 2011; Hoskins *et al.*, 2008), Atlantic cod (Xu and Volkoff, 2007), Nile tilapia (Chen *et al.*, 2011), winter flounder (Buckley *et al.*, 2011), and winter skate (MacDonald and Volkoff, 2010). OX-ir cells or mRNA have also been shown in the pituitaries of Atlantic cod (Xu and Volkoff, 2007), medaka (Amiya *et al.*, 2007), Japanese seaperch (Suzuki *et al.*, 2007a), Nile tilapia (Suzuki *et al.*, 2009), goldfish (Abbott and Volkoff, 2011), winter flounder (Buckley *et al.*, 2011), and winter skate (MacDonald and Volkoff, 2010). OX receptors have a widespread distribution in fish brains and are present in most brain regions including telencephalon, hypothalamus, and hindbrain in zebrafish (Yokogawa *et al.*, 2007), goldfish (Abbott and Volkoff, 2011), and ornate wrasse (Facciolo *et al.*, 2009) as well as in the pituitary of goldfish (Abbott and Volkoff, 2011).

OXs regulate feeding in fish as OX treatments have been shown to stimulate food intake in several fish species including goldfish (Nakamachi *et al.*, 2006; Volkoff *et al.*, 1999), ornate wrasse (Facciolo *et al.*, 2009), and zebrafish (Yokobori *et al.*, 2011). Central injections with a selective mammalian OX receptor-1 antagonist at high doses inhibit basal feeding in goldfish (Miura *et al.*, 2007) and orexin A-induced feeding in zebrafish (Yokobori *et al.*, 2011). In addition, brain prepro-OX mRNA is upregulated following food restriction in goldfish (Abbott and Volkoff, 2011), zebrafish (Novak *et al.*, 2005; Yokobori *et al.*, 2011), Nile tilapia (Chen *et al.*, 2011), winter flounder (Buckley *et al.*, 2011), cod (Xu and Volkoff, 2007), and winter skate (MacDonald and Volkoff, 2010). OXs have also been shown to be involved in the regulation of sexual behavior in fish as central injections of orexin A in female goldfish inhibit spawning (Hoskins *et al.*, 2008).

OXs also regulate sleep/wake states, arousal and locomotor behavior in fish. In goldfish (Nakamachi *et al.*, 2006; Volkoff *et al.*, 1999) and ornate wrasse (Facciolo *et al.*, 2009), OX treatments induce increases in locomotor activity and reward-seeking/foraging behavior. In addition, periods of increased locomotor activity are associated with increased activity of hypothalamic OX neurons in zebrafish (Naumann *et al.*, 2010) and in both Atlantic cod and goldfish, brain OX mRNA expression levels are higher during the day, when fish are active, than during the night (Hoskins and Volkoff, H., unpublished data). Zebrafish lacking the OX receptor (Appelbaum *et al.*, 2009; Panula, 2010; Yokogawa *et al.*, 2007) show short and fragmented sleep, and OX-overexpressing zebrafish larvae (Prober *et al.*, 2006) display abnormal sleeping patterns. In addition, in zebrafish, the number of synapses in OX axons follows a circadian rhythm which appears to be controlled by the circadian clock and to be affected by sleep deprivation (Appelbaum *et al.*, 2010). Interestingly, in winter flounder, brain prepro-OX mRNA expression levels are higher in the winter—when animals are in a torpor-like state of inactivity and fasting—than in the summer (Buckley *et al.*, 2011), reiterating the fact that OXs may have multiple physiological functions in fish.

The arousal-stimulating effects of OXs appear to be the result of interactions between OXs and a number of neuromodulators that have been implicated in the regulation of sleep in vertebrates. In zebrafish, similar to mammals, OX neurons express vesicular glutamate transporters (Appelbaum *et al.*, 2009) and are connected to monoaminergic and cholinergic nuclei (Kaslin *et al.*, 2004), and OX receptors are present in gamma-aminobutyric acid (GABA)-ergic neurons of the anterior hypothalamus (Yokogawa *et al.*, 2007). The release of melatonin, a major sleep-inducing hormone in zebrafish, is induced in cultured zebrafish pineal glands perifused with OXs, and mRNA levels of arylalkylamine-*N*-acetyltransferase, a key enzyme of melatonin synthesis, are reduced in the pineal gland of fish lacking OXs during the night, suggesting an interaction between OXs and melatonin in zebrafish (Appelbaum *et al.*, 2009). In goldfish, injections of thyrotropin releasing hormone (TRH) increase locomotor activity as well as the hypothalamic mRNA expression levels of both OX and OX receptor, suggesting that the TRH-induced increase in arousal is mediated by the OX system (Abbott and Volkoff, 2011). In Nile tilapia (*O. niloticus*), whereas no orexin A-ir cells are seen in the pituitary, orexin B-ir cells correspond to luteinizing hormone (LH)- or TSH-containing cells, suggesting that an orexin B-like substance may be secreted from LH- or TSH-containing cells and may regulate pituitary functions (Suzuki *et al.*, 2009). Similarly, in the Japanese seaperch (*Lateolabrax japonicus*) pituitary, an orexin A-like substance and growth hormone coexist in secretory granules in certain hypophyseal cells (Suzuki *et al.*, 2007a).

VII. Conclusions and Future Directions

In comparison to mammals, sleep in lower vertebrates has received little attention. Whereas the criteria for sleep seem relatively well defined in mammals, this is not the case for either birds or ectothermic animals. Although sleep and analogous states seem to be present in all vertebrate groups (Table 17.1), the distinction between true sleep and arousal/vigilance/locomotor activity is sometimes difficult to establish. Whereas sleep in mammals and to some extent in birds is defined by electrophysiological parameters, there is no convincing evidence that such rhythms exist in ectothermic vertebrates. In these animals, the presence of sleep-like behavior is usually associated with a decrease in spontaneous locomotor activity, which might not be an accurate assessment. Indeed, activity levels in ectothermic animals can be highly dependent on environmental parameters such as food availability, environmental conditions (temperature and photoperiod), as well as the presence of predators (Reebs, 2002). For example, during periods of unfavorable conditions of low food availability, several species of fish, amphibians, reptiles, and even birds enter a "sleep-like" state of torpor characterized by inactivity and fasting—estivation is used to survive hot and dry periods (Secor and Lignot, 2010), whereas winter torpor or dormancy is used to survive cold temperature (Campbell *et al.*, 2008; Crawshaw, 1984; Lutterschmidt and Mason, 2009; Rial *et al.*, 2010)—which probably does not correspond to true sleep. In order to better define "sleep" in lower vertebrates, it would be necessary to assess arousal thresholds, circadian cycles, and the effects of the environment as well as brain electrophysiology. Levels of activity might also depend on reproductive stage (e.g., spawning fish and fish guarding their eggs seem to

Table 17.1 Evidence for sleep and its regulation by orexins in lower vertebrates

	Evidence of sleep/rest	Orexin mRNA cloned	Evidence for a role of orexin in the regulation of sleep/rest	Major references
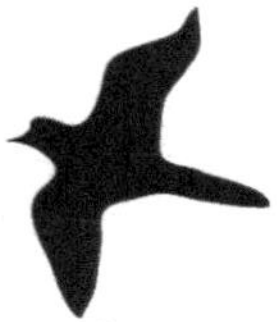 Birds	Evidence of behavioral sleep Evidence of REM sleep and non-REM sleep	Yes (chicken)	Direct evidence Orexins induce arousal in chicks and pigeons Orexins stimulate monoaminergic (norepinephrine, dopamine, and serotonin) pathways	da Silva *et al*. (2008), Katayama *et al*. (2010a,b, 2011)
 Reptiles	Changes in EEG during behavioral sleep/ inactivity	No	No direct evidence Orexin-ir neurons are present in hypothalamus and in regions of the brain that regulate sleep/wake cycles Orexinergic innervation is seen in dopaminergic, noradrenergic, and serotonergic cells	Dominguez *et al*. (2010), Farrell *et al*. (2003)
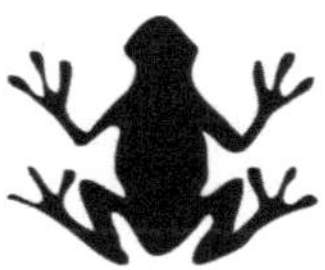 Amphibians	Changes in EEG during behavioral sleep/ inactivity	Yes (Xenopus)	No direct evidence Orexin-ir neurons are located in the diencephalic nuclei, in particular the preoptic area/hypothalamus Orexinergic innervation is present in monoaminergic cell bodies in the midbrain Anesthetics act via the inhibition of OX1R function	Galas *et al*. (2001), Lopez *et al*. (2009a), Minami *et al*. (2007), Singletary *et al*. (2005), Suzuki *et al*. (2008)

(*Continued*)

Table 17.1 *(Continued)*

	Evidence of sleep/rest	Orexin mRNA cloned	Evidence for a role of orexin in the regulation of sleep/rest	Major references
 Fish	Behavioral sleep/ inactivity (lying motionless, reduced respiratory rates) No EEG data	Yes (several species)	Direct evidence Orexin treatments induce increases in locomotor activity Increased locomotor activity is associated with increased activity of hypothalamic orexin neurons Orexin receptor knockouts or overexpression of orexin induces abnormal sleep patterns Wide distributions of orexin neurons within the brain Orexin neurons interact with monoaminergic systems	Facciolo *et al.* (2009), Nakamachi *et al.* (2006), Volkoff *et al.* (1999)

have higher activity levels) and ontogeny (e.g., juvenile and adult fish have different activity phases) (Reebs, 2002). To complicate things, sleep and sleep-like states are highly variable across species.

The question of the function of sleep is also still unclear. If in lower vertebrates, the inactivity periods associated with sleep seem to save energy and also reduce the risk of injury and predation (Siegel, 2009), there is no evidence that they might be needed for purposes such as growth, learning, or memory.

The molecules regulating sleep/wake cycle are also still under scrutiny. Although melatonin and monoamines appear to be major regulators of sleep, recent studies have unveiled the roles of other peptides including OXs. OXs or OX-like molecules have been detected in all vertebrate groups examined to date (Table 17.1). The neuroanatomical distribution of OX neurons appears to be relatively well conserved, although species-specific differences exist, which might indicate that the role of OXs is somewhat conserved among vertebrates. Studies using hormone injections, genetic (OX knockouts) or physiological (e.g., fasting, sleep deprivation) manipulations, and neuroanatomy have shown that in mammals, birds, and fish, OXs show stimulatory effects on feeding and appear to regulate sleep/wake cycles. Although hormone administration experiments have not yet been performed on reptiles or amphibians, the brain distribution of orexinergic neurons and their interactions with monoamine pathways suggest similar role for OXs in the regulation of feeding behavior and arousal in these groups.

ACKNOWLEDGMENT

H. V.'s research is supported by Grants from the Natural Sciences and Engineering Research Council of Canada (NSERC).

REFERENCES

Abbott, M., and Volkoff, H. (2011). Thyrotropin releasing hormone (TRH) in goldfish (*Carassius auratus*): Role in the regulation of feeding and locomotor behaviors and interactions with the orexin system and cocaine- and amphetamine regulated transcript (CART). *Horm. Behav.* **59,** 236–245.

Alvarez, C. E., and Sutcliffe, J. G. (2002). Hypocretin is an early member of the incretin gene family. *Neurosci. Lett.* **324,** 169–172.

Amiya, N., Amano, M., Oka, Y., Iigo, M., Takahashi, A., and Yamamori, K. (2007). Immunohistochemical localization of orexin/hypocretin-like immunoreactive peptides and melanin-concentrating hormone in the brain and pituitary of medaka. *Neurosci. Lett.* **427,** 16–21.

Amlaner, C. J., and Ball, N. J. (1983). A synthesis of sleep in wild birds. *Behaviour* **87,** 85–119.

Appelbaum, L., Wang, G. X., Maro, G. S., Mori, R., Tovin, A., Marin, W., Yokogawa, T., Kawakami, K., Smith, S. J., Gothilf, Y., Mignot, E., and Mourrain, P. (2009). Sleep-wake regulation and hypocretin-melatonin interaction in zebrafish. *Proc. Natl. Acad. Sci. U.S.A.* **106,** 21942–21947.

Appelbaum, L., Wang, G., Yokogawa, T., Skariah, G. M., Smith, S. J., Mourrain, P., and Mignot, E. (2010). Circadian and homeostatic regulation of structural synaptic plasticity in hypocretin neurons. *Neuron* **68,** 87–98.

Ayala-Guerrero, F., and Mexicano, G. (2008). Sleep and wakefulness in the green iguana lizard (*Iguana iguana*). *Comp. Biochem. Physiol. A Mol. Integr. Physiol.* **151,** 305–312.

Azpeleta, C., Martinez-Alvarez, R. M., Delgado, M. J., Isorna, E., and De Pedro, N. (2010). Melatonin reduces locomotor activity and circulating cortisol in goldfish. *Horm. Behav.* **57,** 323–329.

Beauchamp, G. (2011). Collective waves of sleep in gulls (*Larus* spp.). *Ethology* **117,** 326–331.

Bencan, Z., Sledge, D., and Levin, E. D. (2009). Buspirone, chlordiazepoxide and diazepam effects in a zebrafish model of anxiety. *Pharmacol. Biochem. Behav.* **94,** 75–80.

Berger, R. J., and Phillips, N. H. (1994). Constant light suppresses sleep and circadian rhythms in pigeons without consequent sleep rebound in darkness. *Am. J. Physiol.* **267,** R945–R952.

Bobbo, D., Vallortigara, G., and Mascetti, G. G. (2006). Effects of social interaction on monocular/unihemispheric sleep in male and female domestic chicks. *Biol. Psychol.* **73,** 213–219.

Buckley, C., MacDonald, E. E., Tuziak, S. M., and Volkoff, H. (2011). Molecular cloning and characterization of two putative appetite regulators in winter flounder (*Pleuronectes americanus*): Preprothyrotropin-releasing hormone (TRH) and preproorexin (OX). *Peptides* **31,** 1737–1747.

Cakir, Y., and Strauch, S. M. (2005). Tricaine (MS-222) is a safe anesthetic compound compared to benzocaine and pentobarbital to induce anesthesia in leopard frogs (*Rana pipiens*). *Pharmacol. Rep.* **57,** 467–474.

Campbell, S. S., and Tobler, I. (1984). Animal sleep—A review of sleep duration across phylogeny. *Neurosci. Biobehav. Rev.* **8,** 269–300.

Campbell, H. A., Fraser, K. P., Bishop, C. M., Peck, L. S., and Egginton, S. (2008). Hibernation in an Antarctic fish: On ice for winter. *PLoS One* **3,** e1743.

Chang, C. H., Chiao, C. C., and Yan, H. Y. (2009). The structure and possible functions of the milkfish *Chanos chanos* adipose eyelid. *J. Fish Biol.* **75,** 87–99.

Chemelli, R. M., Willie, J. T., Sinton, C. M., Elmquist, J. K., Scammell, T., Lee, C., Richardson, J. A., Williams, S. C., Xiong, Y., Kisanuki, Y., Fitch, T. E., Nakazato, M., *et al.* (1999). Narcolepsy in orexin knockout mice: Molecular genetics of sleep regulation. *Cell* **98,** 437–451.

Chen, W. B., Wang, X., Zhou, Y. L., Dong, H. Y., Lin, H. R., and Li, W. S. (2011). Molecular cloning, tissue distribution and the expression in the regulation of food intake of prepro-orexin in Nile tilapia (*Oreochromis niloticus*). *Zool. Res.* **32,** 285–292.

Cirelli, C., and Tononi, G. (2008). Is sleep essential? *PLoS Biol.* **6,** e216.

Cirelli, C., and Tononi, G. (2011). Molecular neurobiology of sleep. *Handb. Clin. Neurol.* **98,** 191–203.

Cirelli, C., Gutierrez, C. M., and Tononi, G. (2004). Extensive and divergent effects of sleep and wakefulness on brain gene expression. *Neuron* **41,** 35–43.

Clotfelter, E. D., O'Hare, E. P., McNitt, M. M., Carpenter, R. E., and Summers, C. H. (2010). Serotonin decreases aggression via 5-HT1A receptors in the fighting fish *Betta splendens*. *Pharmacol. Biochem. Behav.* **87,** 222–231.

Crawshaw, L. I. (1984). Low-temperature dormancy in fish. *Am. J. Physiol.* **246,** R479–R486.

da Silva, E. S., dos Santos, T. V., Hoeller, A. A., dos Santos, T. S., Pereira, G. V., Meneghelli, C., Pezlin, A. I., dos Santos, M. M., Faria, M. S., Paschoalini, M. A., and Marino-Neto, J. (2008). Behavioral and metabolic effects of central injections of orexins/hypocretins in pigeons (*Columba livia*). *Regul. Pept.* **147,** 9–18.

de Lecea, L., Kilduff, T. S., Peyron, C., Gao, X., Foye, P. E., Danielson, P. E., Fukuhara, C., Battenberg, E. L., Gautvik, V. T., Bartlett, F. S., 2nd, Frankel, W. N., van den Pol, A. N., *et al.* (1998). The hypocretins: Hypothalamus-specific peptides with neuroexcitatory activity. *Proc. Natl. Acad. Sci. U.S.A.* **95,** 322–327.

Dew, C. (1976). A contribution to the life history of the Cunner, Tautogolabrus adspersus, in Fishers Island Sound, Connecticut. *Chesapeake Sci.* **17,** 101–113113.

Dewasmes, G., Cote, S. D., Le Maho, Y., Groscolas, R., Robin, J. P., Vardon, G., and Libert, J. P. (2001). Effects of weather on activity and sleep in brooding king penguins (*Aptenodytes patagonicus*). *Polar Biol.* **24,** 508–511.

Dominguez, L., Morona, R., Joven, A., Gonzalez, A., and Lopez, J. M. (2010). Immunohistochemical localization of orexins (hypocretins) in the brain of reptiles and its relation to monoaminergic systems. *J. Chem. Neuroanat.* **39,** 20–34.

Dridi, S., Swennen, Q., Decuypere, E., and Buyse, J. (2005). Mode of leptin action in chicken hypothalamus. *Brain Res.* **1047,** 214–223.

Dubin, R. E., and Baker, J. D. (1982). Two types of cover-seeking behavior at sunset by the princess parrotfish, Scarus taeniopterus, at Barbados, West Indies. *Bull. Mar. Sci.* **32,** 572–583.

Duboue, E. R., Keene, A. C., and Borowsky, R. L. (2011). Evolutionary convergence on sleep loss in cavefish populations. *Curr. Biol.* **21,** 671–676.

Emran, F., Rihel, J., Adolph, A. R., and Dowling, J. E. (2010). Zebrafish larvae lose vision at night. *Proc. Natl. Acad. Sci. U.S.A.* **107,** 6034–6039.

Eriksson, K. S., Sergeeva, O. A., Haas, H. L., and Selbach, O. (2010). Orexins/hypocretins and aminergic systems. *Acta Physiol. (Oxf.)* **198,** 263–275.

Espana, R. A., and Scammell, T. E. (2011). Sleep neurobiology from a clinical perspective. *Sleep* **34,** 845–858.

Esteban, S., Nicolau, M. C., Gamundí, A., Akaârir, M., and Rial, R. V. (2005). Animal sleep: Phylogenetic correlations. *In* "Evolution of Sleep," (P. L. Parmeggiani and R. Velluti, Eds.), pp. 207–246. Imperial College Press, London.

Facciolo, R. M., Crudo, M., Giusi, G., Alo, R., and Canonaco, M. (2009). Light- and dark-dependent orexinergic neuronal signals promote neurodegenerative phenomena accounting for distinct behavioral responses in the teleost *Thalassoma pavo*. *J. Neurosci. Res.* **87,** 748–757.

Faraco, J. H., Appelbaum, L., Marin, W., Gaus, S. E., Mourrain, P., and Mignot, E. (2006). Regulation of hypocretin (orexin) expression in embryonic zebrafish. *J. Biol. Chem.* **281,** 29753–29761.

Farrell, W., Delville, Y., and Wilczynski, W. (2003). Immunocytochemical localization of orexin in the brain of the green anole lizard (*Anolis carolinensis*). *Soc. Neur. Abstr.* **33,** 828.4.

Furuse, M., Ando, R., Bungo, T., Ao, R., Shimojo, M., and Masuda, Y. (1999). Intracerebroventricular injection of orexins does not stimulate food intake in neonatal chicks. *Br. Poult. Sci.* **40,** 698–700.

Galas, L., Vaudry, H., Braun, B., Van Den Pol, A. N., De Lecea, L., Sutcliffe, J. G., and Chartrel, N. (2001). Immunohistochemical localization and biochemical characterization of hypocretin/orexin-related peptides in the central nervous system of the frog *Rana ridibunda*. *J. Comp. Neurol.* **429,** 242–252.

Gaztelu, J. M., Garciaaustt, E., and Bullock, T. H. (1991). Electrocorticograms of hippocampal and dorsal cortex of two reptiles—Comparison with possible mammalian homologs. *Brain Behav. Evol.* **37,** 144–160.

Gibson, R. N. (1993). Intertidal teleosts: Life in a fluctuating environment. *In* "Behaviour of Teleost Fishes," (T. Pitcher, Ed.), pp. 513–536. Chapman and Hall, London.

Goldshmid, R., Holzman, R., Weihs, D., and Genin, A. (2004). Aeration of corals by sleep-swimming fish. *Limnol. Oceanogr.* **49,** 1832–1839.

Grandner, M. A., Patel, N. P., Gehrman, P. R., Perlis, M. L., and Pack, A. I. (2010). Problems associated with short sleep: Bridging the gap between laboratory and epidemiological studies. *Sleep Med. Rev.* **14,** 239–247.

Grillner, S., Rossignol, S., and Wallen, P. (1977). The adaptation of a reflex response to the ongoing phase of locomotion in fish. *Exp. Brain Res.* **30,** 1–11.

Grutter, A. S., Rumney, J. G., Sinclair-Taylor, T., Waldie, P., and Franklin, C. E. (2011). Fish mucous cocoons: The 'mosquito nets' of the sea. *Biol. Lett.* **7,** 292–294.

Hagan, J. J., Leslie, R. A., Patel, S., Evans, M. L., Wattam, T. A., Holmes, S., Benham, C. D., Taylor, S. G., Routledge, C., Hemmati, P., Munton, R. P., Ashmeade, T. E., *et al.* (1999). Orexin A activates locus coeruleus cell firing and increases arousal in the rat. *Proc. Natl. Acad. Sci. U.S.A.* **96,** 10911–10916.

Harman, N. B. (1899). The palpebral and oculomotor apparatus in fishes: Observations on morphology and development. *J. Anat. Physiol.* **34,** 1–4011.

Hartse, K. M. (1994). Sleep in insects and nonmammalian vertebrates. *In* "Principles and Practice of Sleep Medicine," (M. H. Kryger, T. Roth, and W. C. Dement, Eds.), 1st edn., pp. 95–104. Elsevier Saunders, Philadelphia, PA.

Hartse, K. M. (2011). The phylogeny of sleep. *In* "Handbook of Clinical Neurology," (P. Montagna and S. Chokroverty, Eds.), Vol. 98, pp. 97–109. Elsevier, Amsterdam.

Hobson, J. A. (1967a). Electrographic correlates of behavior in the frog with special reference to sleep. *Electroencephalogr. Clin. Neurophysiol.* **22,** 113–121.

Hobson, J. A. (1967b). Respiration and EEG synchronization in the frog. *Nature* **213,** 988–989.

Hobson, J. A., Goin, O. B., and Goin, C. J. (1968). Electrographic correlates of behaviour in tree frogs. *Nature* **220,** 386–387.

Hoskins, L. J., Xu, M., and Volkoff, H. (2008). Interactions between gonadotropin-releasing hormone (GnRH) and orexin in the regulation of feeding and reproduction in goldfish (*Carassius auratus*). *Horm. Behav.* **54,** 379–385.

Huang, W., Ramsey, K. M., Marcheva, B., and Bass, J. (2011). Circadian rhythms, sleep, and metabolism. *J. Clin. Invest.* **121,** 2133–2141.

Huesa, G., van den Pol, A. N., and Finger, T. E. (2005). Differential distribution of hypocretin (orexin) and melanin-concentrating hormone in the goldfish brain. *J. Comp. Neurol.* **488,** 476–491.

Javůrková, V., Hořák, D., Kreisinger, J., Klvaňa, P., and Albrecht, T. (2011). Factors affecting sleep/vigilance behaviour in incubating mallards. *Ethology* **117,** 345–355.

Jones, S. G., Vyazovskiy, V. V., Cirelli, C., Tononi, G., and Benca, R. M. (2008). Homeostatic regulation of sleep in the white-crowned sparrow (*Zonotrichia leucophrys gambelii*). *BMC Neurosci.* **9,** 47.

Jones, S. G., Paletz, E. M., Obermeyer, W. H., Hannan, C. T., and Benca, R. M. (2010). Seasonal influences on sleep and executive function in the migratory white-crowned sparrow (*Zonotrichia leucophrys gambelii*). *BMC Neurosci.* **11,** 87.

Kamisoyama, H., Honda, K., Saneyasu, T., Sugahara, K., and Hasegawa, S. (2009). Corticotropin-releasing factor is a downstream mediator of the beta-melanocyte-stimulating hormone-induced anorexigenic pathway in chicks. *Neurosci. Lett.* **458,** 102–105.

Kaslin, J., Nystedt, J. M., Ostergard, M., Peitsaro, N., and Panula, P. (2004). The orexin/hypocretin system in zebrafish is connected to the aminergic and cholinergic systems. *J. Neurosci.* **24,** 2678–2689.

Katayama, S., Hamasu, K., Shigemi, K., Cline, M. A., and Furuse, M. (2010a). Intracerebroventricular injection of orexin-A, but not orexin-B, induces arousal of layer-type neonatal chicks. *Comp. Biochem. Physiol. A Mol. Integr. Physiol.* **157,** 132–135.

Katayama, S., Shigemi, K., Cline, M. A., and Furuse, M. (2010b). Intracerebroventricular injection of orexin-A stimulates monoamine metabolism but not HPA axis in neonatal chicks. *Neurosci. Lett.* **484,** 157–161.

Katayama, S., Shigemi, K., Cline, M. A., and Furuse, M. (2011). Clorgyline inhibits orexin-A-induced arousal in layer-type chicks. *J. Vet. Med. Sci.* **73,** 471–474.

Kojima, K., Kamijo, M., Kageyama, H., Uchiyama, M., Shioda, S., and Matsuda, K. (2009). Neuronal relationship between orexin-A- and neuropeptide Y-induced orexigenic actions in goldfish. *Neuropeptides* **43,** 63–71.

Kramer, B. (1990). Electrocommunication in Teleost Fishes: Behavior and Experiments. Springer, Berlin.

Kulikov, A. V., Karmanova, I. G., Kozlachkova, E. Y., Voronova, I. P., and Popova, N. K. (1994). The brain tryptophan hydroxylase activity in the sleep-like states in frog. *Pharmacol. Biochem. Behav.* **49,** 277–279.

Lenke, R. (1988). Hormonal control of sleep-appetitive behaviour and diurnal activity rhythms in the cleaner wrasse *Labroides dimidiatus* (Labridae, Teleostei). *Behav. Brain Res.* **27,** 73–85.

Lenke, R. (1991). The opercular gland of the cleaner-wrasse *Labroides dimidiatus* (Labridae), a light-, electron and scanning electron microscopic investigation. *J. Fish Biol.* **39,** 383–392.

Lesku, J. A., Martinez-Gonzalez, D., and Rattenborg, N. C. (2009a). Ontogeny and phylogeny of sleep. *In* "The Neuroscience of Sleep," (R. Stickgold and M. P. Walker, Eds.), pp. 61–69. Academic Press, Oxford.

Lesku, J. A., Roth Ii, T. C., Rattenborg, N. C., Amlaner, C. J., and Lima, S. L. (2009b). History and future of comparative analyses in sleep research. *Neurosci. Biobehav. Rev.* **33,** 1024–1036.

Lesku, J. A., Vyssotski, A. L., Martinez-Gonzalez, D., Wilzeck, C., and Rattenborg, N. C. (2011). Local sleep homeostasis in the avian brain: Convergence of sleep function in mammals and birds? *Proc. Biol. Sci.* **278,** 2419–2428.

Lima, S. L., Rattenborg, N. C., Lesku, J. A., and Amlaner, C. J. (2005). Sleeping under the risk of predation. *Anim. Behav.* **70,** 723–736.

Lopez, J. M., Dominguez, L., Moreno, N., and Gonzalez, A. (2009a). Comparative immunohistochemical analysis of the distribution of orexins (hypocretins) in the brain of amphibians. *Peptides* **30,** 873–887.

Lopez, J. M., Dominguez, L., Moreno, N., Morona, R., Joven, A., and Gonzalez, A. (2009b). Distribution of orexin/hypocretin immunoreactivity in the brain of the lungfishes *Protopterus dolloi* and *Neoceratodus forsteri*. *Brain Behav. Evol.* **74,** 302–322.

Lopez, M., Tena-Sempere, M., and Dieguez, C. (2010). Cross-talk between orexins (hypocretins) and the neuroendocrine axes (hypothalamic-pituitary axes). *Front. Neuroendocrinol.* **31,** 113–127.

Louisy, P. (1987). Observations dur l'émersion nocturne de deux blennies méditerranéennes: *Coryphoblennius galerita* et *Blennius trigloides* (Pisces, Perciformes). *Cybium* **11,** 55–73.

Lutterschmidt, D. I., and Mason, R. T. (2009). Endocrine mechanisms mediating temperature-induced reproductive behavior in red-sided garter snakes (*Thamnophis sirtalis parietalis*). *J. Exp. Biol.* **212,** 3108–3118.

MacDonald, E. E., and Volkoff, H. (2010). Molecular cloning and characterization of preproorexin in winter skate (*Leucoraja ocellata*). *Gen. Comp. Endocrinol.* **169,** 192–196.

Marshall, N. B. (1972). Sleep in fishes. *Proc. R. Soc. Med.* **65,** 177.

Maruyama, P. K., Cunha, A. F., Tizo-Pedroso, E., and Del-Claro, K. (2010). Relation of group size and daily activity patterns to southern lapwing (*Vanellus chilensis*) behaviour. *J. Ethol.* **28,** 339–344.

Maximino, C., and Herculano, A. M. (2010). A review of monoaminergic neuropsychopharmacology in zebrafish. *Zebrafish* **7,** 359–378.

McCarley, R. W. (2007). Neurobiology of REM and NREM sleep. *Sleep Med.* **8,** 302–330.

McDonald, M. D., Gonzalez, A., and Sloman, K. A. (2011). Higher levels of aggression are observed in socially dominant toadfish treated with the selective serotonin reuptake inhibitor, fluoxetine. *Comp. Biochem. Physiol. C* **153,** 107–112.

Meglasson, M. D., and Huggins, S. E. (1979). Sleep in a crocodilian, *Caiman sclerops. Comp. Biochem. Physiol. A* **63,** 561–567.

Mieda, M., and Sakurai, T. (2009). Integrative physiology of orexins and orexin receptors. *CNS Neurol. Disord. Drug Targets* **8,** 281–295.

Mieda, M., Hasegawa, E., Kisanuki, Y. Y., Sinton, C. M., Yanagisawa, M., and Sakurai, T. (2011). Differential roles of orexin receptor-1 and -2 in the regulation of non-REM and REM sleep. *J. Neurosci.* **31,** 6518–6526.

Mikkelsen, J. D., Hauser, F., deLecea, L., Sutcliffe, J. G., Kilduff, T. S., Calgari, C., Pevet, P., and Simonneaux, V. (2001). Hypocretin (orexin) in the rat pineal gland: A central transmitter with effects on noradrenaline-induced release of melatonin. *Eur. J. Neurosci.* **14,** 419–425.

Minami, K., Uezono, Y., Sakurai, T., Horishita, T., Shiraishi, M., and Ueta, Y. (2007). Effects of anesthetics on the function of orexin-1 receptors expressed in xenopus oocytes. *Pharmacology* **79,** 236–242.

Miura, T., Maruyama, K., Shimakura, S., Kaiya, H., Uchiyama, M., Kangawa, K., Shioda, S., and Matsuda, K. (2007). Regulation of food intake in the goldfish by interaction between ghrelin and orexin. *Peptides* **28,** 1207–1213.

Monti, J. M., and Jantos, H. (2008). The roles of dopamine and serotonin, and of their receptors, in regulating sleep and waking. *Prog. Brain Res.* **172,** 625–646.

Nakamachi, T., Matsuda, K., Maruyama, K., Miura, T., Uchiyama, M., Funahashi, H., Sakurai, T., and Shioda, S. (2006). Regulation by orexin of feeding behaviour and locomotor activity in the goldfish. *J. Neuroendocrinol.* **18,** 290–297.

Naumann, E. A., Kampff, A. R., Prober, D. A., Schier, A. F., and Engert, F. (2010). Monitoring neural activity with bioluminescence during natural behavior. *Nat. Neurosci.* **13,** 513–520.

Nelson, J. S. (2006). Fishes of the World. Wiley, New Jersey, USA.

Newman, S. M., Paletz, E. M., Rattenborg, N. C., Obermeyer, W. H., and Benca, R. M. (2008). Sleep deprivation in the pigeon using the disk-over-water method. *Physiol. Behav.* **93,** 50–58.

Newman, S. M., Paletz, E. M., Obermeyer, W. H., and Benca, R. M. (2009). Sleep deprivation in pigeons and rats using motion detection. *Sleep* **32,** 1299–1312.

Nishino, S. (2011). Hypothalamus, hypocretins/orexin, and vigilance control. *Handb. Clin. Neurol.* **99,** 765–782.

Norton, W., and Bally-Cuif, L. (2010). Adult zebrafish as a model organism for behavioural genetics. *BMC Neurosci.* **11,** 90.

Novak, C. M., Jiang, X., Wang, C., Teske, J. A., Kotz, C. M., and Levine, J. A. (2005). Caloric restriction and physical activity in zebrafish (*Danio rerio*). *Neurosci. Lett.* **383,** 99–104.

Ohkubo, T., Boswell, T., and Lumineau, S. (2002). Molecular cloning of chicken prepro-orexin cDNA and preferential expression in the chicken hypothalamus. *Biochim. Biophys. Acta* **1577,** 476–480.

Ohkubo, T., Tsukada, A., and Shamoto, K. (2003). cDNA cloning of chicken orexin receptor and tissue distribution: Sexually dimorphic expression in chicken gonads. *J. Mol. Endocrinol.* **31,** 499–508.

Olla, B. L., and Studholme, A. L. (1978). Comparative aspects of the activity rhythms of tautog, Tautoga onitis, bluefish, Pomatomus saltatrix, and Atlantic mackerel, Scomber scombrus, as related to their life habits. *In* "Rhythmic Activity of Fishes," (J. E. Thorpe, Ed.), pp. 131–151. Academic Press, London.

Panula, P. (2010). Hypocretin/orexin in fish physiology with emphasis on zebrafish. *Acta Physiol. (Oxf.)* **198,** 381–386.

Parzefall, J. (1993). Behavioral ecology of cave-dwelling fish. *In* "Behaviour of Teleost Fishes," (T. Pitcher, Ed.), pp. 573–606. Chapman and Hall, London.

Peyron, C., Valentin, F., Bayard, S., Hanriot, L., Bedetti, C., Rousset, B., Luppi, P. H., and Dauvilliers, Y. (2011). Melanin concentrating hormone in central hypersomnia. *Sleep Med.* **12,** 768–772.

Phillips-Singh, D., Li, Q., Takeuchi, S., Ohkubo, T., Sharp, P. J., and Boswell, T. (2003). Fasting differentially regulates expression of agouti-related peptide, pro-opiomelanocortin, prepro-orexin, and vasoactive intestinal polypeptide mRNAs in the hypothalamus of Japanese quail. *Cell Tissue Res.* **313,** 217–225.

Prober, D. A., Rihel, J., Onah, A. A., Sung, R. J., and Schier, A. F. (2006). Hypocretin/orexin overexpression induces an insomnia-like phenotype in zebrafish. *J. Neurosci.* **26,** 13400–13410.

Rattenborg, N. C. (2006). Evolution of slow-wave sleep and palliopallial connectivity in mammals and birds: A hypothesis. *Brain Res. Bull.* **69,** 20–29.

Rattenborg, N., and Amlaner, C. (2002). Phylogeny of sleep. *In* "Sleep Medicine," (T. Lee-Chiong, M. Sateia, and M. Carskadon, Eds.), pp. 7–22. Hanley & Belfus, Little Rock.

Rattenborg, N. C., Amlaner, C. J., and Lima, S. L. (2000). Behavioral, neurophysiological and evolutionary perspectives on unihemispheric sleep. *Neurosci. Biobehav. Rev.* **24,** 817–842.

Rattenborg, N. C., Mandt, B. H., Obermeyer, W. H., Winsauer, P. J., Huber, R., Wikelski, M., and Benca, R. M. (2004). Migratory sleeplessness in the white-crowned sparrow (*Zonotrichia leucophrys gambelii*). *PLoS Biol.* **2,** e212.

Rattenborg, N. C., Lesku, J. A., Martinez-Gonzalez, D., and Lima, S. L. (2007). The non-trivial functions of sleep. *Sleep Med. Rev.* **11,** 405–409author reply 411–417.

Rattenborg, N. C., Martinez-Gonzalez, D., and Lesku, J. A. (2009). Avian sleep homeostasis: Convergent evolution of complex brains, cognition and sleep functions in mammals and birds. *Neurosci. Biobehav. Rev.* **33,** 253–270.

Rechtschaffen, A. (1998). Current perspectives on the function of sleep. *Perspect. Biol. Med.* **41,** 359–390.

Reebs, S. G. (2002). Plasticity of diel and circadian activity rhythms in fishes. *Rev. Fish Biol. Fish.* **12,** 349–371.

Revell, T. K., and Hayes, W. K. (2009). Desert iguanas (*Dipsosaurus dorsalis*) sleep less when in close proximity to a rattlesnake predator (*Crotalus cerastes*). *J. Herpetol.* **43,** 29–37.

Rial, R. V., Akaarir, M., Gamundi, A., Nicolau, C., Garau, C., Aparicio, S., Tejada, S., Gene, L., Gonz•lez, J., De Vera, L. M., Coenen, A. M. L., Barcelo, P., *et al.* (2010). Evolution of wakefulness, sleep and hibernation: From reptiles to mammals. *Neurosci. Biobehav. Rev.* **34,** 1144–1160.

Richey, S. M., and Krystal, A. D. (2011). Pharmacological advances in the treatment of insomnia. *Curr. Pharm. Des.* **17,** 1471–1475.

Rolls, A., Schaich Borg, J., and de Lecea, L. (2010). Sleep and metabolism: Role of hypothalamic neuronal circuitry. *Best Pract. Res. Clin. Endocrinol. Metab.* **24,** 817–828.

Roth, A., and Schlegel, P. (1988). Behavioral evidence and supporting electrophysiological observations for electroreception in the blind cave salamander, *Proteus anguinus* (Urodela). *Brain Behav. Evol.* **32,** 277–280.

Roth, T. C., Lesku, J. A., Amlaner, C. J., and Lima, S. L. (2006). A phylogenetic analysis of the correlates of sleep in birds. *J. Sleep Res.* **15,** 395–402.

Roth, T. C., Rattenborg, N. C., and Pravosudov, V. V. (2010). The ecological relevance of sleep: The trade-off between sleep, memory and energy conservation. *Phil. Trans. R. Soc. B* **365,** 945–959.

Sakurai, T., and Mieda, M. (2011). Connectomics of orexin-producing neurons: Interface of systems of emotion, energy homeostasis and arousal. *Trends Pharmacol. Sci.* **32,** 451–462.

Sakurai, T., Amemiya, A., Ishii, M., Matsuzaki, I., Chemelli, R. M., Tanaka, H., Williams, S. C., Richardson, J. A., Kozlowski, G. P., Wilson, S., Arch, J. R., Buckingham, R. E., *et al.* (1998).

Orexins and orexin receptors: A family of hypothalamic neuropeptides and G protein-coupled receptors that regulate feeding behavior. *Cell* **92,** 573–585.

Satake, N. (1979). Melatonin mediation in sedative effect of serotonin in goldfish. *Physiol. Behav.* **22,** 817–819.

Secor, S. M., and Lignot, J. H. (2010). Morphological plasticity of vertebrate aestivation. *Prog. Mol. Subcell. Biol.* **49,** 183–208.

Shamoun-Baranes, J., Bouten, W., Camphuysen, C. J., and Baaij, E. (2011). Riding the tide: Intriguing observations of gulls resting at sea during breeding. *Ibis* **153,** 411–415.

Shapiro, C. M., and Hepburn, H. R. (1976). Sleep in a schooling fish, Tilapia mossambica. *Physiol. Behav.* **16,** 613–615.

Shibahara, M., Sakurai, T., Nambu, T., Takenouchi, T., Iwaasa, H., Egashira, S. I., Ihara, M., and Goto, K. (1999). Structure, tissue distribution, and pharmacological characterization of xenopus orexins. *Peptides* **20,** 1169–1176.

Sidis, B. (1909). An Experimental Study of Sleep (from the Physiological Laboratory of the Harvard Medical School and from Sidis Laboratory). Badger, Boston.

Siegel, J. M. (2009). Sleep viewed as a state of adaptive inactivity. *Nat. Rev. Neurosci.* **10,** 747–753.

Singletary, K. G., Delville, Y., Farrell, W. J., and Wilczynski, W. (2005). Distribution of orexin/hypocretin immunoreactivity in the nervous system of the green treefrog, *Hyla cinerea*. *Brain Res.* **1041,** 231–236.

Singletary, K. G., Deviche, P., Strand, C., and Delville, Y. (2006). Distribution of orexin/hypocretin immunoreactivity in the brain of a male songbird, the house finch, *Carpodacus mexicanus*. *J. Chem. Neuroanat.* **32,** 81–89.

Smith, J. M., and Stump, K. C. (2000). Isoflurane anesthesia in the African clawed frog (*Xenopus laevis*). *Contemp. Top. Lab. Anim. Sci.* **39,** 39–42.

Steward, C. A., Horan, T. L., Schuhler, S., Bennett, G. W., and Ebling, F. J. P. (2003). Central administration of thyrotropin releasing hormone (TRH) and related peptides inhibits feeding behavior in the Siberian hamster. *Neuroreport* **14,** 687–691.

Stopa, R. M., and Hoshino, K. (1999). Electrolocation-communication discharges of the fish *Gymnotus carapo* L. (Gymnotidae:Gymnotiformes) during behavioral sleep. *Braz. J. Med. Biol. Res.* **32,** 1223–1228.

Suzuki, H., Miyoshi, Y., and Yamamoto, T. (2007a). Orexin-A (hypocretin 1)-like immunoreactivity in growth hormone-containing cells of the Japanese seaperch (*Lateolabrax japonicus*) pituitary. *Gen. Comp. Endocrinol.* **150,** 205–211.

Suzuki, H., Takemoto, Y., and Yamamoto, T. (2007b). Differential distribution of orexin-A-like and orexin receptor 1 (OX1R)-like immunoreactivities in the Xenopus pituitary. *Tissue Cell* **39,** 423–430.

Suzuki, H., Kubo, Y., and Yamamoto, T. (2008). Orexin-A immunoreactive cells and fibers in the central nervous system of the axolotl brain and their association with tyrosine hydroxylase and serotonin immunoreactive somata. *J. Chem. Neuroanat.* **35,** 295–305.

Suzuki, H., Matsumoto, A., and Yamamoto, T. (2009). Orexin-B-like immunoreactivity localized in both luteinizing hormone- and thyroid-stimulating hormone-containing cells in the Nile tilapia (*Oreochromis niloticus*) pituitary. *Tissue Cell* **41,** 75–78.

Szymczak, J. T. (1989). Influence of environmental-temperature and photoperiod on temporal structure of sleep in corvids. *Acta Neurobiol. Exp.* **49,** 359–366.

Szymczak, J. T., Kaiser, W., Helb, H. W., and Beszczynska, B. (1996). A study of sleep in the European blackbird. *Physiol. Behav.* **60,** 1115–1120.

Takizuka, A., Minami, K., Uezono, Y., Horishita, T., Yokoyama, T., Shiraishi, M., Sakurai, T., Shigematsu, A., and Ueta, Y. (2007). Dexmedetomidine inhibits muscarinic type 3 receptors expressed in Xenopus oocytes and muscarine-induced intracellular Ca2+ elevation in cultured rat dorsal root ganglia cells. *Naunyn Schmiedebergs Arch. Pharmacol.* **375,** 293–301.

Tam, J. K. V., Lau, K. W., Lee, L. T. O., Chu, J. Y. S., Ng, K. M., Fournier, A., Vaudry, H., and Chow, B. K. C. (2011). Origin of secretin receptor precedes the advent of tetrapoda: Evidence on the separated origins of secretin and orexin. *PLoS One* **6,** e19384.

Tata, J. R. (2006). Amphibian metamorphosis as a model for the developmental actions of thyroid hormone. *Mol. Cell. Endocrinol.* **246,** 10–20.

Tauber, E. S., Rojas-Ramirez, J., and Peon, R. H. (1968). Electrophysiological and behavioral correlates of wakefulness and sleep in the lizard, *Ctenosaura pectinata. Electroencephalogr. Clin. Neurophysiol.* **24,** 424–433.

Tejada, S., Rial, R. V., Gamundi, A., and Esteban, S. (2011). Effects of serotonergic drugs on locomotor activity and vigilance states in ring doves. *Behav. Brain Res.* **216,** 238–246.

Teske, J. A., Billington, C. J., and Kotz, C. M. (2010). Hypocretin/orexin and energy expenditure. *Acta Physiol. (Oxf.)* **198,** 303–312.

Tobler, I. (1995). Is sleep fundamentally different between mammalian-species. *Behav. Brain Res.* **69,** 35–41.

Tobler, I., and Borbely, A. A. (1985). Effect of rest deprivation on motor activity of fish. *J. Comp. Physiol. A* **157,** 817–822.

Torterolo, P., Lagos, P., and Monti, J. M. (2011). Melanin-concentrating hormone: A new sleep factor? *Front. Neurol.* **2,** 14.

Volkoff, H., Bjorklund, J. M., and Peter, R. E. (1999). Stimulation of feeding behavior and food consumption in the goldfish, *Carassius auratus*, by orexin-A and orexin-B. *Brain Res.* **846,** 204–209.

Walker, J. M., and Berger, R. J. (1973). A polygraphic study of the tortoise (*Testudo denticulata*): Absence of electrophysiological signs of sleep. *Brain Behav. Evol.* **8,** 453–467.

Wong, K. K., Ng, S. Y., Lee, L. T., Ng, H. K., and Chow, B. K. (2011). Orexins and their receptors from fish to mammals: A comparative approach. *Gen. Comp. Endocrinol.* **171,** 124–130.

Xu, M., and Volkoff, H. (2007). Molecular characterization of prepro-orexin in Atlantic cod (*Gadus morhua*): Cloning, localization, developmental profile and role in food intake regulation. *Mol. Cell. Endocrinol.* **271,** 28–37.

Yamamoto, T., Suzuki, H., Uemura, H., Yamamoto, K., and Kikuyama, S. (2004). Localization of orexin-A-like immunoreactivity in prolactin cells in the bullfrog (*Rana catesbeiana*) pituitary. *Gen. Comp. Endocrinol.* **135,** 186–192.

Yan, A., Zhang, L., Tang, Z., Zhang, Y., Qin, C., Li, B., Li, W., and Lin, H. (2011). Orange-spotted grouper (*Epinephelus coioides*) orexin: Molecular cloning, tissue expression, ontogeny, daily rhythm and regulation of NPY gene expression. *Peptides* **32,** 1363–1370.

Yokobori, E., Kojima, K., Azuma, M., Kang, K. S., Maejima, S., Uchiyama, M., and Matsuda, K. (2011). Stimulatory effect of intracerebroventricular administration of orexin A on food intake in the zebrafish, *Danio rerio. Peptides* **32,** 1357–1362.

Yokogawa, T., Marin, W., Faraco, J., Pezeron, G., Appelbaum, L., Zhang, J., Rosa, F., Mourrain, P., and Mignot, E. (2007). Characterization of sleep in zebrafish and insomnia in hypocretin receptor mutants. *PLoS Biol.* **5,** 2379–2397.

Zhdanova, I. V. (2009). Fishing for sleep. *In* "Evolution of Sleep," (P. McNamara, R. Barton, and C. L. Nunn, Eds.), pp. 238–265. Cambridge University Press, Cambridge, UK.

Zhdanova, I. V. (2011). Sleep and its regulation in zebrafish. *Rev. Neurosci.* **22,** 27–36.

Zhdanova, I. V., Wang, S. Y., Leclair, O. U., and Danilova, N. P. (2001). Melatonin promotes sleep-like state in zebrafish. *Brain Res.* **903,** 263–268.

Zieba, D. A., Kirsz, K., Molik, E., Romanowicz, K., and Wojtowicz, A. K. (2011). Effects of orexigenic peptides and leptin on melatonin secretion during different photoperiods in seasonal breeding ewes: An in vitro study. *Domest. Anim. Endocrinol.* **40,** 139–146.

CHAPTER EIGHTEEN

Orexin System in Teleost Fish

Kouhei Matsuda,*,† Morio Azuma,* *and* Ki Sung Kang‡,1

Contents

Abstract

Orexin is a neuropeptide distributed widely among vertebrates. In mammals, orexin and its receptor system are involved in the regulation of food intake, locomotion, and psychomotor activities including the sleep/wakefulness cycle. With regard to nonmammalian vertebrates, there has also been intensive study aimed at the identification and functional characterization of orexin and its receptor, and recent investigations of the role of orexin have revealed that it exerts behavioral effects in teleost fish. Goldfish and zebrafish are excellent teleost fish models, and in these species it has been demonstrated that orexin increases food consumption as an orexigenic factor and enhances locomotor

* Laboratory of Regulatory Biology, Graduate School of Science and Engineering, University of Toyama, Toyama, Japan
† Laboratory of Regulatory Biology, Graduate School of Innovative Life Science, University of Toyama, Toyama, Japan
‡ Department of Anatomy, Showa University School of Medicine, Tokyo, Japan
[1] Present address: Natural Products Research Center, Korea Institute of Science and Technology, Gangneung, Gangwon-do, South Korea

Vitamins and Hormones, Volume 89
ISSN 0083-6729, http://dx.doi.org/10.1016/B978-0-12-394623-2.00018-4

activity, as well as being involved in the regulation of active and rest status (circadian rhythmicity and the sleep/wakefulness cycle), as is the case in mammals. This chapter reviews current knowledge of orexin derived from studies of teleost fish, as representative nonmammals, focusing particularly on the role of the orexin system, and examines its significance from a comparative viewpoint.

I. Introduction

Orexin (or hypocretin, as it is sometime known) is a neuropeptide that was first identified as an orphan-receptor ligand, and subsequently as an appetite regulator (Sakurai *et al.*, 1998). Orexin exists as two molecular forms derived from the same precursor: a 33-residue peptide known as orexin A, and a 28-residue peptide known as orexin B. Although it was thought originally that orexin has no functional or structural identity with any other known regulatory peptide, one notable exception is hypocretin, which has been considered to belong to the incretin gene family of peptides, including members of the secretin–glucagon superfamily such as growth hormone releasing hormone, pituitary adenylate cyclase-activating polypeptide, vasoactive intestinal peptide, and glucagon-like peptides (Alvarez and Sutcliffe, 2002; Tam *et al.*, 2011). Subsequently, the orexin receptor was found to have two forms: orexin receptors 1 and 2 (OX1R and OX2R) (Sakurai *et al.*, 1998; Tam *et al.*, 2011; Wong *et al.*, 2011). In mammals, neuronal cell bodies containing orexin-like immunoreactivity are located in the lateral hypothalamus, which is referred to as the "orexigenic center," and nerve fibers containing orexin-like immunoreactivity are widely distributed in various regions including the cerebral cortex, hippocampus, limbic system, and brainstem, suggesting that orexin controls multiple brain functions such as emotional regulation (de Lecea *et al.*, 1998; Sakurai and Mieda, 2011; Thannickal *et al.*, 2000). Consistent with this observation, orexin has been found to regulate the sleep–wakefulness cycle and to suppress the gonadotropin-producing cells in the hypothalamus (Kilduff and Peyron, 2000; Kohsaka *et al.*, 2001; Porkka-Heiskanen *et al.*, 2004; Sakurai, 2005; Sakurai *et al.*, 1998).

The orexin gene or cDNA has also been characterized in nonmammalian species. The structure of fish orexin appears to be less conserved (Kaslin *et al.*, 2004; Tam *et al.*, 2011; Wong *et al.*, 2011). Recent studies indicate that some neuropeptides influence food consumption and related behavior in nonmammalian vertebrates, notably in teleost fish (Kang *et al.*, 2011b; Lin *et al.*, 2000; Matsuda *et al.*, 2011a). Orexin is distributed in the brain of teleost fish and exerts central and neuroendocrine functions (Huesa *et al.*, 2005; Kaslin *et al.*, 2004). In particular, the effect of orexin on feeding behavior has been studied in teleost fish. In the goldfish, intracerebroventricular (ICV) administration of orexin A stimulates food intake, and the orexin A-induced orexigenic action is mediated via the orexin receptor, subsequently leading to activation of the neuropeptide Y (NPY) Y1 receptor (Matsuda, 2009; Matsuda *et al.*, 2011a; Nakamachi *et al.*, 2006; Volkoff *et al.*, 1999). In this species, the orexigenic response to orexin A is also modulated by cocaine- and amphetamine-regulated transcript peptides and leptin (Abbott and Volkoff, 2011; Volkoff *et al.*, 1999). ICV injection of orexin A also stimulates locomotor activity in the goldfish (Matsuda, 2009; Nakamachi *et al.*, 2006). In the zebrafish, ICV injection of orexin A induces an orexigenic action and hypermotility (Yokobori *et al.*, 2011), and overexpression of orexin promotes wakefulness and inhibits rest (Prober *et al.*, 2006). Taken together, these observations indicate that, in Cypriniformes (including the zebrafish and goldfish), orexin not only regulates energy homeostasis by stimulating food consumption but also involved in the regulation of psychophysiology in teleost fish by enhancing locomotor and psychomotor activities, suggesting that it is involved in multiple brain functions in teleosts (Appelbaum *et al.*, 2009; Rihel *et al.*, 2010). However, except for the case of goldfish and zebrafish, there is no information about the involvement of orexin in feeding and emotional behavior, or other physiological processes, in teleost fish, and the function of the orexin system in fish has not been well studied. Therefore, this chapter focuses on the characterization of orexin and its receptor system, the distribution of the orexin transcript and orexin-like immunoreactivity, and the effect of orexin on food intake, locomotor, and psychomotor activities in teleost fish, especially the goldfish and zebrafish, which have been overlooked hitherto.

II. Orexin and Its Receptor in Teleost Fish

The orexin gene or cDNA has also been characterized in nonmammalian species such as the chicken (*Gallus gallus*), clawed toad (*Xenopus laevis*), zebrafish (*Danio rerio*), tiger puffer (*Takifugu rubripes*), Atlantic cod (*Gadus morhua*), goldfish (*Carassius auratus*), medaka (*Oryzias latipes*), winter flounder (*Pleuronectes americanus*) and winter skate (*Leucoraja ocellata*) (Alvarez and Sutcliffe, 2002; Buckley *et al.*, 2010; Faraco *et al.*, 2006; Kaslin *et al.*, 2004; MacDonald and Volkoff, 2010; Nakamachi *et al.*, 2006; Ohkubo *et al.*, 2002; Shibahara *et al.*, 1999; Xu and Volkoff, 2007). The primary structure of the orexin precursor is conserved among mammals (Tam *et al.*, 2011; Wong *et al.*, 2011). However, as shown in Fig. 18.1A, phylogenetic analysis using the amino acid sequences of the orexin precursor by the neighbor-joining method has revealed that the structures identified in

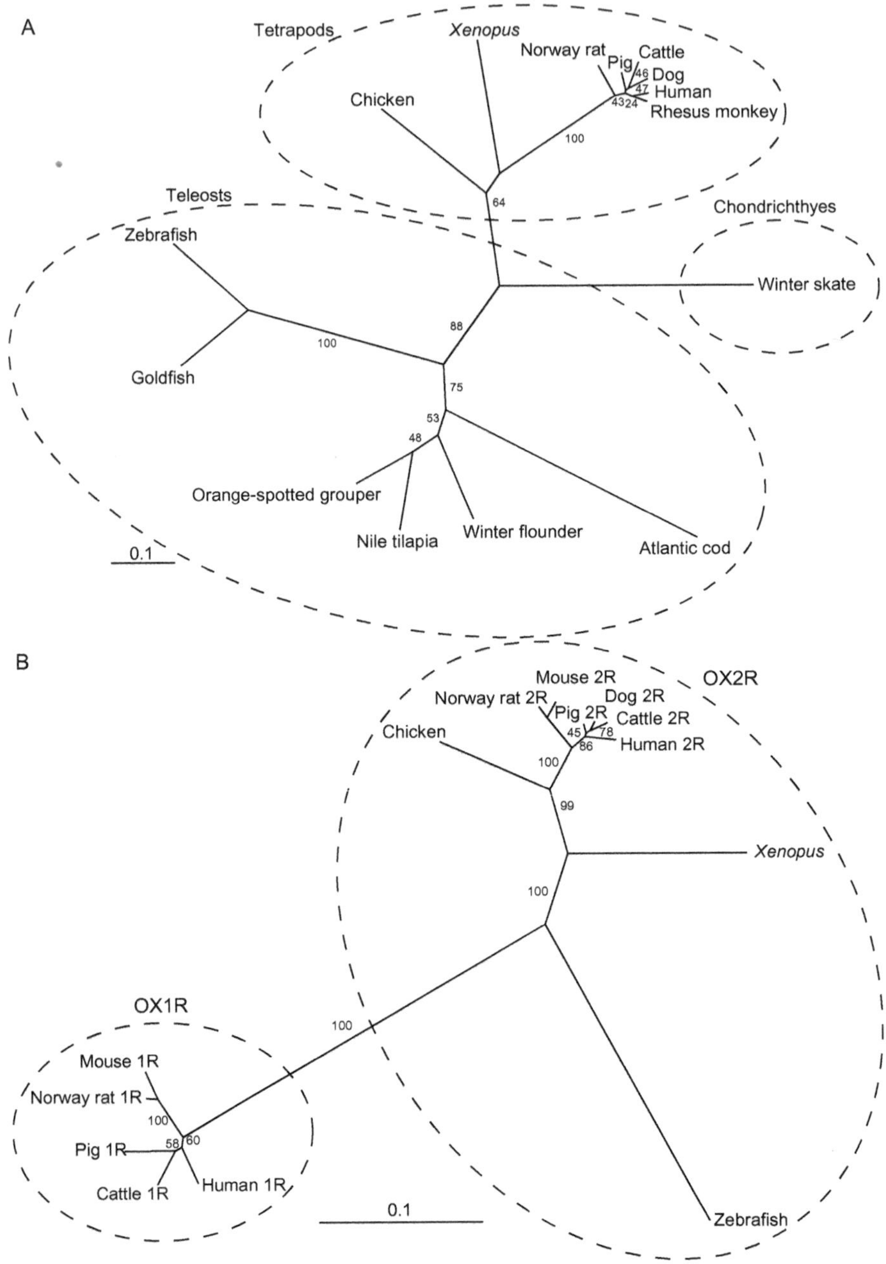

Figure 18.1 (A) A phylogenetic tree of the primary structure of the orexin precursor inferred by the neighbor-joining method using ClustalW. The numbers at the branch points are derived from bootstrap analysis (100 repetitions). The scale bar represents a phylogenetic distance of 0.1 amino acid substitutions per site. GenBank IDs: human

tetrapods are slightly similar to that of the mammalian orexin precursor, whereas the structure of the fish orexin precursor appears to be less conserved (Kaslin *et al.*, 2004; Wong *et al.*, 2011). Two forms of orexin, orexin A and orexin B, are derived from a common precursor encoded by the orexin gene, in which loci have been shown to be conserved throughout vertebrate evolution (Alvarez and Sutcliffe, 2002).

Orexins A and B bind to two orexin receptors, OX1R and OX2R, which belong to members of class B of mammalian G-protein-coupled receptors (Wong *et al.*, 2011). However, information about the orexin receptor in nonmammals, including birds, amphibians, and teleost fish, has been insufficient. To date, one receptor for orexin has been identified in chicken, *Xenopus*, and zebrafish (Ohkubo *et al.*, 2003; Tam *et al.*, 2011; Yokogawa *et al.*, 2007), and this receptor corresponds structurally to mammalian OX2R (Wong *et al.*, 2011). On the other hand, recent studies have failed to identify the gene encoding the OX1R in nonmammals, including zebrafish (Panula, 2010; Wong *et al.*, 2011). Molecular information about the fish OX1R is lacking. From an evolutionary and comparative viewpoint, the OX2R is likely to be a more ancient receptor form in vertebrates. Phylogenetic analyses of the chicken and *Xenopus* orexin receptors by the neighbor-joining method using the amino acid sequences of mammalian OX1R and OX2R have revealed that the nonmammalian orexin receptors may be classified into the mammalian OX2R group. However, in the tree, the zebrafish orexin receptor appears to form a separate cluster (Fig. 18.1B). Further investigations to clarify the relationship between mammalian and nonmammalian orexin receptors, especially the fish receptor, would be warranted.

prepro-orexin, NM_001524; Rhesus monkey prepro-orexin NM_001194432; Norway rat prepro-orexin, AF019565.1; dog prepro-orexin, NM_001033994.1; pig prepro-orexin, MN_214156.2, EF434655.1; bovine prepro-orexin, NM_001166520; chicken prepro-orexin, NM_204185.1, AB056748.1; *Xenopus* prepro-orexin, Shibahara *et al.*, 1999; Atlantic cod prepro-orexin, DQ486137.1, EU096315.1; goldfish prepro-orexin, DQ923590.1; zebrafish prepro-orexin, NM_001077392, DQ831346; Nile tilapia prepro-orexin, FJ871159.1; winter flounder prepro-orexin, GQ397970.1; orange-spotted grouper prepro-orexin, HM992945.1; winter skate prepro-orexin, HM367085.1. (B) A phylogenetic tree of the primary structure of orexin receptors inferred by the neighbor-joining method using ClustalW. The numbers at the branch points are derived from bootstrap analysis (1000 repetitions). The scale bar represents a phylogenetic distance of 0.1 amino acid substitutions per site. GenBank IDs: human OX1R, NM_001525; human OX2R, NM_001526; Norway rat OX1R, NM_013064.1; Norway rat OX2R, NM_013074; mouse OX1R, AY336083.1; mouse OX2R, NM_198962; dog OX2R, NM_001002933; pig OX1R, NM_001043346, DQ321701.1; pig OX2R, NM_001129951, DQ321702.1; cattle OX1R, NM_001048182; cattle OX2R, NM_001192677; chicken orexin receptor, NM_001024584, AB110634.1; *Xenopus* orexin receptor, HQ242647.1; zebrafish orexin receptor, NM_001079868.

III. Distribution of Orexin Precursor Transcript and Orexin-Like Immunoreactivity in Teleost Fish

cDNAs encoding the orexin precursors were isolated from goldfish and zebrafish and cloned as described above (see the Section II). Subsequently, the distribution of the orexin precursor transcript in the central nervous system and peripheral tissues of those species was examined using *in situ* hybridization or RT-PCR. Expression of orexin receptor mRNA was observed in the periventricular regions of the brain (Yokogawa *et al.*, 2007). Figure 18.2 shows the distribution of the orexin precursor transcript in the central and peripheral tissues of the goldfish. Orexin precursor mRNA is strongly expressed in the brain, pituitary, and gonads and is moderately expressed in the other tissues. In the winter flounder, the distribution of the orexin precursor transcript has also been observed (Buckley *et al.*, 2010). The expression of mRNA for the orexin precursor is distributed in the brain, including the telencephalon, mesencephalon, diencephalon, cerebellum, medulla oblongata, and spinal cord. In addition, RT-PCR has indicated that the orexin precursor transcript is present in peripheral tissues such as gill, liver, gut, stomach, spleen, kidney, and gonad.

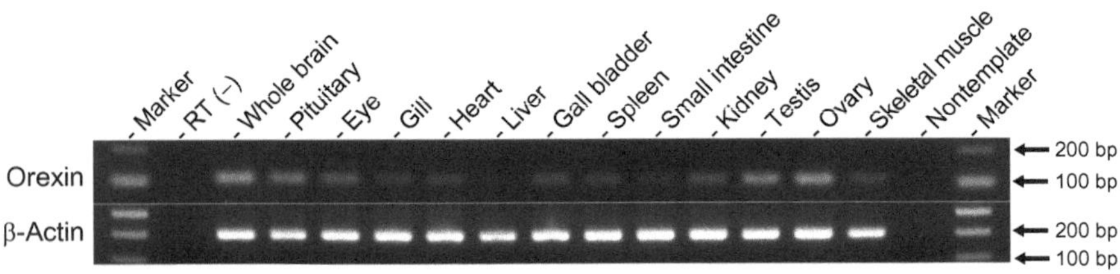

Figure 18.2 Reverse transcriptase (RT)-polymerase chain reaction (PCR) analysis of orexin precursor mRNA in the goldfish tissues. Total RNA was extracted from various tissues including the whole brain, pituitary, eye, gill, heart, liver, gall bladder, spleen, small intestine, kidney, testis, ovary, skeletal muscle. For amplification and quantitation of the cDNA fragments encoding the orexin precursor and β-actin, the two-step RT-PCR method was used. Reverse transcription was carried out at 50 °C for 60 min, and the resulting cDNA was subsequently amplified using 35 cycles for orexin and 23 cycles for β-actin of 94 °C for 40 s and 60 °C for 40 s followed by 72 °C for 30 s. Gene-specific primers for amplification of the orexin cDNA fragment were based on the nucleotide sequence of goldfish orexin precursor (GenBank ID, DQ923590.1). PCR with the sense primer (5′-CGT CAA GGT CCT GCA AAT TAT ACG-3′) and antisense primer (5′-CTG CCG CGT CGT TAT TAA AGC-3′) yielded a 102-bp product encoding part of the goldfish orexin precursor cDNA. Goldfish β-actin-specific primers were used as the internal control for PCR amplification (goldfish, GenBank ID, AB039726.2). Using these primers (sense primer, 5′-CTA GGT ATG GAA TCT TGC GGT A-3′; antisense primer, 5′-TAC TCC TGC TTG CTG ATC CA-3′) a 287-bp product corresponding to a region in the part of the β-actin cDNA for goldfish was obtained.

Orexin-like immunoreactivity was first observed in the brain of the zebrafish (Kaslin *et al.*, 2004), indicating that the major population of neuronal cell bodies possessing orexin-like immunoreactivity is located in the hypothalamic area including the gigantocellular part of the magnocellular preoptic nucleus, the posterior tuberal nucleus, and the lateral recessus in the hypothalamus (Kaslin *et al.*, 2004). Subsequently, it was reported that the goldfish brain contained neuronal cell bodies and fibers showing orexin-like immunoreactivity (Huesa *et al.*, 2005). Schematic drawings of orexin-like immunoreactivity in the brains of the goldfish and zebrafish are illustrated in Figs. 18.3 and 18.4. In these species, the neuronal cell bodies containing orexin-like immunoreactivity are located highly specifically in two regions of the hypothalamus: the preoptic area, including the magnocellular nucleus, and the area bordering the third ventricle, including the nucleus posterioris periventricularis (goldfish) or posterior tuberal nucleus (zebrafish), and the nucleus recessus lateralis. Nerve fibers containing orexin-like immunoreactivity are located mainly in the midbrain and various other regions. The localization of orexin-like immunoreactivity has also been examined in the medaka, and orexin-like immunoreactivity is widely detected throughout the brain (Amiya *et al.*, 2007). In this species, neuronal cells showing orexin-like immunoreactivity are located mainly in the hypothalamic area along the third ventricle, including the nucleus posterioris periventricularis, as is the case in goldfish. In addition, the distribution of orexin-like immunoreactivity has also been examined in the brains of the African and Australian lungfish, *Protopterus dolloi* and *Neoceratodus forsteri* (López *et al.*, 2009). In both the species, the most immunoreactive neurons are present in the suprachiasmatic nucleus and dorsal hypothalamus. Only in *Neoceratodus*, however, important cell populations are located in the preoptic area and infundibular hypothalamus, whereas small numbers of faintly reactive neurons are present in the lateral septum and ventral striatum. Fiber labeling has been shown to be widely distributed in all main brain subdivisions but is more abundant in regions such as the septum, preoptic area, suprachiasmatic nucleus, lateral hypothalamic area, thalamus, pretectum, and tegmentum. Less conspicuous was the innervation is evident in the pallial regions, habenula, optic tectum, rhombencephalic reticular formation, and spinal cord (López *et al.*, 2009).

IV. Effect of Orexin on Food Intake in Teleost Fish

A. Goldfish

Feeding conditions affect the levels of expression of orexin precursor mRNA and orexin synthesis in the hypothalamus of fish. In goldfish that have been fasted for two or more days, the number of neuronal cell bodies

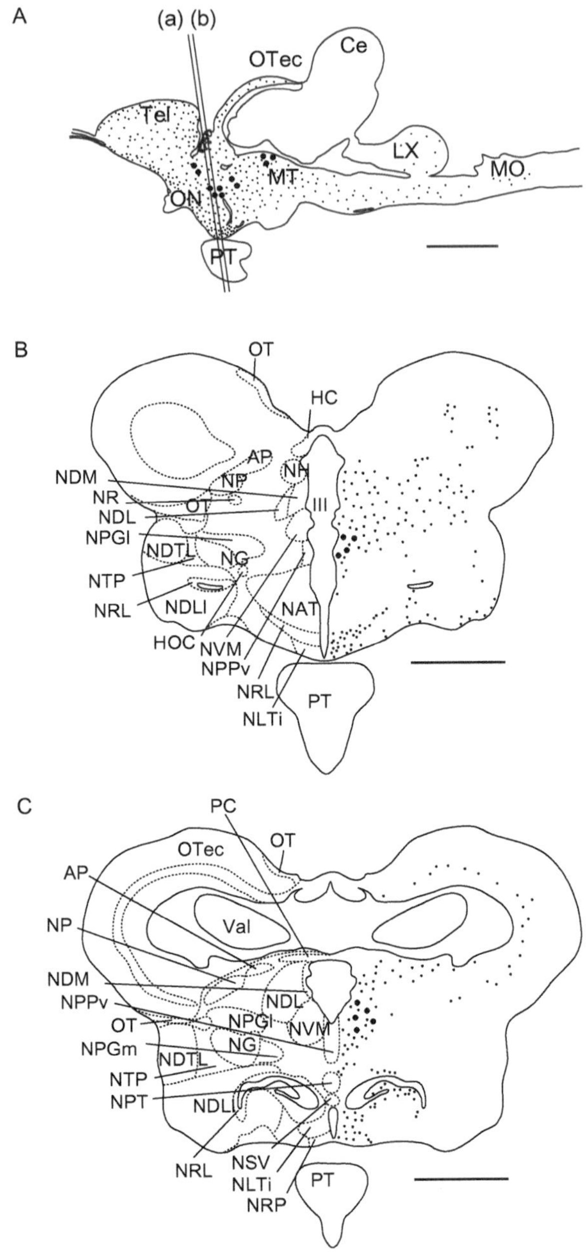

Figure 18.3 Schematic drawings of the distribution of orexin A-like immunoreactivity in the brain of the goldfish (A) is a sagittal section view, and (B) and (C) are cross-sectional views at levels (a) and (b), as indicated by the respective lines in the sagittal section view. Neuronal cell bodies and fibers with orexin-like immunoreactivity are

containing orexin-like immunoreactivity in the hypothalamus is significantly increased in comparison with that in normally fed fish (Nakamachi *et al.*, 2006). Moreover, intraperitoneal (IP) administration of glucose for 12 h induces a significant decrease in the number of neuronal cell bodies showing orexin-like immunoreactivity in the brain. Expression of orexin precursor mRNA in the brain changes according to feeding status: fasting for 7 days induces a significant increase in the levels of expression of orexin precursor mRNA (Nakamachi *et al.*, 2006). These results suggest that fasting enhances orexin-like immunoreactivity and the expression of orexin precursor mRNA in neuronal cells in the hypothalamus, indicating that a relationship exists between the density of orexin-like immunoreactivity and orexin synthesis, or its functional state, in the goldfish brain.

There is a direct evidence that orexin enhances food intake in goldfish. ICV administration of human orexin A at 0.28–2.8 pmol/g body weight (BW) and orexin B at 0.34–3.4 pmol/g BW stimulates food consumption (Volkoff *et al.*, 1999). A subsequent study using goldfish has indicated that ICV administration of orexin A antiserum decreases food intake, that the orexigenic action of human orexin A is more potent than that of human orexin B (Nakamachi *et al.*, 2006), and that the orexigenic action of orexin A at 2.8 pmol/g BW is blocked by treatment with SB334867—an OX1R antagonist in mammals—at 10 pmol/g BW (Miura *et al.*, 2007). However, as described above (see the Section II), there is no evidence that the OX1R is present in teleost fish (Wong *et al.*, 2011). Therefore, SB334867 may antagonize orexin A at the goldfish orexin receptor, which belongs to the OX2R family. Interestingly, the orexigenic action of orexin A at 2.8 pmol/g BW is attenuated by treatment with the growth hormone secretagogue-receptor antagonist, [D-Lys3]-GHRP-6, at 10 pmol/g BW, and the orexigenic action of ghrelin at 1 pmol/g BW is blocked by treatment with SB334867 at 10 pmol/g BW, suggesting that, in goldfish, orexin A and ghrelin have interacting orexigenic effects on the central nervous system

indicated by filled circles and dots, respectively. Scale bar = 1 mm. Abbreviations: AP, area pretectalis; Ce, cerebellum; HC, habenular commissure; HOC, horizontal commissure; LX, vagal nerve; MO, medulla oblongata; MT, midbrain tegmentum; NAT, nucleus anterior tuberis; NDL, nucleus dorsolateralis thalami; NDLI, nucleus diffusus lobi inferior; NDM, nucleus dorsomedialis thalami; NDTL, nucleus diffusus tori inferior; NG, nucleus glomerulosus; NH, nucleus habenularis; NLTi, inferior part of nucleus lateralis tuberis; NP, nucleus pretectalis; NPGl, nucleus preglomerulosus pars lateralis; NPGm, nucleus preglomerulosus pars medialis; NPPv, nucleus posterior periventricularis; NPT, nucleus posterior tuberis; NR, nucleus rotundus; NRL, nucleus recessus lateralis; NRP, nucleus recessus posterioris; NSV, nucleus saccus vasculosus; NTP, nucleus posterioris thalami; NVM, nucleus ventromedialis thalami; ON, optic nerve; OT, optic tract; OTec, optic tectum; PC, posterior commissure; PT, pituitary; Tel, telencephalon; Val, lateral lobe of valvula cerebella; III, third ventricle. The nomenclature used for brain nuclei was based on the brain atlas for goldfish (Peter and Gill, 1975) and for carp (Pirone *et al.*, 2004).

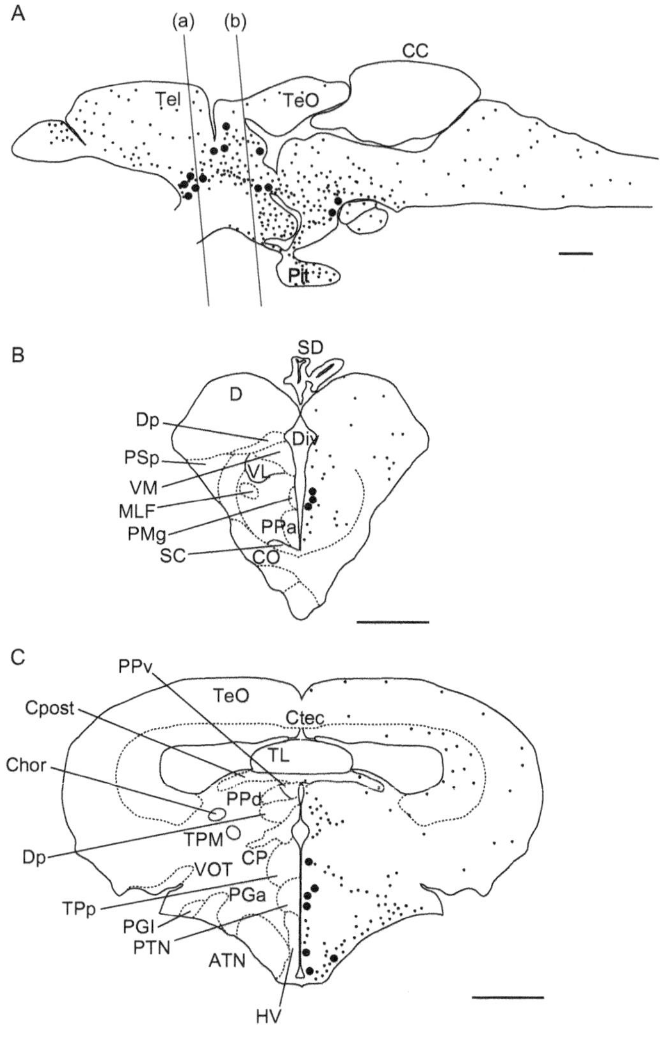

Figure 18.4 Schematic drawings of the distribution of orexin A-like immunoreactivity in the brain of the zebrafish (A) is a sagittal section view, and (B) and (C) are cross-sectional views at levels (a), and (b) as indicated by the respective lines in the sagittal section view. Neuronal cell bodies and fibers with orexin-like immunoreactivity are indicated by filled circles and dots, respectively. Scale bar = 0.2 mm. Abbreviations: ATN, anterior tuberal nucleus; CC, cerebellar crest; Chor, horizontal commissure; CO, optic chiasm; CP, central posterior thalamic nucleus; Cpost, posterior commissure; Ctec, tectal commissure; D, dorsal telencephalic area; Div, diencephalic ventricle; Dp, posterior zone of dorsal telencephalic area; Hv, ventral zone of periventricular hypothalamus; MLF, medial longitudinal fascicle; PGa, anterior preglomerular nucleus; PGI, lateral preglomerular nucleus; Pit, pituitary gland; PMg, gigantocellular part of magnocellular preoptic nucleus; PPa, parvocellular preoptic

(Miura *et al.*, 2007). In goldfish, the orexigenic action of orexin A is also inhibited by treatment with the NPY Y1 receptor antagonist, BIBP-3226, at 100 pmol/g BW, and the action of NPY at 1 pmol/g BW is abolished by treatment with SB334867 at 10 pmol/g BW (Kojima *et al.*, 2009). These data indicate that the orexigenic actions of orexin A and NPY are mediated by mutual signaling pathways in goldfish (Matsuda, 2009). Interestingly, gonadotropin-releasing hormone 2 (GnRH2; chicken GnRH II, another name for GnRH2) mediates the anorexigenic actions of α-melanocyte-stimulating hormone and subsequent corticotropin-releasing hormone, and GnRH2 is known as a potent anorexigenic neuropeptides in goldfish (Kang *et al.*, 2011a; Matsuda *et al.*, 2008). GnRH2 also suppresses expression of orexin precursor mRNA, and orexin inhibits GnRH2-induced reproductive behavior (Hoskins *et al.*, 2008), suggesting the involvement of orexin in the reproduction in fish. In mammals, orexin participates in the regulation of reproduction via the hypothalamo–pituitary–gonadal relationship (Nurmio *et al.*, 2010; Silveyra *et al.*, 2010).

B. Zebrafish

To date, most of the data pertaining to the regulation of food intake by orexin in teleost fish have been obtained using goldfish, as described above (see the Section IV, A) (Kojima *et al.*, 2009; Matsuda, 2009; Miura *et al.*, 2007; Nakamachi *et al.*, 2006; Volkoff, 2006; Volkoff *et al.*, 1999, 2005), and the situation in other teleosts has remained unclear. Recent data have indicated that the number of neuronal cell bodies showing orexin-like immunoreactivity in the posterior tuberal nucleus, but not in the gigantocellular part of the magnocellular preoptic nucleus of the hypothalamus is increased in zebrafish fasted for 7 days (Yokobori *et al.*, 2011), suggesting that orexin-like immunoreactivity in the posterior tuberal nucleus is related to feeding status, and that fasting for 7–14 days induces a significant increase in the orexin precursor mRNA levels in the zebrafish brain (Novak *et al.*, 2005; Yokobori *et al.*, 2011).

So far, in zebrafish, there has been no direct evidence for the involvement of orexin in appetite regulation. However, a method has been developed for measuring the food intake in this species (Piccinetti *et al.*, 2010; Yokobori *et al.*, 2011) by directly observing and recording the number of food pellets eaten by an individual fish, as in the case of the goldfish.

---

nucleus; PPd, periventricular pretectal nucleus sorsal part; PPv, periventricular pretectal nucleus ventral part; PSp, paravocellular superficial pretectal nucleus; PTN, posterior tuberal nucleus; SC, suprachiasmic nucleus; SD, sorsal sac; Tel, telencephalon; TeO, optic tectum; TL, longitudinal torus; TPM, pretecto-mammillary tract; TPp, periventricular nucleus of posterior tuberculum; VL, ventrolateral thalamic nucleus; VM, ventromedial thalamic nucleus; VOT, ventrolateral optic tract. The nomenclature used for brain nuclei was based on the brain atlas for zebrafish (Wullimann *et al.*, 1996).

A recent study has demonstrated for the first time the stimulatory effect of ICV-administrated human orexin A on food intake in the zebrafish (Yokobori *et al.*, 2011). In that study, ICV administration of orexin A at 0.3 and 3 pmol/g BW induced a significant increase of cumulative food intake during 60 min after treatment. ICV administration of orexin A at 30 pmol/g BW did not stimulate the food intake, being possibly indicative of an overdose effect, receptor downregulation, or receptor desensitization, as is the case in goldfish (Nakamachi *et al.*, 2006; Fig. 18.5). Although the synthetic orexin A employed was of heterologous origin, ICV administration

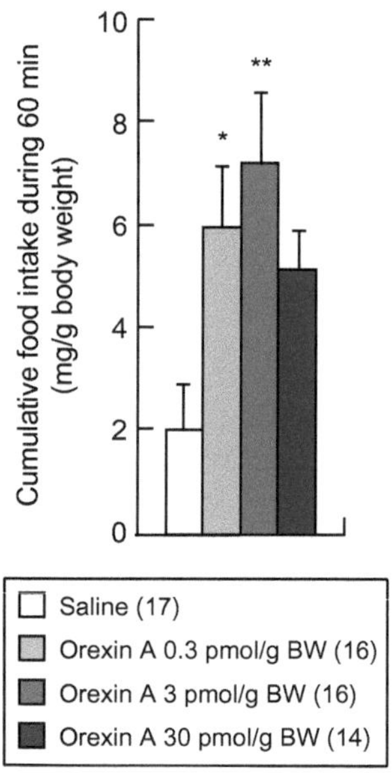

Figure 18.5 Effect of ICV administration of orexin A on food intake in the zebrafish. Zebrafish (0.3–0.6 g body weight, BW) of both sexes were purchased commercially and kept for 2 weeks under controlled light–dark conditions (12 L/12 D) with the room temperature regulated to 20–24 °C. Two hours before the experiments began at 10:00 a.m., each fish was supplied with food at 3% of its BW. In order to examine the effect of orexin A on food intake, ICV administration was carried out as described previously (Yokogawa *et al.*, 2007) with minor modifications for our laboratory (Yokobori *et al.*, 2011). Each fish was placed in wet tissue paper under anesthesia with MS-222 (3-aminobenzoic acid ethyl ester, Sigma-Aldrich Co., St. Louis, MO, USA). A small part of the parietal bone was carefully removed using a surgical blade, and 0.5 μL of test solution containing Evans Blue dye was delivered into the third ventricle of the brain of each fish using a microinjecter-holding system designed for small fish and a small Hamilton syringe with 0.1-μL graduations and a disposable fine needle. Correct placement of the injection was confirmed by the presence of Evans Blue dye in the ventricle. Fish were then injected with synthetic orexin A at 0.3, 3, or 30 pmol/g BW. Fish in the control group were given injections of the same volume of saline. After ICV injection, the bone gap was filled with a surgical bonding agent.

of human orexin A enhanced food intake in the zebrafish. The primary structure of orexin precursors has been conserved during evolution among the vertebrates (Wong *et al.*, 2011). However, the amino acid sequence of zebrafish orexin A shows 32% identity with that of human orexin A (Wong *et al.*, 2011). Synthetic human orexin A shows effective physiological activity in zebrafish and goldfish (Nakamachi *et al.*, 2006; Volkoff and Peter, 2000, 2001; Volkoff *et al.*, 1999, 2003; Yokogawa *et al.*, 2007). The orexigenic action of orexin A is blocked by treatment with SB334867 in zebrafish (Yokobori *et al.*, 2011). However, as described above (see the Section II), there is no evidence that the OX1R is present in teleost fish (Wong *et al.*, 2011). Therefore, SB334867 may also antagonize orexin at the zebrafish orexin receptor, which belongs to the OX2R family (Wong *et al.*, 2011).

C. Other fish

In a marine teleost fish, the ornate wrasse (*Thalassoma pavo*), IP injection of orexin A at a high dose of28 pmol/g BW stimulates the food intake (Facciolo *et al.*, 2009). In the winter flounder and winter skate, fasting stimulates the expression of orexin precursor mRNA in the hypothalamus (Buckley *et al.*, 2010; MacDonald and Volkoff, 2010), suggesting that orexin might play a role in feeding regulation in these species. To date, however, except for the goldfish and zebrafish as described above (see the Section IV), there is no information about the orexin function, and the involvement of orexin in feeding regulation has not been well studied in fish. Further study will be required to elucidate the function of orexin in appetite control in fish.

V. Effect of Orexin on Locomotor and Psychomotor Activities and the Sleep/Wakefulness Cycle in Teleost Fish

A. Goldfish

Orexin exerts locomotor and psychophysiological function in teleost fish. Recent studies have revealed that ICV administration of orexin A at 2–2.8 pmol/g BW stimulates the locomotor activity in goldfish (Fig. 18.6; Matsuda *et al.*, 2011a; Nakamachi *et al.*, 2006). Regarding the mechanism of

Recording of food intake was started 10 min after ICV injection. Each fish received food at 3% per g BW and food intake was measured directly by recording the number of diet pellets eaten by individual fish during the 60 min after treatment. The results are expressed as the mean ± SEM, and the number of fish per group is indicated in parentheses. Significance of differences was evaluated by one-way ANOVA with Bonferroni's method, as compared with a saline-injected group (*$P < 0.05$, **$P < 0.01$).

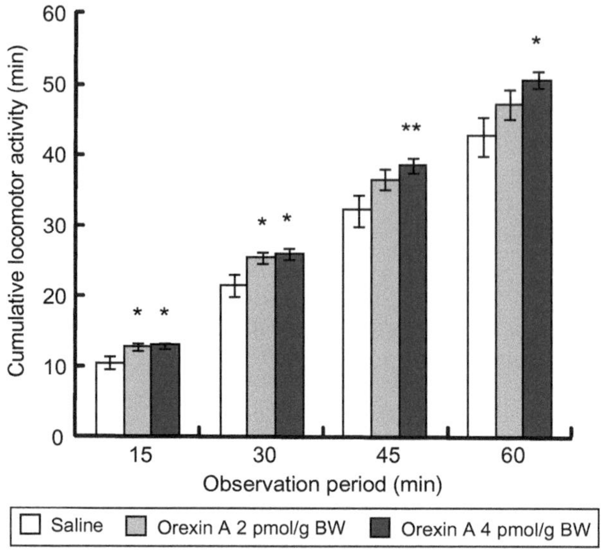

Figure 18.6 Effect of ICV administration of orexin A on locomotor activity in goldfish. Young goldfish (7–10 g body weight, BW) of both sexes were kept under controlled light/dark conditions (12 L/12 D) in a temperature-regulated water tank (20–24 °C) for 2 weeks before use in the experiments. Two hours prior to starting the experiments, at noon, each fish was supplied with food equivalent to at least 2% of its BW. For ICV administration of orexin A, fish were anesthetized in water containing 2 mM MS-222. The animals were then placed in a stereotaxic apparatus and a small part of the parietal bone was carefully removed using a surgical blade. One microliter of test solution was injected into the third ventricle, and the gap was then filled with a surgical bonding agent. Injection into the correct site was verified by the appearance in the ventricle of concomitantly injected Evans blue dye. The fish in the experimental groups were injected with orexin A at 2 and 4 pmol/g BW. The fish in the control group were injected with the same volume of saline. Each fish that had received ICV injection of orexin A or saline was placed in a small white experimental tank filled with tap water. Recording of locomotor activity (swimming time), which was started 15 min after ICV injection and continued for 60 min, was performed with a video-tracking system for automatic recording of goldfish behavior (EthoVision Color Pro, Noldus Information Technology, Wageningen, Netherlands). The results are expressed as the mean ± SEM, and 6–15 fish were used in the experiment. Significance of differences was evaluated by one-way ANOVA with Bonferroni's method, as compared with a saline-injected group (*$P<0.05$, **$P<0.01$).

the increased locomotor activity of teleosts by orexin, there is virtually no report. The plausible mechanistic pathways can be discussed from the studies with rodent models. Dopamine has been importantly implicated in the central nervous control of motor activity (Alachkar *et al.*, 2010; Rizzolatti and Luppino, 2001). The tyrosine hydroxylase-immunoreactive cells as a marker of dopaminergic system in the ventral tegmental area received innervation from the orexin immunoreactive fibers. In behavioral studies, orexin A-induced hyperlocomotion, stereotypy, and grooming behavior when administered centrally in rats, and these effects were abolished by dopamine antagonists (Nakamura *et al.*, 2000). These results suggest that the involvement of the ventral tegmental area dopaminergic system in orexin-induced locomotor activity.

Recent reports also indicate that the scototaxis protocol (a test to ascertain the preference for light/dark background areas) can be used to evaluate the psychomotor activity of teleost fish, notably anxiety-like behavior (Faganello and Mattioli, 2007; Matsuda *et al.*, 2011b; Maximino *et al.*, 2010). For example, it has been reported that when goldfish are initially kept in a small tank, and then placed in a small rectangular experimental tank with black and white background areas, the locomotor activity is affected (Matsuda *et al.*, 2011a,b). Intact fish transferred to the second tank shows a preference for the black, rather than the white, background area: the average time spent in the black background area is two to three times longer than that spent in the white background area (Matsuda *et al.*, 2011a,b). This scototaxis test appears to be suitable for evaluating the effect of pharmacological compounds on the psychomotor activity in teleost fish. Thus, ICV injection of the mild tranquilizer diazepam, a central-type benzodiazepine receptor agonist, reduces the time taken to move from the black to the white background area, whereas the anxiogenic agent FG-7142, an inverse agonist of the central-type benzodiazepine receptor, prolongs the time spent by the fish in the black background area (Matsuda *et al.*, 2011b). These observations validate the use of this behavioral test for the evaluation of the anxiolytic and anxiogenic properties of pharmacological compounds. In fact, the scototaxis test has recently been employed in fish to investigate the anxiolytic- and anxiogenic-like activities of neuropeptides such as NPY and octadecaneuropeptide in relation to feeding regulation (Matsuda *et al.*, 2011a,b).

B. Zebrafish

The zebrafish has been widely adopted as a model for the studies of sleep and related brain function (Rihel *et al.*, 2010; Zhdanova, 2011), because it has been shown to be a useful laboratory animal in the fields of comparative genomics, developmental biology, endocrinology, neuroscience, and behavioral biology (Faraco *et al.*, 2006). In this species, large populations of γ-aminobutyric acid (GABA)-ergic neurons in the hypothalamus express the orexin receptor (Yokogawa *et al.*, 2007). Overexpression of orexin in this species is reportedly associated with insomnia-like behavior, promoting and consolidating wakefulness, and suppressing a resting status (Prober *et al.*, 2006). On the other hand, zebrafish lacking the orexin receptor exhibits short and fragmented sleep under dark conditions (Yokogawa *et al.*, 2007). In the study of zebrafish hypocretin/orexin receptor mutant (hcrtr−/−), the level of expression of mRNA for arylalkylamine-*N*-acetyltransferase, an enzyme involved in melatonin synthesis, is reduced in hcrtr −/− pineal gland during the night. Moreover, hypocretin/orexin perfusion of cultured zebrafish pineal glands induces melatonin release, suggesting the regulation of sleep/wakefulness condition by hypocretin–melatonin interaction in zebrafish (Appelbaum *et al.*, 2009). These data suggest that orexin is involved in the regulation of sleep/wakefulness in fish, as is the case in mammals.

C. Other fish

IP injection of orexin A at a high dose of 28 pmol/g BW stimulates locomotor activity in the ornate wrasse (Facciolo *et al.*, 2009), and treatment with a $GABA_A$ receptor antagonist, bicuculline, at 1 μg/g BW reduces the locomotor activity with convulsive behavior in this species, suggesting the involvement of $GABA_A$ and orexin receptor systems in the regulation of motor behaviors (Facciolo *et al.*, 2010).

VI. Conclusions

There is reliable information to indicate that orexin exerts an orexigenic action in goldfish and zebrafish. In other fish, orexin may also be involved in appetite control, since it is expressed mainly in hypothalamic regions, and feeding or fasting conditions affect the expression and synthesis of orexin precursor mRNA.

Recently, behavioral studies have indicated that tests of preference and activity can provide valuable models for evaluating the psychophysiological effects of neuropeptides such as orexin. Such tests in goldfish and zebrafish have shown that orexin induces an increase of locomotor activity. These data indicate that, in fish as in rodents, as well as being implicated in the regulation of food intake, orexin is also involved in the control of locomotor or psychomotor activity in fish. Indeed, orexin regulates the rest and activity (sleep/wakefulness) in zebrafish. It is of considerable interest that the orexin system and its function might be conserved among vertebrates, but that its molecular basis may differ somewhat from the tetrapod system: in teleost fish, there is only one receptor for orexin, and OX1R has not yet evolved. In the zebrafish, the OX1R locus is missing from the chromosome.

It is likely that orexin-induced actions are responsible for energy homeostasis, including food intake, locomotor and psychomotor activities, reproduction, and sleep/wakefulness cycle in teleost fish (Fig. 18.7). However, further study will be required to elucidate the molecular mechanisms underlying the function of orexin in teleosts.

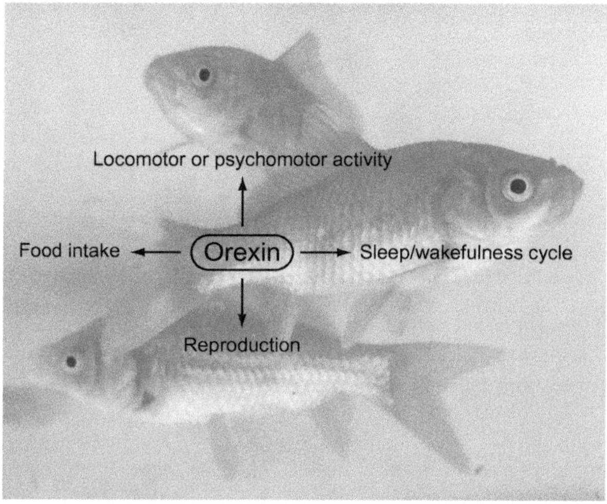

Figure 18.7 Schematic drawing depicting the role of orexin in teleost fish. Orexin-induced actions are responsible for energy homeostasis, including food intake, locomotor and psychomotor activities, reproduction, and the sleep/wakefulness cycle in teleost fish.

ACKNOWLEDGMENTS

This study was supported by a Grant-in-Aid from the Japan Society for the Promotion of Science (21370025 to K. M.).
Conflicts of Interest. The authors declare no conflicts of interest.

REFERENCES

Abbott, M., and Volkoff, H. (2011). Thyrotropin releasing hormone (TRH) in goldfish (*Carassius auratus*): Role in the regulation of feeding and locomotor behaviors and interactions with the orexin system and cocaine- and amphetamine regulated transcript (CART). *Horm. Behav.* **59,** 236–245.

Alachkar, A., Brotchie, J. M., and Jones, O. T. (2010). Locomotor response to L-DOPA in reserpine-treated rats following central inhibition of aromatic L-amino acid decarboxylase: Further evidence for non-dopaminergic actions of L-DOPA and its metabolites. *Neurosci. Res.* **68,** 44–50.

Alvarez, C. E., and Sutcliffe, J. G. (2002). Hypocretin is an early member of the incretin gene family. *Neurosci. Lett.* **324,** 169–172.

Amiya, N., Amano, M., Oka, Y., Iigo, M., Takahashi, A., and Yamamori, K. (2007). Immunohistochemical localization of orexin/hypocretin-like immunoreactive peptides and melanin-concentrating hormone in the brain and pituitary of medaka. *Neurosci. Lett.* **427,** 16–21.

Appelbaum, L., Wang, G. X., Maro, G. S., Mori, R., Tovin, A., Marin, W., Yokogawa, T., Kawakami, K., Smith, S. J., Gothilf, Y., Mignot, E., and Mourrain, P. (2009). Sleep-wake regulation and hypocretin–melatonin interaction in zebrafish. *Proc. Natl. Acad. Sci. U.S.A.* **106,** 21942–21947.

Buckley, C., MacDonald, E. E., Tuiak, S. M., and Volkoff, H. (2010). Molecular cloning and characterization of two putative appetite regulators in winter flounder (*Pleuronectes americanus*): Preprothyrotropin-releasing hormone (TRH) and preproorexin (OX). *Peptides* **31,** 1737–1747.

de Lecea, L., Kilduff, T. S., Peyron, C., Gao, X., Foye, P. E., Danielson, P. E., Fukuhara, C., Battenberg, E. L., Gautvik, V. T., Barlett, F. S., Frankel, W. N., van den Pol, A. N., *et al.* (1998). The hypocretins: Hypothalamus-specific peptides with neuroexcitatory activity. *Proc. Natl. Acad. Sci. U.S.A.* **95,** 322–327.

Facciolo, R. M., Crudo, M., Giusi, G., and Canonaco, M. (2009). Light- and dark-dependent orexinergic neuronal signals promote neurodegenerative phenomena accounting for distinct behavioral responses in the teleost *Thalassoma pavo*. *J. Neurosci. Res.* **87,** 748–757.

Facciolo, R. M., Crudo, M., Giusi, G., and Canonaco, M. (2010). GABAergic influences on ORX receptor-dependent abnormal motor behaviors and neurodegenerative events in fish. *Toxicol. Appl. Pharmacol.* **243,** 77–86.

Faganello, F. R., and Mattioli, R. (2007). Anxiolytic-like effect of chlorpheniramine in inhibitory avoidance in goldfish submitted to telencephalic ablation. *Prog. Neuropsychopharmacol. Biol. Psychiatry* **31,** 269–274.

Faraco, J. H., Appelbaum, L., Marin, W., Gaus, S. E., Mourrain, P., and Mignot, E. (2006). Regulation of hypocretin (orexin) expression in embryonic zebrafish. *J. Biol. Chem.* **281,** 29753–29761.

Hoskins, L. J., Xu, M., and Volkoff, H. (2008). Interactions between gonadotropin-releasing hormone (GnRH) and orexin in the regulation of feeding and reproduction in goldfish (*Carassius auratus*). *Horm. Behav.* **54,** 379–385.

Huesa, G., van den Pol, A. N., and Finger, T. E. (2005). Differential distribution of hypocretin (orexin) and melanin-concentrating hormone in the goldfish brain. *J. Comp. Neurol.* **488,** 476–491.

Kang, K. S., Shimizu, K., Azuma, M., Ui, Y., Nakamura, K., Uchiyama, M., and Matsuda, K. (2011a). Gonadotropin-releasing hormone II (GnRH II) mediates the anorexigenic actions of α-melanocyte-stimulating hormone (α-MSH) and corticotropin-releasing hormone in goldfish. *Peptides* **32,** 31–35.

Kang, K. S., Yahashi, S., and Matsuda, K. (2011b). The effects of ghrelin on energy balance and psychomotor activity in a goldfish model: An overview. *Int. J. Pept.* **2011,** 171034.

Kaslin, J., Nystedt, J. M., Ostergard, M., Peitsaro, N., and Panula, P. (2004). The orexin/hypocretin system in zebrafish is connected to the aminergic and cholinergic systems. *J. Neurosci.* **24,** 2678–2689.

Kilduff, T. S., and Peyron, C. (2000). The hypocretin/orexin ligand-receptor system: Implications for sleep and sleep disorders. *Trends Neurosci.* **23,** 359–365.

Kohsaka, A., Watanobe, H., Kakizaki, Y., Suda, T., and Schiöth, H. B. (2001). A significant participation of orexin-A, a potent orexigenic peptide, in the preovulatory luteinizing hormone and prolactin surges in the rat. *Brain Res.* **898,** 166–170.

Kojima, K., Kamijo, M., Kageyama, H., Uchiyama, M., Shioda, S., and Matsuda, K. (2009). Neuronal relationship between orexin-A- and neuropeptide Y-induced orexigenic actions in goldfish. *Neuropeptides* **43,** 63–71.

Lin, X., Volkoff, H., Narnaware, Y., Bernier, N. J., Peyon, P., and Peter, R. E. (2000). Brain regulation of feeding behavior and food intake in fish. *Comp. Biochem. Physiol.* **126,** 415–434.

López, J. M., Domínguez, L., Moreno, N., Morona, R., Joven, A., and González, A. (2009). Distribution of orexin/hypocretin immunoreactivity in the brain of the lungfishes *Protopterus dolloi* and *Neoceratodus forsteri*. *Brain Behav. Evol.* **74,** 302–322.

MacDonald, E. E., and Volkoff, H. (2010). Molecular cloning and characterization of preproorexin in winter skate (*Leucorasia ocellata*). *Gen. Comp. Endocrinol.* **169,** 192–196.

Matsuda, K. (2009). Recent advances in the regulation of feeding behavior by neuropeptides in fish. *Ann. N. Y. Acad. Sci.* **1163,** 243–252.

Matsuda, K., Nakamura, K., Shimakura, S. I., Miura, T., Kageyama, H., Uchiyama, M., Shioda, S., and Ando, H. (2008). Inhibitory effect of chicken gonadotropin-releasing hormone II on food intake in the goldfish, *Carassius auratus*. *Horm. Behav.* **54,** 83–89.

Matsuda, K., Kang, K. S., Sakashita, A., Yahashi, S., and Vaudry, H. (2011a). Behavioral effect of neuropeptides related to feeding regulation in fish. *Ann. N. Y. Acad. Sci.* **1220,** 117–126.

Matsuda, K., Wada, K., Azuma, M., Leprince, J., Tonon, M. C., Sakashita, A., Maruyama, K., Uchiyama, M., and Vaudry, H. (2011b). The octadecaneuropeptide exerts an anxiogenic-like action in goldfish. *Neuroscience* **181,** 100–108.

Maximino, C., Marques de Brito, T., Dias, C. A., Gouveia, A. J., and Morato, S. (2010). Scototaxis as anxiety-like behavior in fish. *Nat. Protoc.* **5,** 209–216.

Miura, T., Maruyama, K., Shimakura, S., Kaiya, H., Uchiyama, M., Kangawa, K., Shioda, S., and Matsuda, K. (2007). Regulation of food intake in the goldfish by interaction between ghrelin and orexin. *Peptides* **28,** 1207–1213.

Nakamachi, T., Matsuda, K., Maruyama, K., Miura, T., Uchiyama, M., Funahashi, H., Sakurai, T., and Shioda, S. (2006). Regulation by orexin of feeding behavior and locomotor activity in the goldfish. *J. Neuroendocrinol.* **18,** 290–297.

Nakamura, T., Uramura, K., Nambu, T., Yada, T., Goto, K., Yanagisawa, M., and Sakurai, T. (2000). Orexin-induced hyperlocomotion and stereotypy are mediated by the dopaminergic system. *Brain Res.* **873,** 181–187.

Novak, C. M., Jiang, X., Wang, C., Teske, J. A., Kotz, C. M., and Levine, J. A. (2005). Caloric restriction and physical activity in zebrafish (*Danio rerio*). *Neurosci. Lett.* **383,** 99–104.

Nurmio, M., Tena-Sempere, M., and Toppari, J. (2010). Orexins and the regulation of the hypothalamic-pituitary-testicular axis. *Acta Physiol (Oxf.)* **198,** 349–354.

Ohkubo, T., Boswell, T., and Lumineau, S. (2002). Molecular cloning of chiken prepro-orexin cDNA and preferential expression in the chicken hypothalamus. *Biochim. Biophys. Acta* **1577,** 476–480.

Ohkubo, T., Tsukada, A., and Shamoto, K. (2003). cDNA cloning of chicken orexin receptor and tissue distribution: Sexually dimorphic expression in chicken gonads. *J. Mol. Endocrinol.* **31,** 499–508.

Panula, P. (2010). Hypocretin/orexin in fish physiology with emphasis on zebrafish. *Acta Physiol (Oxf.)* **198,** 381–386.

Peter, R. E., and Gill, V. E. (1975). A stereotaxic atlas and technique for forebrain nuclei of the goldfish, *Carassius auratus*. *J. Comp. Neurol.* **159,** 103–127.

Piccinetti, C. C., Migliarini, B., Olivotto, I., Coletti, G., Amici, A., and Carnevali, O. (2010). Appetite regulation: The central role of melatonin in *Danio rerio*. *Horm. Behav.* **58,** 780–785.

Pirone, A., Lenzi, C., Betti, L., Giannaccini, G., Lucacchini, A., Marroni, P., and Fabiani, O. (2004). Immunohistochemical distribution of neuropeptides Y in the mesencephalon and rhombencephalon of carp, *Cyprinus carpio* L. (Cyprinidae:Teleostei). *Comp. Biochem. Physiol. A Mol. Integr. Physiol.* **138,** 175–185.

Porkka-Heiskanen, T., Kalinchuk, A., Alanko, L., Huhtaniemi, I., and Stenberg, D. (2004). Orexin A and B levels in the hypothalamus of female rats: The effects of the estrous cycle and age. *Eur. J. Endocrinol.* **150,** 737–742.

Prober, D. A., Rihel, J., Onah, A. A., Sung, R. J., and Schier, A. F. (2006). Hypocretin/orexin overexpression induces an insomnia-like phenotype in zebrafish. *J. Neurosci.* **26,** 13400–13410.

Rihel, J., Prober, D. A., and Schier, A. F. (2010). Monitoring sleep and arousal in zebrafish. *Methods Cell Biol.* **100,** 281–294.

Rizzolatti, G., and Luppino, G. (2001). The cortical motor system. *Neuron* **31,** 889–901.

Sakurai, T. (2005). Roles of orexin/hypocretin in regulation of sleep/wakefulness and energy homeostasis. *Sleep Med. Rev.* **9,** 231–241.

Sakurai, T., and Mieda, M. (2011). Connectomics of orexin-producing neurons: Interface of systems of emotion, energy homeostasis and arousal. *Trends Pharmacol. Sci.* **32,** 451–462.

Sakurai, T., Amemiya, A., Ishiim, M., Matsuzaki, I., Chemelli, R. M., Tanaka, H., Williams, S. C., Richardson, J. A., Kozlowski, G. P., Wilson, S., Arch, J. R. S., Buckingham, R. E., *et al.* (1998). Orexins and orexin receptors: A family of hypothalamic neuropeptides and G protein-coupled recetors that regulate feeding behavior. *Cell* **92,** 573–575.

Shibahara, M., Sakurai, T., Nambu, T., Takenouchi, T., Iwaasa, H., Egashira, S. I., Ihara, M., and Goto, K. (1999). Structure, tissue distribution, and pharmacological characterization of *Xenopus* orexins. *Peptides* **20,** 1169–1176.

Silveyra, P., Cataldi, N. I., Lux-Lantos, V. A., and Libertun, C. (2010). Role of orexins in the hypothalamo-pituitary-ovarian relationships. *Acta Physiol. (Oxf.)* **198,** 355–360.

Tam, J. K., Lau, K. W., Lee, L. T., Chu, J. Y., Ng, K. M., Fournier, A., Vaudry, H., and Chow, B. K. (2011). Origin of secretin receptor precedes the advent of tetrapoda: Evidence on the separated origins of secretin and orexin. *PLoS One* **6,** e19384.

Thannickal, T. C., Moore, R. Y., Nienhuis, R., Ramanathan, L., Gulyani, S., Aldrich, M., Cornford, M., and Siegel, J. M. (2000). Reduced number of hypocretin neurons in human narcolepsy. *Neuron* **27,** 469–474.

Volkoff, H. (2006). The role of neuropeptide Y, orexins, cocaine and amphetamine-related transcript, cholecystokinin, amylin and leptin in the regulation of feeding in fish. *Comp. Biochem. Physiol. A Mol. Integr. Physiol.* **144,** 325–331.

Volkoff, H., and Peter, R. E. (2000). Effects of CART peptides on food consumption, feeding and associated behaviors in the goldfish, *Carassius auratus*: Actions on neuropeptide Y- and orexin A-induced feeding. *Brain Res.* **887,** 125–133.

Volkoff, H., and Peter, R. E. (2001). Interactions between orexin A, NPY and galanin in the control of food intake of the goldfish, *Carassius auratus. Regul. Pept.* **101,** 59–72.

Volkoff, H., Bjorklund, J. M., and Peter, R. E. (1999). Stimulation of feeding behavior and food consumption in the goldfish, *Carassius auratus*, by orexin-A and orexin-B. *Brain Res.* **846,** 204–209.

Volkoff, H., Eykelbosh, A. J., and Peter, R. E. (2003). Role of leptin in the control of feeding of goldfish *Carassius auratus*: Interactions with cholecystokinin, neuropeptide Y and orexin A, and modulation by fasting. *Brain Res.* **972,** 90–109.

Volkoff, H., Canosa, L. F., Unniappan, S., Cerdá-Reverter, J. M., Bernier, N. J., Kelly, S. P., and Peter, R. E. (2005). Neuropeptides and the control of food intake in fish. *Gen. Comp. Endocrinol.* **142,** 3–19.

Wong, K. K., Ng, S. Y., Lee, L. T., Ng, H. K., and Chow, B. K. (2011). Orexins and their receptors from fish to mammals: A comparative approach. *Gen. Comp. Endocrinol.* **171,** 124–130.

Wullimann, M., Ruppe, B., and Reichert, H. (1996). Neuroanatomy of the Zebrafish Brain. A Topological Atlas. Birkhäuser Verlag, Basel, Switzerland.

Xu, M., and Volkoff, H. (2007). Molecular characterization of prepro-orexin in Atlantic cod (*Gadus morhua*): Cloning, localization, developmental profile and role in food intake regulation. *Mol. Cell. Endocrinol.* **271,** 28–37.

Yokobori, E., Kojima, K., Azuma, M., Kang, K. S., Maejima, S., Uchiyama, M., and Matsuda, K. (2011). Stimulatory effect of intracerebroventricular administration of orexin A on food intake in the zebrafish, *Danio rerio*. *Peptides* **32,** 1357–1362.
Yokogawa, T., Marin, W., Faraco, J., Pézeron, G., Appelbaum, L., Zhang, J., Rosa, F., Mourrain, P., and Mignot, E. (2007). Characterization of sleep in zebrafish and insomnia in hypocretin receptor mutants. *PLoS Biol.* **5,** e277.
Zhdanova, I. V. (2011). Sleep and its regulation in zebrafish. *Rev. Neurosci.* **22,** 27–36.

Index

Note: Page numbers followed by "*f*" indicate figures, and "*t*" indicate tables.

U

V

W

Z

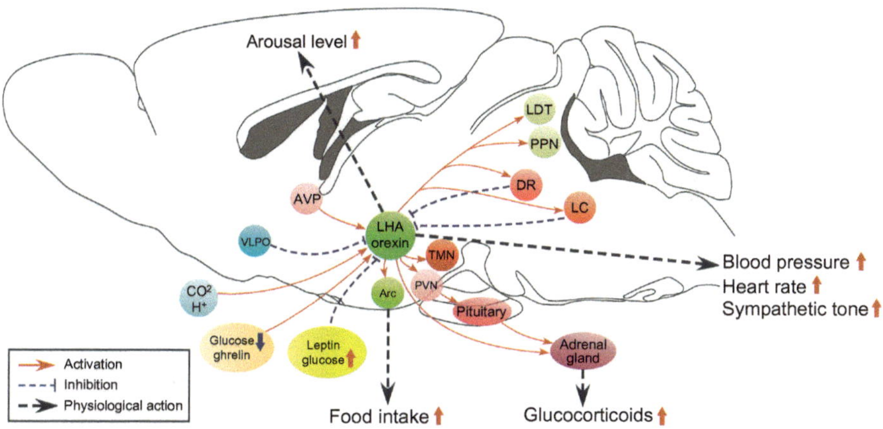

Tomomi Tsunematsu and Akihiro Yamanaka, Figure 2.2 Interaction of orexin neurons with other brain regions and peripheral tissues. Orexin neurons are exclusively located in the lateral hypothalamic area and project throughout the brain. Dashed blue lines show inhibitory projections. Red arrows show excitatory projections. Dashed black arrows show physiological actions of the orexin system. Arc, arcuate nucleus; DR, dorsal raphe nuclei; LC, locus coeruleus; LDT, laterodorsal tegmental nucleus; LHA, lateral hypothalamic area; PPN, pedunculopontine nucleus; PVN, paraventricular nucleus; TMN, tuberomammillary nucleus; VLPO, ventrolateral preoptic nucleus.

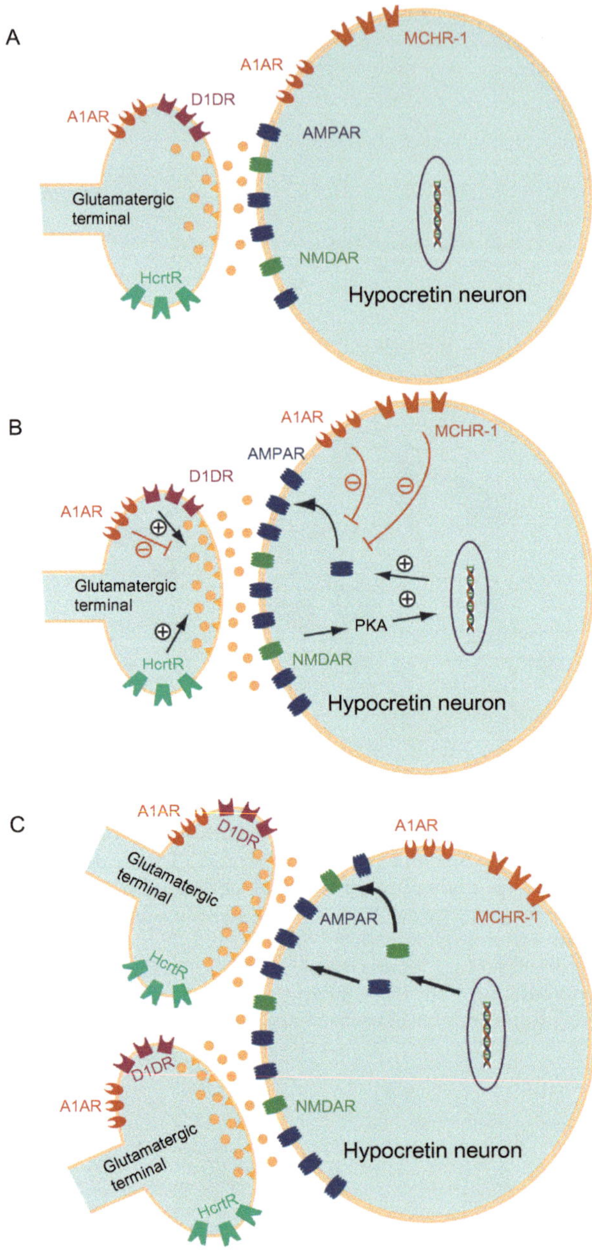

Xiao-Bing Gao, Figure 3.4 Experience-dependent synaptic plasticity in hypocretin/orexin neurons. (A) Glutamatergic synapses on hypocretin/orexin neurons before synaptic potentiation. (B) Synaptic potentiation of glutamatergic synapses on hypocretin/orexin neurons triggered by an acute exposure to environmental factors (food deficiency

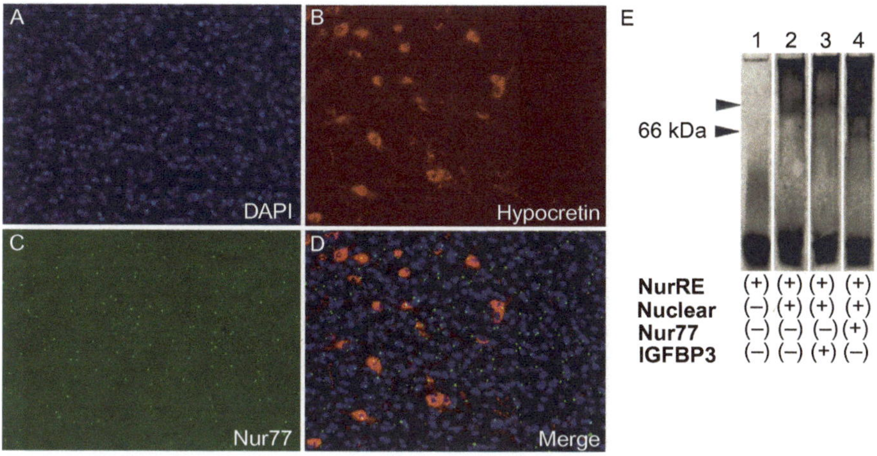

Susumu Tanaka, Figure 5.2 Colocalization of hypocretin with Nur77 in murine hypothalamic hypocretin neurons, and an electromobility shift assay with nuclear receptor subfamily response elements. (A) DAPI-labeled nuclei (blue); (B) hypocretin (red) visualized using Alexa-594; (C) Nur77 (green) visualized using Alexa-488; (D) Merged image of A, B, and C immunofluorescence; (E) electromobility shift assay using HeLa nuclear extract. Triplet NurRE oligonucleotides were subjected to nondenatured 4% PAGE after incubation with nuclear extracts from HeLa cells transfected with pCMVTNT vector (mock) (lane 2), with IGFBP3/TNT expression vector (lane 3), or with Nur77/TNT expression vector (lane 4). No protein was applied to lane 1, so triplet NurRE oligonucleotides maintained their original molecular weights.

---

or sleep restriction) occurs in an activity/experience-dependent manner as reported in the expression of LTP. Synaptic potentiation may occur at both pre- and postsynaptic sites, for example, enhanced release of glutamate from presynaptic terminals and upregulation of glutamate receptors in hypocretin/orexin neurons. (C) Repeated exposure to environmental factors leads to reorganization of synaptic architecture in hypocretin/orexin neurons, including the increased number of excitatory (glutamatergic) synapses on hypocretin/orexin neurons. AMPAR, AMPA receptor; NMDAR, NMDA receptor; D1DR, D1 dopamine receptor; HcrtR, hypocretin/orexin receptor; MCHR-1, MCH receptor-1; A1AR, A1 adenosine receptor; PKA, protein kinase A.

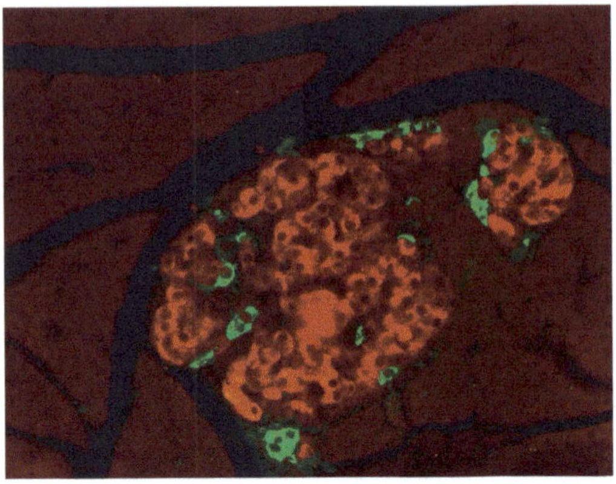

Ernest Adeghate, Figure 7.1 Light micrograph showing OX1R-positive cells (red) in pancreatic islet of cells of Goto-Kakizaki rats. Glucagon-immunopositive cells (green) are located in the periphery of pancreatic islet of Langerhans. Note the large number of islet cells containing OX1R in the central region of the islet. Magnification: 200×.

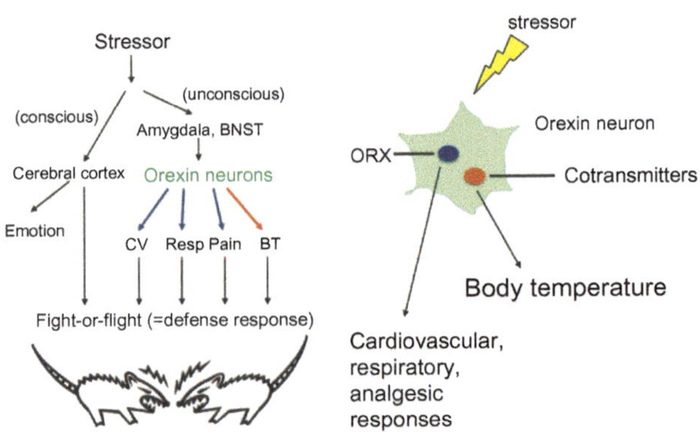

Tomoyuki Kuwaki and Wei Zhang, Figure 8.4 Hypothetical diagram showing the key role of orexin neurons in the fight-or-flight response. When animals confront a stressor, orexin neurons mediate cardiovascular (CV), respiratory (Resp), and analgesic (Pain) responses by using orexin as a transmitter. At the same time, orexin neurons regulate body temperature (BT) by using cotransmitters other than orexin. These responses are collectively called the defense response that prepares the body for the fight-or-flight behavior. Adapted from Kuwaki (2011).

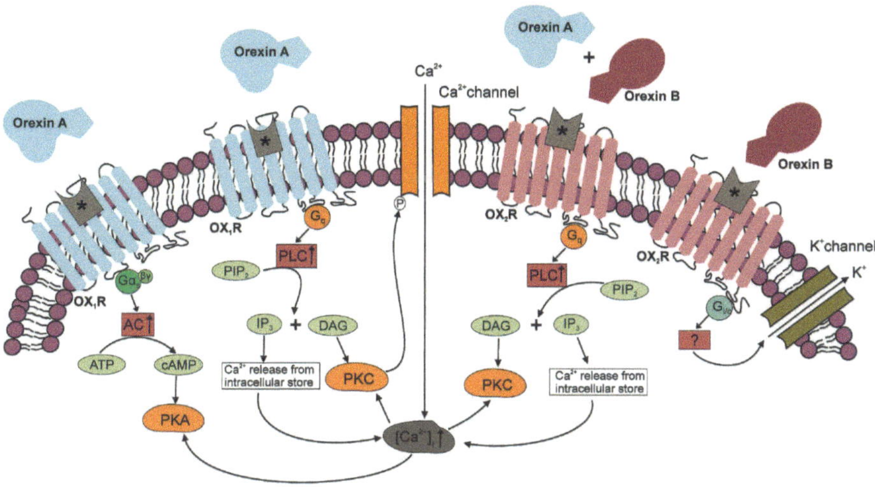

Israt Z. Shahid *et al.*, Figure 9.2 Schematic of the main signaling pathways of OX_1R and OX_2R upon the activation by orexin A and orexin A or orexin B, respectively. AC, adenylate cyclase; cAMP, cyclic adenosine monophosphate; DAG, diacylglycerol; G, G protein; IP_3, inositol triphosphate; P, phosphorylation site; PIP_2, phosphatidylinositol biphosphate; PKA, protein kinase A; PKC, protein kinase C; PLC, phospholipase C. Asterisks mark the orexin-recognizing sites of OX_1R and OX_2R.

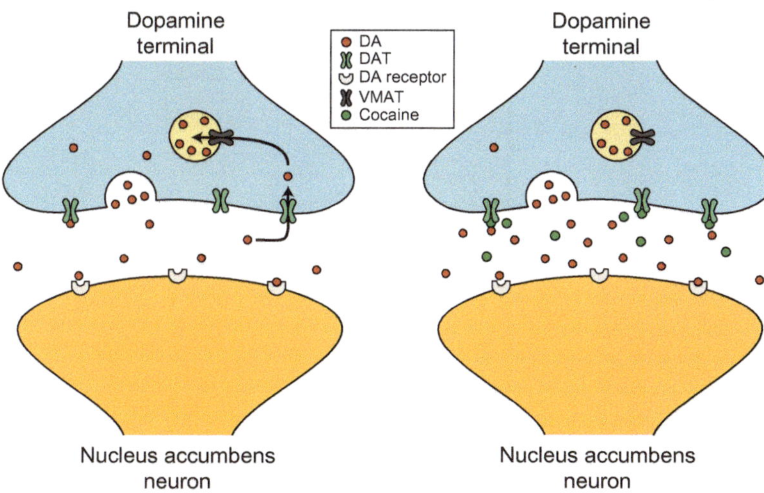

Rodrigo A. España, Figure 10.4 Effects of cocaine at the dopamine transporter. (Left) Under normal conditions, dopamine (DA) neuron firing results in dopamine-filled vesicles to fuse with the presynaptic membrane and subsequently release into the synaptic cleft. Once in the synapse, dopamine can bind to postsynaptic dopamine receptors and then is removed from extracellular space by the dopamine transporter (DAT). Once dopamine is back inside the presynaptic terminal, it is repackaged into synaptic vesicles for future release via the vesicular monoamine transporter (VMAT). (Right) Cocaine increases extracellular levels of dopamine by interacting with the DAT and thereby inhibiting dopamine uptake back into the terminal. As dopamine uptake is reduced, levels accumulate in the synapse and dopamine has a greater opportunity to bind to dopamine receptors.

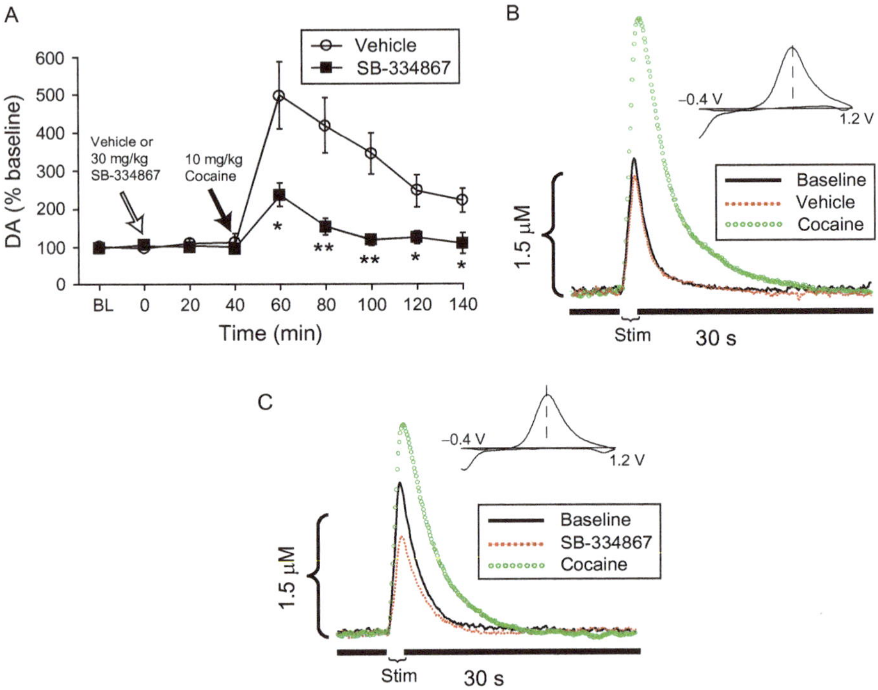

Rodrigo A. España, Figure 10.5 SB-334867 attenuates cocaine-induced elevations in dopamine signaling in the NAc core. (A) The mean ± SEM of extracellular levels of dopamine (DA) within the NAc core following i.p. injection of vehicle ($n=6$) or 30 mg/kg SB-334867 ($n=6$). Representative concentration–time plots and cyclic voltammograms (insets) of dopamine responses from rats that received pretreatment infusions of (B) vehicle or (C) 10 nmol SB-334867 into the VTA. Stim represents the time of electrical stimulation (1 s, 60 Hz pulse). (Insets in B and C) Cyclic voltammograms depict two current peaks, one at 600 mV (positive deflection) for dopamine oxidation and another at -200 mV (negative deflection) for reduction of dopamine-*o*-quinone. The position of the peaks identifies the substance as DA. $^{\star}P<0.05$, $^{\star\star}P<0.01$ relative to vehicle.

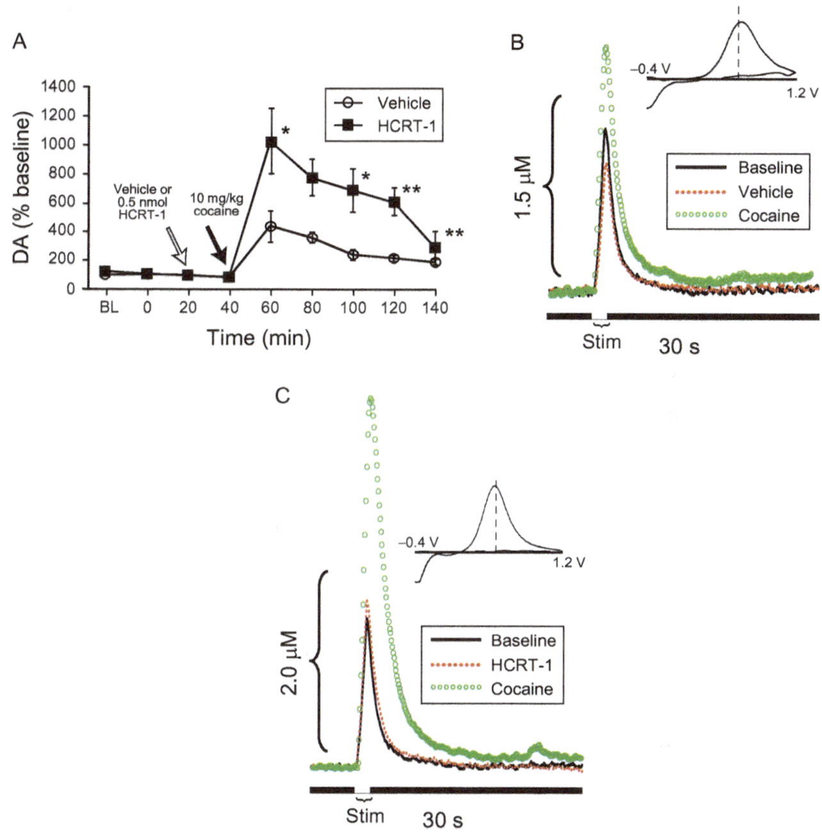

Rodrigo A. España, Figure 10.7 Hypocretin-1 augments cocaine-induced elevations in dopamine signaling in the NAc core. (A) The mean ± SEM of extracellular levels of dopamine (DA) within the NAc core following intra-VTA infusion of vehicle ($n = 6$) or 0.5 nmol hypocretin-1 (HCRT-1; $n = 6$). Representative concentration–time plots and cyclic voltammograms (insets) of dopamine responses from rats that received pretreatment infusions of (B) vehicle or (C) 0.5 nmol hypocretin-1 into the VTA. Stim represents the time of electrical stimulation (1 s, 60 Hz pulse). (Insets in B and C) Cyclic voltammograms depict two current peaks, one at 600 mV (positive deflection) for dopamine oxidation and another at −200 mV (negative deflection) for reduction of dopamine-*o*-quinone. The position of the peaks identifies the substance as DA. $^{*}P < 0.05$, $^{**}P < 0.01$ relative to vehicle.

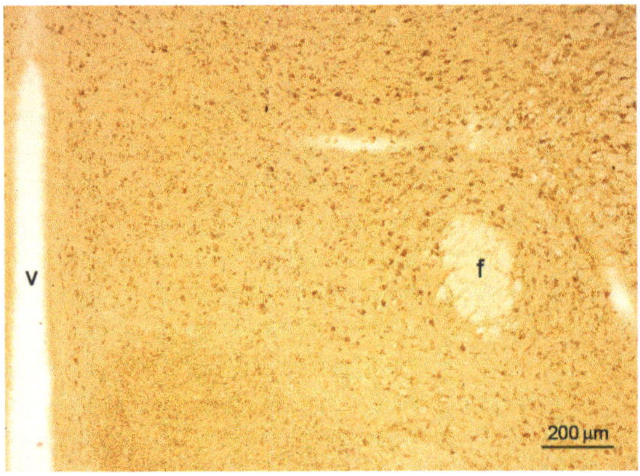

Ozhan Eyigor *et al.*, Figure 11.1 Expression of KA2 subunit of kainate receptors in the lateral hypothalamus. Note the abundance of KA2-immunoreactive perikarya in the perifornical area of the lateral hypothalamus (v, third ventricle; f, fornix). KA2 subunit was labeled with a rabbit anti-KA2 polyclonal antibody (1:2000 dilution, R52-4, Eyigor and Jennes, 2000).

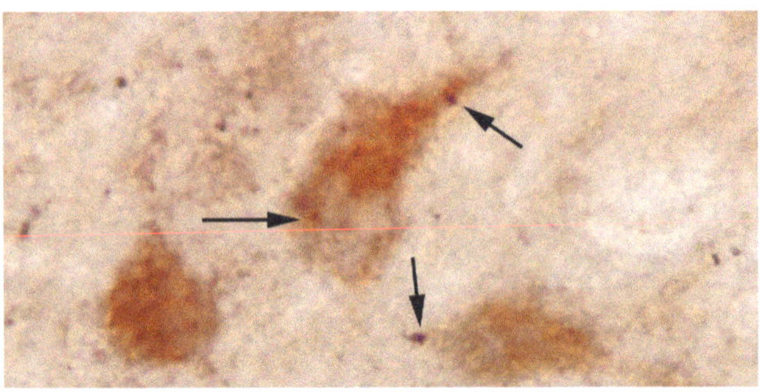

Ozhan Eyigor *et al.*, Figure 11.2 Expression of VGluT3 protein on the orexin neurons. Orexin neurons are seen with the cytoplasmic DAB reaction (gray, actual color is brown). The black puncta on the orexin neurons as well as in the vicinity are the Ni-DAB reaction localizing the VGluT3-positive terminals (arrows). Orexin neurons were labeled with a goat anti-orexin A polyclonal antibody (1:1000 dilution, Santa Cruz Biotechnology, USA), while the glutamatergic terminals were labeled with a guinea pig anti-VGluT3 polyclonal antibody (1:5000 dilution, Chemicon International, USA).

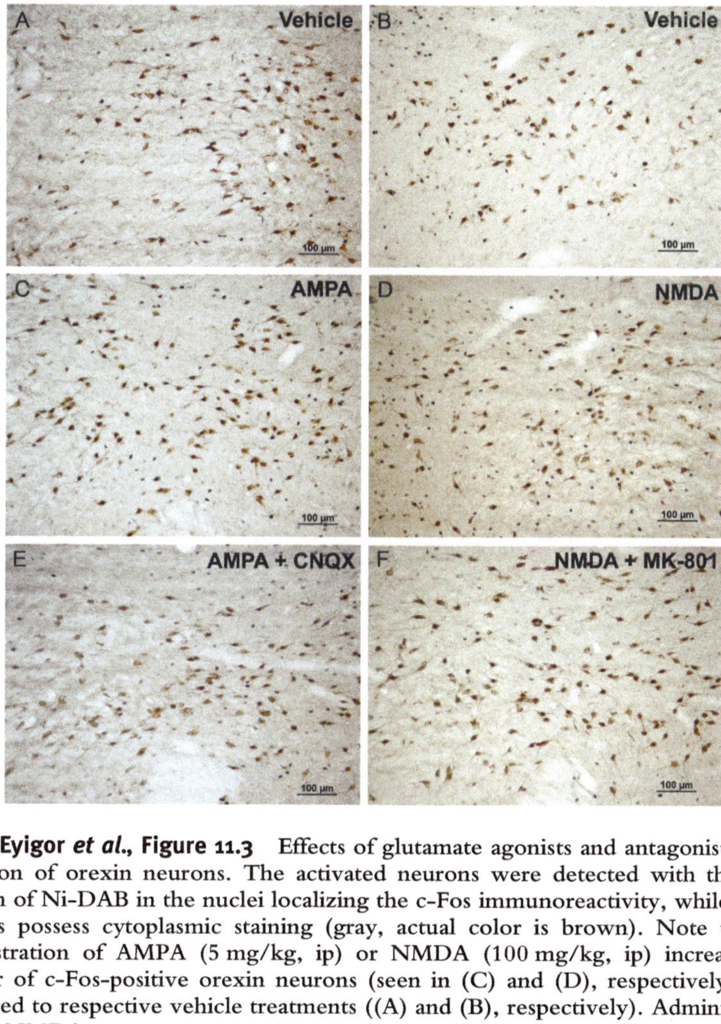

Ozhan Eyigor *et al.*, Figure 11.3 Effects of glutamate agonists and antagonists in the activation of orexin neurons. The activated neurons were detected with the black reaction of Ni-DAB in the nuclei localizing the c-Fos immunoreactivity, while orexin neurons possess cytoplasmic staining (gray, actual color is brown). Note that the administration of AMPA (5 mg/kg, ip) or NMDA (100 mg/kg, ip) increased the number of c-Fos-positive orexin neurons (seen in (C) and (D), respectively) when compared to respective vehicle treatments ((A) and (B), respectively). Administration of non-NMDA receptor antagonist CNQX (5 mg/kg, ip) 15 min prior to AMPA diminished the number of activated neurons (seen in (E)). MK-801 administration decreased the number of c-Fos-expressing orexin neurons (seen in (F)), but statistically, this decrease was not significant. Orexin neurons were labeled with a goat anti-orexin A polyclonal antibody (1:1000 dilution, Santa Cruz Biotechnology, USA), while the c-Fos expression was assessed with a rabbit anti-c-Fos polyclonal antibody (1:20,000 dilution, Oncogene, USA).

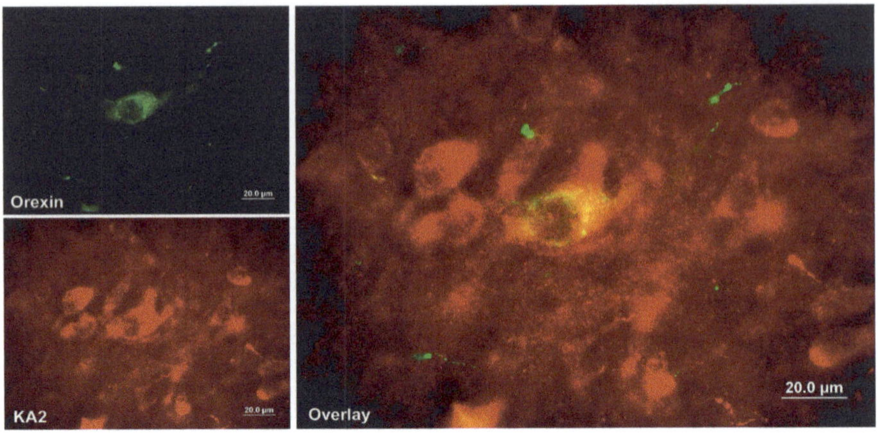

Ozhan Eyigor *et al.*, Figure 11.5 Kainate receptor subunit KA2 expression in orexin neurons. Orexin neurons are seen in green (FITC, left top) and KA2-positive neurons are seen in red (Texas red, left bottom). The overlay on the right shows that the KA2 immunoreactivity is colocalized in the orexin-immunoreactive neuron (yellow color). Note that there are other KA2-positive neurons in the vicinity which lack the immunoreaction for orexin A. Orexin neurons were labeled with a goat anti-orexin A polyclonal antibody (1:500 dilution, Santa Cruz Biotechnology), while the KA2 subunit was labeled with a rabbit anti-KA2 polyclonal antibody (1:2000 dilution, Eyigor and Jennes, 2000).

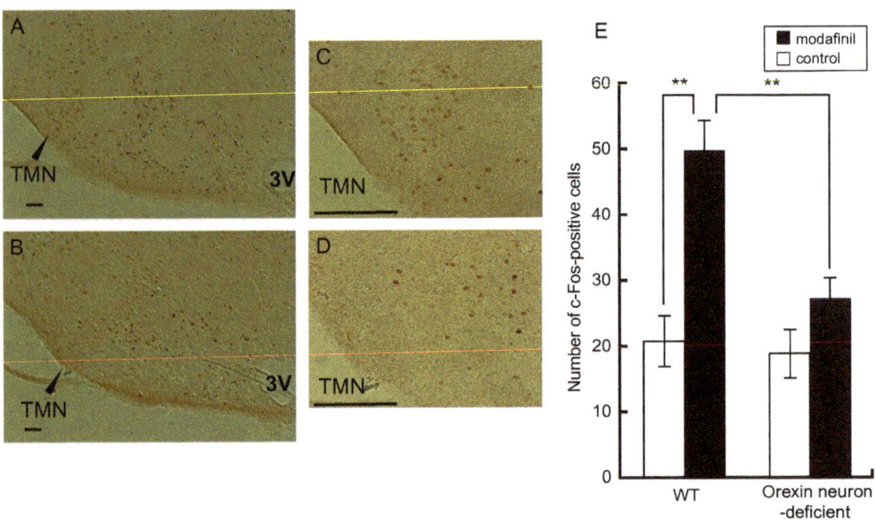

Tomoko Ishizuka *et al.*, Figure 14.8 Representative photomicrographs of c-Fos expression induced by modafinil (150 mg/kg, i.p.) in (A) wild-type and (B) orexin neuron-deficient mice of the TMN (Ishizuka *et al.*, 2010). The magnification of the TMN of (C) wild-type (WT) and (D) orexin neuron-deficient mice. Scale bars, 100 μm; 3V, third ventricle; TMN, the tuberomammillary nucleus. (E) Cell counts of c-Fos-positive cells in the TMN. Each column represents the mean and SEM ($n = 4–5$). $^{**}p < 0.01$.

Kolibri 360 GmbH
Ferdinand-Jühlke-Straße 7
99095 Erfurt, Deutschland
produktsicherheit@kolibri360.de